AGAINST ALL ODDS

(A Look Through the Eyes of a Survivor)

An Autobiography

by

Craig W. Meyers, M.S.

Table of Contents

Overview

In order to benefit those who may be tempted to stray from accepted standards of behavior because fundamental principles of conduct previously adhered to are viewed as primitive and/or counterproductive, I document the detrimental precursors leading to my vehicular tragedy in the first two chapters of my book. Mistakenly thinking that substance use could rid me of my faulty perception that I was somehow a deprived adolescent, I detail my personal escapades experimenting with marijuana and alcohol as an idiotic college freshman, so that the long-term harm of resorting to such means as a "solution" to problems may be highlighted. My clouded teenaged perspective of the world and sequestered presence both contributing to an inaccurate view of my place in the universe, I try to paint a picture with words of how various influences guided the view of myself as inept, with the hopes that aspiring adults who may read this account of my catastrophe don't let impulses and/or crazed hormonal influences impede their development. The opening frames of this personal expose also written with the intent of demonstrating what can result if certain practices of behavior are adopted—incorporating my ensuing understanding as a family therapist and counseling supervisor into my writing—I also attempt to model the importance of reviewing certain dynamics which can commonly occur within different households. Simply put, just try to discourage younger people from living on "The Wild Side" by relaying what could realistically happen to them by making this choice and to stress how the "messages" sent by members within a family system can leave a powerful impact on impressionable minds.

Emphasizing how these different variables led to the accident, the three middle chapters not only detail firsthand this survivor's psychological, cognitive, and physical struggles battling the symptoms of a severe brain injury, but the emotional impact such a condition had on those who cared for me. Providing an example for both the novice and professional, my objective being so specific in these interior chapters was to educate the reader about what exactly one can encounter when the core of the central nervous system has been damaged. Indicating my recognition level at a given time, an appetizing interplay of the first and third persons are utilized to give the reader an authentic "feel" of what exactly I could sense in my environment. Events are conveyed utilizing my perspective in the initial two chapters, however, descriptions of various circumstances assume a narrative format outside of my vantage point during those instances when my mind was incapable of processing my surroundings. Gathered from notes of my state when I was comatose at Allegheny General Hospital in Pittsburgh and an aphasic rehab inpatient, precise dates and occurrences are presented.

Only about five weeks after the surface of my brain was bruised, from admission to discharge, the rehabilitation center I would subsequently be transferred to would begin to videotape my therapies and consequential progress. A patient in Harmarville Rehabilitation Center's brain trauma unit for approximately five months, a series of cognitive and physical therapy sessions would be filmed over time and made into one videotape approximately fifteen minutes in length. Showcasing several of the symptoms noted in my book, amazing everyone who has ever viewed this film because of the healthy manner in which I currently present myself, I had been told that this videotaped depiction of my astounding comeback has been the feature of training sessions in Europe. Used for many years to promote the efficiency of Harmarville's head injury therapy program and as an educational tool for Psychology graduate students at the University of Pittsburgh, this public relation's/instructional tape captures a truly remarkable recovery that anybody could appreciate. Serving as confirmation of my one-time critical condition, this videotaped evidence substantiates the claims that mine is a genuinely different kind of human-interest story.

A symptom of my head injury with which I struggled, agraphia is an aphasic condition where one forgets how to write because of trauma to the mental processes. Not only are there an absence of titles exclusively written by head injury survivors advertised in readers' directories or occupying space on shelves, but absolutely none were ever authored by a one-time critically brain traumatized young adult who once couldn't even remember how to manufacture letters in their mind and replicate these symbols on stationery. A form of amnesia, my acute inability to jot down words on paper and subsequent achievement of writing a book about my trials would appear to be a solid promotional bonus for my one-of-a-kind project.

Unlike most titles in bookstores/libraries and so many other related topics on the market, the fact that my manuscript had been written by someone who had personally endured the terror of a severe head injury disability and recovered so magnificently from this traumatic brain injury that he was capable of earning an advanced Master's-level educational status and work professionally as a therapist, should give this book the quality of validity and authenticity. Not to make light of other written endeavors, this writer accomplishing so much in the face of such a destructive handicap would seem to lend credence and significance to this global memoir's existence. Unfortunately, upon re-entering the real world after being hurt, I would soon discover that negative societal opinions towards those with histories of brain damage would be just as—if not more—difficult than any debilities caused by the injury to my brain.

Upon my pursuits to become a contributing member of society, in addition to underscoring different outpatient efforts and many circumstances surrounding my re-entry into college, the next three chapters deal with my unending attempts to overcome the guarded postures which notoriously accompanies anyone whose thinking at one time wasn't "hitting on all eight cylinders." Even more trying than any physical setbacks or cognitive aphasias experienced, judgments based on assumption—and not fact— have been the most difficult hurdle I've had to overcome since being squashed into that utility pole. Throughout my travels over the years being a survivor of a traumatic brain injury, from job pursuits to interpersonal relationships, I have recorded in my life story some of the less-than-flattering occurrences which are part of my history because of the hesitant position held towards those who once sustained a severe brain contusion.

With the ninth and final chapter summarizing a few aspects of the previous eight, I try to wrap things up and answer as many ambiguous blanks as I possibly can. Finishing with a strong and realistic message, the contents of this nonfiction review would appear to have the potential of being a prominent educational and motivational "voice" for those who decide to absorb its teachings/meaning.

Chapter 1

Covert Tears of One

Whether they awoke by the sound of the thunder or astounded by the quake of the earth—with fearful anxiety—these dark, grim-faced figures approached the metallic mass which embraced the unrelenting structure. Light's glow engulfed the homes of those who would normally be resting for the next day's greeting, but tonight the inhabitants disturbed of their rest would gather outside to see what caused the ground to tremble and the silence to be interrupted. Since there was no storm, thunder could not be a possible explanation for the violent vibration. And being that this was not the rocky coast of California, but the rolling hills of southwestern Pennsylvania, an earthquake could only be the figment of an imaginative mind. Those unfortunate enough to witness what was before them had—only moments earlier—been preparing for the arrival of morning, anticipating the same serenity as every other nightfall. Instead, sirens broke the late night silence.

Their tranquil community was transformed into one where activity and apprehension prevailed. "Stillness" not a quality of this night, minds occupied with a terrifying frenzy and paralyzing numbness focused on the crushed anomaly amongst them. Each passing moment, the loud, penetrating wail was getting nearer, yet distant for those who were tormented by the agonizing visions of what could transpire within the heap of steel pressed against the pole.

Time was of the essence, for the body that lie motionless was gradually deteriorating with each tick of the clock. Blood poured from thc ripped flesh that was once a right ear, and what once supported the weight of a 160-pound youth, was now splintered into fragments——not unlike a stump which fall prey to a wielded axe. Hebetude born from the brain being assaulted of its vitality, the victim's fist clenched with such force under his chin that one could have easily thought he understood his predicament and was incensed that his trust had been violated.

The promise of something which had always seemed to elude his grasp was, paradoxically, the culprit of his current plight. Like a butterfly emerging from its cocoon, this confined youth was taking a step away from his hermit-like existence and was going to do the unthinkable and be amongst peers, enjoying himself.

The uncertainty, confusion, self-doubt, and the accompanying fervor were all characteristic of this youth's adolescence. Leading to the unwanted presence of restricted isolation, interpretations of the spoken word and deductions drawn from actions with no meaning anguished the teen ever taunted by misconstrued assertions. Whether the core of these calculations had deeper roots or was a selfimposed intrusion, feeling emotionally remote hindered fulfillment like a shackle restrains its captive. Accepted as logic by those feeling damned by pubescence, to be in "need" was not allowable, for an admission of such a weakness would not be tolerated.

Believing that divulging conceived distress would not be placed within the boundaries of others' understanding, feeling possessed, the expression of irritants could not possibly be exorcised. The origins of this suffering may never be fully realized, the pain so immersed, its source not within the realm of comprehension. Manifested by pathology, the surroundings, inflicted by self, or induced by measures outside the bounds of control, the evaluations made by a mind in the embryonic stage of development could have no significance as it relates to the ingredients of what actually occurs. Peccant imaginations often complicating a teen's vision of the world, truths not intact, distorted perceptions of self-worth may evolve for a merging adult still toiling with the complexities encountered amidst their fragile circle of experience.

Reluctantly endured, being alone and distant never were questioned, for its onset had been acknowledged as a given. Identified as a symbol of disparagement, tormented covertly with a silent plea that the passing of years not be the only means in which assistance may be rendered, hopes maintained that the root of pain shall be dissolved by more than an outgrowth of enhanced learnings and increasing appreciations. Breaking free from the bondage earmarked by the perceived frustration of being chastised, a young person exploring their new territory needs to overcome assignments of deficiency or else anticipate an existence of conviction. Being sensitive and introspective to anything which resembled criticism, even of the constructive nature, could be gravely internalized and taken as an attack. Allowing for the discomfort of misdirected labels to prevail, hurt and submission inevitably would be projected inward and unjustly owned. Not warranted, to avoid suffocation, denied longings would need to be looked upon as unfortunate and not as an omission of fiber.

Too often fixated on that which is not part of one's possession, juvenile minds have been known to reach for the inaccessible. A young mind not yet programmed to absorb the products of enhancement, often tends to solely monitor elements absent from their holdings. Frequently, not in concert with reality or sensitive to sacrifice, restless tyrants sometimes will strive for the short-term without paying homage to the offerings made on their behalf or property already firmly grasped. Conditioned to respect elders and not question their logic about the realities of the world, paralleling the extreme personality of the young man about to embark on a mission to overcome the demons his injury has left him to extinguish, obedience and respect would silently exceed the limits of healthy seasoning.

With the concentrated involvement required and the never ceasing presentation of dramas over a time-span, parenting is the most difficult job in the world. A fine line exists between being too lenient/permissive and too prohibitive; too far to the left or too far to the right. With no set guideline or rule to follow, there's no way possible a parent could be perfect, as enough mistakes will be made during a child's upbringing. My own parents did many, many amazing things right, teaching me values which would benefit and direct me for the rest of my life.

Kind, hard-working, intelligent, generous, considerate, astute, friendly, striving, and respectful were but a few of the traits which made up their fine character. Rarely even receiving a deserved, light spanking on the buttocks, physical discipline was a form of correction which could not be connected with my parents. Violations of any sort were beyond the scope of imagination. Living in a comfortable home, situated "in the thick of" a nice, middle-class neighborhood, having some money in the bank, food on the table, and clothes on one's back were attributes which I didn't fully appreciate or demonstrate the gratitude that I could have because I'd be so accustomed to gaining from the fruits of my parent's experience and labor. Entities which many people would be eternally grateful for, I practically felt guilty that I could make complaints about any thing. Feeling a sense of shame and selfishness, any "wants" trespassing the fabric of those providing me with this "life of ease" would undergo a guarded examination before being uttered.

My perceived stature of being seen not heard, and chronologically stationed as the youngest of four children (my oldest being eighteen years older than myself, my sister sixteen years my senior, and my youngest brother "only" eight years my elder) possibly were why I wanted to participate and excel in high profile professions where respect/recognition would no longer be traits I believed were absent from my life. With those adolescent hormones of mine leaping about and jumping ever which way not helping to facilitate my outlook of the world, the hunger for this attention and breaking free from the subjugation I thought I detected was intense, but could never be conceded to for fear of being ridiculed. These undercover strivings were part of my silent existence, with this aversive state only manifesting self-doubt and diluting what little confidence existed.

Demonstrating some solid skill and really putting my heart into refining my abilities performing these "hobbies," encouragement would never be forthcoming to develop areas which interested me. Repeatedly stressing that I'd never be able to establish any kind of professional standing if I didn't go to college, I'd more or less be on my own without a whole lot of aid pursuing presumed avocations which tantalized me. Told that the special talent required to excel in the fields of baseball or guitar playing was something that I could never attain, I half-heartedly ceased trying to strive in these activities. Pointing out that my fascination to master these "fun" ventures was only due to being in the adolescent stage of development and nothing else, I grudgingly packed up my dreams and set about on a more conventional course with a heavy heart. Ego getting in the way, I didn't want to be convinced of the rationale.

I really loved baseball, but my exhibition on the field was symbolic of my life in general, for potential never sprouted. When it would be my turn to bat in a game situation, I would step in the batter's box wanting to exude an aura of confidence and competency, however, hidden under this projection was a defeatist attitude which would make success remote. This fake emanation deceived few, as the self-question which developed through years of passivity was just too evident. The obsession with baseball and the subsequent hours of enduring practice resulted in my possessing superb eye-hand coordination and an extraordinarily powerful right throwing arm. Skills that I knew I had, as well as my coaches throughout the years when I would demonstrate this gifted athletic prowess while being comfortable and relaxed during practice. Come game time, however, the comfort and enjoyment were sifted out of me and replaced with uneasiness, tension, suspicion, and mistrust in my abilities.

Every one of my coaches, from Pony League to high school, knew I had the ability, but also realized that—due to some emotional barrier—was being restricted from attaining what I could. My Pony League coach, for example, would become frustrated with my attitude and call me "Tom Dooley" because of my penchant for hanging down my head in dejection after making an error at shortstop in the course of a contest after picking everything in sight during pre-game drills. If someone in the stands would yell a derogatory comment directed at me or the team, I would allow them to be a prophet. There isn't much fight in someone who's been kicked when they're already down.

I can still hear my coaches say, "Why can't you do that in a game?," as I would be stinging the ball during batting practice. Like life was for me, the seed that was potential awaited to be developed, however, the sun and moisture necessary for growth was not to be. Not understanding the self-defamation which I never questioned as anything but the truth, I permitted this to weigh me down.

Like so many other teens, much, if not most of this bloodied adolescent's personality was a facade where being laid-back, pain-free, and conforming were proper because owning these traits as part of one's character was how to be accepted. Asphyxiated by my internal investigation, being overly- sensitive made this enveloping outer wall bring me down to the depths of apathy. Interpretations of how I fit into society's mix being clouded by an obtrusive distortion of concepts, the teen-aged glandular process had a profound influence in the sense that I consistently would view the great majority of difficult circumstances as a battle not to be won. Often feeling as if I were about to fall off the "deep-end" and on the fringe of withdrawal, both the "nature" and "nurture" components had a significant effect on my sustained egocentricity, for I could have trouble acknowledging others' position, not demonstrating a capacity to compromise principles which hadn't previously been recognized. Barely allowing for the appreciation of those substances heretofore disregarded, the promotion of sustained growth could not be possible.

More than a facade, regarded as "in step with" natural progression was a lie. Looking inward and seeing a product of perceived misgivings, created a person wanting to be distant from others where ridicule and the corresponding pain would be as obscure as experiencing pleasure. I wanted attention, yet, did not want to be subjected to being focused upon. Wanting accolades, but unsure how to receive them, confusion's noose tightened and panic had been christened.

Self-persecution making the ultimate goal of accepting myself not possible, my tendency to retreat hindered my search for a definition of purpose. Hardly wanting this concealed existence, but needing it for survival, trapped me in an enclosure of bewilderment, frustration, and resentment. An unhappy loner whose self-imposed pain was intense, I felt I couldn't relinquish the misery. Not corresponding with their make-up, mistakenly not giving my folks the benefit of the doubt that they'd have the sensitivity to respond in a favorable light, I almost made a fatal mistake.

My mom, Gwendolyn Claire Meyers, was forty years old when she had me and my dad, Frank L. Meyers, was forty-three when I was born. Because of their own upbringing practically two generations before in a previous era where rules and discipline were generally adhered to without question, their own parenting style/philosophy naturally was similar to the one which they were exposed. Dad's, "My way or hit the highway" approach to parenting was largely instilled in him by his mother's domineering guidance. The premise, "We are the way we are because that's how our parents made us," evidently influenced dad when he would incorporate a not-too-infrequent dictatorship demeanor when instructing and/or correcting his offspring.

Reinforced later in his life when dad served in the armed forces and worked in the police department, mom not infrequently would have her hands full being a negotiating buffer between her kids and husband. "Compromise" not a word easily found in his vocabulary, having an inclination for getting "hot under the collar" when needing to mediate an issue he'd rather not discuss, dad didn't tolerate his "rule" being challenged. Viewing disagreement as disrespect, unless mom could somehow get a word in, dad would usually have the last say.

Not having the most amiable effect on the newest product of the Meyers' family, to me, dad was an imposing figure. Being that I was a little bit scared of him, I still can get icy chills down my spine thinking of times when dad's been angry, as his face would get as red as Satan's claw and his whole body would appear to steam. Jaws tight and teeth clenched, dad's greenish-brown eyed stare would weaken one to the point where shame was felt for refusing to abide by his word, making the treasonist feel compelled to plead for forgiveness. Dad would assume a posture like that of a gladiator being attacked by his mutinous crew, as a not-so-tender dialogue would shoot from his lips like bullets from a machine-gun on the front line.

When dad was this way, there's no way I would think of making a stand and was reluctant to say anything for fear of being emasculated. Waving a white flag in submission was the only way to maintain a cease fire. Retreating into a fetal position, when dad was mad, it was an event that wouldn't be forgotten soon or something one would want to provoke—especially me because of my subordinate position within the Meyers family. Although he never struck his younger kids, the expression on dad's face and the aggression in his voice reminded one that the potential for physical correction was there. Proud that he could elicit this effect, the fiery expression/image characterizing dad when he got pissed left a lasting impression because when dad exhibited such an extreme mood, the family would need to quickly learn how to maneuver, so as to not "set him off" any further.

Years having developed a growing mellowness in dad and my knowing what eggshells to avoid walking on to preserve this "lovable" stature, dad and I had a strong relationship overall. Being a mistake that wasn't intended to happen—as dad would jokingly say that I was here on this earth because he wasn't quick enough—I knew that there was truth to this statement, despite its funny content intended to make light of the "accident." Having three children before me who weren't exactly angels had taken a toll on mom and dad, for they were tired, wanting a much-needed/deserving break from the rigors of parenting. Because of their advanced age having a newborn and mistakenly assuming the baby factory was inoperable, my parents were not particularly overjoyed when informed "Craig" would be making an appearance and were quite surprised knowing they'd need to put "diapers" on their shopping list again.

Knowing that eventually they would be subjected to the traumas a teen typically present guardians, my parents game plan for life would unexpectedly be modified. With my oldest brother's hellion escapades behind the wheel of a car almost two decades earlier still simmering on the edge of dad's conscious and my need to climb out of the "nest" to find out what life was all about, the yolks once inside of these eggshells would be splattered in every direction. Engaging in a war that would have a staying impact, I would be bombarded.

Turning sixteen, I wanted to see what the world had to offer me outside my four bedroom walls which it seemed I had always been quarantined under the specter of my parents. I wanted to escape my isolation, stop being a loner who felt limited by his perceived subservience, and drive a car so I could do some neat stuff like going on a date or to a Pirates' game at Three Rivers Stadium. Given the opportunity to explore my surroundings, I'd finally be able to take advantage of the many pleasures life has to offer. Going to one of the local malls with friends or maybe to a movie theater with some "honey" from school, I thought I'd be afforded the chance to investigate some unchartered waters.

With the way high school chemical secretions were flowing through my body, my diagnosis of the world felt excessive. Given the flawed manner in which I seemed to dissect events occurring about me, life wasn't something that provided harmony, but merely a framework where one exists and tries to survive. Guarding against the countless ills ready to forsake one, for fear that danger could evolve, deviating from what was known would not come easy. Like pulling teeth, stepping forward into a fresh horizon where the promotion of growth/development occurs would be delayed by ghosts from the past.

Getting my driver's permit and needing to practice with my parents, not really all that thrilled with the prospects of a rookie driver assuming control of their car, they refused. Saying that I first had to have Driver's Ed in high school and get the basic instruction before they'd take me out, stress had been postponed. Just as soon wishing this tension could be alleviated altogether, not looking forward to this dreaded day, the school semester would end before long.

After passing Driver's Ed, it was now time for the most difficult part of the driving process—having my parents undertake an open-minded role as instructors. Being that they had done this automobile training before with their other kids with mixed results prior to my turn, and because of their advanced years/subsequent low stress tolerance—not to mention my oldest brother's troubles—this was a time my parents weren't exactly celebrating and wouldn't be basking with delight knowing that they'd need to endure this experience of soul-testing one more time.

When I'd ask to go out and practice, the veins in my 60-year-old father's forehead would pop out and his arms would flail, looking like a serpent seeking its next prey. Being a real confidence-booster, this stress would be expressed by his impatience when I wouldn't integrate his verbal instruction right away into technique. Paternal anger would arise because I didn't know anything more about a car than where the brake, steering wheel, and radio dial were.

After the practice sessions throughout the area in our old Buick Skylark, I took the driver's test and got my license following the second test (I didn't pass the first one because I didn't park close enough to the curb). Having my license, I incorrectly thought I was free and had the means to see what was out there for me.

Shortly after getting this licensed admission to the real world, however, my dad sold the Buick. An automatic transmission and the only car I'd ever driven with the exception of the one in Driver's Ed, buying a Chevy Citation that dad immediately proclaimed my mom's and off-limits to Craig, I'd basically be back to "Square One." Stuck with having to rely on my challenged mechanical "skill" in order to gain my much sought-after independence, dad "gave me" his beloved puke green Mercury Bobcat which was a standard transmission.

Possessing a teaching style where he'd holler and get angry, dad's intolerance for anything but perfection when we'd go out for practice runs in his "baby" only compounded the problem of my being developmentally delayed whenever it came to anything automotive. The combination of my being anything but intuitive when it came to managing a car and dad screaming in my ear from the passenger seat that I was a "dumb ass" for not being able to simultaneously step down on the clutch, shift to the proper gear on cue, keep my eyes on the road, prevent "taking out" any mailboxes, and check the side/rear view mirrors for surrounding traffic, extreme tension would be manufactured just about every time we'd "buckle up" and head off for the road.

Not knowing if I fell victim to the adolescent stereotype of being a troublemaker, only having the sensitivity to view dad's inhibited decisions about my operating a vehicle as unfair treatment and not a determination based on extensive experience, I merely saw his judgments as a restraint where dad just looked for any excuse to keep me from getting in that driver's seat because that would be one big worry he wouldn't have to contend with. Conflict occurring just mentioning anything about driving, frustration developed for both of us because of our communication breakdown when being "tutored" how to drive a stick-shift.

The difference in generations putting us on incompatible wavelengths, dad made the automobile training experience a miser able one for me. Actually making me afraid to drive a car and almost feeling a sense of "shame" that I was putting my older dad through the nausea of teaching a teenager how to drive, I never learned how to handle the Bobcat. Knowing this was going to happen, I detested dad for this. Being without any kind of transportation, with everyone else around me acquiring the ability to maneuver a car, I was embarrassed and retreated back into my hole of isolation again.

If I didn't live in a big neighborhood of about one-hundred houses where I could walk to friends' homes to get them to play sports of some kind, I'd have been totally reclusive. Every single weekend without fail during the better part of the academic year, if I wouldn't be playing a pick-up sandlot ballgame of some sort, I'd spend the great majority of my time alone, sitting in my room and playing rock 'n' roll albums on my J.C. Penney stereo through headphones. Becoming an awesome "air guitarist" with all the practice, my Friday and Saturday nights would come and go without experiencing the dates, get-togethers, and outings every teenager NEEDS to become acquainted with in order to grow/develop properly.

Getting used to this isolative state and pretending that I was content so I wouldn't make "waves," I really didn't want to be bothered by people anymore because I was so unhappy. Having an increasingly difficult time maintaining a false front that things were just fine, those pubescent hormones were busy making life agonizing for me when I'd go to school on Monday and hear how it seemed everyone else's weekend appeared so eventful/interesting. Strenuously forcing a smile, I'd be able to let the topic brush past me when asked what I did. Knowing how to change the subject, I'd be proceeding on my merry old way.

His occasional tendency to get explosive when things didn't go precisely as planned contributing to my oldest brother's not recognizing his family of origin after he got married, dad knew how to incorporate a teaching modality flaming with volatile overtones. Unbearable reminders from the past helping to foster a rabid perception towards young drivers, by the overall disposition he exhibited when working with me, dad appeared to have difficulty accepting that my individual reserved personality just might result in an outcome characterized by less friction. A relatively trouble-free adolescent driving experience being an impossible concept to visualize, abandonment from those qualities necessary to desert would not occur. A solitary presence at a time when yearnings require investigation, does not reap a fruitful harvest.

Knowing that I never went out, with a narrow circle of friends, I can remember being told that I'm going to be lonely someday because of my inclination not to socialize. Prone to being solitary, concern would be expressed for me. With a manner in which to travel not at my disposal, this situation would be similar to one where a treasure hunter would be encouraged to dig for gold, but not given a shovel. Being a no work, no play entity which merely took up space, I was an alliance of one.

Detached from activity did have one positive aspect—I learned how to play guitar and further develop my love for music. Playing baseball during my three-month break from school and not working summer jobs, I had to rely on good ole mom and dad to get me the electric guitar I've always wanted. Visions of my siblings' past musical failures still very much catalogued in my parent's memory banks, victimized once again by images from yesteryear, I would be told that I didn't possess the mental fortitude to learn how to play the instrument. Similar to my long-running pursuit trying to convince my ultra-conservative parents of my desire to participate in organized baseball, after years of bruised knees pleading, my folks finally came through in November 1979 when I was sixteen and bought me a Les Paul copy. Like their other kids' attempts with their respective instruments years before, figuring I'd get frustrated with the six-string and wouldn't "stick with it," they really weren't intimidated that their dream for me to further my studies would be posed with any kind of threat. Whether childish or I actually had found something which really appealed to me, I'd have other ideas, however.

Hour after hour, I practiced diligently. I loved my guitar and I was beginning to learn fast because of this infatuation. On the brink of obsession, I now didn't care if I were apart from the outside world. I had an excuse for my being removed because acquiring the ability to play music smoothly requires spending an exuberant amount of time "in the woodshed" wrapped around an instrument by yourself in order to gain the necessary skills/dexterity.

To hell with peers. To hell with driving. To hell with schoolwork, especially. I now have the means to retire in my own little world that—oddly enough—allows me to fantasize about being adored by the masses and universally accepted, while still being within my comfort zone of being alone.

When I wasn't blasting my eardrums with my L.P.'s, I spent most of my time by myself either throwing a tennis ball on the side of the house training to be the next great shortstop, playing my guitar, or spending countless hours listening to my Aerosmith albums. Aerosmith came to Pittsburgh's Civic Arena on December 9, 1979 and I was going to my first concert with a long-time neighborhood "buddy" and two other schoolmates. Those hebetic bodily processes playing havoc with my scope of reason, feeling secluded from peers but not having the freedom to express the core of this disdain, had me purposelessly spiraling without any sense of control. Tangled in an entrapment of lost resolution, the resulting sensations of restriction made me feel not unlike a caged animal. Overly-impressionable, that which knows only confinement will become instinctively wild when outside the bars of their domain. Once outside my self-assigned detention, not realizing that my means of "escape" had spawned a cancer, it was during this show that I discovered another "friend"——marijuana.

The reaction from my first experience with weed wouldn't soon be forgotten, for it was one of omnipotent proportions; a response of guilt, excitement, and paranoia. The excitement surfaced because the "real me" came to the front. I no longer was the quiet, shy, introverted follower, rather, the humorous, outgoing, assertive self that I knew was within me, but couldn't unchain. The fear that I wouldn't be accepted was replaced by the knowledge that "I'm okay and you're okay."

And I was embraced. As a matter of fact, I'd be king of the hill. I demanded and received the respect by those that I was with at the concert. When I wanted to be funny, my buddies laughed "with" me hysterically. Getting the respect I desired and being accepted when I wanted were traits I didn't realize that I had. My new "friend" made this awareness possible and the sense that I was inferior to all was sifted out of me like the blood of a corpse before a showing.

It wasn't until my junior year in high school that I discovered this new dimension that my great, new "friend" provided me. With the walls of the self-constructed Hell crumbling, I would no longer be in custody, arrested by constraint. With the liberty I had seized in the course of my endless search, my new vision showed that life needn't be so complicated and desolate, rather, like a flower reaching for the sun, something natural, simple, and joyous. This tiny, "harmless," cannabis seed made this enlightenment possible. Remembering this dangerous mirage as some type of key to expression, a lethal memory had been unearthed.

Because those I had gone to the show with were experienced smoking pot, their high had worn off long before the last note had been picked, while my buzz was hitting its peak on the way home to Washington. During the half-hour drive back, I prayed my parents were asleep, for my eyes were bloodshot and I reeked of reefer. I could imagine my dad meeting me at the front door as I was trying to sneak in and, realizing I was stoned, belting me across the chops that first time. I could see my loving, caring mom standing at the top of the stairs in her nighty, glaring at me as I sprawled to my feet, not saying a word, only looking through me with the ultimate disappointment. Picturing mom not uttering a word to me until the turn of the 21st Century, or a cure for the common cold was found—whichever came last—I'd be petrified with this delusional thought. When I voiced this paranoia, those who had been laughing "with" me only an hour before, were now laughing "at" me.

For a few brief hours, wishing that this heightened metamorphosis would provide me with some kind of resolution to what "ailed" me, I hoped that I had found an answer. However, after the masquerade that I was royalty had dwindled away, I felt guilty because I did something I saw as devious to the two people I love most. Affirmation for me that there is a God in Heaven, when King Arthur got home, my parents were in bed.

Shortly after the smoked alteration had worn off, reality set in again and I was back to my life of solitude. Not evident during its conception, the evolution of a malignancy had formed, believing that a spirited realm could be apprehended beyond the arena of uncolored sensation. Coming at a high price, the abbreviated glimpse into distortion was an exciting transformation, however.

Unfortunately, the legacy I left behind during my secondary education was one based on consecutive days not bringing a book home from school. I despised school, not only because of the boring bookwork required to excel in academics, but also because of the inferior position I assumed when interacting with peers outside of my neighborhood friends. Whether it had something to do with the testosterone spewing throughout my system or simply my irrational viewpoint, assuming others were innately better than me didn't help in my efforts to be included. Having a fair share of acquaintances, thinking that I was unworthy of anyone's time, I really wasn't a member of any type of clique, however. Fearing to be perceived as a desolate soul with no direction, manufacturing a balanced facade was a necessity.

A never-ending cyclic pattern of confusion had been manifested by the perception of messages received about myself and the environment. Developing a standpoint where I seldom wanted bothered by people, I sought select friendships, so I wouldn't be entirely secluded. Confronting the self-defaming thoughts that haunted me, this self-deprived youth would secretly stew in bitterness. Having a musical outlet to explain my separation, I had an alibi to fuel the facade of appearing at ease with my routine.

Capturing what I thought to be the perfect "release" which meshed with my personality, the little utility I saw in classwork went right out the door. Doing just enough to get by, not at all indicative of my potential capabilities, I was only a mediocre "C" student throughout high school. With my class rank being of the three-figured variety, I barely applied myself. Hardly exhilarating, studying the evolution of the Iroquois Indian tribe and memorizing the elements comprising a chemical didn't cause me to froth at the mouth with excitement, so I'd whip my $120 guitar out of its plastic case once I got home from classes and start wailing away through my 30 watt Peavey amplifier when I should have been breaking out my textbooks.

While I was pounding out the barre chords to AC/DC's "Night Prowler" when this tune was reverberating out my speakers, I imagined Bon Scott and Co. calling for me to jam with them in Pittsburgh's Stanley Theatre in front of thousands of screaming fans. As burning sweat was pouring from my brow stinging my eyes, Angus Young and I were bobbing our heads and high-stepping around the stage. With the spotlight shining on us while we were gyrating about, at least a dozen beautiful seventeen-year-old girls were lifting up their tops demonstrating how well-endowed they were before flinging their bras at me, cheering wildly.

Hearing, "Craig, Craig, Craig" and thunderous pounding, my arousal halted because I'd discover it wasn't the crowd chanting my name or the stomp of their feet to the rhythm of the music, rather, the thumping was coming from the bedroom door and the shrieks trespassing my fantasy world originated from just outside this partition. Nor would the bright gleam be emitted from "Bic" lighters held high, waving in unison to the pulsating aggressiveness of the solos, but the silhouette intruding upon my "personal space" had evolved from the hallway light on the other side of this entrance.

Quickly lifting the needle off the record, and leaning my guitar against the bed, I jumped out of my rocking chair and opened up the door. Blinded momentarily, standing there with her penetrating smile was my angelic mother telling me that I had received mail from West Virginia University's Admission and Records. Surrounded by a proud glow with the letter in hand, face twitching from fighting back an anticipatory smile, mom could hardly wait until I opened up the notification.

Frost-bitten by indifference, dark shadows of me stuffing my nose into tantalizing books for at least four more years cutting into my disturbed conscious, I felt hollow inside. Envisioning myself as a permanent "General Studies" major, when I read the contents to mom that I had been accepted at W.V.U., tears filled mom's eyes because she was overjoyed. Tears gathered in my eyes too—-but it wasn't due to being beside myself with joy.

Mom stressed to me time after time after time, the importance of having money and getting the necessary background/experience needed to pocket some cash. Her stance being that education is the key to ultimate happiness/wealth, I could appreciate mom's viewpoint, for she knew what it was like to do without and saw what hardship really was. Getting me some notoriety amongst my fellow classmates when I was in elementary school because my parents were the only ones who could take out their teeth, with my folks "up" in years when I joined the clan, I was one of a very few teenagers during my generation having parents who struggled through the Great Depression. A very intelligent woman, mom never had the opportunity to attend a four-year college because she was devoted to raising a family and provided the necessary support dad required to attain his Bachelor's, then Master's Degree.

Wanting the best for me so I wouldn't have to sacrifice like they did, my parents thought that the only real way to achieve success was to get further education and be buried in books. Like most anything else, taken in doses of moderation and not excess, this school of thought incorporated as part of the sum and not acknowledged as a whole could deliver some prosperous returns. Social and emotional development regarded as a secondary consideration, mom's fundamental philosophy developed its roots from the principle that if one has some dollars in the bank, these necessities for maturation will eventually take care of themselves in time.

Being an only child who had many uncles, aunts, and cousins who would pamper her, mom didn't have to venture far to find companionship. A member of a close family unit as a child, the light of her kin's eyes, mom really had no need or motivation to socialize outside of the family tree. In addition to experiencing the enormous trials of a recession, the importance of seeking friendships beyond relatives not being a learning process mom necessarily felt she had to address during her formative years, very possibly could have influenced her outlook of what factors were essential for healthy blossoming.

Because of the high regard held for mom and dad's understanding of the world, I couldn't bring myself to tell my folks that attending college wasn't foremost on my "to do" list. A combination of this listless soul's having the utmost respect for his parent's experience/knowledge of the world and my petty opinion of myself—without question—I prepared to attend West Virginia University in the fall of 1981, despite my abhorrence of academics.

Repeatedly reminded that I wouldn't have to lift a finger to get the needed money for room, board, tuition, and books—not wanting to be selfish or disrespectful—telling my parents that I didn't feel college was right for me wasn't about to happen. Provided these necessities on a gold platter, unlike a lot of less fortunate students-to-be who flipped burgers at some fast-food joint or sold popcorn at the movie theatre so they'd have a chance at going to school, taking advantage of this shot at furthering my studies which presented itself to me wouldn't be regarded as something necessarily useful. Being a 17-year-old with little exposure to the world, I didn't have much of an idea what in the hell I wanted to do with my life. About to finish thirteen years of school that lacked being noteworthy or exciting in any way, I just knew that I was tired of the scholastic runaround and wanted a break from tests. Possibly senseless and egotistical, the activities I was good at and liked to do were being discarded as a dead-end that few gain any kind of prosperity. Taking life as it came, not armed with any type of set design, my long-range plans being nonexistent, I would be on a course where I could only flounder.

Hinting that I wanted to pursue my interests in music or sports, I'd be told that these were activities that most "bubble gum" adolescents are fascinated with and that this fantasy will pass like any other fling. Suggesting it might be a good idea to take a year off from school so I could "find myself" and/or re-energize, the focus would naturally turn to the monetary aspect of this decision. With inflation and the ensuing higher cost to get an education, an unnecessary expense which would need to be avoided, this alternative wouldn't be considered.

Falling behind the rest of the members of my high school graduating class, cautious never to rub him the wrong way, I could picture dad reaching the boiling point if I told him that I didn't want to go to school and saying, "It'd figure you wouldn't want to do something good for yourself. You just want to sit on your ass and play that ukulele all day."

With life chartered out for me, the backbone of this perfect blueprint was that I go off to college. Because of their selfless effort and incredible sacrifice made on my behalf during my upbringing, the very least I could do for my parents would be to fulfill their dream that I get a degree. Serving as the kerosene for her proud glow, with this course of action strategically mapped out for me, I diligently watched mom expend the effort to prepare me for my freshman year. If it were permitted by the university, I'd have let mom go to orientation for me.

My priority supposedly being that I head off to school to get an advanced education so I could establish a professional standing and earn some bucks, I always just assumed that if one were not in special-ed and could count to fifty without too much trouble, they were college-bound. Besides, anybody who wanted to be more than a custodian at K-Mart was off to some establishment of enhanced learning after receiving their diploma. Not even liking to clean my room, I couldn't begin to fathom mopping up an entire department store.

School administration apparently believing that I had a little academic potential anyhow, I'd be placed in a lot of Phase 4 "brain" classes at Trinity when my schedule wouldn't be filled up with study halls and paint by number classes. A mixture of my solitude character perceived by more than a few as one fueled by alcohol/cannabis herb and it being within my realm of possibility that scholastic achievement may actually exist, because of West Virginia University's reputation of being both "Party School U.S.A." and an institution of high academic principle, my ultimate choice of this school to enroll wouldn't come as total surprise. However, this facade would come back to haunt me.

When one distances themself from others, often a history can be presumed that couldn't be any further from reality. Because of the loud, raucous, heavy metal music I became known to like, it had developed as a given by a tad more than a few senior high circles in school that my antics must've corresponded with these hard core musicians performing this brand of darkness. Essentially being a loner when I wasn't trying to be a "jock" on some ballfield, feeling a need to "live up to" the rock 'n' roll lifestyle and become associated with a social group of some form, I had a ticket to disaster waiting for me with the way I'd attempt to "fit in."

Not contesting this faulty label I would be given by those who didn't realize the absurdity of their generalization, not believing I had an identity throughout my secondary schooling, I wasn't about to proceed through college not being known for anything. Longing to hold a pass to acceptance, truth hardly a prerequisite, I wouldn't object to forfeiting principle. Following a misguided pattern which didn't conform with the depths of my belief system, I'd be putting one foot in the grave.

Not even liking the taste of beer, I might have drank the equivalent of two beers TOTAL during high school. Being the epitome of "red," if I was playing softball with some buddies and one of them brought some suds, I'd take a gulp and hold it in my mouth for an inning, then spit it out when no one was looking. With my middle name being "school spirit," despite the high school football field only a half-mile away from my house, not once did I attend a game. Never going anywhere socially, the only times I'd ever witness dances, dates, or parties was when I'd watch "The Brady Bunch" reruns on T.V. If it weren't for my stroking palm, I'd have been a virgin.

Having the mode of transportation required to be involved amongst peers only a dream, I had to learn to tolerate being alone. Fearful of being judged in anything but a positive light, believing that others could read right through me, I would be able to convince myself that being without company was a desirable option. Looking in the mirror and seeing someone nondescript in every sense of the word, my growing pain itches made it a difficult struggle viewing Craig Meyers as adequate. Trudging along in a lackluster fashion, confronted with an existence of avoidance and perceived condemnation, supposititious abandonment inflicted upon myself, self-imposed isolation would be a Hell I had to teach myself to be comfortable with because I didn't know how to be free. Enduring a censored presence in an environment not conducive to a rich opinion of myself, am I ever ecstatic that the surroundings where I have tasted so much bitterness will soon only be a memory, and not the living suffocation it has come to be. Ungrateful yearnings bred by newfledged biological changes, one ordeal would be set to lead into another.

Many snatches of his personality reminding mom of her cherished father, led to believe that the pathway to success went through a college campus, I would be influenced to accept that the only legitimate option for me after high school was to follow in the footsteps of my enriched brother and go to a school of higher learning. Graduating from W.V.U. magnum caum laude and securing a job immediately after school, my sibling rival would be the perpetrator leading mom to think that it was my turn to set the college training world back on its heels. Making matters all that much worse for the wear, after attaining his sheepskin, my brother had to go off and marry his high school sweetheart—a fellow Mountaineer who also prevailed with high honors. A Rebecca of Sunnybrook Farms type, this marriage made in Heaven only solidified mom's position that I become refined at a university setting and meet a co-ed so sweet. If these relationships are productive and not geared to advance one's own standing by subjecting others to their deficiencies, living with siblings is a learning process that can better teach one how to function in society and get along with people.

Indicative of how our relationship had developed as a chummy one over the years—short for ugly—I have habitually referred to my older brother, Scott as—"Ug." A response to his daily name-calling/disparaging assaults on me since I was a little boy, Ug's ability to express himself verbally and perceive things in a humorous way were two skills utilized as weapons once I was born to enhance his own standing amongst the relatives. Being the youngest of three for eight years until I joined the ranks, Ug felt the need to grab center stage, so he'd have an outlet to display his worth. Not wanting to relinquish "the spotlight" he enjoyed so much, a manner in which Ug's demand for continued attention had presented itself once a younger member of the household inexperienced with the ways of the world and defenseless to the manipulations of those intellectually/emotionally more mature had made his appearance.

Not infrequently, feeling as if they don't "measure up" to their older siblings, a youngest's command for attention will often cause them to be "loud." Because of their more-than-occasionally favored position within a family, the last born are more likely to make major mistakes over and over and over again, for their indiscrepancies are more likely to be overlooked. Spawning impatience and carelessness, having difficulty learning the benefits of "biting their tongue," a most recent born's customary need to over-achieve within a given arena so that they be attended to, can muster circumstances that are inappropriate. Chronologically, I assume the youngest position amongst the Meyers' siblings, but anyone who has heard Ug at a family get-together knows who holds this status emotionally.

Taking reverence in the exploitation of the errors that are part of any development, while using this exposure to heighten own self-worth by means of deflating another, would be a demeaning method of getting laughter. Needing relief from his pressure-packed job, dad wouldn't be opposed to a cackle now and again.

Visions of her father's comic gestures joyfully dancing in her head, with mom's laughter at Ug's demoralizing commentary serving as his encouragement to continue, my role had become defined within the Meyers family. An incredible expense for the sake of jovial cynicism, constant ridicule carving a distressing timidity on many fronts, taking a trampled self-concept into various realms of society wouldn't help me in my interactions with others. Just beginning grade school not making me immune to my high school brother's fists when a difference would occur, with eyes looking the other way, I got the childhood "message" that aggression towards me was an appropriate means of conflict resolution.

Not infrequently displaying an appearance of inadequacy, derisive assaults wounded me in the sense that I accepted my role of being mortified all too readily and without debate. With the intent that I be anchored deep within the bleakness of being subordinate, dwelling on my inability to achieve left me in a position where equality could not be possible. Crippled by persistent taunting, pursuits to attain assertiveness would all but be destroyed. So that dominance may be attained, deficits or items not within a child's sphere of understanding would be focused upon with a magnifying glass and anything less than displaying adult competency/efficiency would subject me to misunderstood criticism that I wouldn't be able to stop or equate its meaning. A follow-up editorial sure to make the airwaves, the core of wisecracks would be assimilated as part of my character and make the elements necessary to be well-adjusted, a remote venture. Insisting this ceaseless scorning would harden me for rough waters which I may encounter in my voyage ahead through life, depreciation would leave a mark.

A part of healthy development is establishing relations with those of the opposite sex. However, if a young female would approach me or if I was just being civil with her—not necessarily friendly—I would be continuously humiliated. Feeling stupid and wanting to maneuver around the abasement that was sure to be waiting for me at home, I'd avoid interactions with girls like a virus. Worshipping the ground that he walked on, images of her father would joyously filter into mom's conscious when she'd laugh at the discomfort Ug created for me during those times when the promise of having a girlfriend was replaced with feelings of foolishness. My maternal support thinking how "cute" my reactions to insults were, my last tier of defense had been sabotaged. With impressions lasting at this young age, I developed an avoidance attitude towards the ladies when I was in school that—like a leech on an open sore—was arduous to discard. Trying to make up for lost time, thank God this early discouragement to make female friends/partners didn't make me "funny."

Symbolic of how we regularly interacted and my ability to command authority within the Meyers' family, when we'd travel about eighty miles to Johnstown, Pa. to visit my grandparents in dad's compact Mercury Bobcat, dad couldn't refrain from smoking his fucking pipe for an hour and a half, despite knowing his way of ridding the tension from his job as the Director of the Western Area Vo-Tech School in Houston, Pa. made me extremely nauseous. Mom sitting passively in the passenger seat, Ug would have a field day on these trips laughing, as I fought back the puke that wanted to spew from my mouth.

Breathing my dad's secondary smoke for a total of sixteen years, doing the unthinkable and speaking up about how his carbon monoxide habit would make me sick, dad would become so vile that he'd tell me that none of their other kids ever caused as much trouble between he and mom as I did. Experiencing incredible pain, when voicing a displeasure or expressing an opinion causes more trouble than some of my siblings' dark indiscretions, I just better pretend everything's alright. Learning the lesson that being heard is disrespectful, I had been trained to shut up and not disagree.

Persistent degradation and feeling frustrated that I could not express myself, assuming a profound inferiority, I would repeatedly bounce my head off the back of our couch resembling what someone with autism does when they've had enough. Possibly questioning in his mind if his advanced age had made a child who was mentally stunted, dad would insist that I stop when I'd spring back and forth, saying that people will think that I'm "retarded." Cleaning up or cooking, undergoing a silent worry, mom wouldn't have much time to comment about my weird recoiling behavior. But when Ug would see me do this, he'd rejoice and make sure to get anyone around to join in the mocking festivities. Entering the freshman collegiate world of Basic Instruction 101 courses and student teachers, not possessing the emotional composition to recognize the commitment before me, my immature development served as the nucleus of my wayward aims in life.

Biding my time, for seventeen-and-one-half years, the day I have prayed would hurry up and get here will soon finally be approaching——graduation from high school. Celebrating this achievement, gathered around friends, reflecting on the years prior to the attainment of the long-awaited diploma would seem to be natural and desirable. Cherishing triumphs in preparation for the growth of a new generation and appreciating the learning experience tribulations play in one's development from a child to a young adult would seem to be something memorable and hailed with joyous anticipation. Ruminating about the first driving experience with a family member who hoped to return not being maimed, that first date, dances, weekend trips with friends, the prom, or the grand slam in the bottom of the last inning with two outs to propel your team from a three-run deficit to victory are things which should put a smile on one's face, not a tear to the eye. But for me, feelings of happiness did not correspond with these thoughts, rather, a deep-seated sense of neglect and deprivation.

During these turbulent years when my libido was being starved, emotional stability could not possibly be a part of my make-up. From where I stood, the maintenance of a facade would be essential and of the utmost importance. Amidst the bonds of torment, but trying to portray an image of being enshrined atop glory, I couldn't escape the futile strivings that reality had become.

Potentials never realized because of ingrained self-doubt and fear of expression, a burgeoning self-confinement made me vulnerable to uninvited devices.

With a perceived cruelty about me, I just wanted to be left alone to escape the hidden barriers which trapped me and left this complex member of the "me" generation thrashing within his Victim Role. Developing a desire to be self-contained, projecting a fallacious image of ignorance and incompetence, an exhibition of truths would not be permissible, for fear of vigilant judgments. Not to be challenged, displaced manipulations integrated as the soul of my poignancy would suppress that which I had harvested. The perverse influence of the organic process in a juvenile mind does not lend itself to junior impulses having any basis with intrinsic acceptance.

On graduation, tossing the tassel on my cap was a symbolic gesture for me. Going from one stage to another, the supposed transition from homebound dependency to independent responsibility was an unwelcome predator. Not ready to stop playing baseball or my guitar, all the other college-bound neighbor kids were aspiring engineers, accountants, lawyers, and teachers. Figuring I could be a rock 'n' roll icon because I could play a dozen power chords flawlessly, I didn't want to go to work and school. But that's exactly what I was preparing to do in the summer of 1981.

A week before Trinity's graduation ceremonies, I secured a summer job at the Floral Hill Greenhouse in town working the 3:00 P.M.-11:00 P.M. shift——the first summertime vacation I'd ever had where I didn't play baseball everyday. And in a couple of weeks, I was destined to go to W.V.U.'s orientation with my best friend from high school and soon to be college roommate, Kevin Brezinski. "Let's go-oooooo, Mountaineers."

Chapter 2

Making of a Nightmare

Down on my luck, the fall semester arrived as scheduled. Preparing to embark on what was supposed to be a mission that would lead to a distinguished career, opting for a pre-journalism course of study, I chose a field where I could put into use The King's English as my major basically because this was the only scholastic subject which sparked any kind of interest for me. The capacity to jot down expressive concepts being the one area I could excel at if the spirit hit me, I have shown some skill dabbling with creative writing. More appealing to me than dissecting frogs or examining rare rock formations found only in remote regions of South Africa, I thought I could at least utilize my faculty for integrating words to convey some sort of picturesque message as a means to sustain a decent livelihood. Having a mind that can stray off the beaten path into a little bit of ingenuity, keeping my fingers crossed that I had the right "stuff," it would require much more than hope to translate academic instruction into a profession where I could command respectable earnings.

The amount of time I spent investigating potential specialties within journalism—or any vocation for that matter—was limited. Instead of "sports writing" where I could at least integrate my interests in athletics and writing, I made a first-rate blunder choosing "Advertising" as the branch within journalism I'd pursue. Knowing that I wouldn't mind having these things too someday, I just knew that Darrin Stevens on the T.V. show, "Bewitched," was in advertising and had a nice house and a skinny wife—research at its finest.

This freshman collegiate semester wouldn't be about the three basic "R's" of reading, writing, and arithmetic, rather, Journalism 1, Humanities, and Political Science, amongst a host of other stimulating courses I couldn't wait to sink my teeth into. Not seeing the practicality of any of these classes as they might apply to my life, I just knew that I wasn't going to be the next Edward Morrow, thought Oedipus and Socrates were sexually transmitted diseases, and might remember that George Bush was the Vice-President on a good day. Not that I was necessarily stupid, rather, the utility of studies had yet to be appreciated. Getting reacquainted with a "friend" I had the pleasure of getting to know once before while a student in high school, the first week of school got underway, and no time was wasted plotting a course which would impact me for the rest of my life.

Overwhelmed by my new surroundings, I was intimidated being in a different state with the anticipation that I excel at and assimilate to this unknown college environment. Never learning to adapt to the high school setting where I had at least attended classes with many students for the better part of a decade, I didn't have any idea how in the hell I was supposed to catch the world on fire and be a success at West Virginia University where I didn't know a soul or have a clue as to what in God's name I was doing. With all the bustling/crazed activity where countless strangers with accents were unpacking and getting situated, the PRT shuttle car zipping around was similar to that of my brain waves which wanted to explode with all the commotion. "Excitement" the order of this inaugural day when students could move into their dorm room, there were so many things to do in such a short period of time. Expected to reach out and explore new territories in Wild, Wonderful, West Virginia when I never really took a look at old frontiers in Laid-back, Typical, Washington, Pa., I felt threatened.

Seeming like light years ago, I would be glad Kevin was here to remind me that I once came from a place where I actually had a vague idea of what was going on and knew a few people. Four high-rise residential complexes designed mostly for freshman who must live on campus, Kevin and I would be living in the Towers. Situated in the Evansdale Campus, the particular story we'd be residing arguably having more derelicts than San Quentin Penitentiary, my roommate and I lived on the zero floor of Towers 4. There were quite a few Trinity Hiller Class of '81 alumni living in the Towers structure whom I was acquainted with, but besides Kevin, I didn't really consider myself good friends with any of them. But that would change in a hurry.

Two guys I knew of during high school, but never associated with, roomed together in one of the other Towers. Possessing traits which corresponded with my coveted desire to "belong," pretty good friends with the long-time neighborhood "buddy" who introduced me to the hemp I thought led to the utopia of freedom and appreciation, "B. 'Boss' Bostko" and the immortal "Paul Michaels" would be my Mountaineer buddies helping me to forge my way to the promised land of high regard. The beginning of a tragedy, ill-advised motivations would siphon me of any existing ambitions.

Describing my life as uneventful would be a gross understatement, excessively dull would be more apropos. My everyday routine not exactly stimulating, in Webster's Dictionary alongside the word, "mundane," lies my senior picture that can also be found in the '81 school yearbook. Analogous to the makeup plastered on my face with a paint brush for this snapshot in order to cover up the multitude of zits resting here, the forced smile that I presented for the camera hid the ugliness my adolescence had strapped me with. Laboring under a false impression sensing that I was by some means muzzled, the thrill of tasting forbidden fruit had oozed from my overbearing conscience into unexplored temptation. Where the excitement of not getting caught begins, a life disregarding conviction shall be one absent of design.

Basically why I had never hung out with them, both Michaels and "Boss" had reputations for being partiers in school. Too enmeshed with sports and music to concern myself with alcohol or drugs, foreign substances were never an enticement. Needing to surrender my fascination for these two glamour occupations, I needed to find some other interest to occupy my fantasy. Approximately forty-five miles away from home, I knew I wouldn't have to worry about getting caught by my parents gallivanting from my customary unaccompanied/reserved demeanor to a little bit of rabble-rousing. Sure to result in me being "tarred and feathered," I wouldn't realize the benefits of such protection.

A popular guitar player in school, known for liking his females, Boss knew how to charm and utilize the comb in his back pocket like a gunslinger uses a six-shooter. Having a silver tongue second to none, Boss knew how to enamor the young girls to slip out of their panties. This gift, as well as his solid ability on the six-string, made Boss an appealing person to develop a friendship with.

Through the long-time neighborhood "buddy" who introduced me to marijuana, amongst a few others, what I had heard about Michaels sounded interesting because I would be on a quasi-recruiting mission in search of as many adventurers as possible to fraternize with while taking a look around this huge university. Never saying so much as a word to him during high school, Michaels appeared to have a certain mystique about him that projected confidence and respect. Wanting to display a real man's man image, Michaels' "kick-back" approach only made his assertive persona that much more likable. With quite a few of my friends being on the "backward" side like myself on many fronts, it was refreshing encountering someone to be pals with who could display an aura of mystery, yet be cool at the same time. A little intriguing coming across someone with such brains, gusto, and spirit, I thought I was making the most of an opportunity.

Adding to the appeal, coming from a background where his parents and older brother were employed as health care professionals, Michaels had the benefits of an upper middle-class support system teaching him values growing up. Supported by this foundation, not allowing his social class to interfere with his natural tendency to be down-to-earth, Michaels seemed to be the kind of guy someone wouldn't mind getting to know. Supposedly operating from the best of both worlds, seeing attributes of Paul's character as interesting and something which wouldn't want to be relinquished, my death certificate had been so close to being signed.

It didn't take long for me to make my way to the other Towers to play some guitar with Boss. As we played some rock 'n' roll tunes, Paul would be sitting on the edge of their bunk bed moving to the infectious beat of the music. Cigarette dangling, with his shoulders swaying and playing his imaginary guitar ever so effectively, Paul got each of us a beer. An offering I accepted as if I were a seasoned pro, while the AC/DC and Judas Priest tunes were pumping from Boss' Marshall amp, a few guys who lived on their floor would pop in and join us, voicing their approval of the music being played. Getting some notoriety and having a good time in the process, maybe this college atmosphere wouldn't be so bad, after all.

After the crowd had dwindled down to where it was just me and the "Dynamic Duo," Paul went to his desk and opened a drawer. Yanking out some "Tip-Top" papers, he then sat down and rolled the perfect joint. Its symmetry was breathtaking. Its texture like that of granite. And its beauty majestic. Only a connoisseur of this art could create such a harmonious configuration.

My having absolutely no objection, when Paul reached into his pocket for his lighter, thoughts of the one and only time I had ever gotten high occupied my conscious. Exhilaration ascending to a fever pitch, recollections of how I had been at peace with myself and tranquil within the world about me that sole instance I had gotten "buzzed," took hold of my awareness. Settling upon me like morning dew on the leaves of a towering oak, a sense always seeming to bypass this forlorn creature, I felt accepted and accomplished.

The light allowing me to discover that the world need not be destitute of freedom and perception, toking this heavenly herb provided me with a new strength, power, and security. Enthralled that I had gained admission to a continuum where solace could be appreciated, I was overjoyed by the comfort knowing that I had the means to access a new recognition.

Obsessing about the wondrous effect pot had on me, my ability to grasp and acknowledge the intricacies of the world provided me with a new respect for all that existed. With this invigorating perspective and cognition being the quintessence of understanding, I couldn't be persuaded that the abilities and power of cannabis weren't boundless. Blossoming strength and endless foresight mine to glean, weakness, submission, and malice no longer would be applied traits of my character or had meaning in the overall truth of my stature. A rebirth of mind and spirit, I had finally arrived!

Having developed as a captivating interest, music was no longer just an assemblance of rhythms, rather, an expression of an idea and emotion via orchestrated harmonies and melodies. Strumming a chord, I'd be Eric Clapton at his finest. Playing my Gibson copy behind my head, I sounded like Jimi Hendrix at Woodstock. I did not come into this world September of '63, but September of '81.

Not needing to answer to anyone but myself, I thought about how the dorm room was my domain and how my outlook had been enhanced with this freedom. A license to rebel, the caged animal knowing limitations and restriction had been set free to his own devices. Seen as the object of obstruction, experimenting without stringent guidance or exploring without fear of prosecution, the prelude to my final chapter had almost been written.

Holding my sensitivity captive, inhaling burnt leaf and venturing into its abstract sensation had helped me to secure two friends tonight in Paul and Boss. And another would be awaiting my return back to our room.

Easy-going, inhibited, family-oriented, and level-headed are but a few of the synonyms descriptive of Kevin Brezinski. Extremely reserved unless members of his familial circle are around, until the ice has undergone an extensive thaw and broken thoroughly, Kevin's unbelievably shy around new acquaintances. However, after Kevin warms up to someone/gets comfortable with them, it would be practically impossible to shut him up once he got going. With all those pistons in his motor eventually starting to heat up and pump rapidly, it would be tough to imagine Kevin being initially introverted. A tremendous family life influencing his involvement, fortunate to be in a "Cleaver" atmosphere, Kevin would be blanketed with security.

Exceptionally fine people, Kevin's bond with his mom, dad, and sister is such that they are inseparable. Operating a family business in Washington, a tight togetherness occurs during both work and play. Splendid role-models, Kevin had been brought up in a loving environment of stability which helped to promote his even-keeled outlook on life.

Attachment and openness not exhibited liberally within the Meyers' clan, a kind of understanding exists not to expose affection too much. Demonstrations of emotion not a regular occurrence, although we get along fine enough, displays of feeling are infrequent. Not exempt from being moody, unsure if the dynamics of the varying family systems play a role, my temperament could generally be less predictable than Kevin's.

Very ordinary in a multitude of ways, Kevin's treatment of those he considers friends is far from typical, however. Going to great lengths for those he likes, Kevin's friendliness is larger than life. The impressive thing about his behavior is that it is 100% pure and natural, no artificial flavoring or coloring.

Because no two people are exactly alike, the sayings, "Birds of a feather flock together" and "Opposites attract" are both descriptive of our friendship. We've had our differences in the past, but the unique interplay of these two spectrums keeps this fellowship firmly intact. With the similarities significant, our association wouldn't be at risk of being severed.

A decent guitar player, Kevin's the one who gave me the final push to be inspired learning the instrument. Our fondness for rock 'n' roll being the foundation of our companionship initially, tipping the scales for me, my evolution from fan to participating musician had started when I'd see Kevin's fingers make their way across the fretboard of his Strat, playing an assortment of familiar rock songs.

Both dateless, our affinity for female buttocks, cleavage, and groin area would therefore be intense. Fantasizing about derobing hot-looking members of the opposite sex and then devouring them, was our favorite pastime and topic of discussion. Our teen-aged sex glands working overtime in overdrive while being tantalized in these frisky collegiate surroundings, replacing hard rock music as a primary passion, hoping to take a whiff of some W.V.U. "skirt" would develop as the backbone of our new enthusiasm. With all the young Mountaineer beauties drawling away in their habitually sexy fashion and seductively running around in tight shorts during this warm phase of the fall semester, I'd be hard-pressed even remembering who guitarist Jimmy Page of Led Zeppelin was. Hell with brains, me and Kevin wanted flesh having our own place amidst co-eds galore.

In the same Webster's Dictionary with my senior picture by the word, "mundane," there's a likeness of Kevin's chubby frame beside the word, "perceptive."

Not too much getting past this guy, Kevin is very keen when it comes to knowing what occurs within the environment. However, the night I had been "recreating" with the Dynamic Duo, Kevin needn't use his Sixth Sense to know that I was at an altitude where nose bleed occurs.

Keys jangling as they hit the floor, I fumbled several times trying to get the opener into that incredibly tiny keyhole. After greeting a few passers by in a "happy" voice, I unsuccessfully attempted to gain passage into my new home one more time. While chuckles echoed off the walls down the hallway at my expense, I struggled to remember which way to turn the key to unlatch the lock. Finally able to jam the key into that minuscule orifice, I turned the wrong way a couple of times before kicking in the door. Flinging this partition open, I crashed my plastic guitar case into the wall. Sporting a shitty grin, Kevin looked up from his scratch pad and proclaimed that I was "fucked up."

Kevin never seeing me in a state like this before, and my thinking that the world was just one massive comedy club, neither of us could stop laughing. Imagining what transpired in the Dynamic Duo's bedroom, I gave Kevin a detailed account of my evening at Paul's and Boss'. Not totally without experience when friends tested the waters of The Great Unknown of Substance Use, Kevin would be accustomed to the various chemical antics of those rock musicians he knew who tried to live up to the lifestyle.

Far from being a puritan, liking to drink his beer in moderation and occasionally exceeding control if the situation presented itself, Kevin knew what getting "toasted" was all about. Since buying our books was about the only real homework up to this point—sure to be a fan favorite of Mr. and Mrs. Brezinski—I would be able to talk Kevin into putting away his loose-leaf notebook and do some barhopping in Sunnyside. Then, we could hit "The Dungeon" near High Street, so we could take advantage of the "drink and drown" pitcher special. On second thought, this college life "IS" awesome.

My first drinking experience where I would be sent reeling would soon follow this marijuana enlightenment. Craving to be accepted and not wanting to be considered a "geek," when the two studs whose room was next to ours had offered me to join them for some screwdrivers, I couldn't say "no" because that would have been a missed opportunity to make some more friends. Analogous to the cowboys refusing to smoke a pipe with a neighboring tribe's chief, in my mind, relenting would have meant being on their social "shit list." Not about to risk foregoing any future good times, with Kevin passing on this invitation because he was reviewing a text, my passion to gain admission into a recreation circle smothered my focus/priorities.

With chest out, gut sucked in, and voice dropping a tone or two, I marched into my neighboring floor buddies' room like the "Master of Merriment" I set out to be. Downing one drink after another, different guys from the floor dropped by to join us. Getting introduced and reintroduced to quite a few convicts-to-be, I'd be one of the boys this night. Chugging away as if I had done this hundreds of times before, I'd be determined to "fit in" and get on a reservation list of any forthcoming festivities. Truthfully knowing that I hadn't had much experience with anything stronger than carbonated cola during my drinking history, Kevin would soon find out just how big of a "lightweight" I actually was.

After the drinking excursion where I hammered countless bottomless glasses, this fallen angel made it back to the room where Kevin was studying. Kevin's desk light would be reflecting a smirk where, if I didn't know him better, I'd have thought he just got laid. With the walls separating the rooms being thin, Kevin could hear every liquor-induced, comic gesture regurgitated in the adjacent room. Funny comments wouldn't be all that would get spewed about.

Throughout the evening, I promptly got sick, leaving the excrements of the infinite number of vodka and orange juice concoctions I had ingested floating in the garbage can strategically placed next to my bed. Kevin's jovial grin turning into a countenance of disgust, thinking that I had only went to the restroom around the corner, my grossed-out roommate would make the claim that I disappeared for an hour or so. Frantically searching for Houdini, Kevin would embark on a detective mission.

Dick Tracy went looking for me in the two floor bathrooms, any apartment where the door was open, and downstairs. Too bashful to check any rooms of those on our floor he didn't know, Kevin would call Paul/Boss and be told that they hadn't seen me and didn't have any idea where I was. Not sure what to make of this mess, shrugging his shoulders, Kevin went about looking for me again.

Hoping that he wouldn't come across an artist's sketch of my face on a "Fugitive Wanted" poster the next day because someone who fit my description had robbed a bank, Kevin returned from his bloodhound expedition and found me sleeping. Drawing a complete blank, not needing to be paranoid about abuses, tragedy would be cast.

The transmogrification of my sense of reality would not be the only new experience that occurred during those first few days of school. Having very little experience and no luck with the young ladies during high school, it took all the energy I could muster to keep my tongue in my mouth when a beautiful feline gift from Heaven sat down right next to me during my English 1 class in Hodges Hall and smiled. Eyes about to bulge out of my head, I could feel cold sweat trickling down the back of my spine. For fear that I had suddenly become mute, I dare not open my mouth to say anything because I wouldn't exactly be sure what sound might come out. With goose bumps popping up all over the skin of my arms, it took some effort to keep my "stiffy" from standing at attention, too.

Besides being pretty with a fantastic body, it turned out she was nice and didn't appear to be dense. Hesitating and groping for words after a conversation had finally gotten started, my inexperience "rapping" with the opposite sex had to have been quite evident. With her bright smile and pursuit to keep talking serving as signals, apparently my relative innocence had been found to be at least a little appealing. An attractive girl seeming to be legitimately interested, come to think of it, this college environment really wasn't looking so bad.

Talk about striking gold, along with a corresponding interest in music so profound leading this to be her major, she was a fellow freshman who also lived in the Towers. Not only did we reside in the same dorm complex, "proximity" being a subjective term, but this gem "only" lived about 50 miles from Washington in a community east of Pittsburgh called Penn Hills. Residing in this huge suburb near Monroeville—if we should "hit it off" reasonably well as the semester progresses—an observer not realizing a source of travel wouldn't be available to me or that driving Pittsburgh was prohibited in the Meyers' family, might think the locales of our hometowns were almost ideal. Smitten beyond belief, I was going to propose to her when she said she liked the spectacular rock guitarist, Eddie Van Halen, and could play two musical instruments, but I didn't want to look too anxious.

Asking me where I was from, when I told her "Washington," getting wide-eyed and excitement coloring her voice, this princess wondered if I knew this guy, "Alan," who graduated from Trinity a year or so ahead of me. A combination of my knowing Alan had an iffy reputation and her apparent interest in him by the tone of pleasure in her words when referring to him, made me somewhat questionable of her. But I didn't let that discourage me too much because she had a great ass.

Because of my growing tendency to be chemically altered, I had begun to be identified as a partier. Believing that I had never had any kind of identity before, although taking mind alterers into my system didn't require any special type of talent, I thought being noticed for something and admitted into a quasi-fellowship club was great. Meeting people and making new acquaintances left and right, along with my former high school sidekick Kevin, I thought my days of singularity were over. Convenience adding fuel to the fire, if I wanted reefer, it would be easy because I had heard that two dealers lived a couple of doors down on our floor. Thinking that it was a stroke of luck that all I needed to do was walk down the hallway to get my "fix," the seeds of disaster had been planted.

Bored to tears reading my Poli Sci text, when one of my new floor buddies came into our room asking me if I wanted to sit in and smoke a bong with a group of fellow rejects down the hall, I put the book down after glancing over three pages because the new understanding of self and all creation marijuana gave me was more alluring than reading about the duties of the Secretary of Defense. Scanning notes for class the next day with his boyish simper, I didn't bother to extend the courtesy of asking Kevin to come along because he wouldn't ever get high.

A few doors down, we got the water bubbling and the steam rising. A half-hour and several tokes later, with the bong passed round and round for our inhaling pleasure, I experienced the same sensational ascent I had the two previous times I'd gotten high. Not quite "wasted," believing that fortune had smiled upon me, among my doobie associates I had become acquainted with were the two pre-engineering majors who sold herb. Having worked in the greenhouse over the summer, I had some cash at my disposal to buy some dope of my very own. Armed with a twenty-dollar bill, I purchased a dime bag of marijuana.

Studies placing a distant second, all I could think about was bouncing over to the local mini-mart and getting some "Tip Top" papers, so I could roll my first joint. Given to me by Ug's wife as a high school graduation present, after I used my "Cross" pen to sort the seeds from the leaves, I'd put the finishing touches on my wrap. Its symmetry was sickening. Its texture like that of a sponge. And its beauty non-existent. Only a novice could create such a spectacle.

After rolling several of these marijuana cigarettes which looked like pregnant worms, an invitation they gladly accepted, I informed Paul and Boss of my purchase and asked them over to help me smoke the pot after dinner. Quickly jamming the food down our throats, after the four of us ate supper together in the cafeteria, the Dynamic Duo and myself started firing up the first deformed joint I had bought. While Kevin sat at his desk doing an assignment, my two new Mountaineer buddies and myself anxiously awaited to start flying.

Having the means to taste life a little bit, the freedom one has in college away from home wasn't a totally virgin situation for Kevin, so his adjustment to W.V.U. was a smoother adaptation. Knowing how to separate work and play, Kevin could bring into focus what needed to be done in order to excel. But this night, Kevin would half-heartedly be doing his homework, with the other 50% absorbed how me and the Dynamic Duo were ascending to a higher elevation. Enjoying the college life to the fullest, I'd be sorry to see this first week come to an end.

For the first handful of weeks, I went home every weekend with Kevin. Not elaborating much, I would feed my parents the same line that classes were going fine and I was doing okay with my studies. Usually bringing a lot of books home, I thought that if the motivation struck me to do some classwork, I'd at least have my stuff there. Giving the cosmetic quality that I had finally discovered the importance of academics, rarely would the moment hit when I'd be tempted to even take a look at what I brought home.

Not able to go for a ride anywhere, hardly a break, I'd be sitting in my room Friday night, throughout the afternoon on Saturday and Sunday, not doing much besides listening to my static-laden, secondhand phonograph and playing my guitar. All the while, I'd anxiously await returning to Morgantown on Sunday night, so I could get stoned again. Rarely even bothering to pay any neighborhood chums a visit, my psychological preoccupation with marijuana had grips on me so tightly, I really didn't care about anything else.

After being dropped off at college by whoever would be car pooling us, I'd almost immediately call Paul and Boss to come over and smoke weed. Likely floating before my dad or Kevin's sister even got back to Washington, going home would be a double-edged sword, for I missed levitating about the clouds, yet, still liked the dependability mom and dad would provide me. Returning to a home environment for two days—away from one which subjected me to unwanted responsibility—would be the booster shot that I needed, so I could survive the next week of going to class.

Staying in Morgantown every weekend, I really admired Paul because he never went home. Displaying an outward show of confidence, Paul would be of his own freewill and apparently thriving in the process. Refining his autonomy in West Virginia, I really thought a lot of Paul. Pipeline to Washington still very much in operation, even Boss would pop home occasionally to check on his harem.

Well-rounded and only eighteen, after getting out of the Jacuzzi, Paul would be the type to tie a couple of flies for his tackle box before heading off to Canonsburg Lake to reel in some trout. Paul's ability to socialize and be independent were but two attributes with which he would be blessed.

Able to play quarter-bounce with an incomparable flair, Paul would make his opponent drink beer after beer after beer. As spectacular as Old Faithful's proudest and most magnificent spurt of nature's moisture, the splash the coin made in the glass of brew after Paul had it repel off the tabletop would be striking. Impressed, with finger rigid and targeted in the direction of the hapless underdog who dared compete against this wunderkind, Paul would announce who was to drink next. With bodies lying at his feet after this grained annihilation, Paul assumed his distinction of victor which was the style he was tailored.

Causing anyone to witness this prized contest of raw-edged nerves to spurt out a deafening, "Wow!," on those rare moments when Paul's coin missed its target, he'd empty his mug with only a few breathless swigs. Amazingly, when this youthful prodigy would be selected to drink, Paul not only downed the beer, but left the quarter in the glass, as it slid into his mouth.

Ever-so-casually withdrawing the twenty-five cent piece, Paul had demonstrated his mastery of this game of skill, meaning, and importance. While waiting his turn to conquer those who would risk challenging him, Paul would drag on his cigarette before exhaling and simultaneously inhaling the smoke through his nose, creating an unbelievable ferris wheel type of effect. Able to down malt with the best of them, it would be tough to imagine Paul ever letting drinks get the better of him. Fascinating to see such advanced maturation, Paul was only a teenager and growing a beard. Incredible.

Having a presence about him which commanded respect, not knowing anybody who didn't like Paul, one felt comfortable being around this winner. His suave demeanor leaving me a little bit in awe, with little effort, Paul let one know that he liked and accepted them. Putting those around him at ease, Paul appeared to be a good-natured guy who wanted people to feel good about themselves. Projecting an image of security, Paul left those near him inexplicably feeling a sense of trust. And it would be here that the mask would ultimately become unveiled.

Feeling good about myself would be something that I had a good bit of difficulty with, but being away at school around peers who seemed to like me, I'd be getting better at accepting Craig Meyers. Trying not to be smothered by insecurities about who I was or what I wasn't, I wanted to know how to establish some kind of framework where I could begin constructing pillars of mental fortitude.

Owned misgivings not quite dismantled, I wouldn't be immune to falling into some of the same ruts I had been choked with my entire adolescence.

However, Paul just being Paul, he unwittingly helped make me feel better about things during different intervals throughout the semester. Not feeling worthy, I wouldn't think of going over to Paul's and Boss' room without an invitation or a reason to visit like playing guitar or smoking some pot. Not wanting to be an intrusion, I wouldn't stop just to say "Hi" or to bullshit. Encouraging me to drop by, Paul said that I didn't come over enough and that he'd like to see me more. Pitifully reserved and doubtful of my place in this world, Paul's openness made me feel great about what I represented.

Like Kevin, Paul's penchant of doing right by those he liked was genuine. For instance, if me or Boss would be playing our guitars in front of some guys who were impressed with what they heard and one of us didn't have our instrument, Paul would feel bad for the one excluded from the adoration and say something like, "Boss plays too" or "Craig can play that song pretty good." Possibly considered trivial, the meaning of this message would have significance.

Thinking that Paul was super, I really liked him. I thought the feeling was mutual.

In the same boat as far as girls were concerned, Paul came over to the dorm room one weekend when Kevin went home and wanted to talk about how troubling it was for him not having a female to spend some time with. Being Boss' roommate, Paul witnessed how a guy can get something when that testosterone level rises. Confiding in me that not having a girlfriend bothered him, seeing firsthand that Boss' gonads made their rounds with different girls throughout the Towers didn't make matters any easier for Paul. With guys, Paul had a wit as quick as a rattlesnake's bite, an approach as smooth as a fine Chablis, and a delivery like that of a Rhodes Scholar. However, because females usually don't hunt muskrat or know the best bait for bass fishing, Paul was at a loss for words with them.

Hoping for a better tomorrow with the ladies, Paul and I reflected about our struggles getting some kitty to pet. Relief gained just talking about our lack of fortune, we could then joke about how our single lives hadn't exactly been overflowing with much intimate female activity. To top off this afternoon of male bonding, I reached into my Cheap Trick "Live at Buddokan" album sleeve where I hid my pot and we proceeded to smoke the remainder of the weed before Paul left.

A little while later, I called Paul to see if he wanted to do some "hound dogging" for chicks, but he had plans to go to a party with some guys on his floor. With both of our roommates going home for the weekend, incentive for work all but depleted, I had absolutely nothing to do. Blinded by flattery, I thought being omitted was no big deal because the widely-respected Paul Michaels chose me above all others to talk about some problems he was having. Glad to have gotten to know Paul and discover why he was so well-liked, being much too intimidated and timid to ever attempt developing anything with the beauty in my English class, I thought this new friendship with Paul was the best thing that happened at school thus far. If I only had foresight.

Dinner time approached and since the three guys I ordinarily "chowed down" with in the cafeteria weren't around, I picked up some food at the nearby McDonald's and ate by myself in the dorm room because I didn't want to be seen in this mess hall eating alone. Weekends being a time when normal people are out socializing with friends or doing something to have a good time, teenagers absent of peers are assumed to have something wrong with them. With the exception of Kevin and a few others—outside of some guys I played baseball with and a couple of neighborhood pals—most of the people I knew were more acquaintances than good friends. Not wanting to relinquish my facade that I was conforming, I never really learned how to get involved with others, surrounding myself with quality activity. The scenery might be different, but the circumstance of being a one-man army hadn't really changed much being in college.

Such acts of higher learning not a reflection of my personal identity, I wouldn't be joining a fraternity and engaging in any initiation rituals of significance like defecating in the Mountainlair parking garage. Despite her apparent interest, the Ice Age would occur before I would ever ask that princess music major from Penn Hills even to do something as benign as have lunch with me, although I longed for this. Being my own worst enemy habitually assuming that I'd be a pest, concealed struggles harbored within myself were contributors to my starting to feel down again. Using a variety of masterful approaches to give the impression that life was just fine, this wayward creature would need to escape the laborious conflict of unfounded discernment in order to be content.

An unmistakable sound that I hadn't heard since being in the Towers filled the weekend air this Friday night—it was quiet. Dead silent, there were no stereos blaring or tackle football games in the hallway. Not that I had ever tried this, but a book could be heard opening. No one around, everybody but me seemed to be out doing something. Rejection not being something I wanted to experience, unless I would be absolutely certain to get an affirmative answer or positive feedback of some kind, I wouldn't dare ask someone if I could tag along and join in on the fun.

Unsure of how to handle any response or reaction flavored with the slightest seasoning that I wasn't welcome, I wouldn't chance hinting for an invitation. Figuring that they either had just forgotten or were just too busy with other concerns, I would still be "bummed out" that none of the guys on the floor who would help me smoke my pot hadn't stopped by the room to ask me if I'd like to go out with them. Pretending that I really didn't give a damn and was content "sticking by my lonesome," I'd try to tell myself that I was happy to have my bag of weed all to myself to enjoy. Danger sparked viewing escape as resolution, continuing to be apart from others and separated from activity, ongoing dread would be ignited.

Still creating unsightly forms even after all the practice, I rolled another misproportioned joint and fired the "baby" up. Five minutes and several puffs later, the ill-shaped marijuana cigarette I assembled was gone. Waiting to go up, up, and away, I never left ground. With nothing happening after about fifteen minutes, I rolled another disfigured joint.

Halfway through the second creation, dabbling with my new hobby at least three times a week, about all I felt after smoking midway through a reefer stogie would be a little “contact high.” My body having built a resistance to these cylindrical little bastards with all the use, it would take about a joint-and-a-half before I’d finally get going, entering Planet Zeon’s solar system. Floating in this cosmic sensation, limitations would seem foreign and pleasures as bountiful as stars in the universe. Infinite acceptance and universal comfort would embrace me in my recently discovered habitat of perverted honesty.

Barely feeling any change, in no time, my modified atmosphere would be invaded by truths not welcome. Becoming less and less of a prized displacement from actuality, I customarily had to relinquish my valued state of twisted consciousness to that of logic and veracity long before I’d be ready. Battling this prematurity, so that time traveling the distance from the pains of reality may be prolonged, I rolled and inhaled another joint because the duration with which I had been away seemed to dissolve much too early and rapidly. Numb to the world around me, with peace being the rule and not forgotten, the master would once again return to an existence seemingly void of hardship or sacrifice. Being an omnipotent force commanding obedience, I shall return to my throne for yet another reign.

Listening to my music, I’d stare into space, seeing nothing, feeling less. Liberated from perceived cruelties, my novel vision could open vast frontiers which would provide me with a touch of grace. Grasping elegance and dreams once fleeting, dissatisfied when the moment this condition would remit, I could capture detail and appreciate the unknown when submerged in vapor. Once enjoying serenity and basking in its warmth with a limited quantity, I could no longer cruise in my rocket ship smoking just a half of a joint.

Needing to light up two to get the same effect, not seeing the trap I had set for myself, I really didn’t care that I had to put away about four times as much dope to get light-headed because I figured it just went with the territory. Needing more weed to put me in a catatonic trance, with everyone I knew out and about doing something, I’d be able to sell myself on the idea that I preferred getting high alone anyway. Not ready or willing to see the broader picture that maybe I hadn’t been received like I wanted to believe, to preserve my mythical front, I’d adopt the position that I basically couldn’t afford providing people with a festive trip smoking my hemp all the time. Reefer costing too much to be giving it away, I’d come to accept that the advantages of getting high alone outweigh group dynamics simply because I wouldn’t have to worry about other people.

Despite his parents surely having their fair share of loot being professionals within the health care field, Paul would be tight with weed during one of our gatherings, so no one could bitch about my planned new position of being frugal in any upcoming sittings. Inching closer and closer to total disgust, feeling that a sense of omission always seemed to follow me wherever this aimless nomad may drift, my dejection would descend to a drastic low. Deviating from truth utilized as a means of rescue, one day not too far off, I'd find myself living on borrowed time.

Come morning, I realized that I had committed the cardinal sin by sleeping off my buzz. Granted a reprieve having my senses be dormant for several hours, lying in bed, I foolishly took in a sense of gratification and satisfaction thinking that I had rid myself of the troubles which had burdened me. Feeling a diversion from exhausting oppression, I had subjected myself to deeper distress hailing marijuana as some key to unlocking this joyless soul from discontent. After this brief moment of lucidity had passed, I realized that I knew of another Trinity grad who went to W.V.U. and liked to party, "Matt Wright."

Like Paul and Boss, the old Craig Meyers never associated much with Matt because he was a reknowned partier who had a reputation of getting "crazy." Looking up his phone number in the student directory, the new Craig Meyers made arrangements to party with Matt and his roommate in the bar district of Sunnyside where they lived, however. Upon my calling him, Matt said that he didn't think that I partied, but he hadn't met the new version. Only kidding myself that partying alone was the best way, I had two more hooligan buddies to enter "la la" land with. Misery enjoying company, I thought I'd be set for a merry semester.

A sophomore, Matt had been experienced with the Morgantown party scene for a little over a year and introduced me to more of the hot spots the town had to offer in the coming weeks. Mid-term grades about inebriated, when I hadn't been getting stoned at the Towers with whoever, I'd catch the PRT to the Beechurst Campus and meet with Matt in Sunnyside. Either to drag some reefer or drink a little, sometimes I'd go to Matt's apartment or he'd come to the Towers. With Kevin doing his homework in a haze during these instances, occasionally calling Paul and/or Boss to come over and join us, we'd all be soaring.

On one occasion, prior to heading to glorious room 4012 in the Towers to continue our hell-raising, my Sunnyside party comrades and I got so blitzed in their apartment that Matt didn't think twice when he discharged the fire extinguisher in the PRT between the Beechurst and Engineering Stations. Probably not caring being so aloft, what Matt didn't realize was that he unknowingly set off some sort of alarm at the transportation center that the extinguisher had been moved from its designated area. Signaling to the PRT headquarters that prompt action may need to be taken to safeguard against a potential fire on the car, I should have acted on my paranoia, for my instincts told me to persuade my fellow dean's list student pals to get off at the Engineering Station before the shuttle reached the Towers. Mistakenly keeping my mouth shut because I didn't want to be perceived as a nerd, some authorities would be waiting for us at the next stop.

When the fog-laden PRT reached the Towers Station, several uniformed officers were awaiting our arrival. Feeling like I was starring as a bad guy in an episode of the "Untouchables," in another galaxy, we said that the car was like that when we got on. Not buying that keen-witted explanation, within a few days, we had an appointment with the dean in charge of discipline. In deep trouble, this wouldn't be the last time one of my new recreation associates hurt me.

Knowing we couldn't concede that the cause of our stupor wasn't alcohol, identifying myself as some sort of desperado, the three of us met to get our story "straight" before the hearing. Praying to God that this college administrator would be sensible to those not involved directly with this fire stifling apparatus getting set off, we planned to tell this authority figure who had the power to levy a severe punishment that we drank too much and got carried away. Not able to eat at the dorm cafeteria all that week because my Towers I.D. card had been confiscated, realizing that he had put his fellow Washingtonian through enough anguish, Matt would ultimately confess to his delinquency and said nothing would ever happen again.

Issuing me a stern warning before returning my card, this dean responsible for correcting those who got "out of line" would tell me that he better not ever see me in his office again because that would result in expulsion. With those college walls closing in on me, going home the upcoming weekend, I would tell my parents that things were going great at school.

Finals' week upon us, with reality having started to sink in, the college life had lost a lot of its "zing." Getting kind of scary, essential that coursework gets focused upon, fun and excitement would be things of the past. Not likely that even a wing and a prayer could help me, because the most pronounced difficulty of my collegiate day would be which album I'd listen to next, my grades were horrid and I needed to pull off a miracle during this testing period, if I wanted to salvage the semester. I had prepared to undertake the daunting task of getting caught up, until I looked at my different syllabuses and discovered that I would need to read 273 pages in my Poli Sci book, take a look for the first time at three-quarters of the notes for my Geology class, and 12 chapters in my Humanities text—within 72 hours. Feeling pressured, tense, and a sense of futility, I smoked some pot to stop feeling so bad.

Academically, the only course I knew that I would do well in was my English 1 Composition class. Socially, however, I'd be hard-pressed to find a setting where I had failed so miserably.

Being proud of my newfound identity as a partier, I idiotically and egocentrically assumed all would be impressed by my role as a hood. Based on her reaction after telling her of my pot-smoking exploits, the knockout music major who took the seat right next to me the first day of class was hardly thrilled. Having always secretly set my eyes on a female to be significant in my life—miles from disparagement—I not only had the freedom to proceed independent of interference, but the opportunity to highlight my strengths had presented itself to no avail.

With my untainted posture apparently appealing to her, with those perky adolescent hormones still contributing to my belief that the old Craig Meyers couldn't possibly be liked, I blew my chance trying to develop some kind of friendship. The first semester almost over and the second a Christmas break away from rearing its ugly head, with W.V.U. and the Towers being humungous places, it would be unlikely that I'd ever see her again. Becoming infatuated with and fixating on marijuana to the point where little else mattered, my long sought-after fantasy of establishing a female relationship of some sort literally went up in smoke.

The pattern of getting high non-stop, drinking increasingly more, and not dedicating the time to learn/understand my subject matter put me in a dank, black hole I couldn't get out of. Everything having a price, I could see that using cannabis to escape the truth had made all that exists a misery that didn't have to be. Perched on an erroneous perception of my position in this world, this king hadn't fallen from his throne, but a foundation of illusion.

Not doing either, I had strayed believing marijuana would serve as some sort of answer to being more accepted and accomplished. Not mature or enlightened enough to face the difficult transition from being a "dud" to someone needing to achieve responsibility, my preoccupation and use of this narcotic plant did nothing for me long-term, but to rob me of those things I could have enjoyed and mutilated what little self-respect I had captured. Setting an all-time record, motivation had been sifted from me to such a degree that I lost most of my incentive to do most everything, but find out when the next shipment of dope would be arriving for retail.

If Kevin wasn't such a good friend and decent human being, he would have said "sayonara" to me a long time ago. He had ridden out this phase with me knowing that when I'd hit the wall that was reality, I'd open my eyes and realize that I had been chasing a mirage. Telling me of the impending destruction I was to encounter, I wouldn't have believed it, for I was riding the majestic white stallion.

On weekends in both Morgantown or Washington, I would usually be by myself, desiring to be around good people, instead. Swamped with despondent images of my purpose and what I was to be, my insularity trapped me with a fury I wouldn't know how to be freed from. Besides those guys I had gotten to know from home, rarely would anyone I had gotten high with have anything to do with me when they weren't smoking my grass. Like it was in high school, I never attended a football game, never went on a date, or took advantage of the many extracurricular activities the school offered which might have interested me. My academic and social life truly in shambles, I hated just about everything about me.

Come Saturday afternoon, despite loving football, I'd sit in my room alone at the Towers watching the hordes of fans file past the dormitory complex up to new Mountaineer Field preparing to tailgate. Three-quarters of a mile or so from my dorm room, there were going to be about 50,000 screaming, spirited, Mountaineer fanatics having the time of their life cheering Darryl Talley, Oliver Luck, and Company. Wishing, but not knowing how to be part of the festivities, I'd be solitude within the confines of our rock 'n' roll postered room sucking in some fumes. Eerily similar to the situation back home, impossible to take in stride, being on the outside looking in was that much more of a harrowing penalty because the opportunity for happiness was so near and well within reach.

Tears filled mom's eyes as they had five months ago when learning that I had been accepted at W.V.U., but they wouldn't be of the overjoyed variety like at the beginning of the school year. Dad stood in the living room speechless, head down, staring at the dark piece of paper. My grade report had arrived.

Reading this document exposing how I did not apply myself, wishing that I were invisible, I witnessed the pain I had inflicted on my parents. Wasting their hard-earned money and disregarding their dutiful planning, feeling shame for being so spoiled and selfish, I couldn't look at myself in the mirror. Seeing the heart-broken disappointment on their faces, not appreciating the sacrifice deposited on my behalf or the investment they had made in me, I could have crawled under a rock. Rewarding them with minimal effort after they had toiled for years, so the chance at going to college wouldn't pass me by, I almost wished that they'd have it in them to slap me around a little bit.

Doing just enough to get by during high school, it had become quite apparent to me that I could no longer just go through the motions in college, if I was to get that degree. A grade point average of 1.7 staring me in the face, below the minimum requirement of a 2.0 G.P.A., I would be put on academic probation. Not improving substantially next semester, I'd be kicked out of school for at least a year. Merry Christmas, mom and dad.

A formula not making it so ironic that Boss also had a stellar 1.7 G.P.A. as well, when we wouldn't be hovering about the stratosphere together, we'd be playing our guitars. Not surprisingly, Kevin had a respectable first semester grade-wise because of his commitment to breaking out the books and heading off to the library to get away from me. Deserving of the utmost respect and only strengthening the confidence I had for him, Paul not only stood out in the crowd when it came to partying, but did well in his classes, too. Maintaining his stature as a sort of icon, believing this to be one of the few positives of the academic year, I actually had regretted not getting to know Paul earlier when we were high schoolers.

In January 1982, a little more than a week before the second semester would be getting underway, my beloved maternal grandmother slipped and fell in a department store in Johnstown. Breaking her right shoulder a day or so after spending the Christmas holiday with us, totally deaf and becoming increasingly more trying to deal with because of her senility/demandedness, this would be a very difficult time for my parents. In addition to being burdened with my widowed grandma's failing health having to serve as her primary caretaker, my folks would be frightfully concerned about their youngest son's upcoming performance in college, for this would have an impact on my immediate future.

Back against the wall, realizing what was at stake, I know I'd have to get serious with the studies and work hard this spring semester. Partying and playing guitar on the verge of extinction, time to "put up or shut up," I would be committed to keeping up with my reading and studying. Not fully aware at the time just how significant this aspect of my character would soon reap massive rewards for me, if I'd be determined to do something, there would be a good chance that I'd get it done.

The second semester would be but two weeks old when Kevin would tell me about a weird experience he had when alone in our room. Saying that a really pretty girl with a nice body came in uninvited when the door was cracked open, sitting at his desk doing some introductory business coursework, Kevin probably thought he had died and went to heaven when this babe came catwalking in. Wanting a closer look at our room decorated with the rock posters, this brunette said she was a music major and that the room looked really cool. While pointing to the Van Halen poster, she told Kevin that she really liked this innovative guitarist. Heart excitedly thumping in my chest, I had asked Kevin specifically what this visitor looked like and it sounded like he had been describing the angel who was in my English 1 Comp class who I had been obsessing about all year.

Stunned by what I had heard Kevin tell me, because I could not fathom a nice-looking female ever wanting to engage in a premeditated course of action hoping to construct any kind of friendship with me, I would reluctantly accept that this either had to be just a coincidence, she had been visiting with someone else on the floor, or was a different girl altogether who merely resembled the vixen I knew. Not likely to be attracted to Kevin's robust, gorilla hair body, although there wouldn't be any alligator clips/roaches scattered about anymore because I'd be smoke-free, I would wonder if this welcomed guest noticed the tiny burn holes in my bedspread caused by popping seeds or the dark ash marks imprinted in the carpet.

Wanting to turn over a new leaf because the old one hadn't been working for me as far as getting any female companionship was concerned, tired of being mateless and beating up on myself with self-defeating thoughts, I figured what would I have to lose seeing if the fox in my English class wouldn't mind doing something when her schedule permitted. Even if there would be a remote chance the girl popping into our dorm room wasn't the sweetheart I hoped it was, having seemed slightly interested during the fall term, I would decide that I would ask the darling from Penn Hills out after the brief holiday break. Yet another fantasy unfulfilled.

With Presidents' Day '82 upon us, there would be no classes on Monday. Mrs. Bostko—Boss' mom—came to Morgantown to take her son, Kevin, myself, and even Paul back home for the three-day weekend. During the one-hour trip up Interstate 79 North, Paul would ask me if I wanted to go to a party tomorrow night that "Rodney Ilyacoff" was having in Washington. Caught off-guard by the invitation, never having any plans on weekends with the exception of listening to my scratched Alice Cooper albums on my $60.00 record player, I said "Yeah" because I thought a change of scenery besides my four bedroom walls at home might do me some good. Figuring I could have some fun seeing a couple of people from high school too, going to that '81 Trinity alumnus' house could give me a chance to find out what other Hiller alumni think of their respective schools.

Since I didn't go to any high school graduation parties, Ilyacoff's get-together would be the first time that I had seen any non-Mountaineers from my class since Commencement ceremonies. Afforded the opportunity to showcase my new identity as a socializing kind of guy who wasn't a "stick in the mud" any longer, I calculated that attending this celebration would be a good way to do something about my isolated reputation and symbolically enter my name on a waiting list for any forthcoming events which I might enjoy. Besides, reasoning that I just might have a good time for a change, I thought hanging out with Paul a little in Washington would likely secure a friendship with this marvel after the school year ended at W.V.U.

The first one Mrs. Bostko dropped off, only reinforcing my favorable opinion of him that much more and believing this to be a reflection of his status, Paul lived in a beautiful home set atop the crest of a hill. Believing that I was a lucky dude getting to know Paul, seeing his nice residence only added to the growing admiration I had for him.

The next to be dropped off, after I was let out at my modest dwellings, the paranoia would start to surface thinking of how it'd have to be Paul who would transport me to and from the party because I didn't drive and wasn't sure where Ilyacoff lived exactly. Taking after my folks in the sense that I could be overly-cautious, even if I could struggle forming an image in my mental movie screen of Paul not able to manage a car ideally after he had a few, logic would no doubt take over and remind me that the instruction my affluent Mountaineer buddy had to have received during his upper middle-class upbringing must've included subject matter related to the consequences of not abiding by the rules of the road. Gathering that Paul had received substantial parental training not to abuse liquor when operating an automobile, a comforting sense of relief would settle in.

Customarily operating from an excessively wary position, I'd rarely have any fun with fellow alumni who didn't live within walking distance of my house. So strictly conservative, I'd be tired of rejecting approaches which possibly could have provided me with a healthy medium. Extremely moderate, the preservative stance I traditionally assumed hadn't done much to promote my feeling involved. Wanting to spread my wings some, I thought taking in a little life might just help make me a tad more complete and whole. However, old habits are hard to break.

Seeing yellow "caution" lights, my mind's rationale swayed like a pendulum. Swinging from the left wing to the right and then back again, my inclination to do nothing being challenged by the viewpoint that maybe a little alteration in my usual boring way of operation might do me some good, I'd be at odds with myself. Conflict ruling my deliberation, I wouldn't be certain if my examinations were ones based on sound judgments or the irrational fears which always seemed to plague my pursuits. Blistering this internal debate, questions muddled with ambiguity would scorch the decision.

Why did Paul ask me to go to the party with him and not his roommate, Boss? Being around him so much in school, did Boss know something about Paul's demeanor that nobody else did which would make him leery of going out with Paul? Had Boss heard an account of Paul's past escapades/history which nobody else had that would make him afraid of being in a car with Paul? Sharing quarters with him, did Boss consistently witness a particular behavior which would scare him away from his roommate after Paul had been socializing?

Swinging back to the left, after having already agreed to go along with him, I sensed that I could risk losing Paul as a friend, if I would suddenly change my mind and relent going to Ilyacoff's. Not exactly ecstatic being a loner again in the Keystone State, showing any type of hesitancy about attending this quasi-reunion wouldn't help me to establish a network of people to do some stuff with. As far as any reasons would be concerned about Boss not buddying around with Paul to this outing, I'd come to the conclusion that he probably was asked, but had plans with one of his girlfriends and not because he'd be fearful of any of Paul's mannerisms. A smart guy, I'd figure Paul wouldn't exceed his drinking limit when driving a vehicle because he would know what could happen.

Their values surely approximating their resources, living in an attractive/upper middle-class development, Ilyacoff's host parents would certainly have to provide at least a little semi-supervision in order to take protective measures against harmful overindulgence or damage to their nice dwellings. By the same token, I would not be able to fathom Paul ever chancing hurting any human being, especially one he gets along with so well and presumably considers a friend. Considering all the factors, quenched by my lack of experience attending house parties, I'd be able to defuse any anxiety.

On top of all the other reasons which would result in my final determination that I'd indeed go to the party, I concluded that since Paul had brilliant professionals as parents no doubt instilling in him a solid moral fiber, he'd certainly abide by conscientious principles, safeguarding against harm when responsible for others' welfare. Moreover, what would be the chance of anything bad happening, one in a billion?

Chapter 3

Coma's Silent Emptiness

As I stood on the front porch waiting for my ride, I'd rap on the window then duck out of sight as Fritz—our feisty schnauzer—barked and came running to see who dared enter his territory. Relieved to see that the roads were dry and the forecast good, I was in a fired up mood myself. Not only was I going to my first party in Washington since my second grade homeroom had cupcakes and milk celebrating the principal's son's birthday, but when I go back to school, I'm going to do something I've never done before—ask a girl for a date.

Ecstatic about going out and being included for a change, I would be in a playful mood by the time I saw the '68 Beetle appear on the horizon. A few hours earlier, Paul had called designating the time he'd pick me up and that we were also going to get my long-time neighborhood *buddy,* "Sam." As I instructed Paul how to get to Sam's house, I couldn't help but notice how aggressively he shifted the gears. I thought to myself, Paul wouldn't show off behind the wheel of a car, he's too bright for that; this just correlates with how he approaches life—with effervescence and vigor.

After getting Sam, we headed towards the hinterlands about four miles away where Ilyacoff resides. When hearing from Paul some of my party escapades during the first semester shortly after crawling into the cramped car, characteristic of our interactions since junior high, Sam launched another of his cynical assaults against me. Wanting to start off this evening of supposed recreation on a positive note hardly making any difference, I'd be subjected to Sam's insults again. Recognizing that Paul and I had only recently become friends, Sam felt compelled to fill in my new Mountaineer buddy how I never went out or did anything. Having the boringest of lifestyles, just staying home so much of the time, I felt extremely embarrassed that the guy who had known me so well since we were five and whom I blindly considered a friend was so comfortable "ripping" on me in front of somebody I had just gotten to know.

Sensing my discomfort over the direction this exchange was headed, so that any further character assassination may be suppressed in his squashed VW, Paul interjected that W.V.U. was a great school and that we had become friends; letting Sam know that I had an ally and nothing else bad about me needed to be said.

Feeling as though a good deal of my life hadn't exactly been saturated with peer group advocates, Paul sticking up for me would only strengthen my opinion of him that much more.

Arriving at Ilyacoff's, many familiar faces were standing in the front yard. My appearance at these type of events not exactly customary or expected—to this day—I still have a dim picture of some former high school classmates greeting me upon my arrival and expressing disbelief that I was actually attending a social outing. Being seen anywhere but a ballfield came as a shock to everyone there, for the only time I ever really associated with those guys beyond school was when they came to the plan to play some backyard football.

There are few specifics about the party itself in Ilyacoff's house that I can recall, with the most pronounced being that I spent some time talking to an ex-high school football player who was a couple of years older than me, "Larry." A student at the local Washington and Jefferson College, coincidentally, Larry was the brother of the guy who knew the Penn Hills music major goddess I had met in English class at W.V.U. this past fall semester. About the only thing I can remember about our conversation was asking him how his sibling, Alan, got to know her and the nature of their relationship. Because of what was to ensue, Larry's answer—among many other things—would be forever erased.

Tucked away somewhere in my memory chips, I can still retrieve a good feeling about the time I had at Ilyacoff's. Hidden within the dark corners of my data banks, I could fill the blank slate with a few, faint pictorial printouts and being in a generally positive mood at the time I exited the residence. After all, I spent some time with peers doing something other than wishing to be involved. Around people I get along with well enough, met an older ex-high school football star lineman who was pretty friendly, and with a girl back in Morgantown who appears interested in me, things would finally be looking pretty good. This just might be the last Valentine's Day I spend by myself. Walking on Cloud Nine, I could feel happy about who Craig Meyers was, which didn't come all that easy for me.

Feeling jubilant about this phenomenal fate which was developing for me, I left the party in a natural, high-spirited mood with Paul and "Wayne"—another Hiller '81 alumnus. However, I would not realize that a short time after approaching Paul's beat up Volkswagen, another fate would befall me.

Preparing to assume my customary position in the backseat, Wayne insisted he'd sit back there and that I should sit up front in the passenger seat since I was a lot taller than he. We playfully argued where we were to be situated until I concurred with Wayne and held the passenger seat upright as he shuffled into the cramped quarters of the back seat. Unbeknownst to me, if I were a king in the game of chess, this apparent act of innocence would be the move which would lead to my checkmate.

A little under two miles from Ilyacoff's house, Patrolman Kenneth W. Torboli of the East Washington Police Department was traveling east on Route 136—

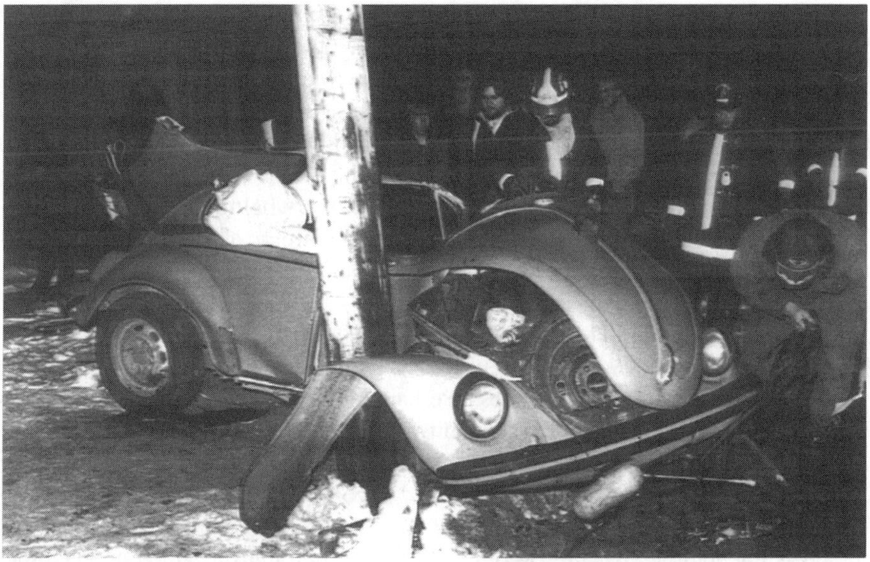

Volkswagen Craig Meyers was a passenger in the night of the accident.

East Beau Street—when an oncoming car was speeding erratically on the opposite side of this winding two lane thoroughfare due West. Upon glancing into his rearview mirror, Patrolman Torboli witnessed sparks shooting from the tires as the Volkswagen Beetle crossed lanes and crashed into a telephone pole about 12:45 A.M. Without hesitation, Patrolman Torboli contacted the local ambulance and fire department services from the City of Washington and South Strabane. Because he not only was a patrolman in this East Washington section of town where the accident occurred, but a Sergeant within the City of Washington Police Department, Officer Torboli knew the procedure which would get an immediate response.

The cans and bottles scattered about the steel carnage which was once an automobile transporting three eighteen-year-old boys celebrating an extended break from college glistened, as the "jaws of life"—the fire department's hurst tool—was cutting its way through the Volkswagen's roof at a fever pitch to the unconscious boy who had been imprisoned within the wreckage for forty-five minutes. For the neighbors huddled about watching and praying, words of concern—not question—filled the air, for the alcoholic contents of the cylinders spread about their feet was no doubt the culprit of the dismay before them. Passersby, in their pursuit to understand, moved onward at a slow pace as officials from the police department and personnel from the fire department urged them to move on. One of those driving by was E. Ronald Salvitti, M.D., who offered to render assistance, if needed. Paramedics waited anxiously either to retrieve life support systems or prepare to get a stretcher for a young corpse.

Nestled in the hills of North Franklin Township in Washington sets a modest home whose senectuous residents' tranquillity would be incessantly shaken that night. Gwen Meyers' (58) sound sleep was disturbed by the ringing phone by the bed at approximately 2 A.M. Wayne's bricklayer mother had called, asking if Craig was in. Yelling out to her husband, who had been up all night caring for his confused mother-in-law, Mrs. Meyers asked Frank (62) if Craig had returned from his outing. Fearful of what was to transpire, an overwhelming feeling of apprehension anguished them with the force of a dagger piercing a heart. What Mr. Meyers was about to see would forever shatter their peace. Craig's bed was empty—he had not returned.

Wayne's mother told Mrs. Meyers that Craig had been in a car accident and that his condition was bad. Why she would ask if Craig were home when she knew he was in the hospital is anybody's guess. Perhaps she wanted to know if Mrs. Meyers had already been informed of the accident and this was her way of ascertaining that. Mr. and Mrs. Meyers contacted Craig's brother, Scott and sister-in-law, telling them what little they knew about the accident and to come watch Grandma Barnhart.

Wasting no time, the elderly couple discarded their nightwear for street clothes and hurried for the Washington Hospital where their son was fighting for his life. Speeding north on Main Street, accelerating through the flashing yellow lights of this early morning trepidation with little regard for any traffic, the ten minute drive to the hospital took what seemed an eternity. With heart racing at the speed that car was moving, his white hair dripping with perspiration, Mr. Meyers was gasping for every breath while trying to make sense the reason for this holocaust.

The haunting memory of Craig lying on the emergency room gurney underneath a white sheet with blood oozing from his inner ear while his head was secured with a neck brace will be imprinted in the mind of Mrs. Meyers until her last breath. When seeing the many nurses saying his name/to "hang in there" loudly over and over to keep Craig stimulated while working frantically to stabilize him, Mrs. Meyers knew the nightmare before her was life-threatening. This was confirmed when the doctor supervising the operation of the trauma unit that night said Craig had sustained a severe head injury that Washington Hospital was not equipped to handle and that Craig would need to be life-flighted to Allegheny General Hospital via helicopter, about thirty-five miles away in Pittsburgh, Pa.

Tears pouring from her eyes, the terror Mrs. Meyers felt at that moment was incredible. Pleading for divine intervention that her son not be a sacrificial lamb because some teens wanted to experience the joys associated with overindulgence, this loving caregiver wouldn't have given it a second thought trading places with her dying boy. She could have never imagined that the evening which began with her son joyously coming home for a holiday weekend, would end up as one where intravenous tubes would feed Craig the shock and pain medicine necessary for survival while an oxygen mask increased his chances another breath would be taken.

Because he knew he might be needed, Mr. Meyers gathered all the strength he could to remain cognizant of what was going on around him. Mrs. Meyers was concerned that her husband was going to pass out from exhaustion, for his face was turning a frightful shade of gray and fearful that the excitement would cause him to go into cardiac arrest. However, Mr. Meyers is a strong-willed man whose astonishing strength enabled him to endure the dread which tormented him. Because expression of emotion, either spoken or acted out was taboo, Mr. Meyers resorted to writing memoirs as a way to exorcise the horror which enveloped him. The following is an excerpt of Mr. Meyers' account of the incidences of February 13, 1982:

> "Craig was home from college for the weekend. It was to be a long weekend and he didn't have to be back to school until Tuesday morning. I was sitting on the couch when Craig came down the stairs from his room and stated he was going out with some of his classmates for awhile that evening.
>
> I was actually glad Craig was going out for once with young people his own age. The first semester of school, Craig would come home and stay the total weekend with his mother and I. I asked him who was going to pick him up. Craig said, "I don't think you know him dad, but I have his picture in our school yearbook." He showed me the picture of the boy. Craig then asked me if I would be up, as he didn't think he would be very late and that he left his keys and money at college. I said I would be up (and) he told me his mother had given him some money and he wouldn't need any more.
>
> When the driver pulled up in an aged Volkswagen, I can remember my thoughts that I was glad it wasn't a "souped up" car. How wrong I was thinking this car to be safe.
>
> As usual, I watched the 11:00 to 11:30 news on television and then went upstairs to prepare for bed. I put on my pajamas and went down to the living room remembering Craig didn't have a key to get in. At about 1 A.M., February 14, 1982, Gwen's mother started her fussing and calling out again so I went to see if she was alright. Some time after that, the phone rang and Gwen called to me and asked if Craig was in. I ran up to his room thinking maybe he had returned when I was preparing for bed—no Craig. As soon as Gwen said "No he isn't," I heard her cry out "Oh no!!" She had just been informed he was in an auto accident and wasn't good.
>
> How I ever got dressed and to Washington Hospital, I'll never remember. How we ever got Scott and (his wife) over to watch Gwen's mother, I'll never know.
>
> The next thing I remember was Gwen asking the mother of the driver if alcohol was involved—the mother said "Yes." They permitted me to go in where Craig was to see him. He was partly cleaned up by then, but still a bloody mess. My first question to the nurse was, "Is there any alcohol on him?" Her reply was, "There is no indication of alcohol."
>
> The hospital had contacted our family doctor and he said he refers all head injuries to Allegheny General Hospital in Pittsburgh and the hospital in turn had ordered Life Flight in to transport Craig to the Pittsburgh hospital. Gwen wanted to go with him, but there wasn't room. This surprised me because I could never get Gwen on an airplane let alone a helicopter
>
> I dislike Pittsburgh traffic with a passion and I did not know how to get to Allegheny General Hospital. But we called Scott, and (his wife's brother) was going to drive us up to AGH because he knew the route. All the time we waited

> for Life Flight and our ride to arrive, the nurses kept saying, "Are you alright Mr. Meyers? Can we get you something?" I was in a fog. All I could do is look at that poor, battered boy and even had the thought if that boy doesn't make it, I don't want to be alright. I wanted to go with him. Driving onto I-79 at Washington, we spotted the helicopter heading north."

In a comatose condition, Craig's diagnosis upon admission to Allegheny General Hospital was Closed Head Injury. Sustaining a basalar skull fracture, Craig was barely hanging onto life. Resulting in his having vascular compromise to the right lower extremity, Craig had a right femoral comminuted fracture which severed his femoral artery. If the arterial occlusion caused by the splintering break of his leg cannot be opened and/or if infection has set in, Craig's leg will need to be amputated. Also, Craig had a serous laceration of the soft tissue of the right ear so severe the ear might have to be removed and replaced with a plastic one. If there are complications, Craig could lose the hearing in that ear.

Together, five surgeons, an anesthesiologist, and a battalion of nurses were gathered about Craig's disfigured body that had been mangled when the Volkswagen's passenger seat was crushed against the utility pole. Performing their heroics masterfully, these miracle workers in the operating room of Allegheny General not only had to work with skill and precision, but with speed, for the swelling of the brain had reached a dangerous level. The longer the lacerations/fractures were exposed and not treated, the greater the likelihood that infection would set in.

The neurosurgeon, E. Richard Prostko, M.D., inserted an intracranial pressure monitor into the body of the right lateral ventricle. This shunt, situated in the middle of Craig's forehead, not only measured the significant cerebral edema (the excessive fluid in the main portion of the brain), but lessened the pressure the brain was pressing on the skull. The brain floats on cerebrospinal fluid within the skull which aids in the protection of the brain by acting as a watery cushion. Absorbing shock, this padding is minimal, however. Since there's only a limited amount of room within the skull, if space for the swelling brain is taken up by fluid, the brain has nowhere to go and presses against the walls of the skull. Possibly resulting in significant damage to the brain, force against a skull can actually be more harmful to this portion of the CNS than the insult itself. Safeguarding against choking the brain off of its space is crucial because the billions of cells and trillions of synapses need room to function properly. Whether it be the point of impact/bruise, being starved of oxygen, or squeezed up against the walls of the skull, if the brain's operation is interfered with in any way, its ability to undertake certain tasks could be permanently lost.

A coma has been defined as a profound state of unconsciousness from which the person cannot be aroused. Even neuroprofessionals have a limited understanding of what exactly happens to the brain when it has been injured and why someone becomes comatose. In layman's terms, the brain can only tolerate a certain amount of painful stimuli when it has been injured or disturbed and when the pain exceeds this level, the brain can't take it and shuts off. When the brain shuts off, one is in a coma.

With a brain contusion, prompt action needs taken in order to minimize the effects of the injury. When damage to the central nervous system occurs, no assurance can be made—not even survival.

After moving to a general waiting area upstairs from a private waiting room on the ground floor when Craig was in the ER, Mr. and Mrs. Meyers waited for somebody—anybody—to provide some encouragement that Craig would be okay. This solace did not occur, for the doctors did not know if Craig would make it, or if he'd ever experience some semblance of normalcy again. To provide this comfort to parents whose mind wavered from visions of Craig sleeping in a crib as a baby to the illuminated X-rays of his fractured skull would be a lie.

The dolar of this Valentine's Day massacre was made even more unbearable when, with the ferocity of acid to an eye, one of the vascular surgeons informed an already distraught Mr. Meyers that if the veins used to replace Craig's right femoral artery fail to function properly and do not feed blood to Craig's lower leg, the limb cannot be saved and would he sign a consent form giving the surgeons permission to cut the leg off. Wide-eyed and jaws clenched that a suggestion like this would even be thought of, Mr. Meyers tearfully protested that Craig's a ballplayer and needs his legs; that there's no way the doctors are going to get off easy by him signing a paper stating that if the surgery is difficult, they have the recourse of severing the leg. No way!! Mr. Meyers would not sign.

Exhausted and ragged, Mr. Meyers dropped his head praying to the Higher Power that life not be sifted from his son nor the strength drained from his body. Normally contained and always practical, Mr. Meyers would have bartered his soul to rid Craig of his agony. He loved that boy.

A rational woman, Mrs. Meyers knew enough about medicine to realize her son might not survive and, if he does, may never live a life free from confinement and limitation. All that existed in her universe at this time in space was her son. Her faith never dwindled nor her spirituality questioned. Her belief in the power of prayer and its direct line to God was the tool she utilized every available moment.

Not knowing if their work would be successful long-term, the vascular surgeons who explored the right femoral artery via an arteriorgram—Daniel L. Diamond, M.D. and Joseph C. Young, M.D.—finished the operation on Craig's severed artery unable to ascertain how the leg would respond. Ultimately requiring an end-to-end anastomoses, these doctors would later report that only time can tell if the open wound in Craig's right leg had been subjected to infection or if the veins that replaced the artery would continue working.

The orthopedic surgeon, Joseph E. Imbriglia, M.D., inserted a seventeen-inch titanium steel rod in the center of Craig's femur to mend the break. The metal used in this open reduction internal fixation procedure will never have to be removed. After the vascular surgeons completed their monumental feat of getting the substitute veins to act as a surrogate artery circulating blood to Craig's lower leg, two dozen staples were embedded in his inner leg to shut the ten inch open wound. A dozen staples were implanted in the outer part of Craig's leg to enclose the opening made when the surgeons' scalpel borrowed the veins which, with God's will, would serve as a passageway for the artery that had fallen prey to the shrapnel of Craig's splintered femur.

Dr. Hankle, the oral maxillofacial surgeon who operated on Craig's right ear which was torn from his head when it penetrated the glass of the passenger door window, reconstructed the ear with the artistry of a Michaelangelo classic. However, one hundred-twenty stitches, not a paint brush, were used for this masterpiece. Despite this work of art, no assurance could be made that the blood flow necessary to maintain the ear would continue.

The ravages of this bewildering decimation left Mr. and Mrs. Meyers paralyzed of little emotion beyond the petrifying fear that their eighteen-year-old son, who was devoid of any sensation while in a fetal-like state, would not live to see morning. Expectations and aspirations of what this boy would someday achieve have now decayed into the most elementary rudiments. An infinite number of questions, but not enough answers. For all intents and purposes, has a life that can experience joy and happiness been replaced by one that may know only despair and restriction. Only the preponderant Lord Almighty could have knowledge of this. Trust that God had worked through the surgeons' hands—answering their prayers—was what the Meyers pleaded for.

Weary from the malevolence of this evening, the gray-haired couple slowly got off the elevator trudging towards the pay phone, so they could call a taxi to take them to the bus station, when Scott appeared in the lobby. The disquietude which possessed him was evident and something Mr. and Mrs. Meyers had never seen, for Scott always projected the image of a stoic and the founder of travesty when it came to interacting with his brother. However, the perniciousness of the past twenty-four hours exposed a side of him which had been hidden so well. Words could not even begin to describe Craig's condition when his brother asked. The harrowing looks on Mr. and Mrs. Meyers' faces telling a story of distress and devastation, Scott could tell just how bad off his brother was.

Upon arriving home, a cooked meal prepared by their daughter-in-law's mother awaited the Meyers. The agonizing feelings repressed by Mrs. Meyers during this night of misery were just too overwhelming not to purge. She needed a cathartic-like expression to rid herself of the demons which taunted her.

With tears flowing, Mrs. Meyers was kept from falling to her knees by the support offered by the family around her. She screamed out how dare someone be so conceited and selfish as to critically injure the son she devoted eighteen years of her life caring and nurturing, for the sake of being social at a party. To have a young life full of promise thrown away by someone's thoughtlessness and irresponsibility was something that could never be forgiven. Knowing that her son was in Allegheny General Hospital struggling to stay alive because of Paul's excessive indulgence, incensed Mrs. Meyers with an inundated feeling of furor. This grieving mother felt regret that she could only imagine standing over a restrained and subdued Paul, burrowing a knife deep within his chest cavity, seeking to remove the lungs which sustained him. Enraged and dumbfounded that Paul's brilliant and worldly parents must not have had the time to provide him with the type of fostering one needs to form moral parameters of conduct, Craig's parents couldn't fully understand how a family could ever refrain from such devotion. Blasphemous or not, Mrs. Meyers damned the souls of Paul and his family for the insensate condition her son was in. Victimized by another family's inability to develop a parent-child bond, for whatever reason(s) healthy development would be stunted, Mr. and Mrs. Meyers wouldn't deserve the consequence.

When a child senses they are not being attended to and are being overlooked, they can feel unimportant and not worthy. And, often because of their inability to communicate effectively, kids will let adults/parents know there is something wrong by their actions. One way young kids show they are disturbed is by smoking and/or drinking at an early age, hoping that a grown-up shows some concern. If nurturing does not occur, the child can feel not cared about. When the child grows to be an adolescent, the teen does not want his peers to realize that he's flooded with insecurities and will go to great lengths to conceal this. Paul's cocksure walk and carefree style were an effective facade, as few questioned his early substance usage escapades beyond being prematurely advanced.

After a sleepless night, while Scott was driving his parents across the Ninth Street Bridge to Allegheny General, an eerie silence lingered, telling a story of three passengers' thoughts that Craig might be dead. Their anxiety rose like the mercury in a thermometer on a scorching summer day as the hospital appeared before them. Did Craig live through the night? Is he overcome with pain? What is he feeling? Can he feel? Questions abound as the Meyers approached the waiting area which was going to be their home for the next eight hours. Between 12–12:30 P.M. and 7–7:30 P.M. they could see Craig twice, thirty minutes in the afternoon and thirty minutes in the evening, while he was in intensive care.

Entering the private ICU room Craig shared with an elderly gentleman who suffered a stroke, Mr. and Mrs. Meyers were relived when they saw the inanimate object which their son now resembled was still breathing. Three trauma nurses, one for each shift, were to be with Craig around the clock. In case something happened, the nurse on duty—dressed for battle—would be right there to render immediate assistance and call for help.

When Scott came into the ICU and saw his comatose brother that first time after the accident, he could feel his stomach tightening and getting sick from the sight of seeing his younger sibling lying motionless; unresponsive to anything or anyone. IV's, monitors, hoses were strewn about Craig measuring his vitals and feeding his body with the medicines and nutrients necessary for survival. Entrenched in his right leg were thick silver staples and wrapped around his head was a sanitary belt holding in place a plastic cup which protected the cauliflower which was his right ear. While the shocked brother stood watching Craig, the trauma nurse was obsessed with the readings of the monitors above Craig's bed, as his blood pressure, heart beat, temperature, and the swelling of his brain were digitally displayed. As urine trickled down a tube from the catheter, Scott needed to excuse himself.

Suffocated by fears of what the next moment may bring, Mr. and Mrs. Meyers spoke to their son and could only hope the sheets covering their boy who had been bludgeoned by the utility pole would continue moving with each respiration. Speaking to a son who could neither hear their words of encouragement or feel the kiss on his bruised face was a task of immense proportions. Encouraged to talk of things which Craig was familiar, the Meyers spoke of what they think the Pirates should do during baseball's interleague trading period, the Steelers' plans for the college draft in two months, and what the critics were saying about Joe Perry's solo project in the papers. They could have been speaking to the lamp by Craig's bedside and gotten the same response, as the only sound coming from Craig's bed was the humming of the motorized oxygen tank and the clicking of the flickering numbers on the many monitors. The only good thing about this perilous morning was that Craig couldn't see his parents' tears of consternation.

Mrs. Meyers gazed at her child's still body hoping and praying that some portion of Craig's personality—no matter how small—would surface, letting the Meyers know that he's still in that body which resembles their son. For Mrs. Meyers, the question and concern were a constant. Was anyone in there? Does he have any life left in him, and if he does, is this what we can expect for the years to come? Or has he already left us and gone to the Afterlife? Wanting to shake him free of this unconscious, Mrs. Meyers would hear herself say, "Where are you? Damn it Craig, wake up and tell us!"

Thoughts about how people in a coma on television just wake up suddenly and say, "Hey, where am I? What happened?" tormented Mrs. Meyers, for she knew this was a scenario conjured by Hollywood and not one based on fact. But just maybe. Leaning on the shoulder of her husband for strength, together they battled the barrage of ominous visions which would overcome most. But because their son needs them, they would become chiseled of valor.

One is supposed to enjoy their retirement, not subjugated by demoralizing thoughts. Retired a little over three years, Mr. Meyers looked down at his son and was being taunted by a myriad of questions about how this tragedy—which left his boy unaware of everything about him—could have been avoided. Languishing from the thoughts that his son's head hit that telephone pole with the force a bat hits a baseball and his lacerated face penetrated the glass window with the power an anchor thrusts into the sea, Mr. Meyers promised Craig that he will do whatever possible to make sure Paul and his family feel repercussions of their actions. Craig's brother-in-law, who served in the infantry during the Vietnam War, wanted five minutes alone with Paul in a locked room.

As their daughter-in-law entered the hospital room, a black gloom beset the Meyers—her arrival meant their half-hour that evening with Craig was over. Mr. and Mrs. Meyers got into an argument over whether or not they were going to rent one of the rooms across the street the hospital reserves for patients' families, or travel the thirty-five miles back to Washington away from the son Mrs. Meyers envisioned would awaken—calling out for them—only to be terrorized thinking he was in this blood-curdling predicament without so much as any support.

Mr. Meyers knew that being vulnerable in the North Side of Pittsburgh could be treacherous and he wasn't prepared to risk the family's well-being, especially when Craig is in a state where he may be dependent on them for his very survival.

Upon their return home, flocks of neighbors told the frazzled seniors that their hopes and prayers were directed toward Craig. Thoughts of Craig's demise lingered, but never conceded to. The pain and worry went beyond description. Images of the phone ringing and a voice saying, "I'm sorry to inform you of this, but Craig's no longer with us," horrified Mr. and Mrs. Meyers.

Consumed by the distance she was from her son and the ravaging perplexity of what—if anything—he is feeling, Mrs. Meyers felt a burning ache in her heart and an icy chill down he spine when the phone rang. Her eyes meeting her husband's, Mrs. Meyers positioned herself ready to leap from her chair and scurry to the phone—only to hesitate. During this momentarily delay, a ghoulish script played in Mrs. Meyers' mind where a surgeon with a blood spotted operating scrub said Craig had suffered some complications during surgery and that a team of doctors tried to stop the hemorrhaging, but couldn't, and that Craig has died. Before the doctor could say "I'm sorry," Mrs. Meyers apprehensively lifted the receiver from its hook—despite its incredible weight—anxiously saying "Hello." Fearful that this script would be played out, the incisive voice of Mr. Michaels corrupted the phone line.

On the one extreme, Mrs. Meyers couldn't have been happier that the Director didn't say "Action," putting into motion the horrid script she conjured, yet, was taken back that she was speaking to the perpetrator of this crime's father. With fingers surely crossed, Mr. Michaels asked the mother of the child his son rendered absent of all sensation how Craig was. When Mrs. Meyers replied that he was alive, the barren trees in the Meyers' backyard swayed ever so gently, as Mr. Michaels must have breathed a shallow sigh of relief. Like a game show host awarding the beaten contestant a consolation prize, Mr. Michaels said that his son would be on crutches for several weeks because he had sustained a cracked pelvis which caused him much pain and that Paul had also lost a contact lens. The pain endured by the Michaels family must be excruciating.

Mrs. Meyers was noncommittal, as she could only picture Paul—realizing the danger of *his* being seriously hurt—veering the driver's side of the car away from the oncoming pole, allowing the pawn in the passenger seat to take the impact caused by his stupor. Possessing the same foresight he had as Paul's guiding influence, Mr. Michaels mistakenly assumed his insurance would cover all Craig's medical expenses, as he assured Mrs. Meyers that his policy was an all-encompassing one. Mr. Meyers, who had picked up the other phone, said little fearing one of his outbursts might result in damaging ramifications later on.

After their grueling day at the hospital, the Meyers needed a sabbatical from this constant overload of disaster, but their calm would be disturbed with the convulsing frequency of a leaking faucet's ever-lasting drip. Crying out how difficult life has been for her—standing in front of the mirror—Grandma Barnhart gazed at her shoulder, wondering how that scar ever got there. Unable to comprehend how badly her youngest grandson had been hurt because her mental capacities had all but deteriorated by now, Mrs. Meyers' mother could not imagine the toxicity her complaints had on those who opened their home up to her. During this time Grandma Barnhart's daughter and son-in-law needed loving care and support themselves, Mr. and Mrs. Meyers had the cumbersome task of trying to persuade this resistant elder that she could no longer live in the home which had been her residence for approximately forty years.

Feeling a surge of energy that she needed to get back home immediately, the eighty-four-year-old woman pointed her crooked forefinger at her daughter demanding to be taken home that very instant, for she was sick and tired of being held hostage against her will. Despite her permanently being unable to lift her arm above shoulder level, Grandma Barnhart scolded Gwen that she doesn't deserve being mistreated and prevented from driving her car to the store where she could get some spring cleaning supplies for the task which lies ahead this upcoming season. Telling Grandma Barnhart that this was against doctor's orders would have been fruitless, for she was intent on resuming her independent life which could no longer be possible.

Not one to handle too much at one time without becoming aggravated, Mr. Meyers' patience with his mother-in-law had evaporated, for he needed time uninterrupted to focus on his son. Screaming how dare she be so selfish when her grandson could be dying that very moment, like Mr. Hyde emerging from Dr. Jeckyll, Mr. Meyers got in the face of his elderly mother-in-law he normally was on cordial terms with. Back-pedaling from this irate father whom she could not hear, Grandma Barnhart and her son-in-law were separated by Scott who put his hands on his grief-stricken father's shoulders and took him downstairs where he could collect himself. Mr. Meyers needed to regain control and rest, for he would go to Pittsburgh once again in the morning.

For five days, from February 14th to February 18th, little changed in the Meyers' routine. They'd arrive at AGH in the morning praying that Craig had made it through the night, and spent one hour total out of the nine or so they were there speaking to their son whom they could not tell whether he could hear them or not. The nurse watching Craig and his older roommate would tell the Meyers that not much has changed in Craig's condition, and that all staff could really do at the time was to continuously monitor him to safeguard against anything happening. To prevent Craig from getting sores and contracting pneumonia, so he'd be as comfortable as possible, staff would gingerly rotate Craig several times a day. For a few hours, Craig would be lying on his back when two nurses would turn his dead weight body on his stomach, before reinserting the many IV's.

When the Meyers returned home, neighbors would want a report on Craig's condition almost the instant they got back. The phone never seeming to stop ringing, consoling friends of the family would offer their encouragement and want updated. On one hand, this was stressful for the Meyers because each time the phone rang, their heart stopped and skin crawled fearing they'd receive news that Craig put up a valiant fight to stay alive, but had sustained too much damage to make it and that it might be better off that he didn't survive. On the other, the offering of prayers, concerns, and sympathy was comforting and greatly appreciated. Mr. Brezinski would call everyday to find out how Craig was doing, expressing his family's sorrow and regard. Mr. and Mrs. Meyers also received calls from the Michaels on a daily basis early on, but for a different reason.

After the Michaels made one of their too frequent inquiries, the trees in the Meyers' backyard always seemed to sway after Paul's folks would find out that Craig hadn't succumbed. Dead leaves, fallen victims of autumn's touch, swirled about destiny unknown with these winds of divided concern. Upon speaking directly to the person responsible for this calamity, Mrs. Meyers admonished Paul for his role in the accident which could have been easily prevented had he been the friend to Craig he professed to be and refrained from drinking when he suspected his coherence and coordination might be compromised. Mrs. Meyers asked Paul if Craig was drinking with Paul saying he wasn't.

After informing Paul that Craig's family did not know the circumstances surrounding the accident or about the details of the party, Paul lied saying the party took place in the nearby community of Canonsburg—about ten miles from Washington—at a residence where he didn't know the family's name. It was only later, during one of her pleasantries with Mr. Michaels, did Mrs. Meyers find out that the party was at the Ilyacoff's in Washington. One would think if Paul truly were a friend of Craig's, he would have been more than willing to help Craig and his family during this dark time when so many questions had so few answers. However, Paul was more concerned with not implicating the Ilyacoff's, than helping Craig. Great guy.

In the morning of February 19th, Mr. and Mrs. Meyers saw no improvement in Craig, as he was still in his aware-free state. Trying their best not to let the constant distress they had been trampled by since Craig's been hurt to show on their face, Mr. and Mrs. Meyers put on their animated expression and approached Craig in a sprightly, optimistic manner; not letting on the sadness with which they were shackled.

During the countless hours at the hospital when they were away from Craig, the Meyers learned from the doctors at AGH as much as they could about head injury. To say the news was encouraging would not be accurate.

Mr. and Mrs. Meyers wanted some answers to the multitude of questions they had. The response they were growing tired of hearing was that there just isn't enough known about the unexplored universe which is the brain to pinpoint what symptoms Craig's going to have and their severity—if he survives. The Meyers were informed that if Craig does live, there is a strong likelihood that there's going to be some permanent damage physically and/or emotionally.

Adding to their tumultuous anxiety, the Meyers were told that the longer Craig remains comatose, the worse off they can expect his symptoms to be. With this information, the thought of Craig's not being responsive was a menacing one, for his awakening from this deep unconscious now took on an element of urgency.

The realization that some people never escape this unknown existence of being comatose was eating away at the Meyers like a burning ulcer. Although they were far from surrendering, each minute it became more and more difficult for Craig's parents to remain optimistic. As the thirty-minute evening visiting time for families to see their loved ones in the ICU approached on February 19th, six days after the accident, the Meyers were about to see something which would provide them with a new confidence.

As the precious half-hour when relatives could see their family member in the ICU grew near, outside the door of the room Craig and the elderly gentleman were in resembled the Parkway West when traffic's bottled up entering the Ft. Pitt Tunnels inbound during rush hour. As Mr. and Mrs. Meyers walked down the hallway from the waiting area to Craig's room staring at the floor beneath them, they were hopeful of—yet not counting on—seeing some improvement from Craig's insensate condition of the morning. As each step brought Mr. and Mrs. Meyers closer to the crowd in the hallway outside the ICU room—this time accompanied by Scott and his wife—the unwelcome predator known as malaise had become a constant.

However, the private nurse's beaming smile greeted the Meyers when the door opened, weakening this intruding menace. Flooded with a sea of hope because this astute medical professional was normally as expressionless as a caretaker of a mortuary, the Meyers rushed to their son's bedside and—bent close to his black and blue face—saw that his eyes were open a quarter of an inch!!

Craig's hospital gown soaked with the tears of joy which fell freely from his father's wrinkled face as Mr. Meyers excitedly exclaimed, "You're gonna make it buddy, you're gonna make it!" Mr. Meyers envisioned his son pounding his glove and chomping on his bubble gum as he positioned himself at shortstop in time for this summer's Thoroughbred League competition. When it was the home team's turn to bat, he could hear his son's name echoing throughout the park as the batting order was announced over the P.A. system. Yep, Mr. Meyers promised himself he wouldn't complain anymore if Craig played his stereo too loud or had his amp turned up too high. Hell, he'd even let it slide when prying loose the Kleenex which stuck to the bottom of the trash can because that's where Craig hawkered. In his mind, it was a given now that Craig was going to pull through this. An impeccable craftsman who has been skillful at constructing things for a half of a century, Mr. Meyers could have never imagined that such a small quarter-inch measurement could have such a massive impact on him.

Mrs. Meyers put her hand in Craig's left one saying, "If you can hear me, squeeze my hand." Ever so gently, like an infant holding its bottle, Mrs. Meyers was overcome with elation when she felt her eighteen-year-old son's hand attempting to grasp her's. Flooded by tears, Mrs. Meyers joyfully said, "He can hear us!!!."

A glimmer of hope in their voices and the slightest flush appearing on their faces, Scott and his wife were ecstatic to witness these caregivers emerge a little from the dark clouds of despair which strangles a parent when they lose a child. Upon his looking at his brother, Scott could see that Craig's eyes were not focusing on anything, rather, staring into nothingness. Like that of a corpse with its eyes open, sight would be void. The family of Craig's roommate were overjoyed that Craig had shown a sign of progress. Seeing Craig's parents' agony when they came in every morning, not knowing if their son's alive, was a grim picture.

Wishes that Armageddon would arrive have been replaced with a rejuvenated spirit and trust that things will work out. Despite not wanting to disrupt their positive outlook which the Meyers feared they would be forever deprived, the nurse was obligated to caution the family that, with brain injury, there will be periods of time when Craig seems alright, only to revert to a less-than-promising state. In order to safeguard against a fall from unyielding jubilation to the murk that is melancholy, the nurse informed the Meyers that Craig's injuries still require close scrutiny because at any given moment, he could regress. While reinforcing the idea that all gains need appreciated, the nurse also knew that to allow Craig's family to revel in what could very well be a mirage, would be sacrileges.

Assuming the insensible state which they have grown all too familiar, Craig would not squeeze or release his parents' hands again this breakthrough day. As the visiting time ended this momentous evening, having witnessed Craig coming in and out of consciousness, the Meyers looked at Craig hoping his eyes opening would be the first step on the road to recovery.

For the first time in what seemed an everlasting deluge of horror, Mr. Meyers was not mired in despondency and swamped with dire portraits of what could become of his youngest. This minuscule opening of the eyes prompted Mr. Meyers to experience an excitement which could not be contained. Although joyful by events of this evening, Mrs. Meyers was more restrained than her husband, not knowing what future dialogue has been written, for head injury can change the calm current the chapter appears destined, into one where rapids become the rule.

The Meyers were home but a few minutes when the phone began ringing. Telling the numerous well-wishers the delightful news of Craig's improvement, these thrilled parents thanked everyone for their prayers and support. A serene comfort warmed the Meyers until the voice of the father, whose son was responsible for their pain, regurgitated from the ear piece of the telephone. A gail force gust of wind uprooted several trees in the Meyers' backyard when informing the caller of the significant gains made by Craig the last twenty-four hours. This driving parental figure fearful of his professional reputation being tarnished if his son would have to go to prison for an accidental slaying, surely would be relieved that an impeding sentence could be avoided for this sinister act of irresponsibility.

Not resulting in a death, the real reason for the accident wouldn't get advertised in the paper and a health care professional wouldn't have to be subjected to explaining how his son had committed vehicular homicide because he was driving under the influence. To conceal the true culprit, a mental itinerary would need to be thought out, so that the blame and focus could be shifted away from Paul and his prominent family. In order to maintain his high status in the community, the company line Mr. Michaels developed would be one where the car his son was driving had skidded on ice, ramming into the utility pole. Part of this story line possibly included Paul risking his own life to save his friend's—after returning home from Bible study. Being that the weather had been mild for a few weeks, Mother Nature was not to blame, rather, Paul's 0.18 blood-alcohol content was the culprit. But that needn't be mentioned.

The trip to Pittsburgh the morning of February 20th was not as bleak as the six other trips, for Craig' eyes opening had instilled a new energy in the Meyers. Wondering what improvement they're going to see today when they get to the hospital, Mr. Meyers' broad smile was indicative of his thrilled mood.

Mr. Meyers pictured a scene where Craig had both his feet underneath the foot of the hospital bed counting sit-ups one-by-one, saying that his busted leg is keeping him from doing as many as he would like and that this hospital stay isn't going to prevent him from staying in shape. Mrs. Meyers would have been happy to see Craig's eyes continuing to open and his spastic right arm loosening from his chin a little.

As the doors to the elevator opened, one of the registered nurses sitting at the nurses' station near Craig's room darted towards the parents. Expecting to hear that their son has made the most miraculous turnaround in the history of neuromedicine, Mr. Meyers surely thought that this white flash rushing towards him was about to inform he and his wife that Craig's complaining of being bored and wants his guitar. However, this was but an illusion, for the RN's stinging words would capsize the Meyers' spirit. Needing to be watched closely—with a doctor on standby—the Meyers would be informed that Craig had been running a dangerously high fever within the past hour.

Embracing one another, hopes trampled, Mr. and Mrs. Meyers were horrified when they saw two nurses working strenuously at Craig's bedside beneath the many additional monitors that had been brought in. The Meyers' fears reached a foreboding level when they could imagine hearing Craig's room being said over the PA system, then the word, "Stat!!," which notifies staff of an emergency situation. As the Meyers stood in the small ICU room watching helplessly—without giving specifics—the nurses quickly changed Craig's bed, putting in a cooling mattress to try to lower his temperature.

Since Craig has been hurt, feelings of helplessness have grasped the Meyers with an overbearing grip. Now all they can do is stand by and watch as these nurses control their destiny. The thought that Craig's leg may have been infiltrated with bacteria after all and that these germs were causing the fever was a demoralizing reality that Mr. and Mrs. Meyers hoped and prayed would not materialize.

Despite the Meyers' desire to be close to Craig in his time of need, their intellect told them to stay out of the way and let the medical professionals do their job. Although it was painful to tolerate, they restrained their maternal/paternal instincts, so Craig could get what he needed. With one hand holding her husband's, while the other guided the kiss she blew to her son, Mrs. Meyers emotions had been running ragged fearing that one of these times Craig just might not be so resilient and come out unscathed.

Within a day's time, their thoughts have changed from one where they were thinking their son was on his way back to one where he was going back—wards. A vicious scene where their boy was lying underneath a blood-soaked sheet with a stump, where his leg used to be, oozing blood ousted the apparition of his fielding grounders and firing strikes. As they would look at Craig, they could only wonder what he was feeling and thinking being in this environment where the numbers on the monitors were clicking as a clock does when time is running out. Strange faces huddling about him like a desperate offense when it's fourth-and-long, the Meyers family's fate was firmly placed in the hands of these professionals "advancing the frontier of medicine."

Craig's eyes were not open and he was as still as the calm, winter evenings of this February 1982. Praying the sheets would continue moving with each respiration, Mr. and Mrs. Meyers were terrified that their son would succumb to this evil where his responsiveness was like that of a cadaver.

The parents of this lifeless youth could imagine Paul, with his broad boyish smile, chug beer after beer in front of his adoring teenaged peers while they patted him on the back following another liquid conquest on the night of the thirteenth. Puffing a stream of smoke from his cigarette, Paul would bark, "Get me another one!," which was met with a roaring chorus of approval. With this attention, Paul undoubtedly felt the warm sense of belonging that all young people strive for, especially those from households where the parent's child-rearing capacities are likely compromised, or not foremost in their list of priorities. How unfair that the Meyers must pay the price because truly important values were not appreciated or instilled.

The Meyers could picture Craig in an adjacent room at Ilyacoff's, not paying mind to any commotion because he'd be engaged in deep conversation about what the Steelers need to do to resurrect the "Steel Curtain" which has decayed due to the age of its members and poor drafts which haven't replenished the line. However, the clapping and hails of acceptance were for Paul's ability to chug down some beer and not for any scouting report or draft analysis. Yeah, Paul was king of the hill this night. Unfortunately, the king's ransom might be their son's life.

During the evening visiting period, Craig showed dramatic improvement. Although the reading on his thermometer was still high, it had fallen a few degrees. And when his father placed his hand in his son's, there was an immediate attempt to clutch it. Mr. Meyers couldn't tell if this was an automatic reflex, or a response to Craig's being terrified. To ease his fears, like a mother reassures her toddler not to be scared of the dark, Mrs. Meyers told Craig that he was running a fever, but that it was coming down and not to be afraid. Like speaking to a small child, she didn't know if she was heard.

Flooded by this sea of havoc, the Meyers were being eaten away inside about how their fortunes have changed within a night's time. Since yesterday, their emotions have shifted 180 degrees. Approaching the day with a seemingly impenetrable optimism, they were devastated to find their son burning with a fever that no one knew why this was occurring. Was his body fighting an infection in his leg, ear, both of them, or has the autonomic nervous system—which controls body temperature—been irreversibly collapsed, thus ending any encore for a Cinderella story? What did the grasping of his father's hand indicate? Was Craig reaching out for someone? Or was the tightening of his hand a biological response sensing the touch of another? Could Craig even sense? If he could, what was he feeling? Questions. So many of them that may never be answered.

As the IV's pumped Craig the medicine needed to prevent his getting an ulcer, Mr. and Mrs. Meyers were excited to see Craig's eyes were open about three-eights of an inch this evening, or a little more than yesterday. They were excited because, little by little, Craig seemed to be "coming to" from the morning, but also wary that this increased conscious might be due to his experiencing unbearable discomfort and sensing a destitute of relief. They didn't know what to think. What did the eyes opening mean? What was the this fever all about; was this a false alarm or a wicked prophecy of what's to come? Did Craig hear and understand when he grasped with his hand? How long will this not knowing what to think last? Will this coming in and out of consciousness be the rule or the exception? This fluctuation of highs and lows was something Dr. Prostko tried to prepare the Meyers for, but words alone cannot possibly describe the diabolical symptoms of this disability which so little is known. They could only hope these peaks and valleys don't deplete them of their will to endure.

Like the sharpened ends of the grave digger's pick, the Meyers subjecting themselves to thoughts of impending upheaval dug a chasm of desolation which they became trapped. Joyous to see Craig going out for once with some peers having fun, the Meyers could not refrain from thinking that only a week ago at this time, their son was alright. In the fourteen years he's lived in Washington, the only time Craig ever went out to a party, he ends up almost getting killed—and that still might happen. How unfair life can be. Who would have thought that within seven days' time, their one-time healthy son could die without warning?

As the Meyers looked out a window from Allegheny General Hospital onto the busy streets and packed sidewalks of downtown Pittsburgh heading towards the elevator going home, they thought that out of all the people in this world, why did their son have to be the one that was hurt so bad? He's only eighteen; why did his number have to come up? Surely, this couldn't be his time. He's a good kid who never caused anybody any trouble, why does he have to be the one that suffers when there's a lot of miserable bastards out on that street that are nothing but trouble and leeches to society? Why? Why? Why?

In the evening of the 20th, the Meyers reflected on the experiences of their day. In this day where there was a surplus of "Why's?" with no answers, the Meyers went from being horrified to happily excited again that Craig's eyes were showing some life. With his lids opening a little more, Mr. and Mrs. Meyers wanted to breathe a deep sigh of relief, but knew now that to become so filled with joy only to have it escape from their grasp was too crushing a blow to endure again. Mercilessly being teased to believe that the light a the end of the tunnel is hope, only to recognize it as merely being a star in the vast unexplored galaxy—light years away—is an unremitting battle that brain injury will wage. To have the air, which was optimism, leak from their balloon was an intolerable hardship that the Meyers have learned to avoid. Just when Mr. and Mrs. Meyers were prepared to take a little time off from this most trying of chapters of the many that have been written in their life and try to unwind some, the phone rang. It was Dr. Prostko.

Fearful of what they were going to hear and with chest burning like the back of a slave who has just been slashed with a cracked whip, the Meyers listened intently as the neurosurgeon told them that sometimes fever occurs when someone has been hurt as critically as their son, and that everything possible is being done to stabilize Craig. Their boy still has a temperature, but it's coming down ever so slowly. Everything about Craig's injury is ever so slowly—especially answers.

To take a respite from the war that Craig's injury declared was impossible for the Meyers because the adrenalin was flowing non-stop with fright about what the future has in store for the family. Fear of the unknown was the wind which guided their sailboat off to a course not known. With head injury, what lies ahead is anybody's guess because no two brain injuries are alike. This was trying for Mr. and Mrs. Meyers because none of their questions could be answered definitively. With the flu, a pulled hamstring, or a torn ligament, doctors basically know that the symptoms will be X-Y-Z and the treatments, A-B-C. But with brain injury, no one knows what's going to happen—and perhaps worse yet—why.

In particular, one unknown haunted Mrs. Meyers. She would wonder, "If and when Craig wakes up, will he remember us?." "Will the son I've spent eighteen years nurturing, caring, and planning for—forget who I am?," "Will he look at me and ask, 'Who are you?'" To think that Mrs. Meyers cleaned up after, bought the things needed in life, doctored, provided a nice home, educated, helped in whatever way possible, prepared meals everyday, etc., etc., etc., for a boy that might not have any idea who she was, would be a horrifying thought for her. If this did happen, she knew that she would just have to start building a new foundation.

Not knowing what to expect in the morning of February 21, Nineteen Hundred and Eighty-Two and learning to approach circumstances which they may encounter with an indifferent attitude, helped the Meyers cope with what they would see today—which wasn't much of anything. As tempting as it was to become elated last evening when Craig's eyes opened their widest since he's been hurt, Mr. and Mrs. Meyers were equally restrained from getting too despondent when Craig assumed the lifeless stature they have become all too accustomed to seeing. Eyes not opening nor hands clutching when feeling his father's, there was no response in either the afternoon or evening visiting periods. With head sunk low, the parents of the boy they thought was "on his way," would continue to talk to their son as if he were at the dinner table after a day at the ballyard.

As Mrs. Meyers told her comatose son that Danny was going to the Air Force, Craig Johnson was accepted at Penn State, and Brian was going to Bringham Young as a pre-med student, the private nurse looked on, feeling remorseful for the woman whose son doesn't likely know that she's even saying anything about his friends. The family of Craig's roommate felt sickened when they saw the comatose boy's strong-willed father let a tear escape, running down to his whiskered jowls.

When the evening visiting period ended, Mr. and Mrs. Meyers slowly walked past the nurses' station. Not letting on he was being emotionally twisted by the events—or rather—lack of events of the day, Mr. Meyers tried his best to smile at the ladies sitting there. With her husband's arm around her shoulder, the devastation Mrs. Meyers was feeling could no longer be suppressed, as her voice cracked like one beaten in battle. Void of strength, when this committed mother said "Goodnight" to the nurses, her tired eyes spoke volumes. Watching the elevator doors close behind the white-haired couple, these hospital professionals wondered how much more Craig's parents could take.

Like every other occasion the phone rang at the Meyers' house, time would stand still and be frozen until Mr. and Mrs. Meyers were assured that the message wasn't to inform them of some mishap involving Craig. When they got a call on the morning of the 22nd, their heart pounded heavy, given Craig's condition of the evening before. When hearing Dr. Prostko's voice, they expected the worst.

Did the fever do what the Volkswagen couldn't and burn Craig to a lifeless crisp? Mr. Meyers turned as white as the hair hanging on his brow, fearing the news was one where plans would need to be made to transport Craig's dead body to Washington. A thought passed by Mrs. Meyers that she will need to contact the funeral home in town and determine where Craig should be buried; either somewhere in the Washington Cemetery near their home or in Johnstown, where the family has a plot.

However, the doctor's voice did not sound like one where arrangements of this kind would need arranged, for it would be one of promise. To their shock, Dr. Prostko informed the Meyers that Craig ate a little ice cream last night!!!

Was this the same boy who did not move or respond at all yesterday? Apparently, the synapses, neurons, lobes, axons, stem, and only God knows what else in Craig's brain decided to get its act together sometime after the Meyers left last night. It would have been fabulous if these drained parents would have been able to see Craig ingest something other than through an IV, even if it was just slivers of ice cream melting on his tongue, but the Meyers didn't care as long as their boy was showing some life and ridding himself of that fever.

Wallowing in disbelief, Mr. and Mrs. Meyers just couldn't figure how one minute Craig's on the edge of leaving this earth and the next, showing signs of making encouraging strides. Because of the unpredictability of head injury, the Meyers were learning that the only way to remain sane was to accept whatever happens and roll with the punches. How many jabs and crosses their older bodies can take remains to be seen, though.

On the morning of 2/22/82, Craig's parents talked to Dr. Prostko in the hospital and the doctor informed them that, provided that no complications develop until then, Craig will be transferred tomorrow from the ICU to the seventh floor head trauma unit where those with neurological impairments are placed. The Meyers weren't sure exactly what this meant, but took it as a turning point for the better because constant observation and limited access to their son would no longer be required. Mr. and Mrs. Meyers were thrilled, for they could spend a good portion of the day with their son from 2:00 P.M. to 8:30 P.M., working on functions Craig's medical team deems necessary for recovery. Being the bearer of more good news, having a difficult time containing his cheer, Dr. Prostko gladly reported once again that Craig swallowed a little ice cream and some juice earlier this morning. Of equal importance was Craig's being able to tolerate sitting in a chair equipped with a chin strap and neck brace while his bed was being changed. Feeling a little nauseous that they should appreciate their husky, eighteen-year-old son being able to let ice cream melt in his mouth before choking it down and sitting on his ass in a chair with a belt wrapped around his forehead to keep his head from falling in his lap, the Meyers kept speaking to their son as if he had just won the lottery to keep his spirits from tumbling.

They talked about what they were going to do once he got better. Mrs. Meyers promised to buy Craig a Fender Stratocaster after he got out of the hospital. With chin quivering and eyes filling with a pool of tears, Mr. Meyers talked of how they're going to have to get their fishing license and go to Dutch Fork Lake this summer. These words were spoken not only to keep Craig stimulated, but to remind themselves what their goal in life is now; what they are subjecting themselves to this hell for—so that a tomorrow isn't out of their son's reach.

During this day where Craig showed his parents none of the magic reported to them by staff, the Meyers cherished the news that the neuro-medical professionals have seen enough improvement in Craig to take him to the next level. Earlier, a representative from the hospital's rehabilitation department told the Meyers that Craig would be starting both cognitive and physical therapy as soon as possible. Although the Meyers understood that it is essential to begin retraining the brain without delay, they couldn't believe their son—who was out of consciousness 99.9% of the time—was even being considered for rehab. Also, Craig's heart rate was still beating incredibly fast, his lungs needed suctioned several times a day, IV's were surrounding him, and a feeding tube was in his nose. To Craig's parents, it was inconceivable that he could begin therapy until the representative told them how basic the work was going to be. Counting, saying his A-B-C's, and following an extended forefinger with his eyes would be the tasks asked of Craig. To think their teen-aged son may find these exercises difficult that any kindergarten student could easily do, enraged the Meyers.

In what has become a common occurrence, the Meyers experienced a maze of punishing emotion which, like a levee breaking, came crashing down upon them with a force not forgiving. All being part of the package when someone you love has had a brain injury, confusion, excitement, thrill, terror, relief, and devastation were but a few of the teasing feelings which stoned this devoted couple each day they were with Craig. Not possible knowing if the carousel of sentiment would ever stop its torment, the Meyers dedication had been rooted for the long haul.

When Craig's parents entered their son's new room on the head trauma unit on February 23, the tenth day of his being hurt, they saw Craig lying on his bed as responsive as a rock in their gravel driveway. When Mr. Meyers said, "Good morning buddy! How you feeling today?," the silence was deafening.

Wearing a smile, Mrs. Meyers told her son devoid of life about him, "Honey, the doctors said you can have this big room all to yourself. A nurse won't be watching you all the time because me and daddy will be here a couple of hours each day."

Taking this Tuesday off to see his brother in his new surroundings, Scott said, "Now that you got this room to yourself, you can fart and nobody will hear you." No response. Nothing. It may have been a different setting, but the results were the same.

Like they heard so many times before, Mr. and Mrs. Meyers were told that when the nurses caught Craig in a conscious moment this morning, they hurriedly gave him juice and ice cream before he slipped into that other world where no one knows where he is—maybe not even Craig himself. Now, because they can spend more than one hour a day with him, Craig's parents might now be able to see for themselves something from Craig other than his unconscious. But that wouldn't be today.

When the nurse knocked on the door and poked her head in saying, "Visiting hours are over," the Meyers couldn't believe 8:30 P.M. had arrived so soon. Trying to gather some salvation from yet another response-free day, Mr. Meyers jokingly asked the nurse if they could spare a few blankets and let them sleep in the corner of Craig's spacious room. The drained father said they wouldn't get in the way and Scott promised he wouldn't feed his brother any more flies. With a smile of her own for the ragged family she admired for their dedication and wit in this incapacitating period in their life, the plump nurse chuckled, saying her supervisor wouldn't go for that, but if she had it her way, they could stay as long as they wanted.

After talking on the phone to their daughter, oldest son, and countless friends and neighbors whose frequent inquiries and encouragement were invaluable, Mr. Meyers looked at Scott and his wife, whose presence and support were vital ingredients to their maintaining the strength needed to withstand this prostration. Thinking how undeserving the family and friends of Craig are going through hell because a boy who has known only a life of privilege needed to be accepted at a party one night, Mr. Meyers tried to acknowledge this as an unfortunate part of history he could not change and would need to tolerate, if he were to proceed in an optimal fashion.

For Mrs. Meyers, hearing from clergy and church members that it is quite natural for a loving mother to have thoughts that a son might be better off dead, rather than suffering through an existence of unfulfilled promise, helped her in the quest to cease feeling overcome with guilt when picturing this alternative. Being a good Christian and an active member of the church, Mrs. Meyers had been burdened with question and self-persecution about this passing image.

Always the optimist, Mr. Meyers would console his wife saying that, because they're not medical professionals, they can't always tell what the signs of improvement are. Stressing that the doctors saw something in Craig that they couldn't see which indicated that some healing had been taking place, Mr. Meyers said encouragingly that Craig being taken out of the ICU and placed in a far less restrictive environment was outstanding. Reminding his wife that Craig's a tough guy who always welcomed a challenge, Mrs. Meyers could only hope that Craig would be on the winning side of this game of survival by the end of the 9th inning. A competitor who abhors losing, Mr. Meyers promised his wife that Craig will win and pull through this; wait and see. As he and his wife discovered the next time they would go to the hospital, Mr. Meyers' words would turn out to be more than wishful thinking.

Although the weather had been dreary most of the week, the mid-day sun of February 24 greeted the Meyers as they pulled out of the tunnel onto the Ft. Pitt Bridge. The slight breeze coupled with the sun's glow made the tiny waves of the Monongahela River beneath them look as if they were the fluttering wings of an angel. The skyline before them glistened with its powerful orange backdrop and the steel pillars of Three Rivers Stadium to their left did not cast the dark shadow it had in days' past. The fountain at The Point seemed to spray water to the heavens with a new strength.

Knowing that hearing is the first sense to return after somebody has been in a coma, Mr. and Mrs. Meyers would talk to Craig about Grandma Barnhart going to a nursing home in Ohio where Claire lives, how Fritz goes in his room everyday looking for his buddy, how the abdominal scan and shoulder X-rays conducted on him yesterday before moving upstairs showed nothing was wrong, and the dust that's collected on the furniture since mom's been going to Pittsburgh everyday.

Allowing a patient to hear a voice which they are familiar facilitates recovery and alleviates any fears they may have that they are alone. Hearing his parents' voice, Craig started to open his eyes gradually. First, a quarter of an inch, then three-eighths of an inch, then a half-inch, three-quarters, and—for what seemed like years—Craig's parents saw his brown eyes open completely!!!

Feeling a warmth throughout his body, Mr. Meyers affectionately shook his son's good arm saying, "Attaboy buddy, attaboy." Mrs. Meyers stood frozen with her hand covering her open mouth looking at the brown, oval iris she was afraid she'd never see again in its entirety. Feeling a rush of adrenalin, the Meyers asked their son if he could see them. Expecting Craig to unilaterally progress and respond, he closed his eyes and fell into the coma again.

The Meyers learned that to prevail through these days where they were unsure of what lurked around the corner, they had to appreciate and remember those precious moments when Craig showed something other than deep unconscious and feed off this. Their hunger for improvement from Craig was insatiable, however, just after the day reached its halfway point, the feast which Craig's parents were to engage would satisfy them this day.

Sometime in late afternoon while she was knelt to his left along Craig's bedside, his eyes gradually opened again and when a few minutes later Mrs. Meyers got up and walked to the foot of the bed to get some water, Craig followed her with his eyes!!! This was the first localized response Craig has had in eleven days where his eyes were focusing on something, not just staring into space. When his father saw this and leaned forward, this movement drew Craig's attention to his dad as Craig slowly moved his head in his dad's direction. Overcome with great joy that their son wasn't blinded, Mr. and Mrs. Meyers hadn't seen each other smile for what seemed an eternity.

Then, just as quickly as he "came to," Craig fell out of consciousness. Several times during this evening, Craig would follow either his mom, dad, or brother with his eyes before slipping from lucidity again, and again, and again. Although not comfortable that their son was unable to remain conscious but for a few minutes, the Meyers were no longer traumatized by this prolonged lack of awareness, for their son was fighting back.

At 1:00 P.M. on February 25th, one hour before visiting hours were to start, the stout RN at the nurses' station looked the other way as the Meyers—fooling absolutely no one—inconspicuously went into Craig's room. Knowing the Meyers have been enduring twelve days of turbulence since their son was almost slaughtered, the nurse wanted Craig's parents to take a break from constant worry and see the good news as soon as possible.

When his parents walked in, Craig was not conscious, but the oxygen mask which had been a fixture on his face for almost two weeks had been removed because Craig was breathing on his own!!! The IV's in Craig's arms which fed him everything from ulcer medication to anti-convulsants to pain killers to everything else under God's sun, were no longer needed and taken away.

At first, the Meyers were bubbling with joy by what they were seeing, but then became absorbed with second thoughts. They wondered if Craig—who had become dependent on the oxygen mask and the IV's for survival—would relapse and stop breathing because something went wrong upstairs in the autonomic nervous system, or some of the nerve cells in his brain would just explode causing God knows what to happen.

Just when Craig's parents were beginning to drown with anxiety, a nurse came in telling the couple who had "worry" stamped all over their faces that Craig's doing well and that their concerns were legitimate but unfounded, and to relax. Instructed to appreciate the immense gains Craig has made, the Meyers took a deep breath hearing these words of encouragement and reassurance from the nurse. Helping to put their minds at ease, when Craig's eyes opened, a warm comfort blanketed them.

Quickly, the nurse went to Craig's side telling him to follow her finger. From side to side then up and down, Craig's eyes went horizontally then vertically watching the nurse's extended forefinger. With his good hand, the nurse asked Craig to raise a finger. Holding one another, the Meyers saw Craig slowly, and with great effort, struggle to pick one finger off his bed. This tiny movement had an impact of the largest magnitude. It showed Craig could hear, understand, and process information. Skills which the Meyers feared Craig may have lost forever because that organ that weighs but a mere five pounds known as the brain, has a bruise on it.

This great day was made even better when the nurse informed the Meyers that the doctor who sewed Craig's ear back together made his rounds this morning and took the stitches out saying Craig's ear was healing remarkably and circulating blood with no problem.

Basking in the good news of this morning, the Meyers couldn't be convinced that Craig would not be able to make a full recovery given the progress made the past forty-eight hours. Despite past head injury cases indicating there will be some permanent disabling condition, the Meyers were trying not to believe this, figuring their son would be the exception. They had to assume this mindset to avoid being an emotional basket case.

For their own protection, the Meyers had to tell themselves that each day that passes now, Craig will be making equally incredible gains until he's back to his old, shitty self. Knowing that youth is on his side, the Meyers were starting to believe the road from here on out would be one of increasing normalcy. This thought would end in but a few moments when the respiratory therapist would come in.

Although Craig didn't need an oxygen mask on his face all the time now, the doctors knew that it was necessary that he still be assisted therapeutically with his breathing until Craig has shown that he's able to do this long-term without any trouble. When he could feel the oxygen mask touching his nose and mouth, making a groaning sound like that of an animal being hurt, Craig would move his head away from this predator. With the respiratory therapist soliciting the help of Craig's dad, Mr. Meyers delicately stabilized Craig's head for the half-hour respiratory treatment while the mask was being applied. Because Craig did not want any foreign objects touching his face, becoming fidgety and cantankerous, this would be a time the Meyers dreaded, for Craig would not sit still long enough to get much done.

Beyond those moments when he would avoid the respiratory therapist's oxygen mask, this day like the many others since he's been hurt, has been very much the same response-wise. When conscious, Craig will swallow some liquid and/or pureed food. And for those brief moments when his eyes are open, would follow his parents' finger. Then, for what seemed like hours eternal, would fall into his deep coma.

Despite the lack of activity from Craig, this was a memorable day for the Meyers. Knowing that Craig's lungs are able to work and that he hasn't lost the ability to breathe was a gift of immeasurable proportions. And seeing Craig's IV's removed, provided the Meyers with a glimmering hope that there will be a better tomorrow for their son. Are those dead leaves ever going to swirl tonight.

When the phone rang in the morning of the 26th, Craig's parents were sedate having been spoiled by the events of yesterday. However, the monotone voice and concerned look on Mrs. Meyers' face spoke volumes that something was wrong to Mr. Meyers who nervously sat on the edge of his chair repeating to his wife, "What is it Gwen? What is it?" Rising this morning with a revitalized confidence and an optimistic outlook, Mr. Meyers' heart sank when his wife said that Craig was running a fever.

Despite having made an unwritten pact not to get too high or too low with any of the news they might receive, assuming that because he was out of intensive care and was more or less disconnected from the life support systems, the Meyers were trounced hearing of this setback. Figuring that Craig was "out of the woods" and was not in any imminent danger of either losing his life or that infection had set in somewhere, the intensity of his parents sadness would be titanic. Like a bacteria left untreated, recurring thoughts of Craig's demise and right leg missing spread rapidly.

Caught in traffic on the Parkway West, the view of the Ft. Pitt Tunnels was a tantalizing one because the cars were entering this black hole single file at a pace slower than one can walk. The orange signs which read "Work Area Ahead" told of the culprit to this jungle of motorized confusion. The quake of the jackhammer's drill and the blowing of the car horns made Mr. Meyers' heart pound with a weighted fury. After thirty minutes of driving a distance that could be walked in three, the rust-colored Citation made it to the crest of Greentree Hill before making its descent towards the tunnel at a speed which made the incline on nearby Mt. Washington look as if it were a stock car at Indy. Although not normally superstitious, Craig's parents couldn't help but to think that this is the thirteenth day Craig's been hurt and that isn't such a good number for him through this whole ordeal which started when he went out Saturday, February 13th.

With heart racing and sweat dripping, the Meyers rushed into their boy's room. Craig unaware that anything was wrong, their son was lying in bed with beads of sweat congregating on his forehead and his sheets puddled with sweat. The cup over his right ear had been removed exposing the scarred, scab-laden appendage which almost ripped off from his head. Armed with coolly dampened wash cloths and Hawaiian Punch Craig loves to guzzle when he's sick, Mrs. Meyers proceeded to nurse her son back to health like she has done hundreds of times before. Placing the moistened wash cloths on his forehead and a flexible tube in his mouth connected to a syringe of the tropical juice, Craig's temperature lowered.

In order to prevent his getting pneumonia, the respiratory therapist put Craig in an upright position in a chair and attempted to give him steam treatments, so fluid would not settle in his chest. Like yesterday, Craig fussed and struggled, refusing to let the therapist get anything near his face. Needing to do his rounds with the other patients, the therapist let Mr. and Mrs. Meyers undertake this enviable duty. Feeling like the pioneers must have during their struggles exploring new frontiers out West in the 1800's, Mr. Meyers held Craig's head still while Mrs. Meyers attempted to apply the mask over her son's nose and mouth. Craig would simultaneously twist his head away and push the cup aside off his face when Mr. Meyers would loosen his grip. As if he could hear, the frustrated father scolded his son, pleading with Craig to leave the mask on. Just when his father's voice took on a tone of urgency and panic, giving his parents the opportunity to finish the steam treatment, Craig lost consciousness, as his head fell limp to the side. This was one of the few times Craig's parents weren't too unhappy of Craig's inability to remain conscious for an extended period of time.

However, when Craig became conscious a little over two hours later, the agitation reared its ugly head to a more pronounced extreme. Moaning as if he was terrified and experiencing unbearable pain, Craig twisted and squirmed in bed thrashing his good arm about as if he had a sword and was fencing a demon happy to see him writhing in misery. The metal frame of his bed squeaked and the guardrails to his side were bending with an uneasy frequency as Craig's arm flung wildly.

Horrified, Mrs. Meyers ran out to the nurses' station to get some help. As Mr. Meyers leaned forward to calm his son, Craig quickly grabbed his dad's tie pulling him down with an unyielding grip. Once again, his father's tears soaked Craig's hospital gown, but this time they weren't tears of joy, rather, tears of suffocation, for Mr. Meyers couldn't breathe. Alarmed, Mr. Meyers put his massive hand around his son's wrist and squeezed tightly before pushing Craig's arm down away from his throat. Tilting his head towards Craig's chest, the noose around Mr. Meyers neck finally loosened when the wrinkled tie eventually became undone.

Upon arriving from the hallway where she retrieved a nurse, before the choked husband could warn his wife not to get too close to Craig, the distraught mother immediately rushed up to his bed and bent over the sideguard rail to console her son. Moaning like an animal that's been hurt, the "brain contused" version of Craig would do something the real Craig couldn't fathom doing in a billion years.

Fist clenched, with a stinging blow, Craig struck his stunned mother just below the neck with such force that she reeled back falling into her husband's arms. Incensed at the sight of Craig punching his mother with such violence, Mr. Meyers pointed his thick forefinger at his son telling him that—hurt or not—he's not going to tolerate watching him hit his mother. Submerged with feelings of grief, pity, and anger, Mr. Meyers looked at his son whose raw elbow was turning red with all this thrashing. Realizing Craig wasn't hearing—and couldn't hear—his admonitions, Mr. Meyers quickly focused his attention to his wife.

Disheartened, struggling to fight back the tears, Mrs. Meyers shook. Being hit by the son she had only shown love for, left her speechless and in shock. Seeing her son toss and turn, moving his left arm forcefully across his body and showing no remorse, Mrs. Meyers could only imagine the suffering Craig was going through. The pain from the punch itself was minor compared to the fire in her heart. Although realizing this was not truly her son, the ache still burned like a blazing inferno.

As Craig started ripping the sheets off his bed, the nurse Mrs. Meyers summoned for help came in. Seeing Craig kick and tear his covers off, the nurse joyfully said this is great and what she's been waiting to see. Mrs. Meyers who was rubbing the welt on her chest and Mr. Meyers whose tie felt like it was stretched to his kneecaps, couldn't believe what they were hearing. A World War II veteran, Mr. Meyers never came so close to dying in his fifteen months overseas, and Mrs. Meyers felt like a captain does when his mutinous crew takes over the ship with an unsuspecting hostility.

Sporting a smile as wide as the Liberty Tubes, the nurse said that Craig realizes something's wrong and will express himself the only way he is capable right now, which is through body motions and groans. The jubilant nurse said because Craig knows that things aren't right, indicates he has the ability to perceive things and make an assessment based on these perceptions. Craig's becoming agitated shows this "realization" process is at least partially intact and is a complex skill which very well could have an immeasurably productive impact on his rehabilitation.

Craig's parents listened intently as this medical professional, who had a hard time controlling her joy, recommended to the Meyers that they read as much as they can about the various stages a comatose patient likely would endure. Reviewing the Ranchos Scale of cognitive/behavioral functioning, the Meyers learned that there are eight levels which help medical professionals and families understand what's going on with a patient who has sustained a traumatic brain injury (TBI) as they go through rehabilitation. These levels apply only to patients with head injuries the first several weeks and months following the injury, not years.

The higher the level, the more functional and responsive the patient is. The Meyers understood that there will be times when Craig appears to be reverting back to a previous level, but not to be alarmed because while the brain is healing, Craig will continue to slip in and out of consciousness, exhibiting a variety of behaviors. Acknowledging that they will see gains occurring rapidly with Craig as the days and weeks go by—but after several months—progress slows at some unpredictable point, the Meyers would prepare themselves for the inevitable stagnation. Bracing themselves for what tomorrow may or may not bring, these trodden caregivers realized that Craig will seem to plateau, not showing the swift, immense gains he had in the first weeks following his injury.

Aware that most of Craig's recovery will take place within two years, these hopeful parents could also hold onto the fact that gains will occur throughout his life. With healthy parts of the brain frequently taking over the functions normally assumed by the damaged sections, the Meyers would never lose faith that Craig would get back on track and be better than ever in some respects. With solemn reservation, the Meyers also gained an understanding that until medical research advances, a contusion on the brain never fully heals, thus rendering the survivor with some permanent disability depending on which function(s) the bruise covers and what signals have been disrupted.

Regarding the Ranchos Scale, the Meyers tried to identify how the different levels may apply to their son. Ranchos #1 is "No Response" where the patient is unresponsive to any stimulus whatsoever. One could jab Craig with a knife when he was at this level and he wouldn't even have known it. Ranchos#2 is "Generalized Response" where the response is limited and consists of basic reactions which are likely to be delayed. If Craig were jabbed with this same knife, he would respond in some elementary form to the pain he was feeling, such as a grimace several seconds after being punctured. Ranchos #3 is "Localized Response" where, if Craig were jabbed, he not only would feel it, but focus where the jab took place either by moving that particular part of his body or—if he could—look where the stab occurred. Possibly, he might be able to nod his head or motion in some way when asked if it hurt.

With his outbursts and other expressions of aggravation, Craig is beginning to show signs of being in Ranchos #4, "Confused, Agitated." Characterized by a heightened state of aggressiveness, activity, and confusion, these traits would normally be viewed as a negative, but with head injury, it's a positive, for it shows the patient is fighting to recover. With such effort being an essential element to any successful rehabilitation, the Meyers viewpoint of Craig's nasty conduct would slowly undergo a transformation.

Most observers likely could understand the Meyers' difficulty accepting Craig's behavior as improvement given his aggressiveness, so Craig's parents would just have to remind themselves that this is much, much, much better than his just lying in bed unaware of everything. Leaping from a Ranchos #1 to a Ranchos #4 in under two weeks' time, the Meyers would be optimistic that many more gains were going to surface, if progress continued on its current course. Not wanting to push their luck and risk minimizing their increasingly jovial mood of the day, because it's impossible to say with any certainty that Craig will advance to the higher levels, class ended for the day.

Despite acquiring a new appreciation that their son's indiscretions were actually an excellent sign, the Meyers had difficulty accepting their luck on Day #13 as anything but bad. Now, Craig's either going to be profoundly unconscious or so restless, he's unapproachable. Just as quickly as Craig awakened from his coma, thrashing his left arm about, he slipped into his deep unconscious. Looking at her still son who only moments before had been as wild as an untamed stallion, Mrs. Meyers felt ill when she saw blood on Craig's sheet. Getting a close inspection, the skin on Craig's left elbow was gone with the continuous thrashing.

In a few minutes, a nurse put a clear bandage on Craig's elbow. Beginning to look like fresh hamburger, this wrapping would only keep germs from entering the wound and not protect the elbow from further injury. The friction of Craig's joint rubbing on his bed when he would tug his arm created the bloody sore, so a nurse brought in a heavy, canvas restraint. Tying this handcuff on his left wrist and securing his leash to a side panel on the frame of the hospital bed would theoretically prevent Craig from moving his good arm.

As she looked at her helpless, unconscious son tied up like a criminal on death row, Mrs. Meyers was approached by another nurse whose husband was a police officer. This Afro-American R.N. who knew that Craig was hurt by a drunk driver, put her arm around Mrs. Meyers and said, "Doesn't that make you mad?"

Hearing from her husband and witnessing too many times herself the tragedy caused by a driver who did not know when to say "When. . . . . . ," this compassionate nurse had plenty of exposure to the crushing dismay families experience when a vehicular operator has "downed" more drinks than they could handle. Sitting to Craig's right and massaging his spastic arm—magically thinking his light touch might loosen his son's contraction—Mr. Meyers always felt he needed to defend his son to those who knew that Craig was at a party where alcohol was consumed and its abuse was the cause of his son's condition. Mr. Meyers would proudly say, "He's a good boy, he never caused us any trouble."

Bound like a flesh-eating carnivore after its capture, the sight of Craig lying in that bed prevented from using his only good limb was an oppressive one for his folks weary of paying the price for Paul's atrocity. Tortured by thoughts that their son might be sentenced to an undeserving conviction of being psychologically slain throughout his life—not appreciated for his virtues, only to have magnified his shortcomings—the Meyers could only look at their son, victim of increduously trusting Paul to be a friend, and hope Craig's will to survive hadn't been sapped.

When Craig "came to" and realized he was restrained, he twisted and turned, trying to free himself to no avail. Attempting to cast out his suffering, Mrs. Meyers explained to Craig that this tie was on to protect himself, but Craig couldn't comprehend what his mom was saying. After several minutes of trying to maneuver himself free, Craig became provoked, squealing and squirming frantically. Rolling to his left, then rolling to his right as far as his paralytic arm would let him, Craig grunted and groaned as if pleading for mercy to take off this straightjacket. With an empathetic voice and a caring touch, Mr. Meyers was eventually able to calm his son. Feeling powerless to rid her boy of that which harassed him, Mrs. Meyers could only look on, wondering what will come of the days ahead.

Not comfortable with Craig's inability to remain conscious very long and fearful his patient might hurt the only functional arm he has, the doctor ordered that Craig start getting used to sitting in a wheelchair for a few hours each day. Theorizing that when Craig's lying in bed, he becomes too sedated due to the many pain-killer medications he takes and loses consciousness, the doctor wanted Craig to be exposed to a stimulating environment, not one where he's unconscious an extended period of time.

With the wheelchair brakes firmly locked, Craig was placed in this seat by the nurses who didn't know how Craig would react to being moved. If they'd have seen beforehand Craig's response to this change of scenery, these nurses would have said, "To hell with the doctors orders."

Becoming dangerously irritated, Craig would get quite upset. Possibly knowing something was "up," unlike when he passively sat in a chair four days ago allowing staff to change his bed, Craig wanted to be left alone lying in the bed which has become his safe haven. Bouncing from one arm of the wheelchair to the other,

Craig's moans of displeasure and the wheelchair crashing against the wall reverberated off the walls of the seventh floor hallway with an eerie resonance. Cries of agony congesting the nurses' station, even the Head Nurse on the unit ceased writing her progress notes for a moment.

The tray resting on the arms of his wheelchair bent like a rubber band does before it's flung when Craig's left fist pounded this tabletop with a murderous force. Weaving from side to side, alternately flinging his arm and hammering his duke on the table, it could not be said for certain if Craig was feeling pain or discomfort in his head, leg, arm, ear, all of the above, or something else. For Craig's parents, the *silence* of not knowing and the *emptiness* of not being able to, were the most horrific traits of Craig's condition.

While lying in bed, Craig would readily lose consciousness hours at a time, not being able to remain alert for very long. If Craig were aware of his surrounding for a ten-minute duration, Craig's parents would count their blessings. If one good thing could be said about this wheelchair experience, it was that Craig stayed conscious longer. When awake, Craig may have been the Tasmanian Devil, but the Meyers tried to revel in what they had heard earlier when informed that Craig being mean and pissy was a sign of growing improvement. Pinching themselves that they were actually believing this, Craig's parents thought it might be good news for the nurse that their son's a living terror, but she's not the one being socked and strangled!

After two hours of almost constant restlessness while sitting in the wheelchair, the nurse finally put Craig back in bed, tying his restraint back on. Because she doesn't like to see anyone constrained in such a way, especially her own flesh and blood, Mrs. Meyers would wait until the nurses left before untying her son. Constant weaving, thrashing, kicking, and pounding exhausted Craig so much that when his head touched the pillow, he usually fell asleep immediately.

The Meyers have been experiencing the hell Craig's been going through every inch of the way—and likely more—because Craig possibly isn't even aware of the dire straits his parents have been witnessing all this time. Coming to the hospital every opportunity they could to see Craig and help whatever way possible, Scott and his wife entered the room. Informing them of the perils of this thirteenth day, Craig's parents cautioned the loving couple of his aggressiveness and unpredictability. After being forewarned not to trust his brother, Scott looked at Craig and said that it's good he's unconscious and numb to everything around him because the pain of everything that's happened to him, physically-mentally-emotionally, would be intolerable to bear.

Being Craig's personal nurse, one of the tasks Mrs. Meyers was asked to undertake was to measure the amount of fluid Craig drinks during the time they're with him in order for the doctors to get an idea of how—and if—Craig's kidneys are functioning. Dutifully following through with all that was asked of her with meticulous precision, Craig's mom was then to record the amount of liquid ingested and give this reading to a nurse before leaving for home. When Craig's eyes opened, Mr. Meyers went out to the nurses' station to inform the staff that Craig was "coming to," so the respiratory therapist could begin doing his thing.

While waiting for the therapy to begin, Mrs. Meyers poured a couple ounces of Hawaiian Punch into a syringe, squirting it into Craig's mouth. Craig worked up quite a sweat from all his bashing about today and was quite thirsty, so his mom prepared a second dose of the fruity red stuff. Before she could finish, however, the respiratory therapist came in donning the look of dreadfulness he seems to have on when working with Craig now.

Not knowing if Craig's temperament was like that of a kitten or an annoyed tiger, the therapist didn't want to take any chances, so he solicited some help from Craig's parents about Craig's mood this day. Finding out that his patient was acting like he thought he was king of the jungle, the therapist swallowed deep, greeting Craig with a smile and a hearty, "And how are we feeling today?" Whoever was in Craig's body didn't buy this "Romper Room" facade for a minute.

When the respiratory therapist placed the oxygen mask over Craig's nose and mouth, Craig violently grabbed the mask, throwing it on the floor. Seeing that Craig didn't want any foreign objects touching his face, the therapist picked up the breathing device, explaining to Craig that if he doesn't get this treatment, he could get very sick and to please allow him to do his job. The encouragement and assurance that came from his parents didn't help either, for Craig reacted with aggressive opposition once more to the therapist's attempts to try again. With shrieking moans of annoyance and rustling about in his bed alerting the therapist that Craig's irritability would require him to operate from the "Be Careful" phase, trying his best to assure that Craig's brain and breathing apparatus work in conjunction with one another, this professional would need to be very mindful of how tactile sensations delivered may be responded to. Not wanting struck or for Craig to hurt himself, the therapist tried to calm the reluctant combatant by telling Craig that there's nothing to fear and that he's just trying to help him. Giving it another go, the therapist's attempts to provide Craig with what he needs for his lungs to function properly were met with even more resistance, as Craig squirmed in bed, shaking his head from side to side. Making a noise as if warning the intruder of the risk being taken—until Craig could be subdued—cooperation wouldn't be forthcoming.

Under normal circumstances, Craig's parents would have been shocked to see their usually mild-mannered son act this way, but these are far from normal conditions, as they have learned not to be overly surprised with any of the tricks Craig might have up his sleeve since his head injury. Usually, one of his mother's threats or his dad's eyes bulging with anger would stop Craig dead in his tracks from misbehaving, however, they had no effect on this new—but not improved—version of their son.

Feeling bad for the therapist engaged in this losing battle, the Meyers made an offer they wish they could have recanted—Craig's family asked if they could be of assistance beyond providing moral support. With a devilish grin, the therapist gladly handed them this responsibility thinking familiar faces would make this task easier. As the worn trooper happily exited the room, the Meyers would have second thoughts about their offer to volunteer.

Looking at each other with mask in hand, standing over Craig, the Meyers weren't sure exactly what they got themselves into. Kicking and tearing the sheets off his bed which would eventually look like Hiroshima right after The Bomb was dropped, his worn parents urging him to "settle down," Craig wasn't exactly in the kind of abiding mood which promotes obedience. The adventure of getting Craig to breathe in his mask proved equally difficult for his family.

Using the team approach, Mrs. Meyers would narrate what Craig's father was going to do. "Now Craig, you lie still while daddy puts this cup over your nose and mouth, so that you can breathe better." Like telling the opposing team's defense what the quarterback was going to do, Craig must have understood because—for the second time today—Craig quickly grabbed his dad's tie, pulling him down and holding him there. Struggling to loosen himself from this death grip until Scott loosened Craig's hand from his dad's newly formed stretch tie, it just might be Mr. Meyers who needs that oxygen mask before this night is over. Standing mistakenly close to his bed, Craig grabbed a hold of his mom's arm and pulled her close to him, before she too was luckily able to free herself.

It didn't seem as if Craig gripped people to be mean or vicious, rather, it appeared he would reach out because he was terrified and wanted to be near someone he recognized. Craig's constant motion and groans of disenchantment must have been his way of expressing the internal confusion and awful pain he was enduring.

On the surface, the luck on this thirteenth day didn't look so hot. The day actually did start off hot, but that being because Craig was running a fever. Occurring almost immediately after his eyes would open, Craig's frequent bouts with restlessness and irritability would be followed by intermittent periods of marked unconsciousness. Choking his father twice today and slugging his mother, Craig's trauma-induced frustration made him absolutely unapproachable. Also, Craig's agitation left him with an elbow as fiery red as his temperament of this day. His unstable demeanor not likely to get him invited to the respiratory therapist's home for dinner anytime soon, Craig's testiness would still be viewed as extremely encouraging by those caring for him, however.

When visiting hours ended, upon leaving, Craig's parents couldn't be certain that their son would stop using them as target practice when they came in tomorrow, but that wouldn't make any difference because their undying obligation was deeper than any bruise they could sustain. Feeling as if they had bull's eyes plastered on them somewhere, still, Craig's parents were bombarded by images of what turmoil tomorrow would bring now that their boy's belligerently operating from this infamous Ranchos #4 Scale. What they did see the next morning would definitely surprise them, though.

Getting off the Pennsylvania Turnpike at Monroeville this Saturday morning—February 27th—not sure exactly where he was, the driver fumbled with the map to see how to get to Pittsburgh from this suburb east of the city. As the cars buzzed about him with what seemed to be the speed of light, having just traveled four hours from Harrisburg, the intimidated man ran his finger along the line on the map which he thought represented the route he was on. Confused and rushed, unsure of where he was headed, a flurry of thoughts about the direction he was going absorbed this traveler's thinking.

"Route 48, that's the road I'm on. No, wait. Yeah, that's it. Hold on a second, what's this Route 22? Maybe that's the route I should be driving. Does this lead straight into Pittsburgh? Then what's this 376—and what the hell's the Parkway East?"

With the drivers behind him hammering on their horns, feeling burning sweat streaming into his eyes like the lava of a volcano, the man who had driven on so many speedways during his days prodded along at a turtle's pace. Not having time to thoroughly review the map strategically planted on his steering wheel, this pressured motorist would soon have to find a restroom as well. As his eyes darted from the road chart to the parade of cars zig-zagging before him—looking for any sign showing the way to Pittsburgh—the thirty-six-year-old stranger not accustomed to a vehicular maze of this magnitude, spotted one pointing to the right. Normally cool under pressure, veering his car sharply and tramping on the accelerator, this lost journeyman wouldn't be at ease when discovering he was in the wrong lane. If the weather hadn't been cold and his window up, the many obscenities shouted his way from those he cut off might have disturbed him had he not seen the sign directing him into town—Pgh. 376 West.

Steering to the right again—but not cutting anyone off this time—getting on the Parkway East, this adventurer felt as if he had rewound the hands of time to the days he sped on different race tracks in his youth. Like Jennerstown Raceway near his boyhood home, cars weaved in and out passing one another, only to be passed later on by someone going even faster.

With jaws dropped at seeing so many cars travel at mach one on an urban highway, the driver tried to spot an exit with the words "Allegheny General Hospital" on it, so he could find his destination. Scanning to his left and scanning to his right, the out-of-towner saw signs which read "Penn Hills," "Churchill," and "Edgewood/Swissvale," but none which read the hospital he was looking for. Coming to a tunnel which seemed to have an apartment on the other side, the exhausted explorer got caught in rush hour traffic, wondering if he should ask for directions at a station somewhere when the congestion dwindles. Thinking better of this foolish idea, he'd tell himself, "Nah, I'll find it."

After being idle on the east side of the Squirrel Hill Tunnels for what appeared to be time unended, as if a starting light had just turned green, the wheels of once stationary cars squealed before traffic thinned and finally got moving. Flying past signs reading "Blvd. of Allies/Liberty Bridge," "Grant Street," and "Stanwix St.," zipping down the parkway, this one-time hellion who used to do some drag-racing in his time, knew he was going the wrong way when he came to another tunnel, OUTBOUND, about fifteen miles from where he got off the turnpike.

Countless U-turns and unnecessary miles later, the lost navigator finally found his pot of gold just about the time acid was starting to eat away at his stomach lining. As the automatic sliding glass doors of the hospital were opening, this determined thrill-seeker mumbled to himself how Pittsburgh's road system is an architectural nightmare. Marching to the information desk, this stranger identified himself as "Craig Meyers' brother" and would like to know what room his hurt sibling's in.

After stepping off the elevator at the seventh floor, Buck told the nurses he understood visiting hours weren't for a while yet, but that he had come a long way to spend some time with his "bro" whom he hadn't seen in four years, since Scott's wedding. Assessing the brother who almost could pass as Craig's dad age-wise, the Head Nurse cautioned this older brother fraught with excitement that what he was about to see was not pleasant. Prepping him how to interact with Craig, the nurse would then try her best to brief Buck about head injury and forewarn him about what he's about to experience. Taking a look at his brother in tatters, Buck would be in for a jolt.

Seeing Craig with his eyes closed, rolling from side to side, groaning as if in excruciating pain, all Buck could do was solemnly gaze at his brother whose grief pervaded the room with a sickening stench. Oppressively, the plea "Oh Jesus, Oh Jesus," kept echoing in Buck's mind as a means to extract the emotional foul which engulfed him. If Buck thought the acid was flowing seeing all those one-way streets pointing in the wrong direction on his way to the hospital, it was gushing now.

Being told what he's about to see and actually seeing the anguish are two different things. However, Buck tried to discard his somber demeanor the best he could and interact with Craig like the nurse instructed him and approach Craig as if things weren't as dismal as they obviously were. But the strength needed to exert this appearance was not humanly possible.

Grappling for the right words to say to his baby brother—eighteen-years his junior—was an immense chore for Buck because—despite being brothers—the two were virtual strangers. Not appreciative of some of his dad's ways with him—deserving and otherwise—Buck married young, stayed in Harrisburg where the family moved after a lifetime in Johnstown, and never came back.

Holding the hand of the brother he barely knew, Buck looked down at Craig not having any idea what to say. Feeling an aching knot in his stomach, Buck looked at his unconscious brother, wondering what kind of personality is Craig going to have when this is all said and done and how this would ultimately play into his future. Knowing how tragic this situation was, made it difficult for Buck to put on the smile that wanted to wither. After several moments of silence, Buck encouraged Craig to fight hard because there's a worker at his auto garage who had the same thing happen to him and that he pulled through it alright after much effort.

After twenty minutes or so of constant talking, Buck knew he wasn't being heard and that Craig probably didn't even know he was there. But still, jabbering on the best he could, Buck told his little brother that mom and dad don't know he's here and that they'll be surprised when they see him. And Buck wasn't mistaken.

When seeing their oldest son holding Craig's hand when they walked into the hospital room, Mr. and Mrs. Meyers had mixed emotions. First, they were happy to see their oldest whom dad Meyers christened with his lasting nickname—"Buck"—which mom Meyers never completely forgave her husband for.

With exuberance, dad Meyers barked, "Buck!" and mom Meyers yiped, "Carson!" However, at the other end of the spectrum was the circumstance leading to this reunion. Craig's moans serving as a backdrop to this grave panorama of wretchedness, the salutations would be short-lived.

Mrs. Meyers, her tired eyes filling with the tears which now seem like they have no end, looked at her unconscious son, softly touching his shoulder and said, "Honey, look who's here; Carson came to see you."

Despite feeling impoverished of strength and sensing little immediate relief from the woes of the past two weeks to the day Craig went out, Mr. Meyers briskly walked up to his unresponsive son. Grinning from ear to ear, saying half in jest, "Buck came all this way to see you; the least you could do is look at him and say, 'Hi!'"

After pausing for several seconds—nothing. The permeative silence to this request which seemed simple enough was just too much for Craig's father to take and—after a few agonizing moments of trying to act as if things weren't so bad—became shaken beyond control. Crying irrepressibly, diluting the facade he was portraying for his oldest that he was an impregnable pillar of strength, Mr. Meyers couldn't take anymore. Never seeing his dad like this before, Buck felt uneasy because he knew that his father would want this exhibit camouflaged and left unexposed. Spawning a growth not benign, harboring emotions would contribute to this icon's tumble.

After returning from lunch where they informed Buck of some of the details of the accident and of Craig's condition, the Meyers saw that staff had moved Craig into his wheelchair. Keeping her distance from the son whom she was not certain would lash out or not, Mrs. Meyers pointed in the direction of Craig's older brother and said once again, "Your older brother came to see you, y'know who that is?"

When Craig slowly lifted his head, letting his chin fall to his chest, brightness penetrated the malicious thunderhead which seemed to hover about their every step since Paul's act of maleficence.

Breathing a gust of relief that Craig responded to a question, a cascade of joy, relief, and excitement fell upon Mrs. Meyers as she said, "Frank!!! Did you see that? Craig nodded his head 'yes.' Did you see that? He recognized Carson."

Thinking that his son might respond in some way to more questions, Mr. Meyers asked Craig if he's hurting anywhere. Heaving his body against the arms of the wheelchair as if trying to break free, Craig didn't say a word or even gave any indication he was aware that he had been spoken to. No eye contact. No facial expression. Nothing. Craig just continued to kick, toss, weave, and swirl in this chair where he felt captive. The *silence* of Craig not responding and the *emptiness* of feeling unable to do more, extinguished the smile on Mr. Meyers' face.

Trying to lighten this mood which was not turning for the better, Buck said with tongue firmly planted in cheek, "Bro, you better let on you know who I am after coming all this way, or I'd have to kick the shit out of you."

Prior to greeting the brother he hadn't seen since exchanging vows with his lovely wife, Scott came walking in and bellowed, "Is he being an asshole again?" For Craig's brothers, they were lucky he didn't hear them, for he was too preoccupied with tearing off his hospital gown and busting his wheelchair.

As the sun was setting on this lackluster day, orange pylons and the splinters of what once was a sawhorse twirled skyward. Not wanting to get chummy with some of the unsavory residents approaching his car, Buck went through a barricade heading home. Drenched with anxiety seeing Buck's car make a wrong turn onto a lane leading towards the West End, Mr. and Mrs. Meyers kept their fingers crossed that Buck would someday find his way back home. Returning to their son's hospital room, Scott was trying to get Craig—who was Mr. Statistic when it came to anything about baseball—to talk about the Pirates. All Craig did, however, was drool on his bib.

Despite floundering in an oasis of ill-fortune which reached malignant proportions, the Meyers went about interacting with Craig and feeding him his perforated dinner with as much vigor as they could muster. Richocheting off the arms of his wheelchair non-stop, it took Mrs. Meyers an hour-and-a-half to spoon-feed her eighteen-year-old infant son his dinner. Making it tedious for his mother to aim the plastic eating utensil for his mouth, Craig's bruised brain wasn't about to allow him to comply. However, Mrs. Meyers would be soaking in a sea of elation that she was able to get Craig to eat a big supper under two hours.

When he would stop swinging his arms long enough, staff placed Craig back in bed where he lost consciousness within minutes. Only moments ago smothered in petulance, Craig would be oblivious to everything and everyone about him once he became comfortably situated for the night. Faithfully holding out hope that an armistice to this assault which had been waged upon them would be declared, even with the incalculable nature of their boy's symptoms, Craig's parents would be far from being gutted of their promise. The *silence* of knowing life was not appreciated to its fullest, and the *emptiness* of it being lost forever, were now all-consuming for Craig's parent as the day came to a close.

Hallelujah!!! The last day of the most hellacious month in Mr. and Mrs. Meyers' life has arrived. Tomorrow a new month begins and a new chapter can be written where prosperity and expectation of fulfillment flourish and abound. If it were only that simple. The passing of time is but one healing agent for those unfortunate ones who have this most complex of debilitating conditions.

Although it's still February, on this 28th day of the month, some definite signs of progress were made. All the staples were taken out of Craig's right leg and the

120 stitches in his right ear were removed. Both were healing exceptionally well. This morning, the doctor ordered that Craig get used to sitting in his wheelchair four hours each day, double the time he had been. The Meyers had mixed reviews about this, for Craig could hardly tolerate sitting two hours without trying to rip the place all to hell. Now, Mr. and Mrs. Meyers can look forward to dodging Craig's attempts to strike them twice the amount of time they had before. However, any change which appeared to be made because Craig was improving, was welcomed by his parents without question. Apparently, Craig was still getting rambunctious in bed, for his nurses fitted him with a heelbo pad to wear in order to protect his elbow from the constant thrashing.

In a few minutes time after being placed in his wheelchair, Craig started getting pissed off that he was taken from his bed and accompanying security blankets. Exhibiting his mood and discomfort over this new position, Craig started to whip his good arm in the air as if trying to swat some flies. The way Craig had been teeter-tottering in his chair, one could have thought a few of these insects flew up his ass.

As Craig was weaving from side to side trying to tip his wheelchair over, he began pulling off his hospital gown. Exposing himself in all his glory, Mrs. Meyers approached Craig saying, "You don't want to do that, someone will see you!"

While Mrs. Meyers was covering up her son, submerged with displeasure that he is expected to withstand the nuisances of sitting and having clothes touch his body, Craig wheeled back and slapped his mother with his open hand. Repairing the guardrail Craig must've broken last night during one of his agitated tirades, Mr. Meyers heard Craig's cracking palm strike his wife's cheek over the clanging metal bars he was trying to fix.

Infuriated, Mr. Meyers approached Craig and reproved him for this baleful act which showed just how much a brain injury can change one's normal personality and alter it into one where desecration is not even noticed. Like the diamondback rattler's strike, Craig snatched at his unsuspecting father's throat, pulling him down by the tie Craig was not about to surrender. Already burning, when Mr. Meyers piercingly looked into his son's eyes, this father saw a boy barren of all awareness of right and wrong. Choked not only of air, but of spirit as well, Mr. Meyers' feelings of fury immediately evolved into one where remorse and sympathy emerged from the anger. When seeing his boy starving to be released from this world of pain, confusion, and torment—after breaking free from his son's grip—Mr. Meyers looked at his son, only able to wonder if life will ever have any meaning for him again. The *silence* of questions left unanswered and the *emptiness* of a future forever altered, would encroach Mr. Meyers' sentiments like a virus insidiously attacks one's body.

Mrs. Meyers, her eyes bloodshot after spending the past half-hour in the ladies' room re-enacting in her mind Craig's palm stinging her jaw, came back into Craig's room feeling as if her heart had been ripped from her chest. Rubbing her red, irritated eyes, Mrs. Meyers looked at Craig feeling pity—not for herself—but for her boy that no one could know the struggle with which he was engaged.

To facilitate Craig's rehabilitation, everyone needs to interact with him as they once did before he was hurt in order for Craig to regain past instruction of what's acceptable behavior and what's not. With this in mind, Mrs. Meyers put her hands on her hips and proceeded to scold Craig in the same manner she did when he was burning the sidewalk along Burd Drive in Camp Hill with his tricycle, trying to run over any little girl that got in his way. "Nobody likes someone who's mean. And if you want me and daddy to stay, you've got to stop being so nasty." Craig did not acknowledge that he understood, or even that he had heard his mother.

Despite being fatigued by the storm of discontent which had showered upon them this dark morning, Mr. and Mrs. Meyers would attempt to spark some kind of memory in the tangled web which was Craig's recollection. Wheeling Craig down the end of the hallway where there was a picture window with an excellent view of Three Rivers Stadium, the Meyers were hoping some fragment of Craig's past would spring forth. Looking at her son, hoping for some kind of response, Mrs. Meyers said, "Do you know what that is? That's Three Rivers Stadium, where the Pirates and Steelers play. That's where Dave Parker goes whenever the Pirates have a game."

"And that's where Bradshaw, Franco, and Lambert always destroyed the Browns," Mr. Meyers said proudly. Apparently, a "connection" had been made, for Craig stopped the constant, random movement of his head and focused his eyes on the concrete ballyard.

Knowing that Craig's attention for a moment had not been fleeting and had been grasped, Mrs. Meyers said, "That's where you would like to work someday. Why you throw the ball against the wall on the side of the house so much; so your arm stays nice and strong, and your fielding continues improving. That's why you're on a ball field sun up to sun down."

"Yeah, and the way the Pirates are looking, Chuck Tanner's gonna want you to hurry up and get better, so he can put you in the lineup," Mr. Meyers said, choking on the emotion this thought kindled.

Eyes riveted on his injured boy who was absent of all expression, while Craig surveyed the scene where his favorite team hosts their opponents, Mr. Meyers visions of his son flashed back to happier times. Hearing, "Craig, Craig. C'mon Craig" chirped by Craig's Colt League teammates, Mr. Meyers could imagine his boy preparing to deliver another pitch. This gnawed at Mr. Meyers like a vulture devouring its capture and clawed at his soul with a viciousness only wished upon by one's worst enemy. The *silence* of "not knowing what you got 'til it's gone," and the *emptiness* realizing life was taken for granted, would clutch the Meyers as the curtain was finally falling on this fiendish month, February 1982.

A new month, a new week, a new day—but not a new beginning greeted the Meyers this Monday, March 1. Seeing her son's only workable arm tied to the bed rail when she came in and Craig—now wearing a diaper—bustling about in his wheelchair later on, made Mrs. Meyers' anger steam like molten lava. Things did not improve when the nurse handed the weary mother, spinning in this whirlwind of regression, a baby bottle to give Craig when he's thirsty. The nurse said this was an improvement over the syringe this matriarch had been using.

Putting aside their anger of what Paul's wanton deed did to their son, the Meyers thought that talking about the accident might help Craig remember things, so they went about telling their son what had happened to him. Leaning slightly forward towards her adolescent toddler, nervously wavering in his wheelchair like a wild animal that's just been caged—making sure she did not get too close to his swinging arm this time—Mrs. Meyers said, "Honey, you were in a real bad car accident and you're in the hospital now, Allegheny General in Pittsburgh. You hit your head pretty hard and broke your leg—but you're getting better. Me and daddy have been here everyday with you and we can see how much you're improving."

Seeing her teen-aged son in Pampers and holding a baby bottle which she was to feed her "bouncing baby" son with, Mrs. Meyers had to turn for a moment to rid herself of the agony that she had to accept what's before her as improvement. Catching her breath, Mrs. Meyers went on, "You were at a party with Paul Michaels, a boy you met at W.V.U. where you were going to college. He was drunk and smashed his Volkswagen into a telephone pole."

"But you weren't drinking," interjected Mr. Meyers, "we checked on that." Craig didn't know what was going on, for he was in his mindless oblivion. All that he knew was that he wanted to bust loose from that damned wheelchair.

During the four-hour adventure Craig was sitting in his wheelchair, there were several signs of improvement that eventually evolved, however. Craig's eyes would open wide and follow his parents as they walked about his room. When they would speak, Craig looked at them. Craig's appetite was good and, for the first time since his injury, he leaned his head toward his plastic fork for his food before taking a bite. Previously, Craig ingested his perforated meals with a food pump, after having been taken off his IV's.

Unfortunately, this dinner wound Craig up with a new energy. The calm having drained from him, a full-throttle testiness would steam. The jovial RN entered the room in the midst of one of Craig's fits and said to the crazed patient's disheartened parents, "He's still at it, huh? Craig's been 'hyped up' for two straight days." Bending towards Craig, the nurse careful not to get nailed in the face, spoke to Craig in a fashion that a mother speaks to a disobedient child.

"Now, you should be ashamed of yourself acting this way. No one's gonna want to be around you, flinging your arms around and smacking your wheelchair with your elbow like that. You better not hurt that arm—it's the only good one you got. Don't you ever get. . . . ."

Before she could say "tired?," the nurse who mistakenly let her guard down for just an instant, had her tray batted on the floor by Craig's flying hand. The surprised—and now "teed off"—nurse felt like an idiot because the metallic tray's crash prompted several staff to rush in, fearing she had been assaulted. Picking up the sedatives and steroids she was going to give Craig, this usually happy-go-lucky nurse turned ogre barked, "If you could hit a baseball that good, you wouldn't have had to have gone to college!" Stooped down and gathering the medication knocked from her hands, the "swoosh" felt by the nurse was Craig's left cross barely missing her cheekbone. Apologetically, Mr. Meyers stepped forward saying, "But he really is a good boy."

As this treaded-upon gladiator brushed the dirt from the knees of her uniform, she got up saying to the parents saddened by this wave of turbulence, "Don't you worry, we're going to do something about this."

No tinge of vindictiveness or sarcasm in her voice, Craig's parents looked at each other, unsure of what she meant by this comment. Hearing everything while standing out in the hallway, Scott came in on cue saying, "Maybe they're going to castrate him like an aggressive dog. Ha Ha Ha Ha Ha Ha Ha Ha Ha Ha Ha Ha Ha Ha Ha Ha Ha Ha Ha Ha Ha Ha Ha Ha Ha Ha Ha Ha Ha Ha Ha Ha Ha Ha Ha Ha Ha Ha Ha Ha Ha Ha Ha Ha Ha Ha Ha Ha Ha Ha Ha Ha Ha Ha Ha Ha Ha Ha Ha Ha Ha Ha Ha Ha Ha Ha Ha Ha Ha Ha Ha Ha Ha Ha Ha."

Late in the afternoon, the doctor informed the Meyers that mattresses will be placed on the floor and lined up along the wall tonight in order to help relieve Craig of some discomfort. Also, reducing the danger to himself and others while he's in this agitated state, staff thought that anything would be worth a try while Craig's in this aggravated stage where it's not easy for him to relax. The doctor said that Craig will be lying on the floor, free from anything that might get in the way of his flailing arm. If he wants to hit something, all he can do is punch the mattresses. After hanging Craig's chart on the side of the bed, the doctor concluded by saying that this might not be the most conservative method to protect someone, but it's an experiment deserving of some consideration.

Mrs. Meyers gazed out the huge window which made up the entire side of Craig's room, and pictured her confused son somehow breaking the glass and rolling to the street below. When the worried mother told the doctor about her concern, Scott chimed, "Yeah, but look at all the gas money we'll save not having to come to Pittsburgh everyday, then. Ha Ha Ha Ha Ha Ha Ha Ha Ha Ha Ha Ha Ha Ha Ha Ha Ha Ha Ha Ha Ha Ha Ha Ha Ha Ha Ha Ha Ha Ha Ha Ha Ha Ha Ha Ha Ha Ha Ha Ha Ha Ha Ha Ha Ha Ha Ha Ha Ha Ha Ha Ha Ha Ha Ha Ha Ha Ha Ha Ha Ha Ha Ha Ha Ha Ha Ha Ha Ha Ha Ha Ha Ha Ha."

After the doctor left, the Meyers used the remainder of the visiting time with Craig telling him about the mattresses staff will be setting up this evening and talking about things already discussed a hundred times before the past two weeks, hoping something would "sink in." While Mrs. Meyers was trying to jar a memory, telling Craig about how he got angry at her for buying the mouthwash she had coupons for—instead of the kind he liked a week or so before the accident—a loud "BANG" could be heard out in the hallway. A voice yelling, "Watch out where you're going, you almost knocked over that cart!," the ruckus outside the door was intense. Not having the skill to ever be employed as haulers by a moving company, catching the "Oversize" load at an awkward angle in the doorway, two grumbling custodians came in.

Grunting to the Meyers, "Is this where the mattresses go?," the family wouldn't be sure how these two cleaning men would react when told that Craig was the one responsible for their annoyance. Fearing for their life after indicating it was, the Meyers felt bad for the struggling janitors they wanted to help, but remembered what happened the last time they offered their services out of sympathy for a hospital employee and put on their jackets when visiting hours ended this evening.

Before exiting the room, catching a glimpse of these disgruntled workers giving Craig "the evil eye," Scott turned and said, "If he's too big of a dweeb, Life Flight him to Iran. They can take him hostage and then he'll be their problem. Ha Ha Ha Ha Ha Ha Ha Ha Ha Ha Ha Ha Ha Ha Ha Ha Ha Ha Ha Ha Ha Ha Ha Ha Ha Ha Ha Ha Ha Ha Ha Ha Ha Ha Ha Ha Ha Ha Ha Ha Ha Ha Ha Ha Ha Ha Ha Ha Ha Ha Ha Ha Ha Ha Ha Ha Ha Ha Ha Ha Ha Ha Ha Ha Ha Ha Ha."

On the afternoon of March 2nd, Mr. and Mrs. Meyers gazed at the spectacle before them that once was a traditional two-person hospital room. When they left Craig last evening, the Meyers had no idea his room would be transformed into one resembling a moon walk found at any carnival. However, for Craig's parents, this setting was far from entertaining.

With the exception of the entry where they were standing and a small area around his bed, the floor of Craig's room was covered by single mattresses, and setting length-wise along the wall were several more underbeddings. The mattresses along the wall were secured by tan duct tape and those on the floor were situated side by side. There were twenty-eight mattresses in all and each had a sheet covering them. For those responsible for changing Craig's bedding every night, you better believe they're hoping for a hasty discharge.

Meanwhile, Craig was slowly rolling in his new playpen, tearing the sheet off the mattress he was lying on—before yanking the sheet off the adjacent mattress. While in this state of not being mindful, Craig would continuously reach out trying to touch anything he could, whether it be human or something as lifeless as a bed covering. While wheeling in this fog of senselessness, Craig would moan as if enduring a terrible torture.

Unable to merely stand at a distance and watch her son battling his demons, Mrs. Meyers took her shoes off and stepped on the mattress towards Craig. Holding her arms parallel to the floor as if walking a tight rope proved to be of no avail, for Mrs. Meyers came crashing to her arthritic knees, unable to master this trampoline. With the "never say die" gumption which takes hold of her when one of her children are in need, Mrs. Meyers crawled on the mattresses to Craig, assuring him everything was alright; that he needn't be scared.

Mom Meyers reminded Craig, "These are the mattresses me and daddy told you about yesterday, so you wouldn't hurt yourself on the bed rail. The doctor was scared you might've fallen out of bed or really hurt your elbow."

Like the days he did "The Jitterbug" with his wife, Mr. Meyers came bouncing over and cracked, "When the doctor saw how many new ties I had to buy, he thought it would be less expensive getting these thirty or so mattresses wholesale."

Craig didn't hear a word said to him, he just kept ripping the sheets off the mattresses quicker than his mom could tuck them in. For a moment, Mr. Meyers was able to detain Craig's rolling and pulling of the sheets, only to have a more energetic encore take place once he loosened his grip. This weary task of trying to contain Craig's agitation forced Mrs. Meyers to think of a way to distract Craig and keep him occupied. What she came up with seemed to have a profound effect on Craig's recovery.

The idea Mrs. Meyers devised to lessen Craig's agitation was to, of all things, put Craig in the source of much of his agitation—his wheelchair—and push him in front of a mirror, so he could examine himself. She theorized that, up until this point, Craig had been told what's wrong with him, but if he could see his image, Craig might be able to at least get an idea of what this stay at the hospital is all about. Actually viewing his bruised face, torn-up ear, and sitting in a wheelchair, Craig just might be able to clear up some of the confusion with which he's been surrounded and allow him to make some sense of things.

Without taking into consideration that Craig might be terrified seeing himself in this way and might suffer a setback, the parents figuring anything's worth a try wheeled an agitated Craig to the entry where a mirror was located above the sink. Seeing the image of himself, Craig stopped shuffling and took note of his appearance. Staring at his face purple from being bruised and cut by glass, an ear red from almost being severed from his head, a black lump on his sore forehead where the shunt was inserted in his skull, and eyes a jaundice yellow from seventeen days of battling this ordeal which had Lucifer basking in merriment, Craig's affect changed from one that was dull, to one which was more alive. As if he had been swallowed by a cognizance of what was going on, a look of comprehension seemed to adorn upon and exude from his understanding.

Wide-eyed, Craig scanned every detail of his swollen face. Laboring with thoughts that her boy may never show any signs of animation again, Mrs. Meyers got her husband's attention with a whisper. Not saying a word, slowly making his way over and witnessing his son's search for answers, Mr. Meyers would be careful not to divert his son's attention away from studying himself in the mirror.

Craig's parents then explained to their son why he was in a wheelchair, what had happened to his ear, and how that lump got on his forehead. Pointing to each, one by one, they told Craig how these hurts came about and of the circumstances surrounding the accident once again. After the Meyers helped their son with some of these questions while he was inspecting himself, Craig appeared to take on a new awareness. He had at least a little zest in his face now, as his affect seemed to brighten with a new aura of life. Seemingly amazed by the reflection before him, Craig looked into his eyes as if seeking a resolution to the suffering which he had been immersed.

Placed back on the mattresses after the period which he was to get accustomed to sitting ended, Craig's parents tried to continue resurrecting some remembrance, before their son tumbled into his deep sleep, not attentive to anything about him.

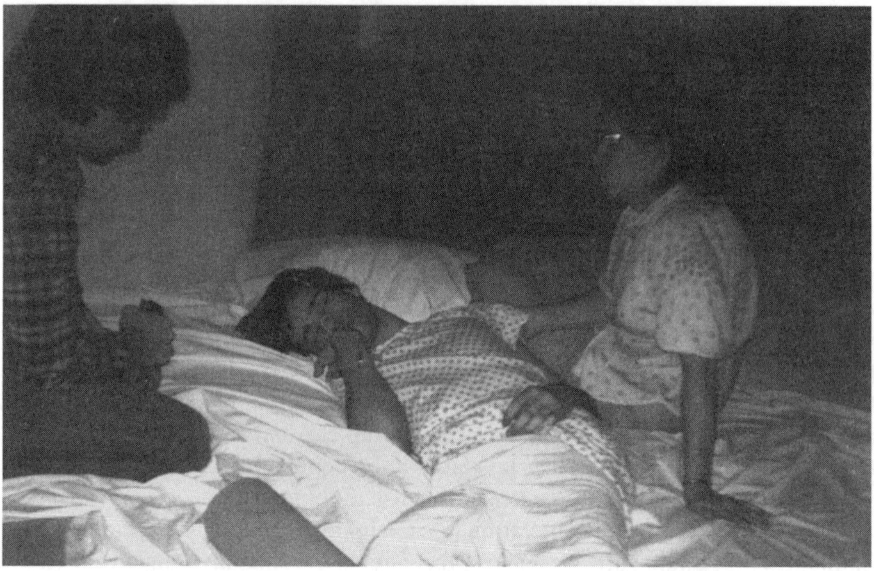

Craig comatose in Pittsburgh's Allegheny General Hospital with his mom and brother keeping vigil.

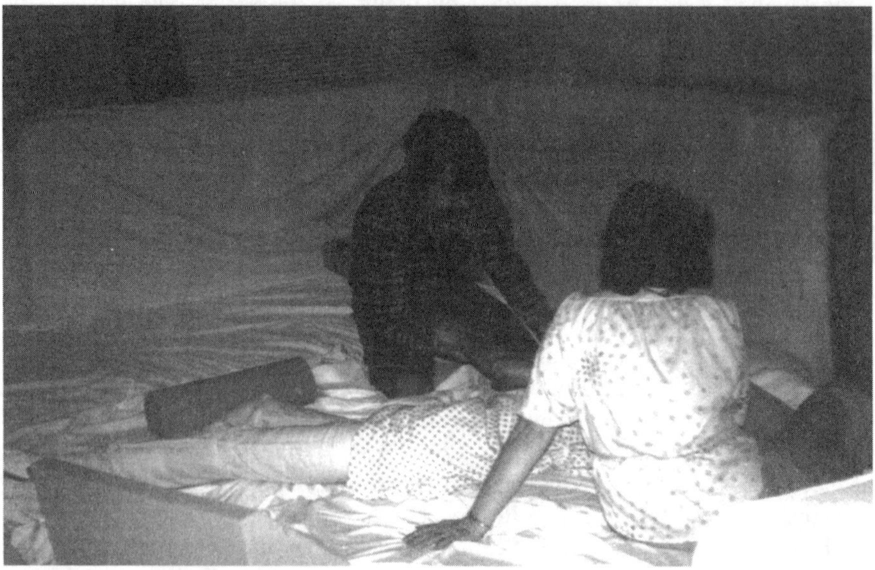

Side view of Craig comatose in A.G.H. bedroom taped with mattresses. These underbeddings were placed here to safeguard against this agitated patient from hurting himself.

Usually, toiling with the burden of snaring Craig's elusive consciousness brought about a torment that's cruelty was not forgiving. However, on this day, this cycle of ups and downs the Meyers have had enough of were more tolerable—for Craig appeared to have turned a corner.

Shortly after arriving home from the hospital, the phone calls started pouring in like they do every night. Always appreciative of the encouragement given, exhausted from their day at the hospital and the drive from Washington to Pittsburgh, the Meyers often found the multitude of phone calls trying. But today, a new effervescence sparkled, making the Meyers more than happy to relive this afternoon's events for the well-wishers who called. With the exception of Mrs. Meyers' unfounded paranoid fear that Craig might break his hospital window—falling seven floors splattering onto the street—and some concerns about the sanitary condition of Craig's lying on a floor of mattresses that people have walked on with their shoes, Mrs. Meyers' glow was filling the phone lines.

Also, Craig's parents were grateful one less call would be coming in. After hearing that Craig was more than likely going to survive, the Michaels stopped calling. That's understandable, hearing the grueling details of Craig's stay at the hospital would spoil their appetite for the after-dinner drink they quite possibly have every evening.

Not saying so much as a peep to the anticipatory parents when they hopped in, as she was scurrying out of the room, the nurse responsible for feeding Craig his lunch while concurrently trying to help him form some words, dejectedly shook her head from side to side indicating she wasn't able to get Craig to speak or eat too much this Wednesday afternoon. With the exception of his inhaling and exhaling, Craig was motionless on his bed of mattresses. Despite knowing head injury doesn't work this way, Craig's parents were secretly counting on Craig making progress from the day before. Heart oozing with optimism, Mr. Meyers said, "You think you're going to start talking to us today, buddy?" Nothing. Wearing a smile the best she could, Mrs. Meyers stood in the background with hands folded about her lap, her eyes blank with disappointment that an epilogue to yesterday's triumph did not greet them upon their return. For the parents who have been let down too many times since Craig's been hospitalized, the *silence* of dreams unfulfilled and the *emptiness* of lost expectation, left the Meyers with a numb hollowness only thwarted hopes can render.

To avoid falling into a cavern of disillusionment, Craig's parents had to remind themselves of what Scott repeatedly emphasized. Scott undertook the role of not letting his parents sink too low by offering encouragement and his rendition of humor. He would say that limitations and a lack of immediate progress from one day to the next can make it difficult to see the entire picture and the improvements being made.

After hour upon unending hour of fruitlessly trying to get Craig to respond in some way, Scott would not allow his folks to have a, "What's the use? He's not hearing us anyhow" attitude when it came to their efforts of revival. Reminding them that addressing the symptoms brain injury can cause is a slow process with many ups and downs that can be worked out better if they stuck together, always provided Craig's parents with a much-needed resurgence of hope and energy. Just two weeks ago, Scott would remind them that they'd have been ecstatic Craig was showing any kind of activity—even if it was agitation. Now, they have some welts, bruises, and ruined neckties showing how well Craig's doing.

This wasn't Craig's preferred way to get celebrity status, but the unique decor of his hospital room with all the mattresses everywhere made Craig the focus of much attention. It was inevitable for those who walked past the open doorway of Craig's hospital room to stop and gape at this "Serta" paradise. With one hand clenched in a fist under his chin and the other hysterically going every which way—or when Craig was simply lying motionless on the floor—the occupant of this padded room was indeed an interesting exhibit on his own merits, no matter the interior decorating. Flustered with anything that touched his body or intruded on his personal space, Craig would be a typhoon-in-waiting.

When one of the older RN's saw Craig in his frenzy, she smiled and said, "This is progress. Craig's fighting because he knows something's wrong and can't do anything about it. He knows he doesn't like feeling this way and is doing what he can to show his frustration. But when he can start taking control, look out! I can tell he's a fighter. Craig isn't going to give up. He's going to beat this thing, you wait and see. You just wait and see."

Long after the nurse had left, those words "Wait and See," continued to play in the Meyers' minds. When Mrs. Meyers commented she knows that they've done a lot of "waiting," but haven't "seen" too much, her husband asked what she's basing this comparison on—the Craig of old or the Craig who was lying in that hospital guerny in a bloody heap just two weeks ago?

As a means to vent the bottled-up harassment which boiled within her, Mrs. Meyers cried, "The Craig of old!! I want him back on that campus at W.V.U. going to class. I want him upstairs playing his guitar. I want him blaring his AC/DC records on his stereo and throwing that tennis ball against the house. I want to see him walking down the street caked in mud after one of his backyard football games."

Her voice broken by gasps to catch her breath, this beleaguered mother screaming to be awakened from the nightmare with which she was trapped sobbed, "I want him back like he was. I want my boy back. I want my boy back."

These words, a creation of repressed mournings, drowned as the mother of seemingly infinite strength cupped her hands over the face which too many tears have rolled. The cold silence which followed spoke tearful volumes that they realized the Craig they knew was forever gone.

Standing in the doorway, looking at the maternal figure draped with sorrow, the older black woman with the deep abiding faith asked, "How is he today?"

Mrs. Meyers turned and glumly muttered, "We thought he'd be doing better than he is."

Dispirited, Mr. Meyers shrugged his shoulders, extending his open hands as if to say, "Here we go again."

Seeing that their confidence was dwarfed by recurring frustrations, the woman who had a family member down the hall said with a doubtless confidence, "He's gonna be alright. God's not gonna take him yet, he'll be just fine."

Impounded in a sea of doubt, the Meyers were happy to hear that someone was so sure Craig would pull through this. Because they can empathize with one another, the words from families of fellow patients can mean so much. And then, just as magically as she appeared, this prophet vanished.

Later in the evening, Craig would become responsive, showing marked improvement. While lying on the floor of mattresses, Craig chewed and swallowed his supper with less assistance from his family. Along with the lessened force-feeding, Craig sucked on a straw for the first time when drinking a can and a half of Hawaiian Punch—instead of the drink being squirted into his mouth via a syringe. Learning to savor every skill Craig has relearned and appreciating any frontier he's trying to master again as a leap of the greatest magnitude, after one's CNS has been damaged, no behavior which resurfaces can be viewed as insignificant or trivial.

Shortly after Mr. and Mrs. Meyers arrived in Craig's empty room on this March 4th afternoon, they heard the metallic squeak of wheels coming down the hallway and a faint feminine voice of a young woman. "So Craig, what did you do in PT this morning? Were they able to get that right arm down any?" This attractive blonde hospital worker's question was met with a mute silence, as Craig's inability to form any clear speech patterns continued. Craig was growing increasingly more frustrated that he couldn't shut his eyes and exit this annoying consciousness, so he started kicking, moaning, and thrusting his body. Making the trip down the hallway feel like a cross-country excursion for this petite nurse expected to transport this patient twice her size, Craig's hyperactivity only worsened.

The one-sided conversation of the nurse's aide and the rusted clamor of a wheelchair that needs oiled were getting nearer. "In Communication Therapy, did you work on. . . . . . . ?" Before the nurse's aide could finish her question, she stopped, becoming startled to hear Craig's parents in the room.

"There he is !!," Mr. Meyers boasted. "Did you work hard today, or did you give the therapists a tough time again?"

After a few moments of this everlasting quiet, Mr. Meyers wishfully looked at the aide, asking her if there has been any progress getting Craig to say something. "No, not today. But we're working on it? Aren't we Craig?," she reported without the slightest hint that a response to her question would be forthcoming.

Pushing Craig to the edge of the mattresses, intending to transfer him onto his peculiar sleeping arrangement, the aide locked the wheels of the wheelchair before putting her arms under Craig's. Tapping her shoes on the bedding to get an idea of the footing, the aide sprung with an uneasy recoil. Answering with a, "Don't worry, transfers in difficult situation were covered in my training,"—sweating blood—the Meyers asked if they could be of assistance.

Before long, the nurse's aide's knees were shaking unable to maintain her balance lifting Craig's dead weight body from his wheelchair. Mrs. Meyers squealed when the aide and Craig went tumbling down. The aide cushioned Craig's fall, as she dutifully made sure she was underneath her patient.

After checking that Craig's broken leg and spastic arm hadn't been hurt in the fall, this cute little nurse's aide scampered out of the room. When the initial shock of seeing his son go down wore off, Mr. Meyers thought if Craig only knew what he was laying on top of, he'd have regained consciousness right away.

The remainder of the afternoon, Craig was in his state where nature shuts off the senses because it doesn't like what it's feeling. But when he regains consciousness a few hours later, the accumulation of effort by the family, doctors, nurses, therapist, and people like the nurse's aide, will begin showing some dividends.

After Craig wolfed down the supper fed to him, the Meyers family worked with him on his various limitations. While lying on the mattresses where he wanted to escape into his ozone of unconsciousness, Craig was stimulated by his family.

Concurrently, Mr. Meyers would rub Craig's contracted arm, while Mrs. Meyers explained what had happened to him for the thousandth time before describing where he is for the hundredth time. Shifting gears, Mr. Meyers would then have Craig follow his finger and Scott—giving his mother a break—would then talk about what was happening throughout spring training camps in the world of Major League Baseball and what the Steelers plan to do in the draft. A home economics teacher at the rival high school, Scott's lovely wife would tell Craig how guys he played baseball against are wishing him well. This therapy—Meyers style—continued until Craig became agitated, trying to grab anybody or anything that was within his range.

The work with Craig was slow, tiresome, sometimes dangerous, and often unrewarding, but if Craig showed any benefit from their presence, the Meyers would be there, giving it their all. To relinquish hope was out of the question and, although their spirits had been shot down too many times to count, giving up the ship would never be considered. They would not and could not permit this treason. Their sanity was often hanging by a thread and their hopes, all too frequently, were like the dying embers of a doused inferno. The Meyers will do everything in their power, so their son will have a life where his constitutional right to pursue happiness will not escape him. This determination preserved the Meyers' willpower to keep going and kept them from falling into the clutches of self-destruction.

The immediate satisfaction from working with a person who has had a head injury is almost nil. The results of many hours of cumbersome effort can, many times, be taking one step forward and two backwards. This is trying on the soul and tests one's fortitude. To help a patient who's had a traumatic brain injury overcome the odds which are stacked against them, it is essential—for optimum recovery to occur—that family and/or friends reach inside themselves and gather the strength which they might not have known they had; making a focused commitment to help in any way possible.

After a seemingly endless struggle where Craig's family tried to instill some idea for him where he was at and what was going on, the Meyers took a much-needed—however brief—break from this exhausting rehab. As they stood in the entry re-energizing for the next round, what the Meyers would hear could only be topped by the blowing of Gabriel's horn.

Piercing the crypt-like stillness of the hospital room was an unintelligible gurgle. Like the parched explorer searching for water in the anhydrous infinitude of sand which is the Sahara, Mr. and Mrs. Meyers crawled to Craig as fast as their worn knees would allow them.

"You want to say something buddy?," an excited Mr. Meyers asked, praying that Craig would utter just one word.

"What is it honey? We can't understand you," Mrs. Meyers pleaded, bebopping on the mattresses just behind her husband.

Such as that devastated explorer who finds a canteen empty from the sun's beating rays next to the skeleton of another adventurer before him, the Meyers hopes were dashed and anxiety returned when—in a matter of seconds—Craig returned to his Twilight Zone. Fraught with eagerness, Mrs. Meyers asked her husband, "What did it sound like he was saying to you, Frank? Was anything clear to you? Were you able to make anything out? Did you happen to. . . . ?"

Tortured by the disappointment of not being able to catch Craig before his grand exit, an angry Mr. Meyers shouted, "No, no, no. I didn't hear a damn thing either."

Hearing the commotion, cutting short his cigarette break, Scott rushed in from the waiting room just down the hall and asked, "Is everything alright? Did something happen?"

"Yeah, Craig tried to say something, but we weren't able to understand him," Mr. Meyers replied. "Craig sounded like a Martian. He was trying to speak a language that didn't sound like anything from this planet. It only lasted a couple of seconds. (It) sounded like a record played backwards at a fraction of the speed it should be."

Pausing for reflection and recall, Mrs. Meyers mused, "Craig sounded scared and as if he were hurting."

Seeing that his parents could use a little lift—and with a pause for effect—Scott quipped, "Damn it, I knew he'd talk again. Ha Ha Ha Ha Ha Ha Ha Ha Ha Ha Ha Ha Ha Ha Ha Ha Ha Ha Ha Ha Ha Ha Ha Ha Ha Ha Ha Ha Ha Ha Ha Ha Ha Ha Ha Ha Ha Ha Ha Ha Ha Ha Ha Ha Ha Ha Ha Ha Ha Ha Ha Ha Ha Ha Ha Ha Ha Ha Ha Ha Ha Ha Ha Ha Ha Ha Ha Ha Ha Ha Ha Ha Ha Ha Ha Ha Ha Ha Ha Ha Ha Ha Ha."

Although what Craig did this afternoon could not be classified as talking, tomorrow is another day.

Craig's parents heard the familiar squeak coming down the hallway this fifth day of March 1982, but there was something different in the voice of the nurse's aide—it was colored with a vibrance and vigor that the Meyers never heard before. With a smile as big as her heart, the nurse's aide came in unable to control her excitement for the parents accustomed to hearing mostly bad news about Craig.

"They were able to get Craig to talk! He counted to five this morning," the aide who looked like she was going to wet herself reported.

Feeling an urge to go herself, Mrs. Meyers asked "What?," not sure whether to believe what she thought she heard.

Adrenalin rushing to his head, flustered by this unexpected surprise and his wife's untimely bout with deafness, Mr. Meyers confirmed, "She said Craig counted to 'five' this morning in therapy. They got him to talk!!!"

Hearing himself say this, a smile that lighted up the room came from this father treaded upon too many times to recall since his son could have been incinerated. As the aide was giving the details of the speech therapy session which had Craig say something for the first time since he probably screamed, "Oh my God!!!!!,—Paul!!!!" just before hitting the telephone pole twenty days ago, the Meyers looked at their son feeling as though God just might pull off a miracle for him. Later this evening, the sense Craig had been touched would blanket the Meyers.

Any progress witnessed or heard would be savored in order for the Meyers to be able to face the next day without going crazy. Although the situation had improved tremendously, the vast majority of the time Craig usually wasn't doing anything, but lying on his mattresses unconscious. Try watching someone sleep most of the day everyday for almost three weeks and you'll get an idea of what the Meyers' days are like.

In order to keep from climbing the walls, the family must find some way to distract themselves from the barrage of decrepid thoughts which want to take refuge in their conscious every waking hour. To focus on a patient's condition twenty-four hours each day does no one, neither the patient nor their family, any good. To worry, feel anxious or distraught isn't going to speed up the healing process. With God's will, the brain's healing and the repetition of therapy over time are what's going to make a difference in one's recovery, not beating yourself up with dysfunctional thoughts. Sometimes, all one can do is take it a day at a time; trying to find some positive in each; no matter how difficult this might be.

It is natural for a patient and those close to him or her to feel as if the world's coming down on them, fearing what news tomorrow will bring. But in order for the patient to benefit, the family and/or friends must find some way to productively cope. Falling victim to the deluge of horrific visions which will occur with any dehabilitating condition does nothing to help. In order to provide the best for a family member or friend, those rendering assistance need to be at their best possible condition and try their utmost not to be consumed by misery, so they can think with a clear head what needs done to help the patient.

This is not to say that people shouldn't grieve, for it is absolutely, positively essential to express the loss any disabling condition creates. However, there comes a point when this grieving process has to be put aside and the physical/emotional/cognitive work begins. Unfortunately, because the majority of recovery occurs within the first two years of the brain being injured, those experiencing the symptoms of head injury may feel the grieving process has not been completed before the work NEEDS to begin. But that's a fact that isn't going to change, so one needs to ACCEPT it and move on the best they can.

One may ask, "But how does one move on and go about the grieving process?" Talk and learn. Find someone who is not only going to hear what's being said, but is listening too. Family, friends, neighbors, medical professionals, clergy, counselors, and other people who want to understand and can empathize, need to be utilized. The *silence* of pain withheld and the *emptiness* of feeling alone can do substantial damage to the psyche.

Acquire as much information possible. Find out what head injury actually is. What happens to the brain, what the patient and the family needs to do to maximize recovery, discover productive coping strategies which will work for you, learn the basic principles of Rational Emotive Therapy, and locate resources in the community which may someday help the person surviving a head injury.

Notice the words. Person surviving a head injury. Even the term "head injury survivor" can have negative connotations, for it labels the person with the disability instead of recognizing the person as an individual. One may argue this is only semantics, but one's perceptions are vitally crucial to how one handles things. A person has thoughts which create feelings and these feelings precede behaviors. In essence, one's actions at any given time can be attributed to how they're thinking at the time. If one's thoughts are irrational or counterproductive, their actions will correspond with these perceptions. Not to say there won't be circumstances that legitimately will be negative in nature (such as the death of someone close), but to lessen the impact these situations have on one is within control, for people feel how they think.

The positive thing to remember about this is that the person having the thought(s) can control whether or not they keep these perceptions. A person has the control of replacing bad thoughts with more functional ones. And, because thoughts ultimately result in feelings and subsequently behavior, one has control of these as well. This could be viewed as a "Mumbo Jumbo" psycho-babble psychological principle, but it can work. Unless someone's been "brainwashed"—to use a cliche—no other person or thing can completely control how you think, feel, or behave—not even a brain injury.

The Meyers used this power of control in a variety of ways. During those all too frequent times when Craig was "out of it" in his realm of misplaced consciousness, in order to pass the time, the fatigued father would capture a little peace sitting out in the waiting room talking with other family members and the nurses. A very personable man, Mr. Meyers needed to talk to people, so as to remind himself that there really was a world outside of the four walls of Craig's hospital room.

Rarely leaving Craig's side, Mrs. Meyers would often find herself passing the time by doing trivial things. Counting the cars crossing the Sixth and Ninth Street bridges, as well as watching the Life Flight helicopter land and take off were but two ways this ragged mom would use to free herself from the boredom of watching her boy during one of his endless brain contusion-induced siestas. In case she'd be needed or saw Craig show a glimmer of consciousness, this vigilant matriarch was never too far physically. After those inevitable times when her mind would wander, she would quickly assume her sentry-like role with a refreshed dedication.

The all-important Meyers family therapy was also utilized with discretion when needed. If Mrs. Meyers would be caught in the doldrums, Mr. Meyers would remind his wife of the gains made, no matter how minuscule. Whether it was drinking one more sip of Hawaiian Punch than the day before or keeping his eyes open thirty seconds longer than last week, the positives would need accentuated. If Mr. Meyers—the eternal optimist—needed a rare "pick-me-up," all Mrs. Meyers would need to do was tell her husband how Craig might need him in some way, and he'd "snap to." During those not-too-infrequent occasions when both were not at their best, Scott would encourage them, highlighting the improvements Craig's made and to hang tough; that together they'll beat this thing.

Head injury has many peaks and valleys, with those pits being easier to climb out of, if someone's there to give a hand. The trials that will occur after the onset of a disabling injury are going to test the backbone of those it afflicts. Forever seeing a friend or family member different than the way they once were is something one has got to ACCEPT, if they are to continue in a healthy manner. If they can't, the road ahead will be a rough one. Having a strong, resilient support system goes a long way towards a successful rehabilitation effort. And the Meyers are going to make sure Craig gets all the backing he needs.

When Craig returned from wherever he was, supported by two walls, he'd be placed in the corner of his room because this was the best location for him to be fed. Time to eat not making any difference, Craig was not cooperative, as he tried to return to his comfort zone of unconsciousness.

While Mrs. Meyers would attempt to get the plastic spoon in her sedated son's mouth, Craig would slide down wanting to go to sleep. Panicking, Mr. Meyers would prop Craig back up and—despite knowing that he probably wasn't going to be heard—told his son to please stay put, so he could be fed. Seconds after Mr. Meyers said this, Craig was on his way back down again.

It was critical that Craig begin eating, for he was losing weight at an alarming rate. Having lost at least twenty-five pounds, Craig's cheeks were starting to sink in and his legs were thinning. Being able to make out the skeletal features of Craig's face was a sight that Mrs. Meyers could never forget.

After over an hour of this dining experience where Craig's posture was like that of a "Slinky," he was put in his wheelchair and his parents would commence therapy with him. Wanting to hear something from Craig other than moans and groans, Mr. and Mrs. Meyers asked their son if he would look at them. Moving his head ever so slowly towards these parents who never in a millennium would have thought they'd be spoon-feeding their son again, Craig had a look in his eyes where his parents knew they had his attention and were—incredibly—in the same stratosphere.

Without hesitation, Mrs. Meyers spoke to Craig in her soft, persuading voice saying, "Me and daddy were told you counted this morning; let's keep working on that. See if you can count for us."

With his left arm resting on his thigh and his right contracted under his chin ala a poor imitation of Auguste Rodin's "The Thinker," Craig moved his upper torso in his chair as if positioning himself to make a speech. Taking a deep breath of air and rocking in his chair with a methodical precision, Craig leaned forward and—shut his eyes, trying to elude his tormenting consciousness.

Being so close to "making contact," the Meyers would not allow Craig to disappear. With an encouraging perseverance, the Meyers continued their pursuits to get Craig to utter something. Able to get Craig to look at her and hold his head up, instead of slouching and gazing into space, Mrs. Meyers thought that asking Craig about music might get him to respond. After several questions about some of his favorite rock bands with no response but an agitated moan and a ruffled squirming in his wheelchair, knowing that she was so close yet so far, Mrs. Meyers came up with a gem.

Knowing his love for guitar and getting him to talk about some of his favorite types might stimulate some neurons to connect with each other, Mrs. Meyers asked her son, "Can you tell me what a Fender is? I promised to get you one, once you got better."

With head tilted back and gazing towards the ceiling, Craig gasped, seemingly to gather a lung full of air. Eyes glazed, Craig exhaled a quick, barely discernible, "Guitar."

Feeling a tingling electricity throughout his body—normally one to look down on public displays of emotion—Craig's dad had yet more tears roll from his eyes, wetting the sleeves of Craig's hospital gown. As this grateful father bowed his head in his boy's chest, he would cry out, "That's right buddy, it's a guitar. A Fender's a guitar."

Her heart warmed by these two syllables, Mrs. Meyers sat smiling, paralyzed with a feeling of ecstasy words alone couldn't possibly describe.

While they got him going, these overjoyed parents didn't want to stop. "Craig, count to five for us," an elated Mr. Meyers asked of his son.

With the words falling from his mouth slow and to the point, pronounced in a jumbled fashion, Craig reeled off the numbers, "2-3-4-5."

With magazine in hand and in-between sobs, Mrs. Meyers quizzed her son, asking him to identify different pictures. Pointing to different objects in a picture ad of a kitchen for Frigidare, Mrs. Meyers had Craig correctly respond "chair" and "refrigerator" in the nasal twang that sounded nothing like the Craig she knew. With no elaboration whatsoever, Craig's one-word response may have been short, but Mrs. Meyers never heard anything so brief, sound so great.

This therapy continued until Craig became restless and was placed back on the floor of mattresses where he resumed his state of unconsciousness once his head touched the pillow. Preparing to take a break themselves and process the joyful events of the day, the chaplain of the hospital rushed in. Reverend Hugh Crawford emphatically proclaimed, "I heard the news that Craig spoke today. My oh my, that's wonderful. You folks must be thrilled. Let's have a word of prayer. Dear Heavenly Father, ..."

Rejoicing with the minister and hearing this clergyman's words of hope, the Meyers felt more at ease that Craig would travel on the road to recovery.

Shortly after the minister left, a Rehabilitation Nurse from Mr. and Mrs. Meyers' auto insurance company came in, telling Craig's parents that they need to start considering rehabilitation centers which to place Craig. Looking at her son unconscious on the sea of bedding beneath them, Mrs. Meyers was shocked to hear that a transfer was being considered so soon. Craig's condition was still "touch and go" and Mrs. Meyers was fearful that if an emergency arose, which is definitely possible in the early stages of the brain being damaged, Craig would not be getting the constant medical attention he may need.

"Besides," this doubtful mother added, "Craig responds better and is more secure working with his family than staff. And I know whatever rehab center he's at, they aren't going to let us be with him as much."

With this cue, the nurse recommended Harmarville Rehabilitation Center over the other possibility, and emphasized the importance of the brain being retrained at this stage of the ballgame over the risks of anything happening to Craig medically. Empathizing with this anxious mother, this prognosticator assured Mrs. Meyers that Harmarville would be suitably equipped to handle any type of neuromedical emergencies which Craig might have. Lump growing in her throat, mom Meyers would be delivered a punishing blow hearing how her son will always be at risk of having a seizure since his brain had been severely injured. Told that Craig will need to take anti-convulsant medication all his life in order to prevent having one of these uncontrollable spasms, Mrs. Meyers became raving mad that a well-to-do boy didn't think anything of disposing her son's welfare.

Since Craig's been in the hospital, regarding the limitations her teenaged son is going to have for the rest of his days, Mr. Meyers has heard those words, "all his life," too many times to count. Seeing Craig go from W.V.U. to "Sesame Street" in under three weeks time was insidiously taking its toll on Mr. Meyers.

Eyes fixed on his boy who was about to embark on a long rehabilitation journey of unknown territory where seemingly insurmountable crests and enduring plateaus would besiege him, Mr. Meyers fumed, "I wish that drunken bastard Paul were standing right here; I'd kill that son of a bitch."

There's no way this could happen, for Paul has been out of state, back in Morgantown.

Told of Paul's return to his home turf of cold ones on tap, teasing their emotions, the Meyers could picture Paul playing his role to a tee. After heedfully placing his crutches on the carpet, the Meyers could almost hear a dialogue where Paul would tell his audience of floormate admirers how his car hit a patch of ice on a blind corner before colliding into the telephone pole. Seconds being of the essence not withstanding, this envisioned portrayal burning their senses, the Meyers could visualize Paul standing in the dorm's hallway detailing his imagined heroics.

Conjuring this lifelike scenario and viewing their boy's lifeless body everyday sparked an unparalleled anger for this older couple who'd be weary of suffering. Practically feeling the thump of the drum roll, with the culprit of this catastrophe highlighting how he ignored personal pain, Craig's folks believed it wouldn't be beneath Paul to say he had no regard for his own safety while under the twisted metal, because he wasn't about to abandon his unresponsive friend. Not even having the depth to refrain from lying to them after he had almost killed their son, liable to explain to this collegiate assembly that he waited until the last possible moment before ceasing attempts at reviving Craig, these victimized parents could imagine Paul basking with the roaring cheers of approval made by his gullible listeners.

With his paternal guiding force knowing all too well, Sigmund Freud once said, "Dreams are the royal road to the discovery of the unconscious." However, for some strange reason, Paul wouldn't mention anything about how his drinking was the road leading to Craig's unconscious. If and when Craig's awareness ever rekindles, so that the "space in time" void he is surely going to experience one day may be filled, the Meyers would proceed to take some pictures of their comatose son when he was dangling onto life.

Although not apparent at first, Saturday March 6th would be a day further conquests would be made. Mr. Meyers reached into the deep pocket of his sport coat and pulled out his camera. Believing that the hospital's policy was one where pictures were not permitted when someone's in as bad a state as Craig, the Meyers would just as soon keep this under their hat. Operating from his optimistic view, down the line, Mr. Meyers thought that if the family ever gets discouraged with the progress Craig's making, they will have a tangible snapshot to remind them just how badly Craig was at one time.

While lying on his back on top of the mattresses, adorned in a hospital gown top, pajama bottoms, and sneakers to restrain his "drop foot," Mrs. Meyers continuously spoke to Craig while Scott would try to push his brother's contracted arm to the ground. As this therapy was taking place just in front of where Craig would be propped-up to eat, Mr. Meyers snapped a picture.

To get a closer snapshot of his comatose son, the jingling keys in his pocket making it difficult to be inconspicuous, Mr. Meyers bounced over to Craig. Standing above Craig at his son's feet, Mr. Meyers leaned a little to the left, then a little to the right, trying to get the picture centered the best he could. Just when this sly fox was positioned to flick himself a snapshot, interrupting this photo shoot, footsteps would be heard coming towards the door.

With one quick motion, the camera would be concealed again. Armed with the tools of her trade, preparing to take his pulse and blood pressure, the Registered Nurse hip-hoppetyed over to Craig. While holding Craig's left wrist and peering at her watch, this R.N. said to no one in particular, "Yeah, this boy's come a long way. I can remember shining my pen light right in his eyes and they wouldn't dilate. Now look at him, I hear he's starting to talk and it looks like that right arm's coming down a little bit."

In his bullfrog voice, Scott replied, "Yeah, we're working on it. Now if we can only do something about his face. Ha Ha Ha H Ha Ha Ha Ha Ha Ha Ha Ha Ha Ha Ha Ha Ha Ha Ha Ha Ha Ha Ha Ha Ha Ha Ha Ha Ha Ha Ha Ha Ha Ha Ha Ha Ha Ha Ha Ha Ha Ha Ha Ha Ha Ha Ha Ha Ha Ha Ha Ha Ha Ha Ha Ha Ha Ha Ha Ha Ha Ha Ha Ha Ha Ha Ha Ha Ha Ha Ha Ha Ha Ha Ha Ha Ha Ha Ha Ha Ha Ha Ha Ha Ha Ha Ha Ha Ha Ha Ha Ha Ha Ha Ha."

Following this afternoon edition of "Saturday Night Live," after the nurse had left the room, Mr. Meyers would take the picture of his unconscious son lying on the "Sealy Posturepedics" and "Sertas." Fearful that the camera might somehow cause the electrical monitors around Craig's empty bed to malfunction, stuffing the camera away, these would be the only two pictures Mr. Meyers would take of his comatose boy. Making for another dull afternoon for the Meyers, Craig would be "out cold" most of this dreary March day while atop these cloth pads. However, once placed in his wheelchair, Craig would be anything but boring.

After a resistant Craig was placed in his wheelchair for the delightful four-hour period he was not to be lying down, Craig carried on like he always does when he's first put in; heaving against the chair not being able to sit still. As if he can't find a spot in his chair which suits him, not able to sit still, Craig would heave against the chair with a wicked force. Knowing they'd have a fight on their hands once Craig was put in his love seat, the Meyers would usually be fearfully amazed just how cranky their son could get. With his left hand braced on the arm of his chair, Craig shimmied from side to side. Putting his hands on Craig's shoulders, Mr. Meyers shouted, "That's enough, now you settle down."

After a few seconds, Craig would be back at it, going about his business of trying to break his wheelchair again. However, the calm after this storm would be a memorable one.

Up to this point, Craig would respond only to a few of the questions asked of him in brief, direct, one-word answers, never grouping words formulating a sentence—until now. Not at all happy being forced to sit in the wheelchair, Craig stopped his rocking, wishfully looking at his father and said, "Stand me up, dad."

Goose bumps popping, never thinking he'd be so happy telling a family member that they had a fracture, Mr. Meyers said, "You broke your leg, you should stay off of it for awhile."

In Craig's moment of shooting star lucidity, the mother fearful that her son's brain not being operative would forever cause him to be nonsensical and irrational, quickly asked Craig a question which had plagued the Meyers' minds from the beginning. "Are you hurting anywhere?"

With great effort, in a voice sifted of its strength, Craig slowly said, "My head. . . . . Leg."

While Craig showed that he was momentarily cognizant, knowing that repetition is necessary and essential in leaping the canyon which is a brain injury, this injured lad's parents told Craig for the hundred and first time the reason why he's hurting and at the hospital. In the same breath, Mr. Meyers told Craig that he's getting so much better that he'll be going to one of the finest rehab centers in the country, if not THE finest, provided a vacancy at Harmarville becomes available and he's able to be contained in a bed. Employing the calm demeanor he used during his days as a policeman and volunteer fireman/ambulance driver, Mr. Meyers told his son that he would be working in therapy, not only for his physical setbacks, but his thinking as well.

Eyes heavy, wishing to escape consciousness, Craig wanting to put weight on his broken leg which was splintered into many fragments and being held together by a metal rod indicated the degree with which his brain was not working properly. A combination of that bruise on his brain and being bombarded with sedatives turned their son into a person whose ability to sense feeling was distorted. Capacity to comprehend concepts non-existent, Craig's compromised reasoning could not be trusted. Although many abilities have abandoned Craig—possibly never to return—a few would resurface as the day creeped on.

When Craig came out of his arid condition where he was lifeless and lacking any kind of feeling, his parents and Scott grasped the moment. While sitting in his wheelchair, Mr. Meyers showed Craig a dollar bill, asking him what it was. Lacking animation, with a hearty applause coming from Craig's mom and brother, the word "dollar" escaped Craig's lips. Next, Mr. Meyers laid down a five-dollar bill and—after seeming to take a pause to get oriented—Craig correctly identified the money before him with a sort of a "let's get this over with" approach.

After showing Craig a ten and two-dollar bill which were also correctly identified, Mrs. Meyers showed him some family pictures. Holding up a photograph of the family at a picnic in Harrisburg when Craig was just a little boy, Mrs. Meyers asked Craig to pick out his brother Carson, sister Claire, his grandfathers—who both had passed away before Craig was nine years old—and different other family members. With a little hesitation to process who these people were, Craig knew who was being shown.

Before putting the photo back in her purse, Scott contributed, "Yeah Craig, the reason you're making that funny face is because you just drank the worm I put in your Kool-Aid. Ha Ha Ha Ha Ha Ha Ha Ha Ha Ha Ha Ha Ha Ha Ha Ha Ha Ha Ha Ha Ha Ha Ha Ha Ha Ha Ha Ha Ha Ha Ha Ha Ha Ha Ha Ha Ha Ha Ha Ha Ha Ha Ha Ha Ha Ha Ha Ha Ha Ha Ha Ha Ha Ha Ha Ha Ha Ha Ha Ha Ha Ha Ha Ha Ha Ha Ha Ha Ha Ha Ha Ha Ha Ha."

In this identification therapy, since the topic of eating was on his mind, Scott asked his brother what weekly sports magazine Craig read everyday while stuffing his face with food. After a period of silence and a few hints, Craig correctly muttered "Sporting News." After correctly naming for Scott the baseball teams various players played for, not propped in the corner of his room, Craig ate his supper while sitting in his wheelchair for the first time. If Craig was going to go to Harmarville, he'd have to start being able to sit in his chair for extended periods because there won't be a room of mattresses awaiting him there.

The minute-hand seeming as if it would never make its way around, the clock's tick was mesmerizing. Like the clicking fingers of the hypnotist who wants the subject to return, Craig's incomprehensible cry broke the Meyers from their trance. Apparently wanting to tell someone of his discomfort sitting, Craig's speech was like that of a backmasking record once again, as the sound coming from his mouth was like that of a Neanderthal Man in distress.

The Meyers' difficulty understanding what Craig was trying to say, made their son so frustrated that his emotional tone eventually turned into one of pronounced irritability. Realizing his speech wasn't being unscrambled, not able to figure out what his parents' problem was, the volume of Craig's angry voice increased to an alarming decibel level.

Upon hearing the ruckus, one of the evening shift's Registered Nurses entered the room and couldn't help but notice the disappointment on these exhausted parents' faces. Surprised their son's speaking capacity had regressed to its earlier form, from reasonable clarity to becoming incomprehensible, Craig's parents would be informed of the effects an injured brain can have on speech. Distraught that Craig's ability to talk had not progressed as it had earlier in the day, the nurse tried her best to console these tired troopers.

"Now don't you folks worry yourself sick, your boy's making some fine progress. This hasn't been Craig's first setback and likely won't be his last. It's like his 'in and out of consciousness,' sometimes Craig has an idea of what's happening, sometimes he doesn't even know who he is. But don't get yourself too down, Craig'll be talking again. You can count on that."

The Meyers wondered if they'll be able to count on anything again. To be primed for victory only to be shot down time and time again, takes a lot out of someone. Knowing that Craig is going to have setback after setback until this is over, if it's ever going to be over, is something that must be endured. And, if one is to persevere, they need to find the strength to grasp hope and not let it escape. Hope is the key to withstanding the unrelenting punishment a head injury will deliver. If one lets this slip away, there is nothing. Because of the events of the next two days, the Meyers would need to summon all their stamina in order to keep from tumbling into that hole which is evanescent promise.

Sunday, March 7th was not a day of rest for the Meyers—far from it. Clanging the foot plate on his wheelchair with the violence of his mood this day, Craig must really know what kind of shape he's in now, for he couldn't sit still. Cautiously approaching his son who was peeved about only God knows what exactly, Mr. Meyers pleaded outloud, "When's this agitated state he's in ever going to end?"

Contained for a moment by his father's grasp, Craig let out a muffled moan letting his dad know he wasn't pleased being kept from thrashing his arm north, south, east, and west. Recklessly wobbling his chair, Craig moaned as if he'd been stabbed. Needing to get accustomed doing things that aren't real comfortable at first, Craig wouldn't be returning to the mattresses anytime soon because he had to tolerate sitting in his wheelchair longer, if he was going to Harmarville. No telling when a bed may become available for him at the rehab center, Craig would just have to be tough and endure the prolonged agony.

As she looked at her boy cuffed with misery, Mrs. Meyers couldn't believe Craig will be leaving the hospital once a bed is ready at Harmarville. Babbling like an infant and irritably thumping the back of the wheelchair with his left elbow which still looked like hamburger, Craig was in another galaxy unknown to man. Wanting to talk when he would jabber, Craig must have realized the words weren't coming out like he wanted them to. Not able to communicate because the ability to talk had been forgotten, this frustration made Craig mad as hell.

Despite the never-ending encouragement and optimistic efforts by her husband, Mrs. Meyers could not be convinced her baby would be able to benefit from the rigors of rehabilitation. Shaking her head in disbelief, Mrs. Meyers uttered in a tone of submission, "He isn't ready, there's no way he's ready. Craig's not going to be able to go to a rehab yet. He can't even hold his head up on his own. He can't remain conscious but a few hours, so how's he going to be able to do the work therapy requires. He can't walk, talk, and hasn't moved his right arm in almost a month."

Seeing his wife work herself up in a full-blown "tizzy," Mr. Meyers would remind her that this is why Craig's going to rehab—so that he can work on these things. He pointed out the gargantuan gains Craig's has made already and of the potential he's showing for staff to even consider transferring him to a rehabilitation center.

Pressed into service as psychotherapist, Mr. Meyers said, "When a brain's been hurt, they don't waste any time trying to get it to work again."

Despite this father's words of comfort, empathizing with Mrs. Meyers' doubt wouldn't be difficult given Craig's rambunctious history while at Allegheny General. With the exception of those few brief moments when he showed a glimmer of being mildly coherent, Craig was restless and agitated all day. Being that every precious ounce of energy Craig's parents deposited had been siphoned from them this day, their need to refuel for tomorrow's events was essential, if they were to rise above the anxiety which would not be denied.

Their bodies succumbed to the chill when the phone rang this March 8th morning. Hoping it was a wrong number, the Meyers wouldn't be so lucky.

In a few moments after answering the phone, Mrs. Meyers asked, "And when's this to take place?"

Standing a few feet from the phone, twisted with nervous excitement, Mr. Meyers became unnerved after his wife eventually hung up the phone and said, "That was the social worker at Allegheny General; Craig's being transferred to Harmarville tomorrow morning, about ten."

Anytime he's called upon to drive an unfamiliar area of Pittsburgh, Mr. Meyers becomes fanatical. Like bullets shooting from a machine gun, this hyper father asked, "How's he going to get there?" "Where is Harmarville? Is it off 79 or do you have to take the turnpike? I forgot to look at a map last night; I was too bushed." "Do they have people there to watch Craig? Y'know he can't be left alone." "Will he be able to continue seeing Dr. Prostko? We like him." "What time did you say he was going, again?"

Seeing that her husband was working himself into a frenzy, her turn to use some psychology, Mrs. Meyers praised her partner's driving up to this point when they go to Allegheny General everyday and calmly attempted to soothe this terrorized driver by encouraging him to simply "take it slow" until he becomes acquainted with the route. Battling her own uneasiness, Mrs. Meyers replied as quietly as she could that they would be told the specific arrangements which would need to be made upon arriving at the hospital later in the afternoon.

After learning that they'd have to bring some of Craig's clothes, insurance verification, a jacket, and a picture or two of something which Craig was familiar to set on his nightstand from home to Harmarville, Craig's parents went to their boy's room. About to endure more of what they had seen enough of yesterday, the Meyers could only hope that things would be different with the change of settings.

Having just been put on his mattresses after his morning therapy, an unconscious Craig would not respond when his parents said, "Hi" to him this afternoon.

With the jubilation they show every afternoon they come in, Mr. and Mrs. Meyers spoke spiritedly, telling their boy that he's going to be moved to a different place tomorrow and not to be scared; that they'll be there with him too. Upper lip quivering, Mr. Meyers said, "You're going to a rehab center where they're going to get you on your feet again and that right arm playing that ukele of yours. You'll be on that ballfield again in no time."

Knowing his condition is not one where a "kiss and a BandAid" will serve as a remedy this time, Mrs. Meyers could only hope Craig would be able to get something out of rehabilitation and not aimlessly flounder because his brain cannot cooperate. Ragged from three weeks of battling the furor associated with head injury, Craig's mom has been in a hailstorm of panic and disarray since Paul hurt her son. Only able to capture a few fleeting moments where Craig could tell them what he was feeling and thinking, left this mother paranoid with fear, as she could merely guess what was going on in his head.

The Meyers' minds were not put at ease when they were informed that Craig will not be sleeping on his mattresses tonight, rather, he will be returning to his bed that agitates him so much. In order to prepare Craig for his admission to Harmarville, hospital staff would have to apply some systematic desensitization with their unruly patient.

Mrs. Meyers whispered to her husband, "Here's a boy who needs handcuffed while lying in bed, so he doesn't hurt himself. I can see him lying in his bed at Harmarville, not supervised, ripping his elbow up. How do they expect him to benefit from rehab when he's 'fit to be tied.'"

Only adding fuel to Mrs. Meyers' fire that her son was not ready for the move, in a little while, Craig would be in his wheelchair fighting his enemy with a renewed vitality.

The squeak heard by Craig's parents was not that of the rusted wheels of his chair being pushed down the hallway, but Craig abusing the sideplates of his wheelchair like that of a deranged, criminally insane sociopath on a mindless agenda to lash out at anyone or anything. Cautious not to escalate this tirade, the Meyers stood helplessly, watching their son go through the motions of his agitated state. Not wanting to provoke him in any way—not that they'd have to do anything to get him on his warpath—all these parental saints could really do was let Craig "ride out" his aggravation, and safeguard against him seriously hurting himself.

Crying out in a muffled moan as if wanting to be put out of his misery, Craig rustled in his wheelchair like that of one being tortured by a pain only Beelzebub could contrive. Seemingly overwhelmed being prisoner in a haze of misery, Craig would unrelentlessly tug at his hospital gown. As if freeing himself from that which covered his body would allow him to escape the petrifying Hell with which he felt enclosed, like the cell of a convict who has committed a crime punishable by death, freedom from horror would be restrained by walls of confinement.

With his contracted right arm, shredded ear, fractured leg, the large lump in the middle of his forehead, a face purple from being bruised, and gazed eyes, Mrs. Meyers could barely recognize her son. Looking like he'd been spun in a blender after having been chopped and diced, making it virtually impossible imagining Craig ever being whole, this victim's appearance would never be the same. As bad as this accident has left Craig physically, the most difficult aspect his parents have to deal with is how his brain being injured has changed his personality from being mild-mannered to someone they didn't know as their son. Since his brain had been bruised, Craig's banging-clawing-kicking-thrashing led Mrs. Meyers to believe that Craig has been struck down by the worst affliction, for it not only affects one physically, but alters the personality as well. With the exception of those times few and far between when Craig momentarily showed a semblance of his old self, the Meyers had no idea who was in that wheelchair. Perhaps, the one sitting in the wheelchair didn't know who was there either.

Ruffled by their son's agony, the disconcerted expression on these seniors' faces told a story of cyclical frustrations and shattered aspirations this afternoon. It was only the day before yesterday that Craig was able to identify some of the players in the Pirates' lineup, but today, doesn't know what the game of baseball is. Such is the case when one has suffered trauma to the brain which affects not only one's physical abilities, but emotional and cognitive ones as well.

The fear that Craig might always fluctuate from one extreme on the spectrum to the other, occupied the Meyers' thinking. Would Craig's coherence and sensibility always be dependent on whether those brain waves decide to work or not?

Or will he one day be able to have some control? And if Craig will have to live a life where independence is a painful reminder of what he had taken away from him, would he want to survive?

It would *have to* be this way, for these parents forever disturbed from their routine could not fathom their son being gone and would do what they could to make Craig's life as tolerable as possible. Preserving what emotional balance remained, these warriors would tell themselves that the Afterlife will just have to wait before their son takes up residency there because Craig has a lot more living to do here on earth. With all the plans made, nurturing given, and time invested in Craig's development, the Meyers wouldn't be going down without a fight. Although this afternoon was an aphasic one, as the day lurked into evening, the hypothalamus and company worked in concert with one another, so Craig could go about his business of showing why Harmarville would be the next logical step in this leg of the mission.

After Craig devoured his gourmet pureed delicacy at dinnertime, not a willing participant this afternoon, the Meyers went about their therapy with Craig. Mrs. Meyers talked to Craig about what's going on in the neighborhood with his friends, Mr. Meyers had Craig follow his floating finger which swung like a clock's pendulum, and Scott worked on getting his brother's right arm down a little more. This therapy was identical to what these instructors did with Craig last evening, the evening before that, and the evenings prior to that. Retraining that brain requires hard work that is continuous, monotonous, usually boring, frequently painful, and always difficult.

Sticking with Craig like his shadow, the Meyers have been on an emotional roller coaster, praying their car does not derail. Their dedication and commitment doing what they could so Craig would progress was impeccable, as his last day at Allegheny General was on the horizon.

Beyond the horizon, the mist of this March 9th morning made it impossible to ascertain whether the day would be one where the sun would rise to the heavens above or be vanquished by black clouds, threatening to make everything dark. No matter, the Meyers prepared to leave for the hospital one last time on this Tuesday; a morning that was thick with tension.

Entangled by a web of uncertainty when they arrived at Allegheny General, informed that Craig did just fine tolerating his bed last night, the doubt which shrouded the Meyers would be lifted somewhat.

After filling out the necessary papers for discharge, the Meyers walked into their son's room, seeing that Craig had already been dressed by staff in the one set of clothes Mrs. Meyers brought in yesterday from home. Seeing Craig in jeans and a flannel shirt brought smiles to his parents' faces.

"There's our old slob," Mr. Meyers said, feeling boyish himself that his son was at least resembling himself from an attire standpoint.

Never believing that she'd be so happy seeing Craig decked out in his customary "Oscar Madison" garb, Mrs. Meyers was absolutely gleeful that Craig looked like himself clothes-wise, not draped in pajamas and hospital gown around the clock. However, seeing that Craig's jeans were several sizes too large because of all the weight he had lost and his uneasiness sitting in his wheelchair brought reality crashing down again.

As he was trying to rip apart his shirt, before retreating hastily so she wouldn't get in the way of his hand which sought anything to latch onto, Mrs. Meyers bent over to Craig to stop him from breaking off his buttons. Yelling at Craig that he better not lay a hand on his mother, while trying to avoid his rowdy son's airborne arm himself, Mr. Meyers told his soon-to-be- discharged boy not to leave Allegheny General on such bad terms.

After Craig toned-down some, aided by his dad holding down his arm, Mrs. Meyers told her enraged son that he will be put in an ambulance in a little while and transferred to the rehabilitation center "me and daddy told you about." However, Craig's state of mind was once again one where he didn't even know he was being spoken to.

Unfortunately for the Meyers, "a little while" had arrived and it was time to take Craig down to the ambulance in a gurney. With smiles disguising their somber expectation that the future will be one absent of normalcy for Craig, the staff bid farewell to their trooper, wishing he and his parents the best on their walk to the elevator one last time. All the while, Craig laid surprisingly content in his gurney the ambulance personnel were pushing down the hallway. Talking to him in a relaxed fashion, the ambulance driver and his attendant moved hastily along, not about to waste any time while Craig laid there pleasantly passive. This relaxed/non-combative demeanor lasted until the driver started the engine. Then, all hell broke loose.

March 9, 1982 was D-Day for the Meyers, not only because it was discharge day, but because of the battle Craig would put up in the ambulance. Something very disturbing was going on inside Craig's head, for being transported in the ambulance was interpreted as a threat. Thinking that a familiar face traveling with Craig would put him more at ease on his trip in the ambulance, Mrs. Meyers had requested, and was granted, permission to accompany her son. However, this didn't seem to make much difference.

As Mrs. Meyers looked at her frightened son wailing as loud as his bruised brain would allow him to, Craig's agitation and resistance grew more intense. Mrs. Meyers and the empathetic attendant tried to calm Craig by reassuring him that things were alright and that they'll be at the rehab in no time, being that it was only a fifteen-mile drive. The attendant commented to Mrs. Meyers that maybe Craig, sensing his being in a moving vehicle, was terrorized given what had happened to him the last time he was transported by someone.

Pulling onto Route 28 North, the ambulance whisked past the Heinz Factory and by the time it was bypassing such exits as the ones in Millvale, Etna, and Blawnox, Craig was lying in his gurney in the rear of the ambulance dripping with sweat as a result of his being stricken with terror. Slowed by the midday traffic, the ambulance trudged along, passing the Highland Park Bridge to the right. Before coming to the RIDC Park exit which was where they were to get off, Craig's tolerance made its descent to the point where it took the efforts of both Craig's mom and the attendant to keep him from falling prey to his excessive fear.

Following the ambulance in the family car, Mr. Meyers had no idea that the inside of the ambulance had become like the zoo they were not too far away from. As nerve-racking as the trip was at the beginning, it got worse as the miles accumulated. Like the safaris where the inhabitants of the nearby Pittsburgh Zoo were caught, Mrs. Meyers' and the attendant's expedition was to capture some order, as the ambulance made its way onto Freeport Road.

Trying to pacify Craig, letting out muted screams by now and rolling from side to side, the ambulance attendant told his patient that they're almost there and to "hang tough." By the time they made the turn at Eat 'n' Park onto the narrow, winding, pothole-laden, uphill street known as Guys Run Road leading to their destination, Craig was paralyzed with fear. Because of the traumatized unrest occurring within the ambulance, the past twenty or so minutes with Craig have been some of Mrs. Meyers' longest, as she could sense how Sir Edmund Hillary must have felt nearing the crest on Mt. Everest.

As the driver arrived at this pinnacle and made the left onto Harmarville's long driveway, he flipped down his visor because the sun's rays were blinding this afternoon. The powerful glow brightening the earth below, Craig's arrival at this rehabilitation center marked the juncture where the depth of his character would be discovered. After twenty-four agonizing days at the hospital—which seemed like years—the *silence* of needing to appreciate that which shouldn't be, and the *emptiness* treading a path never traveled to a destination not known, would soon make its appearance.

Chapter 4

Turning Point

With the brilliant, orange, sun-glistened, late morning sky serving as its backdrop, Mr. and Mrs. Meyers had no idea that the silhouette before them would be a force which both a resurrection and an awakening would occur for both them and their son. Sweltering with anxiety about how Craig'd react to yet more unfamiliar surroundings and faces, Mrs. Meyers looked at the bold letters on the side of the rehab which read "HARMARVILLE." Mrs. Meyers immediately was impressed with what she saw.

The aesthetic setting and the size of the rehab appealed to this sometimes fastidious critic. Surrounded by many acres of well-manicured/finely landscaped grounds, Harmarville was shaded by many trees and sprinkled with foliage along its driveway and different areas throughout. Mr. Meyers emerged from the parking garage thinking he must have made a wrong turn somewhere and ended up at a resort instead of the rehab center he thought they were going. The gurney being taken out of the ambulance with him aboard and apparently sensing his parents' excitement, Craig could not take in all this stimulation at once. Growling the best he could, this wary admission jerked about his bedded cart, not knowing what fate he was going to be subjected to next.

Trying to calm this shaken patient from his red alert, the Meyers and the attendant soothingly talked to Craig as he was being pushed to the sliding glass door. As Craig was squirming underneath the sheets of the wheeled stretcher, Mrs. Meyers looked at Harmarville's logo displayed on the wall which depicts a person standing of their own free will—crutches discarded—and arms raised triumphantly. She then focused her tired, brown eyes at her son, hoping somehow, some way, that could be Craig one of these days.

Full steam ahead, with nurses, therapists, social workers, clerical personnel, and volunteers all swirling every which way, the attendant pushed Craig to Harmarville's main hallway which was three hundred yards of bustling activity. With some buzzing about and others barely keeping the pace of a crawl, patients in wheelchairs and walkers were also heading in different directions seemingly with no time to spare. Paradoxically, this subway station atmosphere had a calming effect on the easily excitable Mr. Meyers, for it showed this prosaic gentleman that

Harmarville was a no-nonsense place designed with the intent of providing services to those who need the talents of dedicated rehabilitation professionals under the auspices of a businesslike climate.

Having done this many times before, thus knowing the procedure well, the attendant went right to the admissions' desk and the Meyers signed Craig in. The "turning point" was now officially set to begin in this war where the patient and his family not only combat the horrors brain damage will render, but the passing of time, for each moment the clock's hand advances means one breath closer to missed opportunity.

"And now they're off" a little bit further down the hallway to the large black number "3," so distinct resting on its green wall. Unit three was devoted to treating those with neurological impairments, predominantly head injury.

Mrs. Meyers could feel the hair standing on the back of her neck when she heard the yells coming from those eating their lunch at the tables in front of the nurses' station and felt eyes looking at the new patient and his family coming in. The thought that Craig will be around these crazed, sadomasochists nearly twenty-four hours each day struck fear in Mrs. Meyers' heart for her son's safety. Terrified that Craig may fall victim to one of these rationally-impaired, "brain contused" lunatics, Mrs. Meyers was secretly having second thoughts about whether this is the right place for her son. It didn't help her nerves any that, every couple of minutes, someone's name was being barked over the PA system throughout the rehab. As a "Laura Matthews" was being paged to "please contact admissions," Mr. Meyers could see his wife battling this invasion of doubt and tried to console her by saying that this will be the setting "where Craig's comeback will occur."

When a nurse at the station directed the ambulance attendant to where Craig's room assignment was, the Meyers' nerves ascended to perilous heights. The gurney's wheels creaked like shutters of a condemned house subjected to a windstorm's tempestuous fury when pushed down the right hallway to the two-person bedroom that was going to be Craig's new home.

After thanking the attendant for his assistance, the Meyers felt a mix of emotions unpacking Craig's clothes and putting them in the closet. They felt a sense of gratitude that Craig had come this far and were set to read Harmarville's rules/regulations posted on the wall instead of autopsy results on their son. Entrusting Craig's future to people she had merely read a brochure about and heard only through word of mouth as being good, Mrs. Meyers would be fearful for her son. Because this was not a facility geared for medical emergencies, Mrs. Meyers' blood curdled when she imagined Craig having a seizure, swallowing his tongue, lips turning blue, his body violently rolling from side to side, starved of oxygen, unable to call for help because of his inability to communicate. In this script of futility, by the time help arrived, Craig would be as lifeless as a dove dangling from a stray cat's clenched jaw.

Mrs. Meyers had an infinite number of questions with a seemingly finite number of answers. With the time a family can be with their loved one at the center limited, playing over and over in their minds, these worried parents' primary concern was whether or not Craig would continue to be frequently monitored or have to "fend" for himself not being in such "critical" condition anymore. That question was answered by the social worker assigned to Craig's case.

When Laura Matthews, M.S.W. came in, Craig gave her an idea of what his therapists were going to have to deal with. In constant motion with no purpose or direction, Craig rolled around in his gurney, slowing down only to grab something to stick in his mouth or to tear at his clothing. As Craig was gnawing at his shirt sleeve, this social worker explained the mechanics of their son's program to the Meyers.

Taking a burdensome load off their shoulders, until Craig shows it would be safe to discontinue this constant observation, Miss Matthews told the Meyers that their son will have a private nurse watching him in the unit after he finishes his therapy. Miss Matthews said Craig will have Physical Therapy to address his fine and gross motor skill deficits. Psychology to get a baseline where the origin of Craig's difficulties are and regain the ability to use language concepts, Communication Skills to work on both receptive and expressive aphasic symptoms, and Occupational Therapy as a means to work on both his physical and cognitive conditions further.

The social worker told the Meyers that Craig will be given a battery of tests as part of the initial evaluation process, so the therapists can get an idea of what Craig's strengths and weaknesses are. With this information, a strategy of therapies can therefore be planned. She added, promptly getting the medical records detailing the patient's previous hospitalization would be important for both diagnostic and treatment purposes. However, due to bureaucratic obstacles, sometimes this doesn't get done when it should. And Craig's case was one where the patient arrived before the medical records.

When informed specifically that weight-bearing would likely be a course of remedial treatment taken in Physical Therapy in a day or two, alarms went off. After Craig's parents told the misguided social worker that putting weight on his right leg could not occur because it had been broken, Miss Matthews immediately got on the horn and gave the physiatrist supervising Craig's care, Jose G. Amayo, M.D., this information. Not exactly the best way to form a good first impression, the Meyers would gasp a resounding, "Whew, that was a close one." Those medical records best be on their way, for treatment can't be safely conducted until the therapists can review Craig's history.

Upon Miss Matthews' return, the Meyers were given a general idea of how the different programs will be individualized to benefit Craig. Now that it is known that Craig cannot bear any weight on his right leg, during the Physical Therapy initial evaluation, Craig's range of motion, strength, tone, sensation, coordination, and posture will be assessed, as well as his ability to control his head, trunk, and balance himself when sitting. This is so Craig's physical therapist, Janet Alba, LPT, is able to get a baseline idea of what Craig can and cannot do; what Craig can and cannot tolerate.

In Psychology, Mrs. Carolyn Joy, M.S., will conduct an evaluation where an assortment of tests will be applied to determine the degree to which Craig's cognitive limitations are caused by the brain's being damaged (cerebral organic involvement). This psychologist will then outline a program designed to address this organically-induced dysphasia.

In the Communication Skills Diagnostic Evaluation, Diane Rosato, M.A.—the therapist fortunate enough to be assigned to work with Craig on his various language deficits—will determine the extent Craig's ability to understand words/pictures (receptive language) and speech/writing (expressive language) had been affected due to his brain being injured. Identifying the difficulties Craig has with his ability to speak, read, and write would give his therapist an impression of the remedial treatments needed to correct what Craig had—in essence—forgotten, due to his brain being jiggled around in his skull. That is, if those parts of the brain which still work permit Craig to regain some of the language concepts he lost after being kamikazed into that telephone pole.

Occupational Therapy will have Craig work on getting that right arm down and reducing the spasticity of those fingers, so Craig can achieve functional use of his right arm and hand. One of the primary objectives of OT is to work with the patient on the various physical and cognitive limitations, so as much self-care independence as possible may be attained. Therefore, activities of daily living (ADL's) fall into this department's list of many responsibilities. During the initial evaluation process, it will be the job of Craig's therapist—Wendy Wood, OTR—to gauge the barriers which can impede independence and formulate strategies, so improved function and understanding may occur.

After explaining the program to the parents of the son who was fleeced of a life free from physical and cognitive obstacle, Miss Matthews found a nurse to watch Craig while she gave Mr. and Mrs. Meyers a tour of the huge facility where their boy will attempt to rid himself of the crippling conditions Paul's malefic action of drinking and driving created.

Making a left onto the long hallway, the Meyers first came upon the Communications Skills area where Craig will be working, then the Psychology department where he will be tested and practicing to resolve whatever deficits are pin-pointed. Across the hall, to the left, was a gift shop and the doors to the courtyard. A little further down the hallway, to the right, was the massive cafeteria and to the left, the unit where people with spinal cord injuries are treated. At the end of the hallway is one large Physical Therapy gymnasium with another—where Craig will be—adjacent to it; both equipped with parallel bars, mats, pads, stationary bikes, physical torture machinery on the walls, etc.

After viewing the upstairs Vocational Department they could only hope Craig advances to, the Meyers returned to Craig's room. Upon seeing the weary nurse trying to calm their distressed son, the Meyers relieved the private nurse of her duty before Craig made an enemy before even being here an hour.

"You're really going to like it here, buddy," Mr. Meyers claimed, "they have some real fine-looking lady therapists and nurses here that're going to be working with you. You're not going to want to leave!"

Craig's skeptical mom was more at ease and having less doubts after seeing the facility. "This looks like a real good place, honey," Mrs. Meyers said with a rare hint of optimism in her voice before she went about preparing to feed Craig his lunch that had been put through a blender first. Normally the responsibility of a nurse or an aide, Harmarville's staff figured that since Craig was accustomed to his mom feeding him and she was more than willing to do this, they would allow this for a short time until Craig relearns how to feed himself without assistance.

As she fed her son his pureed meal, Mrs. Meyers had a momentary lapse of sickness when she came to grips with the reality of this situation. This was 1982 and she was spoon-feeding her eighteen-year-old son—not 1963—when she did the same thing for Craig as a baby. With this thought, tears began to collect in Mrs. Meyers' eyes because her son was a victim of a miscarriage of trust which caused a regression of almost two decades. Thinking about how the epicenter of this whole tragedy—Paul's lack of a strong, conscientious backbone—got Mrs. Meyers' blood boiling.

Feeling uneasy about this avalanche of emotion, Mr. Meyers changed the flow of passion without delay, "Buddy, this is a top-notch place," this encouraged father said with his characteristic bright outlook since Craig came up the loser in Paul's act of malfeasance, "but you're going to have to work hard for all your therapists; don't give anybody trouble."

If Craig could have assured his dad somehow that he would not give anybody any flak, he'd have been telling an awful lie.

Getting off the turnpike at the Mars, Pa. exit, which was the route Mr. Meyers took on the way back to Washington from Harmarville despite being longer time-wise and mileage-wise in order to avoid downtown Pittsburgh, the Meyers had a good feeling about the care their son was going to receive at Harmarville. The professional atmosphere and the setting itself all seemed to be conducive to optimum care.

Once again, like every other night since Craig's been hurt, the Meyers received a multitude of calls from family, friends, and neighbors wanting updated. When telling someone they hadn't spoken to since Craig's transfer that he'd be treated at Harmarville, these hopeful parents were either reminded by well-wishers of this rehab's excellent reputation or to "hang in there" because Craig's coming back.

Despite being assured that Craig would be watched continuously by staff, Mrs. Meyers' trademark fear and doubt made its appearance again when she questioned in her mind whether her agitated, common sensically-impaired son could sleep in a bed two nights in a row and from here on out. Mrs. Meyers left no stone unturned when it came to assuring her son got the utmost in care. Sometimes the mental anguish she put herself through was not necessary, mostly however, keeping tabs on those rendering treatment was productive and earned her the respect of those around her.

Despite his own inner melee of grief, Mr. Meyers would not allow himself or his wife to be butchered by desolation's insatiable appetite for those not able to endure the havoc a brain injury will deliver. In order to keep going and not be ambushed by ruin, the Meyers made a commitment to work as a team for Craig's betterment. The Meyers were always told that if they need something, they have the backing and to not give up the ship, for calmer waters lie ahead. The Meyers better savor the spark lit by this encouragement, for Craig's second day at the rehab was not one where the seas were gentle.

Choking on foregone hopes' strangling grip which yields no compromise, the Meyers tried to make the most of Craig's second day at Harmarville. Being that Craig's neurological functioning was not going to permit him to cooperate in any way, shape, or form and because his medical records hadn't arrived, these parents who have been by Craig's side every minute since he was pounded against that pole would have to—once again—put aside their hopes that progress would commence.

This perversion of prompt care was made all the more difficult for these parents to put up with when they'd look into their son's mystic eyes. Serving as a window to the upheaval with which Craig was being harassed, these eyes told the story of torment and a world masked with confusion. Hearing Craig's attempts to extract this misery, these parents who time after time have had their hopes crushed one moment only to be replenished with something to cherish the next, wondered why their son was the object of this juggernaut.

Like he was at Allegheny General, when Craig's sedatives and pain killers were wearing off and his brain became ridden with havoc, he couldn't lie still in his bed, as he would roll from side to side fidgeting with his hair, clothing, and anything he could get a hold of. When he'd be in his wheelchair this second day, March 10, Craig couldn't sit still. It was almost like if Craig were motionless, he'd have felt he were a sitting duck for whatever his brain injury wanted to take aim at; be it pain in his head, contracted right arm, busted right leg, or hallucinations. Only God knows for sure. Craig's gazing eyes told a story of a young man traumatized; aloof to that around him.

Craig's parents never saw their son make an effort to communicate; he would only respond in an elementary fashion to stimuli presented to him. That is, if he would react at all. During those rare occasions of showing a trace of someone being in his body, Craig would give a hint that there was reason to keep plowing ahead. Despite countless times when they were frustrated, disappointed, and ridden with pain, Mr. and Mrs. Meyers would never give up. Seeing some positive in a situation, whether it be some expression in Craig's face or another breath being taken, is what kept the Meyers going. More times than not, this was all they had.

Because his records did not arrive, therapy was conducted in Craig's room by his family. Mom and dad Meyers worked with Craig's right arm which was held rigid at an angle that hasn't changed in a month. Mr. Meyers had Craig follow his finger left and right, right and left. Craig was continuously stimulated to speak in his two- or three- word phrases, if at all possible. Later, Scott and his lovely wife repeated this therapy during their round. If this all sounds like a broken record, as if it's been heard before, that's because it has. With TBI, symptoms will play over and over with treatments needing repeated until the brain. . . . .Until the brain does whatever the brain's going to do. That is, of course, if the brain's going to do anything at all.

The family coming in everyday was not only a costly venture on their emotions, but on their billfolds and time as well. When Mr. Meyers took the turnpike to see Craig, this route was sixty-five miles one-way. And about forty-five miles one-way if he cut through the Fort Pitt Tunnels and caught Rt. 28 North. When traveling to and from Allegheny General, this was approximately seventy miles round trip. Being a stickler for keeping accurate data, Mr. Meyers kept a perfect record of meal money spent, parking costs, and other travel expenses including mileage; hoping to be reimbursed by the insurance company.

For example, since Craig's been hurt, the Meyers paid $4.20 each day for parking and an arm and a leg for the minuscule meals at Allegheny General. At Harmarville, the costs were more reasonable. Parking was free and the cost of a meal ticket for one of Harmarville's tasty meals cost $2.50. The toll to use the turnpike round trip would be a dollar a day. Harmarville's visiting hours were Tuesday and Thursday from 6:00 P.M. to 8:45 P.M., and Saturday/Sunday from 10 A.M. to 8:45 P.M. The Meyers, however, were granted permission to come about an hour or two early because of the therapeutic benefits for Craig. Because of Harmarville's distance from Washington, the Meyers planned to spend some nights at one of the cheap motels at the bottom of the hill at a cost of $27 a night.

This has become an expensive venture on Mr. Meyers' fixed retirement income. But no complaints will be heard coming from the Meyers, for no expenditure could provide them with as much value as the one that allows them to see their son who needs them so badly. If they hadn't had the foresight to save for a rainy day, the financial straits could have left them penniless. It doesn't look like the sun's going to shine anytime soon either, for the thunderhead on the horizon doesn't look like it's going anywhere right now.

By evening's end, Harmarville had Craig's medical records, so Craig would be starting therapy tomorrow after he drinks his breakfast. Being that tomorrow is Thursday, visiting hours will begin at 6:00 P.M. That will be the first time in twenty-five days that one of Craig's parents will not be eyeballing him every minute that passes. Talk about devotion.

Wednesday night, lying awake battling insomnia, Mrs. Meyers' tormenting thoughts of not being with her stricken son the majority of the day tomorrow could not be put away. What will Craig think being in this strange place he does not know, many miles from home in another county? What if he needs us and we're not there; will he think we've abandoned him? What if he suddenly becomes coherent and we're not around to see this immaculate progress? What if he expires?

Not able to fall asleep because of his wife's rustling, Mr. Meyers tried to calm this fearful mother, assuring her that Craig's going to be alright. That now is the time Craig starts working independently to regain some of the things that were taken away from him in the accident, that Craig needs the skills of his therapists during the day. And for them to stay out of the way until visiting hours, when *they* can do their work.

When Mr. Meyers finished with how Craig seems to excel when he's by himself anyway, Mrs. Meyers rolled to her side, gazing at the digital clock. Wide-eyed, she stared as the numbers change every minute. . . . . then every hour. . . . . thinking. . . . . worrying. . . . . wondering

The morning of March 11, 1982 would be one where Craig would begin the marathon which is rehabilitation. The rehabilitation would take place not only in the Physical Therapy gymnasium and the cognitive professionals' offices, but throughout the rehab where Craig would need to interact with professionals and patients. The stimulation of collecting thoughts before expressing oneself and receiving input from others provides a person with a sense of reality which is what the individual with a head injury needs because they have been polarized from "what is" and "what never was" or "will be." And on this morning, it was evident that Craig will need to get in better touch with what's true.

The nurses' aide assigned to watch Craig today was only able to get him to chew a few bites of his grinded-up breakfast. This stunned aide had to weave and back off while she was feeding Craig because he would take a few swipes at her with his good arm. Looking as if he were scared and laden with anxiety, it didn't appear Craig was trying to hurt her, but just wanted a person to latch himself onto. Pushing away the arm that was holding this menacing eating utensil, when he wasn't swinging his arm, Craig would lean away from the spoon that was headed for his mouth. Despite his inability and lack of cooperation, this aide got back in the firing line and gave it another "go," without much success.

Whether Craig didn't trust the aide because he didn't know her, or this was his way of showing he didn't find the clump of pureed yummies on the spoon to his liking, or was suspicious of everything and everyone, or was paranoid about what this feeding business was all about, or just felt miserable that being "racked around" prevented him from doing anything but sit still, will never be known. Putting Craig's breakfast tray away, what this aide did know was that she will have to do the same thing in a few hours at lunchtime. One could be certain she'd warn her cohorts about the "Patient from Hell."

In his spirited voice, the volunteer asked Craig why he was at Harmarville. Was it a car accident? Was alcohol involved? Tom, not allowing himself to be discouraged by Craig's lack of a response, went on to explain that most of the younger people in the Head Injury Unit were there because of an automobile accident where the driver had been drinking.

Despite Craig's slouched position in the wheelchair—unaware that he was being spoken to—the volunteer continued talking to Craig in his "happy-go-lucky" tone, for the guy he wheeled down the hallway looked as if he could use a pick-me-up and a smile. Seeing someone so young left in shambles made it a difficult task to conceal the long face that wanted to overtake him, but Tom was able to hold back and give his escortee what he could.

As he was being pushed down the hallway in his wheelchair, Craig was the focus of many eyes, for he was beginning to get annoyed with this motion. Not wanting any part of this transportation experience, Craig's therapists-to-be and fellow "bruised brainers" on his unit all looked at the new kid on the block. Letting out a muted howl, Craig gave those that were to work with him an idea of the struggle that lie ahead for them. And Craig wasted no time showcasing his belligerence.

After Tom locked the brakes on Craig's wheelchair in the Physical Therapy gymnasium and wished him "Good luck" on his first day of rehab, Craig's physical therapist approached her new patient. Despite a friendly smile and a, "How you doin'? I'm Jan Alba, I'm going to be your physical therapist," Craig would be in no shape to reciprocate the greeting.

Letting Jan know she just better watch her step because he's in no mood to be messed with, in his now customary irritated demeanor, Craig started grabbing at his clothing and kicking about in his wheelchair with his good leg. Jan wouldn't have any of this, so she proceeded to unlock the brakes on Craig's wheelchair and wheeled her new patient to the elevated mats, so she could begin the initial evaluation.

Not ready to relent his position as the boss, Craig would not sit still long enough for Jan to perform her magic. Craig didn't know "what" exactly, but he must have known something was up. Always having been suspicious in nature, Craig wasn't about to let this female manipulate his aching body in any way or try to push him around.

When the psychology of calmly talking to Craig and assuring him everything she does is for his benefit didn't work, Jan proceeded to test what Craig would allow her to do; which didn't amount to much at all. Feeling Jan touch his arm or sensing her getting close to his wheelchair, made Craig resist all that much more. Surely, Craig could sense that moving, stretching, and twisting that right arm would result in excruciating pain and he wasn't in any frame of mind to be hurt anymore.

When Craig's hand whisked over her head, John Sirianni, LPT, and Mary Smith, PTA, came running over to help Jan in case her agitated patient tried to tag her again. Scolding Craig for being naughty, Jan's billion dollar personality was slowly sifting out of her. With head injury, often it would be essential that appropriate behavior be spelled out for the patient because it can be dangerous to assume that the person who has had a brain contusion can remember what's acceptable conduct and what isn't. Sometimes, even the most obvious actions need corrected.

Going on to work with one of her other patients, Jan would not tolerate Craig's antics anymore. Although therapists know it can be part of the territory with the work they do, it's still not pleasant being swatted by someone—whether the patient is aware of what they're doing or not. A fist is a fist.

Sitting in his wheelchair amidst the many patients in the back gymnasium who were either lying on mats, paired with physical terrorists doing laps about the gym, or working on exercises of some kind, Craig was trying to tear off his clothes until someone stopped him from showing up every male in the place. Craig then started looking from side to side, as if trying to look for an escape route, so he could flee. Not knowing how to get his wheelchair to move would foil this caper, however. If he could, Craig would have been scooting out of the PT gym, or at least yelling, "Get me the hell out of here."

The clanging of Nautilus machines and the sounds of anguish coming from those put through the living hell that is physical therapy would not stop Craig from sliding deep in his wheelchair to elude the uncomfortable condition of being asked to stay awake and maintain good posture.

In about the time it would take for the Michaels to digest a burgundy nightcap, Jan returned from her "time out" and barked, "Get back up there!! What do you think you're doing?"

Coaxing Craig to sit with back straight and head up, Jan tried to tell Craig the importance of maintaining good posture. Craig didn't want to hear this shit and slid back down.

With her hands open wide, Jan lifted Craig by the arm pits and placed her disgruntled patient at a position she could almost live with until he went down again like a child playing on a sliding board.

With a, "What did I just tell you about that?," Jan yanked Craig back up again despite his desire to be someplace else. Tough gal, that Jan Alba.

Although Jan didn't get much done in the way of assessing her new patient, she did at least let Craig know that he couldn't get "bad" with her without a fight. When someone's had a severe head injury, all behaviors not conducive to what is acceptable must be corrected by appropriate measures, so the patient may relearn how to behave properly. "Time out" and scolding might seem like grade school tactics, but this eighteen-year-old had done to him something that would seem impossible: Craig had reverted back to his "terrible twos."

After the conclusion of his "physical" therapy session, which was a "whimsical" therapy session for all involved, the volunteer looked at Craig's schedule tied to the wheelchair's side panel with yarn, and wheeled Craig to his next program, so he could bless the next therapist with his testiness.

A professional's professional, Carolyn Anne Joy, was preparing to evaluate Craig on this inaugural day by means of seeing whether he might respond to some inquiries. Well, Craig was revved-up and ready to go too—but not to answer questions. Rather, he wanted to "book" out of this Psychology office as quickly as the wheels on his chair could spin him away. However, Craig just better be content where he's at, for his ultimate destination would be one of struggle and devastation, if he'd not be able to meet the challenge that rehabilitation presents those unfortunate enough to experience this test of the soul.

Wanting to establish herself as the ruler of this court, Mrs. Joy found that concurrently cataloging how she wanted to proceed and distracting Craig from his ritual of tearing at his clothing would be a task which would encounter too many road blocks. Therefore, the testing which had been planned for Craig this day would not be feasible because his brain had something else in mind it wanted to do. Namely, to fidget with his clothing and be downright disagreeable.

Mrs. Joy is the type of staff psychologist every facility needs to have. She's a no-nonsense, all-business professional who demands results. Anything less will not be tolerated. The patient with a severe head injury needs this push to excel. Mrs. Joy's requirement that her patients need to "give their all," if they're going to overcome their various limitations, provides those with a brain injury the belief that recovery is more than a fictional venture. Rather, it's something that can be attained as long as one is motivated and focused. Mrs. Joy's stature of not "beating around the bush" and "shooting straight from the hip" masks her heart of gold. It's doubtful she'd want it any other way, though.

After Craig's psychological evaluation proved to be as fruitless as the initial evaluation conducted in physical therapy, the volunteer wheeled this mischievous patient back to the unit where lunch was being served. Patients who pose a risk either to themselves or others must eat on their unit under the watchful eye of staff at the nurses' station. So confused and agitated, Craig wasn't even stable enough to eat with patients, so he was taken to his room where he could slurp down his blended lunch. However, Craig would do more than eat this afternoon.

The overwhelmed nurses' aide gasped, "Oh my God, Lord have mercy!!!," when Craig peeled off his pants, displaying his massive jewels. Taking a quick second peek, the thrilled aide told Craig that doing this burlesque act wasn't proper because there's old ladies on the unit and would cause the young engaged girls visiting their fiancees to have second thoughts. Craig didn't care what she was saying, as he started to pull his Aerosmith "Draw the Line" T-shirt over his head.

Why Craig felt the need to crawl out of his clothing could only be left to speculation. More than likely, it was a response to his mind perceiving reality as a kaleidoscope of confusion, a mounting frenzy, and something no longer understood. Craig didn't know what anything was or meant, he didn't have any idea what was going on. Most everything he had learned and experienced before the accident was now gone. It was an amnesia caused by his brain being bounced around in his skull. Craig's eyes told the haunting story of one who could sense that things were turned upside down and was terrified by this state of lost comprehension.

For those in Ranchos Scale #4, the world is a confusing place where sparsely anything is known or remembered; but still the person wrapped in this torment senses that things are gravely wrong with them. And it's this realization that things aren't right and the inability to do anything about it which manufactures this scale's characteristic agitation. It's this very process of realization, however, that shows the brain still has capability. And possibly one capability will be to reprogram the brain to find that which it has been robbed.

Despite a lack of cooperation, the aide was able to reprogram Craig's brain to the point where he ate a pretty big lunch, which was a satisfactory accomplishment despite Craig's less-than-amiable table manners. Not much else was, but at least Craig's appetite showed spurts of returning. Hopefully, Craig's Communication Skills therapist had a refreshing break as well, for Craig's agitation showed no signs of letting up anytime soon. As a matter of fact, it seemed to escalate as the day progressed.

A short jaunt down the hallway, the volunteer gladly dropped his "peeved" passenger off in front of the Communication Skills offices where Craig's communicative abilities were supposed to be gauged. Supposed to be.

After Vicki phoned once from the reception desk—signaling that the patient has arrived, Diane Rosato came out of her office and felt a sickening twinge of remorse when she saw the young man she was scheduled to work with slumped in his wheelchair, not cognizant of anything. In her soft-spoken, yet persuasive voice, Diane introduced herself and invited Craig into her office, so that they could begin their work.

Humming one of his favorite tunes from the 60's, Bob Jacisin, the Director of the Communication Skills Department, came high-stepping out of his office. In his patented, high-spirited/good-natured fashion, said, "Hi, I'm Bob," to the patient who would be participating in his program. Assuring Craig of his luck having a therapist of Diane's excellence working with him, this affable director tried to put Craig at ease. However, as was the case in his two previously scheduled programs, what Craig would do this day could hardly be classified as "work."

In a voice colored with empathy, Diane placed a book full of pictures on the tabletop of Craig's wheelchair, asking him to identify what the objects were. Having had enough of "Think and Do" books in grammar school, Craig promptly swiped the book to the floor, looking through Diane with his harrowing gaze as if to send the message, "Leave me alone."

Immediately, Diane told Craig how improper this was, but Craig couldn't care less, as he swished back his bangs before falling forward mumbling something which sounded like, "No." In response to Diane's reprimand, Craig restlessly started kicking and tugging at his restraints.

Hearing Craig speak that one word showed Diane someone once was in that broken body, but her attempts to have Craig elicit anything more was met with increasing rowdiness.

Seeing that it doesn't take much to provoke Craig, Diane didn't want to push her luck on this first day she had with him, so her initial evaluation with the Patient from Hell concluded without much fanfare. Craig's inability/lack of cooperation working with Diane was indicative of just how deranged his thought processes had become for, if Diane is not the most quality-laden human being on the planet, she's at the very least in the Top Ten. She's one of those rare breeds who's as gorgeous on the inside as she is out.

Putting her materials away, Diane also let Craig know they would resume this testing whenever he settles down. No one knows when, or even if that will occur, but his next scheduled therapist would soon find out that the mellowing process was not going to evolve in her time with Craig, either.

Craig made his entrance into Occupational Therapy unable to sit still; reminiscent of when he was a little boy and his first grade teacher used to get irritated with him for having "ants in his pants." As if trying to get the message across that he doesn't want bothered anymore, just left alone, Craig cried out in an irritated fashion just like one would expect a person with an emotional maturity of a five-year old to behave when they don't get their way.

Despite his way of pleading to get away from him, Craig's therapist—Wendy Wood—rolled up her sleeves like a surgeon might in the operating room and approached her patient with caution, for this patient's agitation was not showing any signs of easing any and had been documented in the medical records as being unpredictable. After Wendy's brief introduction of herself, Ann Stuart, OTR, and Stephanie Waclo, COTA, the task of measuring the angle which Craig's right arm was rigidly contracted was set to begin. However, with the condition Craig's in now, being "set to begin" and actually beginning are two different things.

In a not-too-passive manner, Craig started yanking at the restraints on his wheelchair and in a tone smutted with anger, mumbled something not in accord with the English language. Craig's attempts to escape from his wheelchair and out from under his clothing proved to be a frustrating experience, making him that much more irritable.

Wendy rushed over to her crazed patient when Craig decided to stick some unattended crayons in his mouth, left there earlier by another patient. By rapidly tossing and turning, Craig let Wendy know he didn't approve of his personal space being invaded when she approached him.

Regardless, Wendy didn't want any blue, green, red, and purple drawing pencils clogging Craig's digestive system, so she took them from his weakened grip. Craig couldn't defecate on his own as it was, and having a couple of Crayolas caught in the wrong angle on their way out might cause him to pass an interesting colored gas, but wouldn't do anything for his irregularity. Being that the Occupational Therapy room was on the unit, those sitting at the nurses' station got a bird's eye view of the terror Craig's head injury has turned him into.

Ranting and raving with a fury normally reserved for a vagrant denied, Craig just would not listen to his therapists as they attempted to stop this hiatus of sanity. All these professionals could do with this thundering bull was keep their fingers crossed the posey on Craig's wheelchair wouldn't come off somehow. If that were to happen, Craig wouldn't be a threat so much to those around him, rather, to himself, for he couldn't stand and would fall, possibly snapping his broken leg again.

Wendy, who looks at least ten years younger that her age, has this feature about her face where it looks as if she's going to break down in tears any second. This look is deceiving, however, for her approach to treatment and the work she does with her patients is one where she not only is sincere and knowledgeable, but also easily made to smile and can laugh with the best of them. However, no cackling would be heard this day for Craig's conduct was no laughing matter. Maybe that was a tear sneaking down Wendy's face after all. Nah, just sweat from an honest day's work.

The RN came in prepared to give Craig his prescribed medications—Dilantin 100 mg TID—already diluted in water, when Craig took a swing and knocked the plastic cup from her hands after he managed to break from the posey which strapped him in. When the cup hit the floor and water splashed on this older nurse's leg, she didn't let Craig get away with this without a good lecture about how he needs this medicine to calm his brain down, so that he doesn't have a seizure and can be more tolerant to those who want to help him.

Not listening, Craig was off in his other realm, a conscience deflated of any conception of what's proper and what isn't. The acrimony born by this medley of puzzling perceptions had a damning hold of Craig, as it was screaming inside of him to be unleashed from the struggle within. Not having the capability to cast out these demons, Craig's agitation was the response of a mind looted of all understanding.

On this day where Craig made a debacle of his initial evals, he must have been smudged with suffering being unable to do the simplistic tasks asked of him and not knowing why. Despite their calm and understanding approach with him, Craig's resistance towards his therapists got worse after apparently identifying these strangers as responsible for his pain. Associating his maze of heightened frustration with these professionals who made him realize basic tasks were impossible, Craig would be steaming.

Like a haunted house where each step brings one closer to an unknown terror, Craig's rehabilitation would be an expedition where a discovery of limitations would abound from out of nowhere. Emotions darkening as if the candle of bright expectations had been blown out and relegated to a wick dying a smoldering demise, Craig would need to reach deep within himself to prevail.

Clinging to an illusion of a spirit not eroded, the Meyers felt as if they were being singed by the licking flames of Hell when they saw Craig hunched over in his wheelchair. Devastated from not knowing what anything represented or how he came about being exposed to this state, Craig's mind and its functions have been erased by attrition. Amazed at the power the brain has over every function in the body, Mr. and Mrs. Meyers looked at their non-responsive boy, unsure of how to properly go about withstanding the oscillation characteristic of this disability. When a single passageway of the many networks within the brain has been disrupted, one's physical, emotional, and cognitive self atrophies; leaving the person with the severe head injury experiencing utter destruction. As well as the family.

Feeling every ounce of his son's pain, Mr. Meyers went over to Craig and delicately tried to loosen the spasticity of his right arm, and have Craig open his hand up from the clenched fist he always holds it in. Both Craig's right elbow and fingers were like they had been set in cement. Because of this, Craig has to use his unaffected, non-dominant left hand for everything.

Eyes half-shut, tired from this first day of rehabilitation where a rude awakening of some of his symptoms had occurred, Craig flinched and let out a moan after his dad spread the fingers on his right hand ever so slightly. It was clear to this tearful father that therapy was going to take its toll on Craig and the family.

Craig would soon learn this rehabilitation is a painful process on the body, soul, and mind. The old adage, "No pain, no gain," is something Craig's going to learn all too well. By dusk, Craig will also be reminded just how humiliating being rendered helpless can be.

Rolled to his side posing in the Sim's left lateral posterior position, Craig's eyes bulged as the cold Fleet fluid was squirted, hitting its target with marksman's accuracy. Even with the curtain drawn, the Meyers could barely stomach what was happening to their son whose bowels were singing the parsimonious blues. The sound emanating from behind the cloak was similar to that of pistons pumping in an engine not in need of lubrication.

This slurping, swishing noise told the story of plastic gloves digging deeper in the anal canal searching for feces that are not going to be pushed out by the bowels because the brain isn't getting the signal that it's time to go. Subsequently, the brain should send a message to the bowels that it's time to disperse the troops and empty out. However, if a bruise on the brain inhibits this message from being received and sent, the bowels will need some help getting this poison out. It's essential that the body regularly gets rid of its waste by whatever means necessary. Craig being subjected to this once a day was a humbling experience to say the least.

An adolescent, in particular, is very conscientious of their body image and demands anything done to or with their body remain private. Whether it be a Fleet enema that gets squirted up his asshole by a stranger or his inability to make sense of a puzzle any four-year-old could piece together, knowing him like they do, the Meyers had no doubt Craig's helplessness made him feel disgraceful. This was one reason why, when they worked with Craig on the fundamental tasks of speech, memory, and recognition, Mr. and Mrs. Meyers were very careful not to further humiliate him, for these symptomatic incapabilites surely are seeds to his irritability.

The Meyers, held hostage by the fear that Craig's struggle with his cognitive lapses will stalemate—leaving him with the functional abilities of a fetus—interpreted the abbreviated animation in his face to mean that he would be capable of answering a few questions. After spending a least a couple hours every day with his parents since being hurt, surely a part of Craig's increased alertness was due to seeing his parents at 5:00 P.M. for the first time today. For sure, Craig knows there's no way on God's good earth he's ever going to be abandoned by those who would sacrifice everything to have a fraction of Craig's old self return.

The Meyers asked Craig how his first day of rehab went, with Craig letting this question pass by without so much as a gesture he heard them. And an answer would not be forthcoming when they asked what he worked on today in therapy. Craig not saying anything might have well have been his answer.

Because he's hardly a wizard when it comes to remembering names, Mr. Meyers allowed his wife to quiz Craig about who his therapists are. "Craig, today was your first day of rehab at Harmarville," Mrs. Meyers said, "tell me who your Communication Skills therapist is, she's real nice."

"And a real 'looker' too," Mr. Meyers interjected, "I'd never forget her name."

Sitting up a little more in his wheelchair and giving the footplate a little kick, Craig seemed to be processing what was asked of him. Craig pushed back his straight hair and then gazed towards the window, fixating on nothing in particular outside for several moments before assuming his state where it almost seemed like he was in a trance. Apparently, Craig forgot he had been asked a question.

Not allowing Craig to vanish from this state where his attention—momentarily at least—seemed to be directed in the "Here and Now," Mrs. Meyers gave it another shot. "Honey, who's the therapist that is going to work with you on your speech and writing? She's real pleasant."

"She's a real pretty Italian," Mr. Meyers reiterated right before his wife elbowed him.

Inhaling lightly, Craig muttered in a voice deserted of its strength, "Diehn." Sporting broad smiles, Mr. and Mrs. Meyers ecstatically let Craig know he was right.

Waiting for Craig to catch his breath, Mrs. Meyers then asked, "Now, who's your physical therapist? She's real nice too."

With the welt on his chest still smarting, Mr. Meyers knew he wasn't about to comment anymore about Craig's therapists' looks so he added, "She seems to be someone you can have fun with; easy to make laugh. I see her in the hallway, and she's always smiling."

Taking another shallow breath, Craig let the name, "Jahn," roll from his lips.

With sheer excitement, Mrs. Meyers applauded enthusiastically, letting Craig know he was on the money again. Holding a pop can he used as a makeshift spittoon, Mr. Meyers celebrated by delivering a splashing, spirited shot of chaw in the tobacco stained saliva which floated about in the container.

With heart racing, Mrs. Meyers asked, "Can you tell me the name of your psychologist? She's real smart and wears glasses. She really seems to know her stuff."

"You better listen to her or you'll catch hell," Mr. Meyers alluded.

Looking at his parents as if to say, "Enough is enough," Craig said in the tone of a whisper, "Missuhs Joi."

With a flurry of adrenalin rushing through her body, an ecstatic Mrs. Meyers cried out, "That's right Craig!! Mrs. Joy's your psychologist!!"

Entering the room amid the excitement, Scott made his solo appearance this day quizzing Craig further. "I don't care who Mrs. Joy is," Scott said in his foghorn voice, "but who's that real pretty nurse with the healthy body pushing the food cart, Craig?" As was the case when he was healthy, Craig didn't pay any mind to his brother.

Before they got to asking Craig about his Occupational Therapist, the Meyers stopped because Craig was beginning to get fussy in his wheelchair, indicating he had had enough for today. He'd had a long day, but there was more to come. A lot more.

After eating only a few bites of his dinner, Craig looked like he was preparing to mount an attack. Shelled by a fusillade of chaos, Craig started shuffling violently from side to side in his wheelchair, slowing down only because his father was able to stabilize him by the shoulders. But Craig didn't give up without a counterattack.

With his only good arm, for but a few seconds, Craig was able to break free from his dad's stronghold, resuming his wavering as if to avoid being captured again. Craig's combativeness, triggered by a brain which perceives everything as a threat, was a response to his being flanked by misery when kept from his perceptual motion.

In these instances when Craig would swell with emotion, his parents wanted to throw a net over him. Until he was given his sedatives, Mr. and Mrs. Meyers knew things would get worse before they got better, as Craig would get more irritable as the day progressed. Possibly, this is the brain's way of showing it wants its sedatives, for it had been awhile since the last one went through Craig's system.

Besieged by his world of delusion, Craig would erupt with the speed and fury of a blitzkrieg. The emotional demolition of Craig's parents left them feeling as if they had been stoned by an enfilade of rancor terrorists.

But as they always had, these fighters were able to get back up after this failed lapidation of their will, and brush themselves off for the next duel. With life as they once knew it hijacked by Craig's need for them, the Meyers devotion and commitment had long ago transformed into one where they were prisoners of their own obligation.

Seeing Craig's aggressive reaction to being trapped in a cage of infirmities where his emotions have been ruthlessly transfixed, the nurses' aide made a suggestion that will live in infamy. She erroneously believed that the warm water of the shower would have a soothing effect on Craig; that the pulsating streams of water coupled with his feeling clean would calm him. It did nothing of the sort.

Never satisfied with how he was situated, whether it be the way he was sitting in his wheelchair or lying in bed, Craig started scattering "this way and that" when the nurses' aides—in unison—let the guardrails down on both sides of his bed. Leery from experience, this battered patient must have known he was about to be pounced upon. Craig had been given sponge baths when he was at Allegheny General and these first days at Harmarville, but "zero-hour" had arrived for that first shower.

With a tad bit of hesitation on Craig's part and difficulty on theirs, the nurses' aides were able to get the suspicious patient out of his street clothes and into a gown. Because the chore of unbuckling Craig's pants, whipping down his fly, and sliding his jeans over that colossal bulge would be time-consuming, Mrs. Meyers was told to bring sweat pants for Craig tomorrow when they come in.

Because of the unrelieved weight of Craig's body, it always took two people to transfer him. After Craig was placed on the shower chair—which looked like a toilet seat with wheels—one of the nurses' aides had to attend to her other patients, leaving Mrs. Meyers as the "Chosen One" for shower duty.

It wasn't long after the warm water poured on his naked body that Craig reacted to this perceived incursion in a manner which one would think he was being impaled by a bayonet, and not gently sprayed with warm water which normally has a relaxing effect on somebody. But the perceptions of an injured brain are anything but normal.

Choking, coughing, and gagging on the streams of water, Craig was told to hold his breath while his hair was being washed. But he couldn't, he didn't know how. Craig actually forgot how to do something as simple as holding his breath. Asking an injured brain to recall things it used to do automatically is anything but simple.

Surely feeling embarrassed that two women were with him in the shower seeing him in his birthday suit while spitting up water, Craig took the offensive. For Craig, it was more like a counteroffensive. Being seized by these droplets of water, Craig's mission was to fight off these watery predators until they stopped their irruptive siege.

Like the "Wicked Witch of the West" in the Wizard of Oz, Craig must have felt like he was melting in this soapy bastille, as his vexation reached unruly proportions. Not expecting to do a Jacques Cousteau impersonation on her visit with Craig this day, Mrs. Meyers' nice blouse got drenched when—during this shower assignment she got volunteered for—her uluating son would fling his arm at the water which then splashed all over her and the nurses' aide. All decked out and soaked to the bone, this waterlogged mother would have an idea how those on the Titanic must have felt on that last fateful luxury cruise.

For two and one-half weeks, very little changed in Craig's condition, as the vice grip Ranchos #4 had on him made it impossible for Craig to do the computer work and physical exercises necessary to reprogram his brain. During this time, Craig continued to be subordinate to the confusion and agitation which infiltrated his mind.

In Occupational Therapy for instance, Craig would continually stick puzzle pieces, sugar packs, and his favorite snack—crayons—in his mouth, chewing on these items as if trying to eat them. As if a hole had been drilled in his conscience and drained of its recognition of proper conduct, Craig's attempts at striptease in Physical Therapy, Psychology, and Communication Skills were not welcome and all too frequent, as was his tendency to float off into the "Great Beyond."

In his bedroom, Craig engaged in a variety of strange behaviors which indicated just how agitated he was. When asked to withstand sitting in his wheelchair, Craig would become irritably restless; weaving from side to side and then back and forth, kicking his footplate the whole time. On at least one occasion, Craig tore down the draperies from its rod. Unable to lie in one set position for more than a few seconds at a time, twisting and turning in his bed had become one of Craig's favorite pastimes since his senses had been taken from him. Participating in sports must have been something Craig was missing, for when he would be handed a cup of water to take with his Dilantin, he would play "Punt, Pass, and Kick." And, of course, Craig wouldn't limit his stripping to times when he was supposed to.

This was a time when, on Craig's first weekend at the rehab, obviously not doing her homework by reading the medical records, a substitute nurses' aide got upset with Craig for some reason and angrily demanded that he stand up. If Mrs. Meyers hadn't been there to inform her of Craig's fractured femur when this aide was "laying the law," Craig would have snapped his leg again. Possibly losing it, if the artery had split open.

Harmarville stresses to the family of the patient who has had a head injury not to baby them, allow them to try things without maximum assistance, so independence may be facilitated. There's going to be times when Craig fails and he'll get frustrated, but this trial and error learning is part of the process when retraining the brain how to do things again.

Wanting to see how much athleticism Craig had left in him, Mr. Meyers rolled up a sock and started tossing Craig this improvised ball. Not positioned in the infield, rather in his wheelchair, Craig caught the sock with surprising consistency. His ability to catch was unexpected, for Craig's coordination had been erratic—at best—in most everything else he did since the accident. Overall, his movements looked as if they were played in slow motion and required a lot of concentration. But the relative ease with which Craig caught the sock with his left hand was astounding. If you got it, you got it.

This sock-tossing was not only something Craig seemed to enjoy, but distracted him from that which was annoying him. Lessening his agitation, this diversion tactic—as well as the interactions with his family—at least brightened Craig's spirits some. Maybe Craig's better mood had something to do with his improved formation of sentences.

One month after he was hurt—March 14—Craig coaxed, "Stand me up, dad." This was indicative of Craig's being so heavily sedated he could not feel that his leg had been broken as well as just how poorly his thinking and memory were, for it had been explained to Craig not all that long ago why he couldn't bear weight on his right leg. Despite this irrational request where their son was devoid of any memory, the Meyers were ecstatic that what came out of Craig's mouth was something other than moans of pain. Maybe staff here at Harmarville have been getting through to Craig somewhat.

Also on this day, Craig's attempts to feed himself were not successful. Although not comfortable seeing their son struggle while he tried to get some food in his rapidly thinning body, the Meyers abided by Harmarville staff's instructions not to do everything for Craig, as they would watch him labor with his silverware. This was the first time Craig tried to eat solid food, and his initial attempt to feed himself without being guided step-by-step. The Meyers couldn't believe what they were about to see.

Holding his fork or spoon with his left hand, sometimes Craig would do okay. But on others, he'd take the food up to his mouth without opening it and ram the food into his closed lips or just beneath his nose. When this didn't work, Craig'd try again doing the exact same thing with identical results.

Other times, Craig would scoop up his food with great difficulty, only to dump it either on the floor or on his lap. At least on these occasions, Craig had his mouth open.

There were times when Craig would take a swipe at an empty space on the plate or make a stab at some meat, when there was no meat to be stabbed. On other occasions, Craig would take his silverware loaded with food and hold it at eye level and just leave it there in mid-air as if contemplating what to do next. And there would be instances when Craig would not chew his food thoroughly enough and when he'd swallow, he would choke then hiccup for what seemed forever.

Bringing the eating utensil towards the top of his head as if to dump it, Craig would then stop knowing this wasn't what he wanted to do. Despite being obviously flustered by his inability to do something he was trained to do as a toddler, always having been the type of person not opposed to a challenge, Craig would take another crack at getting something in his belly. Usually, to no avail, however.

With a look of anger, Craig would try again to master this complicated sequence of events where he is to get the food on the silverware, bring the food up to his mouth, open his mouth, put the food in his mouth, clamp his mouth shut, slide the silverware out while the closed passageway dumps the food on his tongue, situate the food over his teeth, and chew the food before swallowing. Then, taking the silverware down and repeating this chain of events. Unbelievably, Craig had more difficulty doing this than he had taking the S.A.T. a year earlier.

Craig's brain being injured actually made him forget the process of how to go about "munching" down some food. The steps for eating normally come automatically, but for Craig, his automatic pilot must have ejected when it saw the Volkswagen heading for the telephone pole. In the meantime, Craig's mom was going to inconspicuously slip her son a few bites until he learns how to chew and swallow all over again.

"All over again." These words would be heard time and time and time again by Mr. and Mrs. Meyers when they'd ask at what level was Craig going to have to relearn many of the tasks which he—only a month ago—took for granted and did without giving it a second thought.

Knowing something wasn't right, for the first time, Craig looked at his parents and asked in a voice tarnished with sorrow, "What's wrong with me?"

Fighting back the tears hearing his son's pain, Mr. Meyers explained to his boy for the one-hundred twenty-fifth time what happened to him. Gazing at the ground with his hollow stare, Craig seemed to be taking in what his father was telling him this time, however.

Much of Craig's ability to grasp and operate in this world now hinged upon the development of neurological connections not yet discovered. The healing of the brain, known as spontaneous recovery, has an immeasurable impact on how well the person rebounds from a brain injury. And this is where the miraculous work of God comes in. And God's switchboard operator was being inundated with prayers on Craig's behalf.

On March 17, Reverend Dennis Davenport—one of the ministers of the Church of the Covenant where Craig's a member—came to Harmarville to see Craig. The reverend had never experienced anything like this in his life.

Seeing people in wheelchairs oblivious to everything around them, screaming out as if an attack had been launched by Hades' demons—even before setting eyes on Craig—the young minister knew that if this youthful member of his congregation was in a facility which treated patients this bad off, Craig must have been pillaged of his health as well.

Swamped by the "get well" cards sent to him by friends and family taped to his closet, Craig bowed his head with Reverend Davenport and—amazingly—remembered the Lord's Prayer, reciting it in his mumbled voice with this clergyman.

God had a task on his hands revitalizing Craig. From Craig's family, friends, and Dr. Harold H. McConnell, Jr.—senior pastor at the church—who saw Craig when he was in intensive care, to the Michaels who didn't want Paul to go to jail, the prayers came pouring in from the very beginning that Craig be spared.

The most difficult thing about this trip to Harmarville for Rev. Davenport was seeing so many young people hurt so badly. From limbs that have been severed to spines that were contorted, viewing so many people with debilitating afflictions made this man of the cloth appreciate what he had that much more.

When Craig would become overly spunky, unable to keep from messing with his clothes and not being able to remain content for more than twenty seconds at a time, that's when Scott would begin throwing Craig a rolled up sock in order to keep Craig's mind from being eaten away with agitation. Although not delirious about his continued irritability, the Meyers were quite pleased with the improvement in Craig's speech, however.

Before they left on the evening of the eighteenth, for example, Craig asked his parents to bring his guitar tomorrow. Seeing the fingers of his right picking hand stiff from paralysis, as if they had been plastered with mortar, Craig's parents had their reservations about this request. Because Craig was adamant that he have his Montayo, Mr. and Mrs. Meyers ran this wish by the nursing staff who said that Craig's inability to even hold a pick will really light his fuse.

But since Craig was so insistent, the nurses thought that maybe bringing it for one day and letting Craig see that he doesn't have the dexterity to play effectively anymore might just be the spark he needs to get him working in therapy. Craig's parents were just hoping this spark wouldn't ignite an inferno of dismay which could not be put out.

With the sand of the hourglass their menacing foe, the Meyers were not yet ready to read an elegy where their son had perished to the villain which is time.

These bruised, but not beaten, knights were not about to lament the loss of a battle where those that stand triumphantly in the winner's circle have yet to be determined.

Boring a hole in their hopes of a retirement blossoming with serenity, the Meyers' grief was fueled by the thought of what a boy's warped self- deception that invincibility was a given had done to their lives and their son's. After Craig's pursuit of happiness was ransacked, the Meyers' life has been thoroughly wrung of any pleasure.

Since Craig's cataclysmal brush with death, his irascibility and ability to make sense of things were spinning in a state of quandary. But the thing about Harmarville which sets it apart from your average rehabilitation center is its people. The therapists, nurses, doctors, administrators, receptionists, and volunteers all wanted to do what they could to help Craig feel as good about himself as he possibly could, and tried their best to understand what he was going through.

Usually greeted with a smile and always treated with respect, these professionals took an authentic interest in Craig. Seeing that Mr. and Mrs. Meyers were quality people and reading the brief—yet concise—scrapbook Mrs. Meyers took the time to put together about Craig, those at Harmarville knew they had something to work with. Because of staff's legitimate concern, patients being treated by these caring professionals normally wouldn't want to disappoint their therapists and will therefore bust their tail in order to progress.

Despite the only thing Craig wanted to bust at this time was everyone's jaw, those that worked with him did not approach Craig in a fashion where he was a master of mutilation and dean of destruction, rather, in a way where Craig could sense he was accepted. Needing work, but accepted.

This feeling of acceptance that Craig had fruitlessly sought for so long and wanted so badly was finally captured. Albeit, a lot of it was unconditional positive regard being that Craig was a chore to be around. But these experienced professionals knew that this wasn't the real Craig; that the real Craig was somebody that could be approached and a person one could be friendly with.

And the fascinating part was Craig didn't have to act like someone he wasn't to be liked by these therapists. You couldn't convince Craig of this, but there wasn't anything about him that you wouldn't like up until he was hurt—except maybe the multitude of pimples which painted his face for so many years. But even the zits were now gone because something in the intravenous medications Craig was taking while in a coma somehow dried these molehills up. Now, if someone could clear up his right hemiparesis, the various aphasias, and his agitation; that would be an accomplishment!!! Well, at least they're working on it.

These rehabilitation craftsmen were empathetic, yet, knew where the line was to be drawn as far as what they would put up with. Children need the security and WANT the security of knowing who the boss is. If kids sense their caregiver is not in charge—that they are the ones running the show —limits are never going to stop being tested then.

And those with a severe head injury are—in many ways—just like children, for they too frequently need definition of what they should and shouldn't do/what they can and can't get away with. Proceeding with their ever-present professionalism, Harmarville's staff not only was going to attempt to re-educate Craig's mind cognitively and body motor skills-wise, but needed to demonstrate proper social etiquette by instruction and being an example for Craig.

From the guilt one felt for crossing the always smiling/radiant Diane Rosato, to the embarrassment one would experience making Wendy Wood's laugh a growl, patients with a head injury would know their actions were not appropriate based on these role models' reactions. When Jan Alba's voice dropped an octave, one knew that they better run for cover or—at the very least—get their wheelchair rolling, if running's not possible. When Mrs. Joy's eyebrows raised, the person with that head injury knew that they had done something that wasn't right, and just better hope she's in a good mood and doesn't torture them with one of her timed tests.

Despite Craig's inability to do much in the way of participating in the various therapies, he was still progressing. Being bombarded with positive interactions by the therapists during rehabilitation and the nurses when Craig was back in his room was very therapeutic, for it brought a sense of reality to him that was eradicated. Also, because Craig is young, his brain upstairs is working as hard as it can to heal. For the Meyers, who have had their optimism obliterated too many times to keep score, the return of functions that were undone couldn't happen quick enough.

The remainder of the month of March would be one where the brightness of anticipation would be darkened by the hemorrhaging of forfeited dreams. Greeted by light's promising glow the next moment, this cycle appeared as if it would bleed eternal. Such is the case when one has had a severe closed head injury. And Craig was no different.

As promised, the Meyers did bring Craig's guitar the next day and—as they expected—this one-time solid musician became distraught when discovering he had forgotten how to play. Playing the easiest of songs would have been an achievement of immaculate proportions for Craig now. Confused, Craig looked at the fingerboard as if he had never seen a guitar before in his life. Not only did he not know how to finger any chords and was unable to strike single notes because of his wrist's rigidity, Craig could not even pinch his pick. Seeing his struggling son drop his pick to the floor repeatedly, a jack of all trades and master of most, Mr. Meyers got an idea for an invention.

One day during this fateful month, Craig was so insistent he and the family go to Myrtle Beach, he was getting mad they couldn't go at that very moment, leaving behind this rehab bullshit. Because Craig had never been there before, therefore, didn't have any prior eventful experience there, the Meyers could only guess that he heard someone talk about going and decided he wanted to go, too.

On another day, Craig begged one of the volunteers to push his wheelchair to Canonsburg where, supposedly, Craig would hitch a ride the rest of the way to Washington. Now, that would be an interesting sight for someone going down Route 79; seeing a rowdy patient being pushed fifty miles along the highway by a guy in a red blazer.

Craig told his mom one night that a fellow patient on the unit was a "grouch" because "he never talks to me." Craig didn't understand when his mom told him that this older man had a stroke and couldn't talk. And the reason it looks like he always has a scowl on his face is because the stroke atrophied his facial muscles.

Because he'd traditionally draw attention to himself after being pushed to the T.V. room where several other patients would already be sitting in front of the sets, these "couch potatoes" wouldn't exactly be gleeful that Craig had arrived. As the television's flickering light would reflect off his face—in a few minutes' time—Craig would either become such a disturbance, that one of the more functional patients would wheel him back to his room because they couldn't hear their program. Either that, or Craig would become so sedated, he'd fall asleep right away.

Countless Fleet enemas and bed pans full of enema-induced fecal matter later, Craig's bowels were still not working on their own. Mom and Dad Meyers' clothing would continue to be vandalized on a regular basis, as Craig wouldn't stop yanking them down towards him on their visits. The horde of ties Mr. Meyers got for Christmas were sure coming in handy now and Mrs. Meyers started digging in the spare closet for some backup blouses, for the necks of all her good ones had been stretched beyond repair.

Being that Craig's roommate wasn't nearly as critical as he was and didn't want bothered, Craig's exposure to this dark-haired West Virginian was minimal. Craig discovered soon after his admission that if he wanted to move his spastic right hand, he'd have to lift it with his left. And Craig's physical problems weren't only limited to those that had been diagnosed at Washington and Allegheny General Hospitals for—during his examination of Craig—Harmarville's internist, Dr. Milas Zernich, discovered Craig had a "spiked" liver. And, socially, Craig was still acting as if he were a Hell's Angel.

Craig's head injury didn't prevent him from knowing every vulgarity in the book, however. Being that Craig never swore in front of his parents, his cussing antics came as a surprise to them. If and when Craig was disturbed by a sound sleep, told to go to therapy, or to bend over because it was enema time, it would not be beneath him to tell the person to go "Fuck off" or to call them a "Son of a Bitch." Taunted with hatred, anger, and fear, Craig would often just be sitting in his wheelchair out in the nurses' station and slingshot his tasteless/foul language until one of the nurses wheeled him back to his room away from people who have some couth.

Not all was bad for Craig, however. Craig's speech was continually improving and he got to urinate on Scott. Craig was forming sentences more spontaneously with the clarity of his speech being adequate until he got tired at night. When Scott tried to help his brother guide his missile into the hand held urinal one evening when Craig was starting to soak himself, he discovered that Craig's Herculean genitals were impossible for one mere mortal to control and got an urethra shower. "Ha Ha Ha Ha Ha Ha Ha Ha Ha Ha Ha Ha Ha Ha Ha Ha Ha Ha Ha Ha Ha Ha Ha Ha Ha Ha Ha Ha Ha Ha Ha Ha Ha Ha Ha Ha Ha Ha Ha Ha Ha Ha Ha Ha Ha Ha Ha Ha Ha Ha Ha Ha Ha Ha Ha".

Rosemary, a kind-hearted, older nurses' aide whose heart went out to Craig and his family, was not immune to Craig's barrage of filth which would spew from his mouth when his brain dictated it was time to be agitated. One evening when Rosemary came in Craig's room to check on the patient she had done so much for, Craig shouted to his family who were visiting, "There's crow face!" Wanting to crawl under a rock, Mr. and Mrs. Meyers immediately apologized to this verbally abused saint who said that their apologies weren't necessary for, those who have to work with them, know that people with head injuries are bound to say anything at anytime.

With his parents staring him down, Craig knew he was in trouble, so he did what came naturally. Pointing his finger straight at Scott, Craig said to Rosemary, "He told me to say that!!"

The look in Craig's eyes, the increased clarity in his speech—and most importantly—his improved ability to express himself when he spoke, all were cues that his mind was starting to take in some of the information relayed his way and was being processed. Still drifting in and out of consciousness, the amount of time Craig was "in" was slowly increasing. Like a ship lost in the fog, the journey that is head injury rehabilitation is one where perils ahead are unforeseen and waters traveled, hazed with mystery. Since being twisted and purged of his senses, all Craig knew, understood, and remembered was clouded by this opaque mist. However, the ghostly curtain of vertigo which blanketed him was starting to rise.

Craig had improved to the point where he now was eating in the nurses' station. Although not yet in good enough condition to eat in the cafeteria, this was a big step from having his meals brought to his room.

It was suppertime and Craig was wheeled to a table where an older woman who had a stroke was sitting. Craig was but a few feet across from this patient who was going to explode any minute in a volatile rage. She couldn't have known her displaced agitation would become embedded in Craig's memory, instead of just another fleeting image in his world of translucent perceptions.

How's come this old. . . . . crazy. . . . . lady's yelling?. . . . . It looks like. . . . . she's mad. . . . . Why's she. . . . keep saying. . . . . "Christ's son,. . . . Christ's son," and. . . . pointing at me? . . . She's got a problem. . . .

I think. . . . ..she's mad at me!!. . . . I didn. . . . I didn't do anything . . . Jus' sittin' here. . . . trying to eat. . . . Never saw her . . . . . . before . . . in my life. . . . She's gonna throw. . . . her fork at me!!.. . . . . ..Oh God . . . hope somebody stops her. . . . .don't want hurt. . . .

After trying unsuccessfully to hit Craig with her silverware, this lady was stopped by the nurse, Jan Goga, LPN, before getting a chance to reload. In the short time he's been at Harmarville, Craig had formed a real nice kinship with this attractive, blonde nurse who came to his rescue on the first sign her buddy was in trouble. Jan, not wanting Craig to be a dart board anymore, wheeled the lady whose stroke-induced agitation got the better of her someplace where she couldn't crucify Christ's son. If the poor woman tormented by the CVA truly believed that Craig was who she claimed, one would think that—considering who Craig's grandfather would be then—she'd want to get on his good side and not try to use him as target practice. However, there are few on this unit who possess this type of rational thinking.

Maybe because of its heightened anxiety, this would be the first thing stored in Craig's memory banks since joshing with Wayne who would sit in the bull's-eye passenger seat that fateful February night. And/or is a sign that Craig's mind might just pull off a miracle.

The bruise on Craig's brain must be shrinking some, for Craig had the capacity to realize he had been uprooted from that which he knows and is comfortable—home.

In the long run, this is spectacular because it shows that the brain is capable of recovering. Over time, functions lost due to the contusion on the brain can be restored when—and if—healing occurs. However, it is the short-term which can push the patient to the brink of insanity.

The torture of realizing the most basic cognitive and physical functions are no longer there is unbearable and why a patient will get agitated. While the brain is in this state of inoperability, the patient is clawed by living misery. This is why, when professionals see a patient getting mean, they become paradoxically encouraged because it shows the advanced process of realization is coming back; with the definite possibility other processes will follow.

Being a patient in a rehabilitation center where disability and sickness are around every corner is not the most pleasant situation to be in. From Craig's perspective, therapy was for exposing weaknesses and humiliating the person for their shortcomings.

Craig couldn't understand why he had to be subjected to those computer games when it made him so irritable being unable to concentrate for very long. Having significant trouble tracking the horizontal and vertical lines of the simple addition and subtraction problems he couldn't figure out, Craig would get perturbed not being able to "line up" numbers and then follow them with his eyes because they'd wiggle around. Why, in PT, do they ask him to do cognitive exercises he had difficulty with—such as counting backwards and recognizing red from green—when it irks him not being able to do these things? Why don't they just teach him physical motor skills like they're supposed to, so he could walk out of this place and could catch a ride back to Washington from Canonsburg? This rehabilitation is really getting under Craig's skin. And he's going to do what he can to get out.

Trying to play on their sympathy, Craig would call his parents on the days they weren't to visit, pleading with them to please take him home away from these "meanies" who are trying to hurt him. Being a skillful arbitrator, Mrs. Meyers would try to convince her homesick son that if he wants to get better, he needs to stick where he's at and listen to his therapists, for they know how to help him with his problems.

"If you want to play that ukulele or get on the ballfield again," Mr. Meyers would say, "being here with me and your mother isn't going to help you get better. We're flattered you like us so much, but the best thing for you is to stay where you're at. You'll be back home before you know it, better than ever."

Using the psychology she'd developed in her thirty-seven years being a parent, Mrs. Meyers added, "We're not going to get you a Fender guitar, if you're not going to be able to pick it. That'd be too much money to waste."

Despite their pleas to work hard in therapy and their efforts to negotiate a treaty, Craig threatened to bust out of there and go home anyhow. And that's exactly what he tried to do—kind of.

Nobody's around. . . . .'cept my roommate . . . 'an he's sleeping.. . . . I gotta get this rail down. . . . . so I can get out. . . . .

Not being gifted mechanically—to put it mildly—interfered with Craig's attempt to get the bed rail down, so he could then hop on the get-away wheelchair in this attempt to escape. Craig did manage to get the part of the rail down nearest the head of his bed, however, but to get it unlatched at the foot of the bed was another story.

Why won't this loosen?. . . . I'm trying. . . . as hard as I can . . . . . . Need to get this down. . . . Want to go home. . . . .Don't need this place. . . . . . .

When Craig was yanking on these bars, trying to loosen them, this awakened his roommate. Amused, Craig's roommate watched, as Craig was trying to escape from his Alcatraz.

What's he laughin' about?. . . . I'm gettin' out of here. . . . He better not yell for someone. . . . What's he think's so funny?. . . . .

No, Craig's roommate wouldn't yell for anybody, but he did push the call button, so a nurse would come in the room. Obviously, even if Craig had gotten out of his bed and somehow made it to his wheelchair, what then?

Although Craig didn't know it at the time, his roommate did him a big favor by contacting the nurse. So bound and determined to get out of Harmarville, Craig forgot to take into account that he couldn't walk and—even if he could—wouldn't get far on a broken leg. Such is the jumbled rationale and decision-making of a patient who has sustained a severe head injury.

Very few things in and about this world were clear to Craig, but the fact that his vision had been affected by the head injury was a stark reality that he had to contend with every passing moment. Craig had double vision.

As the name implies, when Craig would look at a single object, he'd see two distinct, separate entities. The only way Craig could see objects as they were would be to close his left eye. He couldn't close the other because of his right hemiparesis. What was once Craig's eyesight is now the debris of a mind forever darkened.

Seeing Craig in his wheelchair or sprawled out lying in bed with his one eye closed when he wanted to look at something was a mirthless agony for his parents. Sickened by thoughts that Craig's view of the world would be forever distorted, the calamitous effects of Craig's head injury grappled the Meyers' consciousness with the control of a tyrannical ruler.

By the third week of March, Craig was just starting to feed himself solid foods and had become more amiable with many of the nurses on the unit. Although still not very cooperative in therapy much of the time because of his agitation still lingering, something must be getting through to Craig, for the frequency of his eruptions was tapering. Craig could probably sense that the people at Harmarville were special and that their objective was not to stomp on his ego or bring him to ruin, but to help him.

The rapid improvement in Craig's speech and orientation were evident to anyone who had seen the pulverized boy who was first admitted. However, there would still be days where Craig would go from Dr. Jeckyll to Mr. Hyde with little warning.

One Sunday evening, Craig's parents, brother, and lovely sister-in-law were with Craig having a nice visit. It was during this time that the Meyers saw Craig do something for the first time since he was hurt and something that they were afraid he'd never do again—he laughed.

Mr. Meyers' demeanor when he got angry was a source of humor within the family for, when he got ticked about something, he became quite animated. And animation makes for good imitation, which is what the Meyers family did when its elder statesman was less-than-mild-mannered.

When the Meyers were conducting their cognitive therapy with Craig by quizzing him about different topics—operating from his "everything has a funny angle" position—Scott asked Craig what noise dad makes when he's mad. With jaws dropped, body rigid, and eyes sternly in place, Craig growled in a pit bull-like tone, "ROAR, ROAR, ROAR, ROAR, ROAR" like the family does when they imitate his dad when he's in a sour mood. The chorus of laughter which followed was not only an expression of how funny it was seeing Craig rib his dad, but a sigh of relief that the hell Craig's going through hasn't totally annihilated his sense of humor and all his memories about the family. Despite a tangible reminder that Craig is seizure prone, a tongue depressor taped to the wall behind his bed, this was an afternoon full of joy and merriment for the Meyers.

Craig's continued improvement in his speech and recollection reassured the Meyers that their son was in the right place. Although covert, the Meyers experienced more humor this mid-day when Craig talked seriously about forming a rock band with another patient whose musical talent was as good as Craig's ability to hold a pick.

"When me and you. . . . . get outta here . . . we should form. . . . . we should form a heavy metal group. . . . .When my hand gets better in a month or so. . . . . I'll be able to jam. . . . . If you can sing. . . . if you can sing as good as you say. . . . we'll be pretty good. . . ."

Grateful for any improvement they see in Craig, the Meyers also knew that a lot more work and healing had to occur before those brain circuits would work properly. But there'd be one thing the Meyers could be sure of: Whatever force would be behind Craig's moodiness and agitation, was working just fine.

Craig was pleasant as could be during the day, but the part of the brain which activates the agitation switch decided it was time to flick this lever on come evening. Whether it was because it was later in the evening and Craig hadn't taken his brain-calming sedatives in a while, or he was tired—not wanting any kind of stimulation—the Meyers wished they would have had a restraining jacket.

Any talk or activity seemed to be disturbing Craig. When someone would move or begin speaking to Craig, this must have sent the electric currents in his brain shooting every which way in a confusing, flaming fury.

When Mr. Meyers came up to his son, Craig would push him away—saying an assortment of vulgarities—so his father wouldn't get so close. Without warning or provocation, Craig struck his mother and said in a voice blackened with spite, "I'm gonna make you bleed." In his flurry of disorientation, Craig had transformed into a disciple of hatred.

Knowing that Craig's brain injury has altered his thoughts, emotions, and perceptions to the point where he will have these spurts where he behaves like a heathen still did not alleviate Mrs. Meyers' mental anguish being hit by the son she has made countless sacrifices for. Because she mistakenly correlated Craig's improved appearance with heightened awareness of what was going on, those blows cut much deeper than the ones delivered in the hospital.

Mr. Meyers refrained from any kind of confrontation with his son, for he now has an understanding that the turbulence storming Craig's mind is not within Craig's control and that this convulsion of moral restraint is not of his own doing.

Still, based on Harmarville's recommendation that the family not spoil Craig because he's hurt and allow him to get away with inappropriate behavior, Mrs. Meyers and her lovely daughter-in-law left the room to allow Craig to think about what he did and the consequences of his action. Mr. Meyers simply let Craig know that his assault on motherhood would not be tolerated and was not appreciated.

On their "time out" from Craig, Scott's lovely wife commiserated with Mrs. Meyers to keep this trampled mother-in-law's strength from collapsing. As if held captive in the lot of perdition, Mrs. Meyers cried out how the worst thing about brain injury is the unknown and the misunderstanding.

With most other types of afflictions, what's wrong with the person is a given. However, with head injury, the behavioral aspects and the personality changes make it impossible to predict what is going to happen next when one has been cursed with this malady. This is one reason proper etiquette needs to be taught again and again. With Craig, this "time out" worked to a tee, for after pleading with the family not to go and promising to behave, Craig acted like a little angel.

Playing in the Meyers' minds is a ballad where the "ups and downs"/"downs and ups" of head injury are going to occur whether they're prepared or not. So, if they are to survive this attack when things are not as they appear, their shields of adaptation will need to be held thusly. And through it all, the Meyers have endured and adjusted the only way humanly possible to avoid having that ballad metamorphosed into a dirge which rings out their final chapter.

Craig's cognitive abilities and mood would fluctuate between the good, the bad, and the indifferent at any given moment. Sometimes his demeanor would change in a matter of a few minutes. One moment, Craig might be as passive as a cuddly kitten, the next, he thinks he's Julius Caesar.

Craig's ability to do the cognitive exercises of matching, discerning, counting, etc. would occasionally show some signs of life, only to die from expunction by the time he got to his next program because his ability to concentrate had evaporated. However, Craig's recognition of his parents and some of their hardships was floating to the surface of his consciousness from the dark fathoms of the deep unknown.

Showing the advanced process of empathy, where one is able to comprehend another person's feelings and/or situation, Craig asked one of the nurses if his dad would have to bear the brunt of all costs of his rehabilitation and hospitalization, or would the insurance pick it up. Because of the extensive health care coverage in his dad's policy, Craig was told that things were being taken care of and not to worry.

When they made their appearance in the lobby for their visit, seeing Mr. and Mrs. Meyers smile when they saw Craig waving to them that first time was a sight the nurses on the unit would cherish. Like their predecessors at Allegheny General, these parents were well-liked and respected for their dedication to their son. Also, it showed Craig's increased sensitivity and recognition to his environment.

Craig's brain being disrupted resulted in his having severe sequential deficits, but this waiting in the lobby for his parents was a sign that this was improving by leaps and bounds.

To be waiting for his folks, the brain has to develop a series of steps which require the advanced process of organization. First, Craig would have to recall the evening when families can visit. Second, Craig'd have to know the day and correlate this with it being a time he gets to spend with his family. Also, he would have to remember what hour the family is to arrive and where they come in. Then Craig would have to plan on allowing enough time to be wheeled to the nurses' station where he would greet his parents. And, if they would be seeing Craig this visiting day—which they always did, guaranteed.

This process, SEQUENCE of events, would occur automatically for someone whose brain had not been shuffled like a lottery ball. But for Craig, whose jackpot number came up 9-1-1 one night in the middle of February, his waiting for his parents was indicative that his brain was doing some remarkable things up there. However, not all was going according to plan. It rarely does with head injury.

Unbelievably, a brain injury will cause certain body parts to assume an unnatural position. Like Craig's upper arm contracted under his chin, his right heel cord was starting to bend in the opposite direction it should. It goes without saying that if the angle of Craig's toes are beneath his heel—which is exactly where they were headed—he not only couldn't walk, but couldn't stand either. This is a condition which would restrict Craig to a bed for the rest of his life. Anybody who knew Craig, realized this would not be an option.

Sometimes this unnatural physiological bend requires a doctor to purposely break a bone, so that the limb can be reset. Fortunately for Craig, this was caught in time, so he would not have to have his right ankle popped by having the top of his foot—in essence—sledgehammered.

A physical examination was conducted and it was determined that Craig needed to wear a splint on his right leg all night, every night when he went to bed. The purpose of this hard plastic splint which extends from about the middle of his thigh to underneath his heel was to prevent Craig's foot from sinking anymore than it already had.

This condition that could have an everlasting impact on Craig is known as "drop foot," where the muscles in the foot quickly atrophy which results in the toe of the foot pointing downward and is common to those who have been in a coma. Later in life, this muscle weakness makes it difficult for the person to place their heel on the ground before the anterior part of the foot which creates a "slapping" type of effect when the person walks. Both the front and back portions of the foot hit the ground at the same time because the muscles have little strength to lift the front of the foot up, undertaking the action needed for rolling on the ball of the foot. But Craig's foot descent was far from the Meyers' greatest concern. What they wouldn't give to see Craig hop out of bed right now and slap that right foot while taking a few steps.

Because of the length of the splint, Craig could not bend his knee, making the discomfort impossible for him to fall asleep. The weight, bulk, and heat of the padded splint didn't help matters either. Although his fracture was above the knee, the femur, this added burden on Craig's broken leg was not soothing.

"Please take the splint off . . . . it hurts . . . . . I can't get to sleep . . . . I don't know why I've gotta wear this . . . I can't bend my knee . . . . I need to talk to Amayo . . . get him out of bed!"

Sometimes a compassionate nurse would take off Craig's splint for a couple of minutes to relieve the discomfort, hoping this would help him to get to sleep. Others, going strictly by the book, would tell Craig they can't take it off because this would be against doctor's orders. If Craig didn't get the help he wanted from one nurse, he'd ring in another with the call button, so he could try again.

On this last weekend in March, Craig's lucidity was continuing its ascent. Each time his parents came in now, Craig would smile and wave to them which made their hearts warm.

On Saturday, Craig spoke clearly all day about a variety of meaningful topics. Among them, Craig repeated his desire to go home and learning to drive the Citation. Heart pounding furiously and sweat running down his neck picturing his "head injured" son driving, Mr. Meyers interceded, "Well, first we'll have to, y'know, find out how the eyesight turns out an' uh. . . . . uh . . . how your leg and reflexes respond to therapy."

Although ecstatic about Craig's ability to carry on a conversation when he wasn't Atilla the Hun, this was one topic Mr. Meyers was never in any frame of mind to delve into, so he decided to wheel Craig around the unit for a socialization/diversion spin.

When Mr. Meyers was pushing Craig in his wheelchair out near the nurses' station, an older gentleman started moaning excitedly and waving his hands above his head. Craig saw this.

"Hey dad. . . . I think that guy over there's trying to get your attention . . ."

Looking in the man's direction, Mr. Meyers recognized this patient, for he was a salesman at a clothing shop in the Washington Mall where Mr. Meyers always bought his suits. Having developed a fond acquaintanceship with this businessman, Mr. Meyers felt a painful loss. Because she had applied for work at his school when he was Director, Mr. Meyers also knew this man's wife. Heart-broken and shaken, Mr. Meyers discovered that this fellow Washington Countian had a heart attack and not enough oxygen had gotten to his brain during the cardiac arrest. Leaving him unable to speak or walk, this anoxic condition made this gentleman dependent on his wheelchair to get around. Anything happening to that brain is bad, bad business. By evening, the Meyers' situation would not be good, for Craig's congeniality was—once again—about to disappear with the setting sun.

Craig couldn't have been any more cordial during the morning and afternoon, but the agitation alarm went off in his brain about 6:00 P.M. and he became his irritable "brain contused" self again, talking mean to his parents once he started getting a little bit tired. With the exception of that first time, showers did seem to calm Craig, so he was given one and went to bed at 7:30 P.M.

Sitting by Craig's bedside, the father whose hope always seemed to spring eternal, couldn't fight off the concern which harassed him. Seeing his boy hold his contracted arm under his chin and a splint clinging to his leg was a sight straight from Hell. Knowing that a mind absorbed with bewilderment is one without bountiful tomorrows, Mr. Meyers looked skyward towards the heavenly kingdom and said a silent prayer. The fear of what the future had in store for his son was an obsession which could not be expelled.

The final Sunday of the month—March 28—Craig's sister, brother-in-law, and nephew came in from Niles, Ohio to see Craig. Craig's parents, brother, and lovely sister-in-law were already in the room when they arrived on this visiting day. On the trip to Harmarville, Claire's family had some definite ideas of what Craig would be like. Craig had been hurt forty-three days ago and Claire had called almost every day to get updated on how her brother, fifteen-and-a-half years her junior, was doing. This was the first opportunity Claire got to see Craig because she had been watching Grandma Barnhart all this time, which was quite a load.

In her accounts of things, Mrs. Meyers has always had a tendency to make the "not real good," horrific, and the "fairly interesting," incredible. Because of her characteristic histrionics, Claire and Don were expecting to see Craig in a condition similar to the one he was in while fighting for his next breath in the ICU at Washington Hospital. But one would have to understand that to a mother of a patient with a head injury, anything less than what they were is catastrophic and this is how Mrs. Meyers viewed life this past month and a half.

When the McNaughton's came in, Craig immediately recognized them. Wide-eyed, shaking, and voice cracking, Claire asked her brother how he was feeling and was surprised with how well Craig was able to express himself. When Don asked his brother-in-law how he was doing, Craig greeted his towering fishing companion with an answer which told of his double vision.

> "I see two Dons,. . . . . . one's bad enough!"

Everyone laughed, including Don, who inhaled the sheets off Craig's bed when he sucked in the air needed for his classic laugh. Everybody was more at ease after Craig's crack except his nephew, Little Scotty (age 9). Little Scotty was symbolic of society's viewpoint of brain injury, for he was scared and didn't know what to expect, so he just kept quiet and stayed away, avoiding Craig even after Craig demonstrated his coherence. Told that anything they might be able to contribute to spark a memory would be advantageous to Craig's rehabilitation, Don and Claire began talking with Craig about an assortment of things.

As Craig was telling his sister and Don he has no recollection of the accident or the circumstances leading up to it after they had asked what he could remember, Claire saw her dad, standing in the vestibule by the door, looking up at the ceiling as if analyzing the way Craig was talking and processing things. After this went on for a little while longer, Mr. Meyers pulled his daughter aside.

"Well," this hopeful father said, "what do you think?"

Caught between what she knows her dad wants to hear and the sight of Craig's beaten body, Claire responded, "I didn't think he'd be able to talk and think so well. Me and Don thought Craig'd only be able to look at us and say 'yes' or 'no,' maybe nod his head. This is really a great surprise, dad; the progress Craig's made in such a short time."

Six weeks may not seem like a long time when looked at from a general frame of reference, but when one's child has gone through the evolution process in that span, from sub-human to whatever Craig is now and that parent's been with him every step of the way, that same period of time takes on a whole different perspective. Before they would leave tonight, Craig would give Claire and her family an idea of what Mom and Dad Meyers were talking about when they'd refer to Craig's instability. Maybe Little Scotty knew something nobody else did, after all.

With what seems to be a pattern with him, Craig's tolerance to stimulation went down with the sun. All the people in his room bustling with activity really got Craig's motor running, as he started giving the footplate of his wheelchair a kick and couldn't get comfortable with how he was sitting. Craig's sister adjusted the footplate to his specifications which settled him down some.

For the past few days, Craig's parents were teased into thinking that their son would be able to maintain his good behavior for 24 hours instead of becoming Dracula at night. But this night would be no different, for Craig's mood fluctuation proved to be a continuing saga of premature exhiliration for his parents. However, if there'd be one bright spot about his recent weekend trend to be congenial during the day and less so in the evening, it would be Craig's capability to participate in the exercises planned by the therapists during the day. And tomorrow would be a landmark day.

Monday, March 29, was the first day that Craig went to his day program of Communication Skills, Physical Therapy, Psychology, and Occupational Therapy and did what was asked of him, rather than being a rebel. This marked improvement in his behavior from several days ago was nothing short of incredible.

For the first time, it appeared Craig's true, non-aggressive temperament was surfacing, leaving his therapists feeling reasonably confident that they weren't going to get whacked because they asked Craig to do something his Ranchos #4-infested brain wasn't in the mood for. They were "reasonably" and not totally confident because Craig had come to his therapies before apparently calm, only to avoid participating because he got in such a huff over absolutely nothing. The topsy-turvy emotional changing of the guard that occurs when someone has had a head injury is something these professionals have seen before, so they were not prepared to let down their guard or jump for joy quite yet. But today was different in that Craig's ability to avoid getting irritable lasted all day.

Mrs. Joy dictated in her progress note, dated 3/29/82, that Craig had shown a decrease in his agitated behavior and an increased alertness/tolerance for program since the initial staffing. Although improving, this psychologist described Craig as needing work on his orientation to place and time. Craig's orientation to person was intact.

Craig might be able to say he's at "Harmarville Rehabilitation Center" or was at "Allegheny General Hospital" after being prodded and/or cued, but he still had no real sense of where he'd been or understood why he was at these health care facilities. Craig might be able to say that he was a "freshman at W.V.U.," but he had no "feel" for ever being there.

With a little thought, Craig might know the year of his birth date, but had no tangible experience he could draw from between these years. For example, Craig couldn't say the family moved from Harrisburg to Washington in 1968 shortly before his fifth birthday or that his first year of organized baseball was in 1977 when he was thirteen. If his brain was capable of recall at a given moment, Craig might be able to say that he graduated from high school in 1981, but had no recollection of the school year. Craig was like a computer that had been programmed; he might be able to spit out data, but had no understanding of why or how things had been stored.

Oddly, Craig had no trouble recalling names of family members or friends and could learn and remember who his therapists were. Craig also knew the names of the nurses as well as several of the patients on his unit.

When the brain's been bounced off the walls of the skull like Craig's was, the location(s) of the damage and pathways disturbed which are to follow will determine the physical, emotional, and cognitive deficits/sequela the person will experience. There's a possibility if that bruise on Craig's brain had only been a fraction of a millimeter from where it is now, Craig might have trouble remembering names, but could tell you the details of his first Pony League game and what the weather was like on the day he moved to Washington. Such is the complex system of the brain.

Although still very much frolicking in sadistic delight, the confusion and agitation which seized Craig was improving slowly, but steadily, since his admission. A combination of this improvement, account of how Craig was progressing before coming to Harmarville, Craig's flashes of motivation, and seeing the impeccable character of his family, all were taken into account when staff decided Craig would be a good candidate to do a series of videotapes which would document his condition from admission to discharge. When Craig's parents were approached about this idea, they had some immediate reservations.

Craig's parents experienced joy and fear in one fell swoop. Joy, because Craig's prognosis for recovery must be good, for staff wouldn't waste their time and money on a film production if Craig wasn't going to be a success story promoting the center. Fear, in that if this video would happen to fall in the wrong hands, this could damage Craig's prospects in the future. A film showing Craig's physical disabilities, agitation, confused thinking, slurred speech, that horrific stare, his inability to focus, or any type of aphasia could be infinitely detrimental. So, before they would agree to sign a release, the Meyers made sure that it stipulated that the video could only be used for educational purposes and not wind up on the evening news some night. Truths not defined are but a journey into the perils of chance.

God works through the hands of others here on earth and, fortunately for Craig, a lot of His best crafts/women set up shop at Harmarville. With Craig's co-operation having increased, his physical and occupational therapists could test his range of motion, strength, and flexor abilities in both his right and left/upper and lower extremities. With this information, exercises and strategies can be planned to improve/develop Craig's fine and gross motor skills.

When Craig was profoundly agitated to the point of being weary of anyone who got near him, therapies normally designed for physical restoration had Craig do elementary cognitive exercises like identifying such shapes as a circle, square, and triangle because any manipulation of his arm, leg, or shoulders would be met with hostile resistance. Craig's perceptual abilities are damaged, but not so bad he couldn't associate physical and occupational therapists with physical pain and frustration. This was one circumstance where Craig's being oriented to person was not productive. However, this was about the only thing not productive in relation to these folks, for what they were about to help Craig pull off was nothing short of amazing.

In the cognitive tag team of Psychology and Communication Skills, Craig's mental capacity could be measured with less road blocks, so appropriate perceptual/remedial tests and exercises could be utilized. At first, these were very basic. For example, Miss Rosato and Mrs. Joy would ask Craig simple questions he could answer with one word like naming a person or identifying an object, so an informal assessment could be made to determine the degree which Craig's thinking and memory had been shattered.

Speaking in sentences was something Craig couldn't do with consistency, so several of the questions asked of him were of the closed-ended variety where he could answer either with a 'yes' or a 'no.' When Craig's brain was capable, he could answer a question with a word or two, but he'd never initiate topics to discuss. To start a conversation, one has to take in their environment, process what to say, and deliver the message. This is too complicated of an operation for Craig to undertake at this point. And if Craig was to ever think, speak, or possess any kind of memory again, Diane and Mrs. Joy would sure have to pull some tricks out of their hat. What they were going to help Craig do, would make David Copperfield stand up and take notice.

Withered be the man whose mind cannot explore the world about him and expand with the wisdom it has to offer. Those assigned to work with him would try their best to make sure this didn't happen with Craig. Although greatly improved, Craig was far from being immune to the trespasses which flogged his mind. Cast into a world where one knows not what to expect, these next twenty-eight days would be one where Craig's harvest for tomorrow would begin to be planted. Or would it be reaching for a star impossible to touch?

March didn't ride off into the sunset without a grand finale. Taunted by dreams forever misplaced, Mr. and Mrs. Meyers received a phone call on the last day of the month from a young intern working with Craig in the Physical Therapy department.

Quite upset, she said Craig would not cooperate with her when she'd try to extend his contracted right arm or loosen the fingers of his "crumpled up"/paralytic hand. It was probably evident to Craig that the girl working with him was a rookie therapist with little experience, so he thought using his Ranchos #4 snarl and Ivan the Terrible demeanor would stop her from bending that which didn't want bent. With the hopes that informing his parents of his poor behavior may curtail his devilishness, this University of Pittsburgh student called the Meyers, so they'd relay a message to Craig to stop being so resistant when worked with in P.T. Capsized by a wave of eroded expectation, these seniors weren't happy with their boy when the trainee practically begged them to tell Craig that staff realizes his pain, but that working with his bum arm must be done if he ever wanted to use his dominant upper extremity again.

When Craig made his nightly collect call home on those evenings visitors weren't permitted to be at the rehab, his parents informed their little hellion that they had been notified of his antics this afternoon and went through their "No pain, no gain"/"No, you can't come home" lecture for the umpteenth time. After getting an earful, Craig promised his parents he'd straighten up and work hard. Starved of a life free from decay, Mrs. Meyers hearing reports of Craig's not listening and being uncooperative only confirmed her belief that Craig was not yet ready for rehabilitation.

April Fools is supposed to be only the first day of the month, but this must have been one of the things wiped from Craig's memory for, in the weeks to come, his trickery of showing extraordinary progress/motivation one minute would be followed by an encore of stagnation and hysteria the next. Although little was accomplished these first few weeks Craig was at Harmarville, the groundwork was being laid for bigger and better things to come.

Many mornings, Craig was exhausted because the pain and discomfort caused by that leg brace made it nearly impossible for him to get to sleep when he wanted. The 100 mg of Dilantin Craig would take before he went to bed at night should have helped him get to sleep, but the agony of that brace on his busted leg didn't do much for his insomnia. Counting sheep jumping a fence might work, if only Craig could count beyond the number "seven." The pin in his right leg would bite him with little mercy, if Craig rolled a certain way, so that was a hindrance in his attempts to settle for the night. Also, seeing things as a blurred/distorted perception of two would be a constant, nauseous reminder of the plight which shackled him. Making it more difficult for him to "nod off," Craig's putrid vision not progressing at all left him with some heavy concerns plaguing his mind when he'd try to go to sleep. If seeing things twice what they were and restricted from moving his right lower extremities weren't bad enough in his pursuits to get some rest, Craig's peace was no more, for he had tinnitus.

Craig hears constant ringing in both ears, more pronounced in his right. Although this does not affect Craig's ability to hear because of its low pitch, this brain damaged-induced tinnitus is non-stop and at rare times, without warning, would quadruple in volume/intensity for a few seconds, making it that much more annoying. If one hit a high "A" on an organ and sustains the note, this is the pitch

Craig experiences twenty-four hours, day and night. During the night, when it's quiet and calm, this ring becomes most distinct. Tinnitus has driven more than a few people to insanity and some, to suicide. Maybe if Craig wouldn't be so messed up and preoccupied with every other function of his body, this ear-ringing might just push him over the edge, too. Sweet dreams.

To help him to see things as they are and not double, Craig was to wear a plastic patch taped to his glasses, covering one eye. The eye that gets covered alternates everyday. The brain controls where the eyes focus and the eye then sends an image to the brain. If one eye is focusing on one thing and the other on something else, no matter how slight the differences may be, the brain is receiving TWO images to process. The brain, therefore the person, is seeing two different things. Hence, the words, "double vision."

In Craig's case, because of his right hemiparesis, the paralytic muscle moving his right eye was not responding and his eye would float elsewhere, resulting in two pictures showing on the brain's television monitors. Craig's double vision was a condition known as paralytic strabismus.

The brain controls where the eyes focus and when this optical control system malfunctions and cannot move the muscles behind the eye where it intends, some repairs need conducted. Some ways this can be done are by strengthening the weakened muscle through exercise, turn off one of the optical T.V. monitors—or as a last resort—make a surgical compromise, lessening the dominance of the side not affected with paralysis. Before any surgical procedures are considered to correct this problem, opthalmologists want to give Mother Nature a chance to respond to Father Time. In the meantime, the short-term recourse is to shut off one of the brain's image monitors and this is where the patch comes in. When a brain has been injured, sometimes the only remedy is to trick it.

During the latter part of March, Craig would be administered the Bender-Gestalt Test, so that an assessment could be made the extent with which Craig's mind was fooling him. The Bender is frequently used by clinical psychologists for its diagnostic quality of detecting brain damage. Specifically, it measures perception of spatial relations and memory for material just learned; two functions most sensitive to pathological processes. When used with those that have had a traumatic brain injury, this test is designed in such a way that it can identify disturbances in short-term memory and perception.

The format of this test is one where Craig's shown one card at a time with a specific design on it and asked to copy the design with the card laid out before him. Craig was shown a total of nine cards/designs with the complexity of the sample becoming more difficult as he went along.

The first card had a design of a circle to the left and a diamond-shaped block to the right of equal size, side by side, touching. Underneath the two shapes was the upper-case letter "A," approximately centered between the two shapes. The second had twelve black dots/periods of equal size in a horizontal line, and the third had ten columns of small circles of equal size with diagonal rows of three.

The remaining six designs were abstract shapes which criss-crossed, some within another, others touching and interconnecting. Most preschoolers could replicate these designs, but Craig wasn't at this level yet. To think that only a little over two months ago Craig was compiling a schedule of college courses at a major university for his second semester and now—if he wanted—couldn't get admitted to his grade school's special education program. Catastrophic.

The results of Craig's Bender revealed he had made moderate to marked rotational errors and mistakes of perseveration. An example of a rotational error would be that instead of perceiving that the shapes in the first design he was shown were side by side, the perception function in Craig's bruised brain shifted or "rotated" the designs where he believed they were—for an extreme example—top to bottom.

Perseveration is when a person spontaneously continues an activity and cannot stop, for they have no control. For example, when Craig would try to copy the twelve dots on the second card, he couldn't stop after twelve despite his intention to. Instead, the message his left hand got from his brain was to keep tapping those dots until Craig became aware he had made too many. By that time, Craig might have made fifteen, eighteen, twenty, or twenty-five marks depending when his brain realized it was time to stop. Yeah, some really weird and bizarre things can happen to a person when their brain's been bounced around.

Craig's perseveration made spontaneity difficult for, if he would do something without putting a lot of thought into it first, the consequence would not be what Craig intended. For instance, if Craig was having soup for supper and wanted to pick up his spoon, he would frequently reach for his fork or knife knowing immediately this was not what he wanted to do. Despite this realization, Craig could not consciously move his hand towards the silverware he knew he wanted. Instead of picking up a Dixie Cup full of water on his nightstand that he was to drink with his Dilantin, Craig would lift up his clock, glasses, Sporting News, or whatever else might be laying there until he finally got the cup.

If Craig could only think more clearly, he could have used this perseveration to his advantage. Craig could have wheeled next to that hot-looking nurse with the healthy bod Scott saw pushing the food cart the one night and repeatedly grabbed himself a handful and say, "Damn this perseveration."

By the end of the first week, Craig was showing improvement in both his leg and arm. Mr. Meyers thought Craig's right arm was loosening up a little bit and his fingers looked a little more flexible. This was a good sign for it showed Craig must be doing something in his therapies besides being resistant and that his brain was continuing its attempts to cure itself.

When the brain's been wracked, some nerve cells will survive, others don't. The ones that die, whatever operation they conducted is no more. They are gone—forever. That's why when a function returns, it shows that particular area of the brain is alive and has a chance of becoming operative again. And this is cause for celebration.

On the day following Scott's birthday, April 7th (fifty-three days after they stopped doing their thing), Craig must have been thinking of his brother, for

Craig's bowels moved on their own without an enema. Break out those party horns again, Craig went on his own!!!

When Craig called this ceremonious evening telling them of this feat, his parents were ecstatic. Never did they think that something that's taken for granted, even shunned about for being discussed, could make them so joyful. How something that occurs regularly for most is far from routine with somebody that has had a severe head injury. For those who have had the misfortune of personally being subjected to neurological impairment, the torment that functions will never be normal again has a merciless grip on the conscious.

For many with a brain injury, healing will occur rapidly, with physical and cognitive functions returning at an incredible rate initially. But in time, the rate of recovery slows to the point where one "plateaus"/doesn't experience much in the way of functions returning in the short-term. This does not necessarily mean the functions of a person with a head injury have forever disappeared, rather, instead of weeks and months, the capabilities might go into hibernation for years or decades. Or, very possibly, these functions may never emerge from the dark pit of permanent disability.

In Craig's case, Mr. Meyers would not allow his wife to dwell on what Craig had lost and will lose, rather, this ambassador of optimism would point out that only about fifty days ago they were happy Craig opened his eyes a fraction of an inch and was able to swallow some ice cream. And that this improvement was a clear-cut sign that those interconnecting fibers and network of tiny nerve cells are finding functional passages to travel within Craig's brain.

Mr. Meyers stressed they have to take what progress the brain has to offer and roll with its punches. Taking it step by step, inch by inch, was all they could do and appreciate the astounding progress Craig'd made this past month-and-a-half. This speech as much for him as it was for her, this tested father reminded his wife that some people are in a coma for years and that they have a lot to be thankful for.

Any human being with feeling would grieve for these parents stripped of their golden years where they were to prosper after devoting a lifetime working and responding to the challenges of raising their children. On February 14th, if Craig's parents had been told that their son would be talking and making some sense out of things by the time April rolled around, these saints of devotion would have been eternally grateful. In many ways, the Meyers counted their blessings, but one could not fault them for wanting more from Craig. And more is what they would get.

Now that Craig was not impossible to work with, the "Atari Computer System" can now be employed to help him with his cognitive deficits. The cassettes utilized for these games would not depict intergallactic space wars with the rival galaxy's mother ship trying to defend its planets with space shields and torpedo lasers, rather, the cassettes used within the cognitive therapy realm are designed so the patient with a head injury can relearn basic intellectual functions.

When one has had a head injury, often their ability to focus on something for any length of time has been seriously curtailed. Frequently, the person with this head injury does not have the ability to ignore distraction and keep from becoming preoccupied. When Mrs. Joy or Diane were trying to instruct Craig how to go about using a particular exercise, for example, the majority of the time Craig was either looking around the room, nervously fussing with his hair, or picking at his clothing.

Two prerequisites to learning are concentration and attention span. Without these crucial stepping stones, the ability to process information is non-existent. In Communication Skills and Psychology, under the guidance of his therapists, Craig would work as diligently as his mind infected with bafflement would allow him to. Craig struggled with an "Apple Computer," so that he could maybe regain the basic functions needed—not so much to thrive in society—but to survive.

Although Craig's motivation to do what was asked of him was not a venture he undertook with much understanding, something inside of him sensed that things were not as they should be and that somehow these strangers were trying to help him escape the confoundment which had left him with no idea of his place in the world. Lost is the child who dared not challenge and allowed stagnation to prevail.

The cognitive therapy offices looked like the NASA space programs' headquarters with television screens, computers, keyboards, initialed boxes with cassettes in them, and stacks of reading materials everywhere. Because of their inability to keep the mind from wavering and allowing reality to pass like a shooting star, the patient with a head injury needs something to attract their attention. The computer system used extensively in Psych and CS provided such stimulation.

One computer designed to enhance memory flashes a series of numbers or pictures which Craig must repeat in sequence within a given time. This also required Craig to concentrate on the order the image appeared. After the list of items had finished flashing on the screen, Craig must then recall the order of their appearance, process this stimulation, and then encode what he saw into words. For someone whose chemical and electrical processes have been disturbed within the brain, this task can be a nasty one.

The "Opposum Basic Skills Program" is a computer which helps patients with perception difficulties. This computer game is one where the patient must pair an image on the left side of the screen with its identical image on the right. This task would require Craig to scan what's before him, concentrate on the shape of the figure, pay attention to its twin on the opposite side, and then demonstrate appropriate motor skills when pointing to the shape wanted.

Swarmed with confusion, Craig could sense these were exercises he should be able to do with little difficulty and when he had trouble remembering the order of numbers flashed on the screen, for example, the disgust he had with himself was quite evident. Because of his inability to attend to stimulation, looking around at the walls, ceiling, floor, paper on the desk, or whatever else might catch his fancy, Craig would soon forget what it was he was to remember (amnestic apraxia). What made this all the more tantalizing for Craig was this awareness that things he used to be able to do with no conscious effort were now out of reach. The glazed existence of a brain carved of its functions leaves one to haggle with can blind the spirit and trample one's virtue.

Although they could definitely be drill sergeants, not allowing Craig's frustration to stop them from their pursuits to have him successfully complete their frequently tortuous lessons, Mrs. Joy and Diane kept a healthy balance not to drain Craig of his ability to be productive. These therapists knew what had to be done to bring Craig's world further into focus.

When a jolt to the brain occurs, the more tender sections which contain valuable nerve connections rub against one another, often making a not-too-subtle impact with the more substantial grey matter and the brain's firmer surrounding structures. When this happens, nerve fibers will strain and rip. Blood vessels will then pop and the brain bleeds, swelling within the skull, with this hemorrhaging causing more problems. The brain expanding within this rigid skeletal mass creates pressure and, subsequently, more damage.

With a closed head injury, because the actual insult isn't only localized at the point of impact like an open head injury, the damage can be significantly greater, for the brain often is bruised the opposite side of the impact as well, creating at least two spots that have been affected. The more places that are bruised, the greater the number of functions that will be affected. Craig's brain being juggled about in his head made spatial, sequential, scanning, speech, attention, and concentration exercises a feat of immaculate proportions.

Craig's room and the offices where his therapies took place all had calendars and a large clock, so he could be provided with a visual cue the time of day, which day of the week it was, the month, the date, and even what year it was. Head injured or not, the way people learn best varies from person to person. Some learn better when they see stimuli, as opposed to only hearing it. Others, only need the auditory stimuli for the information to be stored. Some learn best when they kinetically write down what's to be remembered.

With a head injury, stimulation needs presented repeatedly and on a continuous basis, if those stagnant brain waves are going to start jumping anytime soon. Craig was continuously reminded that he was in Harmarville Rehabilitation Center because he had sustained a severe head injury and needs to try his best and work hard, if he wants to return to a lifestyle which resembled the one he was accustomed. When one has had a brain injury, no stone is left unturned when it comes to providing stimulation which may be helpful.

Both Craig's neurosurgeon and physiatrist were pleased with his progress in such a relatively short period of time. The gains Craig was making in therapy were indicative that he and his brain were responding nicely. Because of the healing/spontaneous recovery and the various intangibles which promote a successful rehabilitation effort, several of Craig's sessions had been videotaped.

Despite the obvious improvement in his cognitive and physical processes, Craig was twisted by images of when he was whole, as he could not see beyond what he was like after being hurt and the way he was before the accident. When Craig would say in his now slurred, hypernasal voice, "Why me? Why me?," his father was quick to point out that he and his mother were happy with what they see now, for they can remember—not all that long ago—when a blinking line on a heart monitor was the only indication that there was life in his body.

Craig has come a long way since lying comatose in a bloody heap at Washington Hospital's ER with leg splintered, arm contracted, and ear dangling by a thread of skin. Craig was sure one messed up dude alright, but several aphasias which had yet to be detected would soon make their appearance. Stay tuned for there was more to come.

In Physical and Occupational Therapy, Craig could now understand these professionals working with him are not hurting him to punish him for some reason, rather, this pain is the expensive price one must pay in order to get those body parts and brain in working condition again. While physically testing what they could get away with, occupational and physical therapists would concurrently work with Craig on some of his cognitive reasoning lapses, so that he could better appreciate that no harm was intended. If Craig had not gotten this through his thick, bruised head, they could not have started their work of physical restoration so quickly. And restoring they did.

By Easter Sunday, April 11th, OT had gotten Craig to extend his right arm and hand over his head. This was no small feat. In addition to Craig's brother Scott, his therapists were able to deflect Craig's vulgarities directed towards them and get him to focus on what had to be done to prevent his right arm, hand, and fingers from atrophying. From Craig's vantage point, his right upper extremities were already "dead."

If Craig had to use one of his hands, it would always be his left one which sprung into action. When Craig would want to move his right hand off his wheelchair tray, for example, he'd pick it up with his left. And if he wanted to move his right leg on or off the footplate of his wheelchair, Craig would pick his leg up with his left hand. Craig's left hand was working overtime to compensate for his right side's inability to receive any signals from the brain to move. Craig's right arm would be held closely to his body, just dangling there with his hand only going along for the ride. His fingers would be in a curled position, rigid from spasticity.

When the occupational therapists would pull down the upper part of Craig's arm to straighten it out, the elbow shot with pain as if stung with a high voltage shock and his fingers, when bent, would be overcome with a cracking ache as if being hyperextended. But instead of yelling, "Let go of my fuckin' arm!!" or violently pulling his hand away like he used to, Craig would now allow his therapists to bend, spread, and straighten these limbs which just wanted to be left well enough alone. Craig would soon understand the meaning of, "Hell on Earth."

Craig would no longer need a volunteer to push him to his programs for, in PT, his left footplate was removed and his therapist taught him how to ambulate in his wheelchair. Jan's difficulty teaching Craig how to do this normally simple motor activity of: a) lifting the foot off the floor, b) stretching out the leg, c) placing the heel on the ground, d) dragging the heel back as, e) one leans forward in their chair then, f) repeating, demonstrated just how a brain injury can fog the mind.

To get his wheelchair to propel, Craig had to break down and concentrate on each one of these steps which most people do automatically. And to further complicate this, the cognitive process of concentration is one thing Craig does not have a firm grasp of. It would be improving, yet, light years from being functional. This was yet another way the cognitive and physical therapies work as one.

When trying to put his wheelchair into motion, Craig would look down at his left foot unable to have it do what he wanted it to. He could not move it!! What Jan or Mary had to do then was pick up Craig's left leg repeatedly, so that his brain could relearn what it feels like to lift a leg again.

In time, after Craig got this down, Jan and her assistant would model the motion of stretching the leg. Holding Craig's leg, they would stretch it out, bending his foot up while this was being done and having him land on his heel. Both pointing the foot upward and landing on the hindmost part of the foot had to be shown to Craig as well, so that his brain could get a "feel" of how to do this again. Simple—right? Not for someone whose had an injury to their brain stem like Craig had.

After concentrating strenuously for a few seconds, Craig would lift his foot up and slap it down on the ground quickly, as if not having enough strength to keep it in the air for very long. Sometimes, Craig would twist his foot while it was in the air at such an angle that he would come down, not on his heel, but his ankle. Craig would know immediately this was not what he wanted to do and would give it another shot.

When Jan and Mary would finish physically manipulating Craig's leg/heel cord and modeling the motions he should be undertaking, they would do it again. And following their second round of physical torture and demonstration, around they'd go one more time. And after that, as topping for the cake, Jan would give Craig exercises for him to do when back in the unit. Later in the day, Craig would come back for more drilling in the afternoon PT session.

A mere two weeks ago, Craig couldn't tolerate one session of Physical Therapy, but has improved to the point where he could endure two sessions of this aggravation. To give the definitive answer to why this had occurred could not be possible and would not be important. What would be possible and important was that Craig could go through the rigors of therapy and undergo the work required in order to make some headway.

Whoever came up the saying, "Practice makes perfect," did not sustain a severe head injury. When someone's had a brain contusion, the goal can only be the more modest one of demonstrating some kind of improvement, one agonizingly slow step at a time. In Craig's case, any sign he was showing which indicated he would not have to live in the shadow of what happened to him Valentine's Day 1982, was hailed as an accomplishment of the greatest magnitude. With this, the first steps of many have been taken in the expedition known as recovery.

However, this campaign would take Craig through a jungle of prolonged and extreme cognitive, emotional, and physical agony. The brain's ability to function properly is normally taken for granted, and one can naturally expect that the foundational academic skills learned as a child can be retrieved with no problem. And they usually are, unless of course one has had their brain cells shut down. With paper and pencil, any elementary school child can jot down their name, but Craig couldn't. He had forgotten how to write.

Craig's condition, known as agraphia, is a mental disorder marked by the inability to write. Craig could copy letters, recite the alphabet, identify letters on flash cards, and orally spell words, but was unable to write letters or words from memory. His visual memory of what different letters and numbers looked like was non-existent. When Craig would intend to print a letter he would—99.99% of the time—mistakenly substitute it with another letter he did not want to make or put down a number/symbol from a language not yet developed.

Craig also exhibited perseveration when he'd try to express his thoughts via the written word. For example, he would know there is no circle when printing the lower case letter, "t." Nonetheless, Craig would start off with an oval when asked to write this letter time and time again despite realizing this was incorrect. Craig would immediately identify the letter he mistakenly made, only to repeat the mistake over and over, usually starting off with another wrong symbol. Craig had no control of what his hand wrote. Once that (pen)cil hit the paper, look out, for anything goes.

If Craig were asked to orally spell his name, he could say, "C-R-A-I-G" with no problem. Stick a pencil in his hand and lay a piece of paper in front of him and instruct him to print those same five letters which spell his name without some kind of a cue, and Lord knows what would get on that paper. Maybe "RgXT/," "lM3ev," or possibly the all-time classic, "NzScj."

When a cardboard display with the twenty-six letters of the alphabet printed on it would be within view, Craig could print any word asked of him. Starting with "A" and in order, Craig would point to each letter of the alphabet, saying them, up until he came to the one he wanted. After verbally identifying the letter he was looking for and seeing what it looked like, Craig could replicate its design, printing it on the paper. Going on to the second letter of the word and the rest thereafter, Craig would find the remainder of the letter symbols using the same process.

For instance, if Craig's Communication Skills Therapist, Diane, would want Craig to print her name, she would first ask how it was spelled with her agraphic patient correctly saying, "D-I-A-N-E." Then, Craig would look at the cardboard display with the upper case letters printed in alphabetical order and say out loud—or silently to himself—"A-B-C-D." The auditory cue, "dee," coupled with recognizing the shape his finger was pointed on as the sought-after configuration, Craig knew this was the letter he wanted to print, so he'd copy it onto the paper.

To write the second letter of his therapist's name, Craig looked at his cardboard sample again, uttering and pointing as he went along, "A-B-C-D-E-F-G-H-I," until he heard and saw what he was looking for, and put this down. Craig then found his "A" in no time, the "N" was found somewhere in the middle of the pack, and he quickly got the "E." If Craig were to return to W.V.U. now and had to take an essay test, it would take him the entire semester just to complete a paragraph.

In Mrs. Joy's psychology sessions, more of the same type of writing exercises were practiced. Because of his paralytic dominant right hand, Craig turned into a southpaw overnight and had to learn how to scribble with his left hand. Craig thought that maybe writing with his other hand might have something to do with his inability to produce letters, but was told even if he could hold a pencil or pen with his right hand without dropping it on the floor, the neurological disconnection which took place somewhere between his brain and ultimately what the (pen)cil produced would still be there. Making it impossible for him to write regardless of which hand he used, Craig would have a lot of work ahead.

Because Craig's visual memory was blemished, he not only couldn't picture in his mind the symbols which represented the letters of the alphabet, but had no idea of their size in relation to the context of things. Between the lines of notebook paper and across from left to right, there's only a given amount of SPACE with which to put words and letters. Because this "spatial" function in his brain was nowhere to be found—with a cue in front of him—if Craig were asked to print a three-letter word like "can," he might be able to keep the "C" in the allotted space if lucky, but the "A" and the "N" might take up two or three spaces.

Also, Craig didn't know when one word ended and another should begin. Not that this was tried other than for a baseline purpose, with cardboard cue before him, when Craig would try to write two words together like "red car," his spatial lapse would not permit him to put a space between the first and second word. Something like "rEDcaR," would be produced by his atrocious printing, taking up a varying amount of space.

The deterioration of Craig's spatial ability made it virtually impossible for him to conceptualize words as separate units. The written word and its boundaries meant nothing to Craig. His recollection of letters and words was nothing but an infinite abstraction he no longer understood.

Craig had a difficult time reading as well. Unlike his writing, it wasn't that he totally forgot how to, rather, his ability to scan a line, left to right, was not working. For example, if shown a card with a word on it, Craig could spell the word before him, identifying its letters and say what the word was. But having him read a group of words in a sentence was not a task he did with any ease. Craig would read a couple of words and then—inexplicably—his eyes could no longer follow the horizontal pattern required when reading, shooting down to a sentence or two below the one he was supposed to be tracing.

The different computer programs Craig was working on not only helped him with his attention and concentration, but with this scanning deficit as well. It's absolutely unbelievable what a bruise half the size of a coin does when it gets on either the frontal, parietal, occipital, and/or temporal lobes of the brain. It will forever change the person.

People normally don't have to break basic tasks down into their finer components and thoroughly concentrate because most fundamental undertakings are done instinctively. But, when a brain's been bruised, nothing is fundamental.

For instance, crumpling a piece of paper and tossing it in the trash is no big endeavor, right? For someone that's had a severe head injury, it might not only pose a problem, but be an insurmountable task to ask of someone whose brain waves are irregular. The process of throwing away a piece of paper clumped into a ball requires a series of steps, a SEQUENCE of events.

First, the person has to formulate in their mind what they want to do. Then, the mind dissects the process involved to undertake the task, before actually physically going through the motions. This operation takes a fraction of a second. That is, if one's mind is hitting on all its cylinders. Because his spark plug wasn't working, Craig couldn't do the most elementary of ventures without fumbling.

With the throwing away the paper example, unless the paper were laid before him or pointed to, Craig might not be able to locate the paper due to his scanning and recognition deficiencies. Because of his perseveration, Craig also might not be able to reach for the paper, rather, a pencil, tack, paper clip, or stapler may be reached for instead. Or Craig might take a pen out of the holder and freeze in midair seemingly contemplating what to do with it. Craig might then impulsively reach for a book without thinking and open it, only to slam it shut out of frustration knowing this wasn't what he wanted to do. The apparent simple task of rolling up and disposing of a piece of paper can be far from routine, if the operations within the brain controlling these functions have been rattled in any way.

And because of his distorted perception of the purpose of different objects (sensory apraxia), Craig had lost his ability to make proper use of objects (motor apraxia). Craig just might do his pica routine and start munching on these desk items. Because Craig's sequential ability had been blanketed with a torrent of confusion, if he had been able to find the writing paper he'd been searching, he may, for example, fold the paper into halves and place it on the desk top instead of crumpling it into a ball and dropping it in a garbage can. Craig's mind remembered that he had done this elementary activity of folding paper before, but was unable to differentiate this action from what he currently had been asked to do—rumpling up paper.

Presenting multiple stimuli to Craig was something that confused and frustrated him. Craig couldn't fragment this stimuli into its basic parts and take one step at a time. Rather, his mind took on everything in clusters, making reality nothing but a fleeting impossibility. Perhaps Craig still believed he could still whisk through things he once was able to without giving it any thought, not realizing the true destruction that had occurred.

In the throwing out the paper example, if Craig was asked to put his pencil in the holder and turn off the desk light after throwing the paper away, Craig would sit dumbfounded for a few seconds before throwing the pencil holder in the trash and laying the paper on the floor. When the surface of the brain has been severely marred, the appearance of bizarre behavior is going to occur more times than not.

The frustration came from Craig's inability to purge that which robbed him of his senses. This utter collapse of capability left Craig bruised, but not beaten. Craig somehow sensed that if any remnant of his former self was going to emerge, he was in for a battle. Gone is the hope when a mind has been abandoned.

Not only had Craig's capacity to undertake what his mind intends deserted him, but his memory of specific events during the first eighteen years of his life needed to be unraveled, if he'd ever have any sense of who he was or came to be. It was tragic that Craig was unable to write his name or reaches for a comb in the back pocket of his jeans when he wanted to take a pen out of his shirt pocket, but when Craig's recollection of who certain people were or how he came to know them had decayed, this truly marked the elusiveness his past and much of what was known had become.

Overall, Craig was oriented towards person, however, with many of the "get well" cards, Craig would stare blankly at them, frequently not able to identify who the people were that sent them. And for Craig to read the messages on the cards and the notes from these well-wishers was not possible because his ability to pay attention to any one thing for any length of time was gone. The Meyers would have to read Craig the cards, then tell their "lost" son who they were from. Too often, they'd need to explain to Craig how he knew them. A future without the backbone of a past is the embodiment of a forlorn existence.

However, God's will, the support of his family, the "fight" within him, and the medical/rehabilitation professionals who have worked with Craig all made for a recipe which promotes optimum recovery.

The ingredients for reparability must be in place for, after his parents' Harmarville visit ended on the Easter holiday, Craig's memory had improved to the point where he gave Scott and his childhood friend/next door neighbor, Frank McNamara, a telephone call. To Scott's and the McNamara's surprise and excitement, Craig remembered their phone number respectively. To retrieve these numbers from his memory was a tremendous sign that a renaissance of Craig's mind was occurring and made this Easter celebration one that would have special meaning. Could it be Craig's going to have a resurrection of his own, too?

Physically, the damage to Craig's left portion of his brain caused him to have paralysis on the entire right side of his body (right hemiparesis) which resulted in his having a spastic right hand, arm, and heel cord as well as his five fingers. Craig's right leg and toes were no doubt affected too, but because his leg was broken, no formal determination could be made yet as to what extent. This hemiparesis also had an effect on Craig's eyesight because the muscle behind his right eye was not working, causing him to have double vision.

Craig had a useless side, distorted vision, ringing ears, and busted leg. With these various physical ailments as well as his bruised brain and all its lovely symptoms, if Craig had been hurt ten years ago with these same afflictions, his parents would likely have to be searching for a nursing home to put him in for the rest of his life. Eighteen and rotting in a geriatric facility. The tragedy caused by the evil that is drunk driving is incomprehensible.

The people at Harmarville Rehabilitation Center are what makes that place. No doubt, there are other quality rehabilitation facilities that provide top-of-the-line services in Pittsburgh and the tri-state area of Pennsylvania, West Virginia, and Ohio. But there's no way a better chemistry could have developed at any other facility than the one Craig had formed at Harmarville.

At Harmarville, the quality of care is fabulous and those delivering these inpatient services are a special, caring breed. One can't help but develop a warm rapport with these folks. Craig's association with one of these dedicated employees would have a major impact on him. The rapport developed with this compassionate person would result in an enhanced rehabilitation outcome and an upgraded perception of himself.

Valerie Parke was a full-time nurses' aide who was hired this month and worked the 3-11 P.M. shift on Unit Three. Mrs. Parke had a friendly, bubbly personality which would make her a "hit" with all the patients and their families. Her genuine good naturedness, personable approach, and Valerie being only about a year older than Craig were the ingredients which made for a nice friendship with her new patient. Because Valerie was married, there wasn't the pressure that's involved in a relationship where the goal is intimacy and long-term commitment. This relaxed atmosphere helped Valerie and Craig to "hit it off" right away. They clicked as would a close brother and sister. Being a cute Italian didn't hurt either from Craig's standpoint either. Vertically compromised, but cute.

Since Craig didn't date in high school or never even had anybody he could consider a female friend, this was a welcome, new experience that was too long in coming for him. The only girls Craig knew during his sequestered adolescence were acquaintances who might do his homework for him because they knew he was too busy relaxing. If the phone had rung at the Meyers' residence and a girl on the other end asked to speak with Craig, the earth would have stopped rotating. The timing of Valerie Parke meeting Craig could not have come at a better time for, as badly as he was hurt, Craig needed as many in his Harmarville cheerleading section as possible to keep from falling into the depths of depression. And Valerie emerged as Craig's head cheerleader.

Feeling bad for this guy who was devastated at such an early age, Valerie took a special interest in Craig. During her half-hour break each evening, Valerie would get Craig in his room and away they'd go to the recreation room to hit a ping-pong ball back and forth. It might not have been the same level of competition Craig was used to playing Colt League and high school baseball—with Craig now seated in a wheelchair, wearing a patch over one eye, and tapping a ping-pong ball with his left hand over a net—but he enjoyed it almost as much because of who his opponent was. Valerie was a lot easier on the eyes than Angelo Alberta, Rob Orlosky, Scotty McWreath, Brian Schultz, Steve Oliverio, Fred Schwarz, Scott Staso, Rich Rydzak, Kevin Kelly, Paul Leake, Tim Trusler, Dave Humphreys, Brad Sprowls, John Bednarski, Brian Henry, Vince Knotts, Ron Humphreys, Steve Howe, or Ron Semple. Valerie smelled better, too.

From the therapists to the aides, and the doctors to the volunteers, all played a role of varying degrees in Craig's rehabilitation. Knowing that her ping-pong buddy had forgotten how to write, Valerie made a suggestion that had as much—if not more—to do with Craig's improved writing ability as anything. Correctly assuming that their friendship would motivate Craig that much more to practice his writing, Valerie asked her table tennis buddy if he would write her a couple of letters during the week. Seeing the benefits of this, not only from a therapeutic standpoint, but from a hormonal one as well, Craig took on this project with a passion.

Not wanting to be outdone, it wasn't long before one of Craig's other influential nurses got in on the act, as Jan also wanted some bi- or tri- weekly correspondence from Craig, too. Word travels fast at Harmarville and before long, Craig was writing three or four nurses. All were attractive, but this didn't play a part in his diligently writing every night for a couple of hours, rather, Craig's drive to overcome the tangle which his mind was spun was the sole reason his effort and motivation peaked. Yeah right—and that wasn't all that peaked.

A typical night of printing practice would be one where Craig would wheel himself over to the table at the foot of his bed after eating his supper at the nurses' station and, wanting to open his notebook to the first page so he could begin his letter to Valerie, would instead pick up his glass case. Putting this protective covering down, Craig knew immediately that this wasn't what he wanted to lift up. Like a person with a visual impairment does when they search for something by touch, Craig would pick up everything on the table until he was touching what he wanted. This was similar to his scanning for the letters of the alphabet on the cardboard display where Craig would recite the alphabet and touch each letter as he went along. This same type of tactic had to be employed, if Craig wanted to pick up something.

After finding his notebook and pulling it up towards him so he wouldn't lose track of it again, Craig would then want to reach for his pen, so he could start writing about how trying rehab would be that day. After moving a dixie cup and shuffling papers about the desk, Craig finally had his hand on a pen and recognized instantly that this was what he was looking for. Not daring to let go of it for fear of "losing" it again, just getting set up was a brain teaser. Now for the real misery of getting that brain of Craig's to work when a writing utensil touches paper.

Wanting to start his letter with, "Dear Valerie," Craig would sometimes get cocky and try not to use his cardboard cue, for he wanted to see how much his visual memory could help him. Like the proverbial, "Finding a needle in a haystack," Craig was too far gone to find in his scattered memory what the different letters looked like without some help.

Not only couldn't Craig think of what the various symbols of the alphabet looked like, but his handwriting was absolutely horrid. When writing with the help of the cue, his non-dominant left hand was so uncoordinated, what Craig wrote resembled hieroglyphics and not a symbol of the English language.

The speed and effort which Craig wrote was, needless to say, excruciatingly slow and laborious. The trifecta of his setting up everything so he could begin, the process he had to go through to recognize the letters, and his being uncoordinated left-handed made it nearly impossible for Craig to write a short paragraph in under an hour-and-a-half. When the anger and frustration got to be too much, Craig would need to take a break from writing and, sitting in his wheelchair/harness, off he'd go to tear up some tile.

The encouragement and instruction from staff surely inspired Craig to "give it his all." Not yet oriented to what was going on around him, for his ability to perceive what was transpiring in his world was continuing to be misguided into a haze of not knowing, Craig still recognized that he had a tremendous amount of work ahead and started exercising the only way he could. Powered by the force knowing that being disabled could not be accepted, Craig started doing laps in his wheelchair up and down Harmarville's long three-hundred yard hallway.

With the footplate of his wheelchair removed, Craig could now ambulate and see what this Harmarville place is all about. The freedom to move about is something that's also taken for granted, that is, until one can no longer escape the grasp of being stationary.

Craig wanted to become as proficient as possible at getting around in his wheelchair. Not only did flying about in his new toy he had some control over now work on the movement of various body parts which had basically been in a fixed position for so long, but Craig couldn't be sure this four-wheeled contraption wouldn't be his life-long partner. If this was to be his destiny, Craig wanted to be certain he could master its movements.

Craig was never told that he'd never be able to walk again, but that brain's a funny thing when it's been banged around the head a few times. It can't be said for sure what's going to happen when the central nervous system has been disturbed. What can be ascertained is that Craig wanted to get out of that wheelchair as soon as possible—if possible.

Craig's world these past two months has been viewed within the confines of a hospital bed and a wheelchair that he had no say over its destination. Always a physically active person, being restricted and having no control was a punishment of unbearable cruelty for Craig. Not able to move left Craig dependent on whoever might be around to transport him. At an age where one strives to be independent and break free from the limitations of dependence, this reliance on others for the most basic needs was a torment of the harshest proportions.

From having his ass wiped after taking a "dump," to being showered every evening, to exposing cognitive/physical deficits, not having any privacy and unable to function without the assistance of others robbed Craig of the little self-esteem he might have had. When Craig had the means to explore and move about his environment, he took full advantage of this.

Craig wheeled his wheelchair back and forth so that his left leg, foot, and arm could relearn how to respond to the signal his brain was firing off to "move." Like a toddler, he had to learn the steps involved in order to get from place to place and the only way to (re)learn is to practice. There's no substitute.

However, the difference between the toddler attempting to walk and the patient with a head injury attempting it is different. While the bouncing baby making a stab at taking those first steps will be beaming from ear to ear, the patient with the head injury trying to get from Point A to Point B is going to find it much more difficult to smile. Instead, they'll experience a burning anger what was taken away, and an icy chill fearing that taking steps again will never return. Having something then losing it usually can be more devastating than never having it. Especially if what was possessed was never appreciated for what it meant to the person's life.

Therapists can only show someone the way, it's up to the patient whether or not to listen. Physical and cognitive therapists can be the finest magicians provided the ones worked with do not perceive progress as an illusion. If a person with a disability has the capacity to get better and go about what needs done to improve, they would have to take full advantage of this capability.

Craig was very, very fortunate that his brain allowed him to realize the state he was in required a tireless effort few will ever have to battle. Some people who have had injuries to their brain are hurt so drastically that they do not and will never have any realization of how to go about doing anything, let alone know how to put forth an effort in rehabilitation. Fortunately for a growing number of people who have sustained a severe head injury, the prognosis is getting brighter. Technological advances in medicine are allowing doctors to better help those with head injuries find answers. With his understanding of what needed done to get out of the hole that his brain injury left him to waste away in, Craig was set to embark on a mission that has no end. Exhausted after doing his Indy out in the hallway, Craig returned to his room for yet another round of writing agitation. With a brain injury, eroded becomes the mind when the will no longer triumphs.

On Tuesday, April 13th, Craig graduated from having to eat in the nurses' station and could chow down in the main dining room. A little under a year ago, Craig finished high school, and although there wasn't any commencement ceremony of tassel flipping for this latest accomplishment, its significance was of greater importance. It meant Craig had improved to the point where he could start getting back into the flow of things without being segregated from the mainstream. With the exception of a comment from a guy whose maturity was not advanced, Craig's first day in the dining room went just fine.

Craig could feel that things were falling into place and when Mr. and Mrs. Meyers came in for their Tuesday evening visit, Craig told these heroes that nothing's going to stop him from getting better; that he is trying his best and will continue to work hard. These words gave these strained, but not conquered, parents hope that Craig was going to scratch and claw to get back everything he can.

Since Mr. and Mrs. Meyers didn't see Craig everyday like they did when he was in the hospital, any subtle improvement their son made was noticeable. Looking at their creation all the time, Monday through Friday, it's like when a little kid surrounds a young plant with soil and waters it in Science class everyday, they don't really see how much it's growing as the seedling reaches for the sun. After a weekend home, they come back Monday morning with their mouth dropping open and eyes wide with excitement upon seeing what was before them.

From his speech to his posture, to the clarity of his thinking, Craig's parents were very happy with their little seedling's progress and their decision to bring Craig to Harmarville for rehab. They were able to manage to keep from having their mouths fling open and eyes from protruding too far, but they were unable to hide the joy on their faces or the exuberant tone of their voices upon seeing their boy progress each time they saw him.

One sign of progress was that Craig's digestive system was coming around. Because Craig had lost so much weight when he was in the hospital, Dr. Amayo had ordered that kitchen staff give Craig double portions at mealtime if he wanted, so he could regain the weight he lost. Well, because he likes to eat, Craig took full advantage of this opportunity to make up for lost time and ALWAYS devoured a second helping. This, along with his exercising and brain continuing to get better helped Craig's bowels do their thing, so that by the middle of the month, he was slapping down the toilet seat and going on a regular basis. When the evening nurse would come in Craig's room and ask, "Did your bowels move today?," instead of Craig saying, "No, but I farted twice," he could tell her to put the enema back in her holster, for that wouldn't be needed anymore.

In a little over a month, since his Harmarville admission, Craig has made good progress. Still another galaxy from being physically and cognitively adept, Craig was definitely showing signs of being on the mend. The recent one-way progress which was occurring in the, "Good one minute, bad the next", world of head injury was just too good to be true. Through this whole ordeal, the Meyers have learned—as the old saying goes—"Don't count your chickens before they're hatched." It's a good thing they didn't for Craig had yet to break free from his shell of self-deception. On Sunday the 18th, a week from the day Mr. and Mrs. Meyers wishfully wanted to believe their son's rehabilitation was going to be all downhill after Craig started propelling his wheelchair independently, Craig's brain had found another trick to play on him.

Sometimes people who have lost a limb amazingly feel pain in the limb that is no longer there. Though it wasn't pain, this "phantom sensation" occurred with Craig when his parents were in the bedroom visiting with him. Sitting in his wheelchair, Craig looked at his mom and dad obviously uncomfortable with something. Looking down at the wheelchair tray which obscured his bare right joint, Craig said, "Take this kneepad off."

Mr. and Mrs. Meyers looked at each other not knowing what their son was talking about, uncertain if he was kidding or not.

His parents' hesitation didn't go over too well with Craig, so he annoyingly blurted, "What's that look about? Please take this kneepad off, it's buggin' me!"

"You don't have anything on your knee," Mr. Meyers said, "you must be tired."

In her failed attempt to humor her son teased by this tactile hallucination, Mrs. Meyers then compromised, "If you take my helmet off, I'll take off your kneepad."

Unable to understand his mom's way of trying to get reality to sink in, Craig's easily-induced agitation returned. "Now listen," Craig yelled out fussing with his wheelchair tray, "I'm not tired and you're not wearin' a fuckin' helmet. Stop pissin' around and take it off."

Before he was hurt, Mr. Meyers had never heard filthy language coming from his son's mouth before and—with his adrenalin spewing through his veins—Mr. Meyers shot out of the chair he was seated and removed the tray from Craig's wheelchair, so his hallucinating son could see.

With eyes filling with tears of compassion for his disjointed boy, Mr. Meyers cried out pointing down at his son's kneecap, "Where the hell do you see a kneepad? Show me!"

Voice cracking from both the fear his son was sensing that which was not there and the frustrating reminder Craig was yet suffocating from the trickery a mind shaken plays on one, Mr. Meyers explained, "See? There's nothing there! Your leg's been sliced up pretty bad and nerves have been cut. And you haven't been able to move your leg much because it's been busted."

For fear of Craig's reaction, Mr. Meyers did not say as much as a whimper about how a mind that has skidded along the interior of the skull will feel when nothing's there to be felt. Instead, he explained what Craig could understand and avoided anything which may further muddle his thinking.

"When your leg's been through the hell yours has, it's gonna feel funny for a while. I know it's tough, but all you can really do is wait it out. But don't you worry, sonny boy, we'll be with you when we can if you need us. We'll ride it out together, buddy!"

With his patented optimism, Mr. Meyers concluded, "Don't you fret, once you get up on your feet—and that won't be too far from now—you'll be chasing all these nurses around this place so much, we'll have to bring you another pair of sneakers 'cause you'll have worn your other ones out."

Once again, Mr. Meyers' prophecy was right on the button for, this week in physical therapy, Jan and Co. would be working with Craig on getting him out of his wheelchair.

After a physical examination, it was confirmed that Craig's broken right leg he almost lost had fully healed! With Craig's bum leg now ready for some action—as was the case with the footplate earlier—the right leg rest of his wheelchair could be removed. The dismantling of Craig's wheelchair was a palpable sign that his brain was responding to the work he was putting in.

Although significantly better from when he was at Allegheny General, when Craig first arrived at Harmarville, it had looked like he had been through a slaughter house. Because of this, and seeing the suffering Craig had gone through to get to this point, other therapists not assigned to work with him—but saw Craig everyday in the gymnauseum (sic)—felt tremendous for this patient when he started to work on escaping the confines of his wheelchair. When someone's had a brain injury, this is easier said than done.

On the mats, which Jan and Mary physically helped him descend to, Craig worked on the motions needed to get in an upright position. Rocking back and forth three times to get the momentum going, Jan showed Craig the initial step he would have to undertake to get out of the sitting position.

When modeling this—after placing Craig's paralytic hand on his right knee—Jan said to her wobbly patient that he will have to put the palm of his good hand on his left knee and push down on both his knees at the same time on the third rock when he's leaning forward, so that his legs will straighten and the momentum of his rocking forward will help his upper torso get in a vertical position. After Jan explained what he needs to do and Craig assuring his therapist he understood, it was now time for the big moment when Harmarville's poster child of sorts would stand again.

Momentarily taking a pause from their patients they were working with, Diane Latuska and Theresa Gates looked out the corner of their eyes at Craig hoping they'd witness firsthand the triumphant moment when all of Craig's six-feet would be standing tall. With Jan's hands placed under his pits and Mary bracing his back ready to give him a little push, it was time for countdown.

With nervous anticipation, Jan told her patient, "On three, we'll be going up!"

On the outside, Craig exuded a confidence where it looked like there was no way he was going to be denied, as machoism spilled from every pore. Inside, Craig kept thinking, "Here we go, it's time to die."

Rolling Craig forward the first time, Jan said in a gentle, drawn-out whisper, "One," as Craig's head almost dipped to his shivering knees. With her patient back up, Jan gave Craig the next nudge down, simultaneously saying, "Two!"

Like Dick Clark's Rockin' Eve party on New Year's, the balloons were ready to fall, the non-alcoholic bubbly corks primed to be popped, and the drum roll's build-up reaching its climax marking this accomplishment until Jan barked, "Three!!!" and Craig went back down on his pants again immediately after raising it an inch or two distance off the mat.

Panting from this six-second elevation, the two physical mercenaries asked Craig if he was okay before Jan went about instructing Craig that he needs to utilize his right hand to push down on his knee next time; that she knows it feels awkward right now using this hand he hasn't moved much, but that he has to, if he wants to get on his feet. Jan told Craig the equilibrium has got to be close to being the same as his left side. If Craig's tilted and leaning in one direction too much, her domino patient is just going to tip over.

Tucking the Led Zeppelin shirt in his pants, Craig was ready for the next round of this circus. With the balloons still ready to make their descent, Jan roared without hesitation while rocking her uneasy patient, "One—Two—Three!!! Up we go!!!"

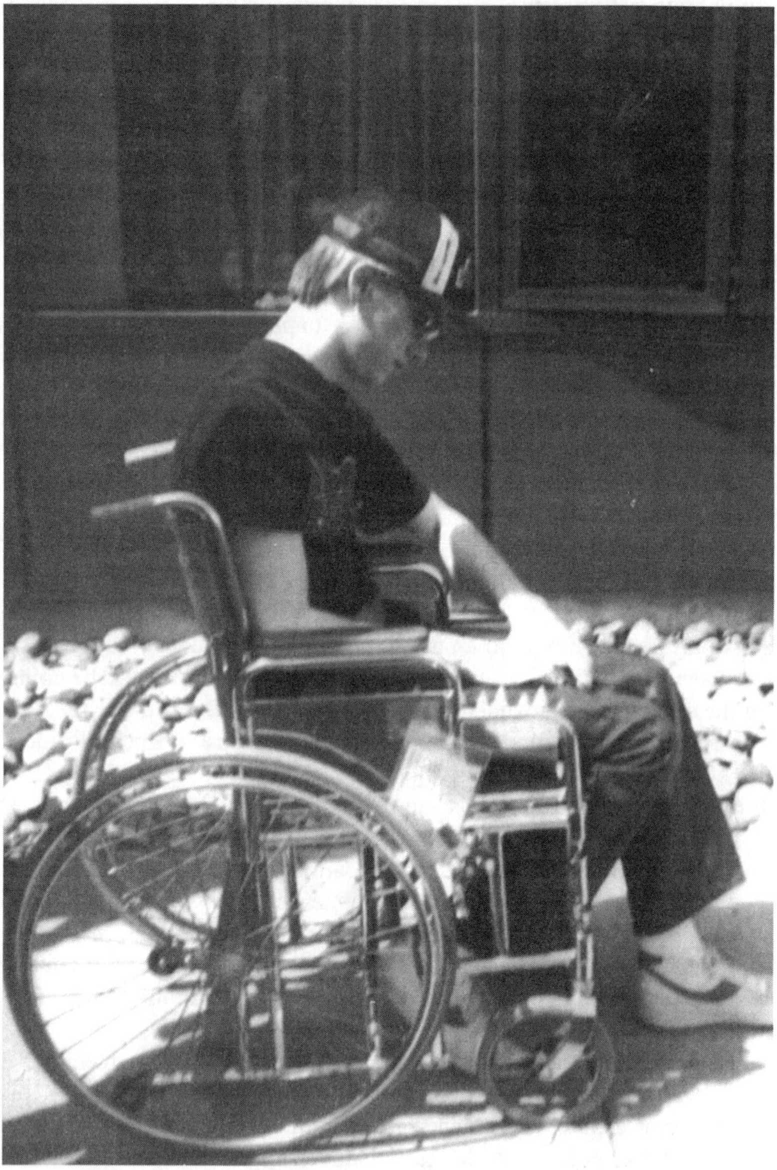

Forgetting how to walk, Craig needed his wheelchair in order to move around. This picture was taken outside of Craig's bedroom at Harmarville Rehabilitation Center.

Cheeks puffed and straining, Mary tried to push this deadweight patient up and Jan, red-eyed from this balancing act, yanked the best she could to get Craig aloft. Knees dipped and thighs rippling, Mary looked like she was catching an extra inning baseball game and Jan was firing off instructions like a captain does when his ship is going down and the distress horn is blaring. Moaning as if in dire need of Kaopectate, Craig rose two inches —four inches—eight inches—ten—eleven—twelve—ten—eight—"May day! May day!"—six—four—two, before going down for the count.

Jan was hunched over and petite Mary now knows what a hernia must feel like. If Craig hadn't developed such a nice rapport with these two young physical terrorists during the weeks he's been at Harmarville, he would have gotten another head injury from them when he started laughing after this failed attempt at standing resulted in his laying sprawled on the mat after his short fall back was valiantly broken by Jan and Mary.

Brushing herself off, Jan said, "So you think that's funny? Tomorrow, we're putting you on The Rack! That'll straighten you up—literally!!"

Running her fingers through her now messed up hair, Mary promised, "You're laughing now Craig, but tomorrow's another day. You'll get yours, don't worry. You better not go to sleep tonight, I may not wait for tomorrow."

It was pleasantries such as these and the personalities of the people who worked with Craig during his rehabilitation that made what should have been an intolerable situation, tolerable. Because of the winning dispositions of Harmarville's staff, this went a long ways towards diluting the effects disability has on the psyche. However, more would be needed if the inadequacies which clasped ahold of Craig were to be dissolved.

Along the walls of the hallway leading to Craig's room in Unit Three were handrails many patients in wheelchairs had to latch onto in order to move about. Craig used these, not only to traipse around in his wheelchair, but to grab onto with his right arm to stretch it out when he would exercise every night. OUCH! OUCH! OUCH!

With an ache shooting from his elbow which would chill a sadist's spine, Craig would use his left hand to grab a hold of his right wrist and pull down his forearm. Then, sliding his left hand off his wrist, Craig would have to separate each finger of his right hand apart before placing his paralytic paw on this titanium guide-rail. Craig would subsequently squeeze the handrail as tight as his right hand could and, in a masochistic-like manner, leaned back causing his elbow to throb with a gnawing pain which shot up to his shoulders and down his fingers. Craig could only tolerate this agony for ten or fifteen seconds a trial and would then have to sit back up.

Preparing himself mentally for the inevitable pain so he wouldn't let out an alarming screech and holding onto the support bar as tightly as he could, Craig would again lean against the back of his wheelchair, straightening out his arm as far as he could. Despite his arm wanting to atrophy at a right angle, Craig was not about to let this happen.

With a look of rage, a teary-eyed Craig would yank on the handrail as if he wanted to tear if off the wall. As the biting twinge went up and down his arm, Craig's anger would escalate and he would say to himself as he continued this self-abusive behavior, "I'm gonna pitch again, I'm gonna play my guitar."

Knowing all too well Craig's tenacity had caused him to overdo it on more than a few occasions when things got him down, nurses would frequently make him stop before he hurt himself. Craig's agitation stemmed from what his life encompassed now and not knowing if he will be submerged by the tears of today in the tomorrows ahead.

Craig's routine was one where he must struggle with things he once had done with ease, so they do not become a lasting reminder of the hand fate had dealt him. Craig's therapies during the day highlight that which he can no longer conceptualize, with this confusion creating the inferno which rages within him. And when therapies were over was when the real work began.

By himself, and for himself, Craig must practice his writing, ambulation, thinking, and stretching on his own, if he's going to withstand the fight of his life. The arm stretching, printing practice, and the drag racing down the main corridor in his wheelchair were not only to revive those skills which Craig's brain can no longer register, but to divert him from the frustration and despondency that wanted to explode inside of him. Because counseling for patients and their loved ones is not a priority at Harmarville, Craig's staying active was how he kept his emotions from being detonated.

Walking along Harmarville's semi-circular hallway leading to Craig's room on the evening of April 20th, Mr. and Mrs. Meyers saw Craig seated in his wheelchair outside of his room where he just finished working on his arm and were sickened by the sight of their boy melting with futility. With his head against the wall, still clinging onto the handrail, the somber look in Craig's eyes told the story of too much pain and no visible sign that his decompensation will do an about-face in this peregrination known as head injury rehabilitation. Because Craig could hold a tight rein on his demonstrativeness, the Meyers were stunned to see Craig stinging with distress.

Beyond a once a week, "life is rosy" group extravaganza held in the cafeteria, no formal psychotherapy would be offered at Harmarville. If it weren't for his parents talking with him over the phone every night and coming on those evenings when families could visit, as well as Valerie's caring involvement during the week, disconsolation would have forged ahead and overtaken Craig.

Struggling on an island of turmoil, degradation, and lost hope where one is oceans away from resolution is something the patient whose mind had been stained with confusion is going to face. When a facility which treats those with neurological impairments does not or cannot allocate the funds needed to exorcise the emotional trauma which accompanies disability, the patient must find other means to rid themselves of this horror, if they are to progress. For Craig, seeing his parents come down the hallway was a relief, for his only resource to discuss that which was eating away at him were now here.

Shortly after they arrived, the Meyers took their boy to the cafeteria for supper and put into action their formula of listening, allowing Craig to talk, and providing encouragement.

"Y'know, my therapists, doctors, nurses, Valerie, everybody; they're all really super. They really know what they're doing, but because they got so many other things to do and so many other people to work with, they don't have time to listen to me talk about how I'm being cut up inside, not knowing how I'm going to turn out. If it wasn't for you, mom and dad, I'd be like those that stay in their rooms all the time crying because they feel no one cares. Their families never come see them, so they have no one to talk to about how horrible it is being disabled. They feel trapped."

Chomping down on his liver and onions as he was talking, Mrs. Meyers couldn't believe that her picky son was eating foods Craig'd always curled his nose up at before and wouldn't touch. Thinking of how her limited choice of what gets prepared for supper could expand, Mrs. Meyers would at least appreciate this one effect of Craig's head injury as not being too bad. However, Craig's expression of feeling as if he was in solitary confinement soon erased any joy the Meyers felt over Craig's eating anything that didn't move.

"Besides Valerie—and I really don't want to dump my problems on her—there's not really anyone to talk to about my troubles, so I just do my own thing 'n rip up the hallway with my wheelchair and write until my hand gets sore. I guess that's good 'cause I'm practicin' stuff I need to and it distracts me from everything, but still there's so much wrong with me."

Feeling as though a spell had been cast upon him, Craig continued in a voice weary from this thought of his being cursed somehow, "I know there's going to be a time when everything's gonna hit me at once; not being able to walk or write. If my memory will ever come back. And then, it'll be tough to ignore. If it weren't for Valerie, I'd be goin' nuts because there wouldn't be anyone to talk to."

Rocking nervously at the dinner table with these thoughts of desertion, Craig said, "I feel so alone. That nothing's going to work again. Here at Harmarville, I know I just gotta suck it up and be tough. It's hard though; sometimes I just want to fuckin' die."

Hearing their son talk of his demise did not go over too well with Craig's parents. Mrs. Meyers reminded Craig that a lot of people worked hard to keep him alive and not to throw away the money that had already been committed on his behalf.

Stressing to his disheartened boy that his time hasn't come yet, Mr. Meyers said, "God must have some big plans for you, son. Or else you would have been left for dead on Beau Street."

Catching his breath during his dad's sermon, Craig took advantage of his only opportunity to unleash the pent up demons which, otherwise, would have fermented within him.

"I was a journalism student a few months ago and writing words was my main tool. Now, I can't even print my damned name unless I have a piece of cardboard with the letters on it in front of me," Craig said at a volume his parents reminded him to lower, for others around might hear despite being situated in a far-off corner of the dining room.

In a tone which started as a whisper, but ended in a roar, feeling as if he'd never break free from this hex that he thinks had been put upon him, Craig said, "I can't even get to the toilet when I need to take a shit 'cause I'm stuck in this fuckin' wheelchair for the rest of my life. And then I need someone to wipe my ass clean. Eighteen-years-old and I can't do a thing for myself. God, why'd You do this to me?"

Craig's parents weren't about to let their son assault the Father so, before Craig could attack his second portion and guzzle down his fruit punch, Mr. Meyers wheeled Craig out to the hallway away from those who could hear him rant and rave.

"Life isn't fair. The one party I go to in Washington in ten years, I end up being messed up. Paul—he's the drunk. He should be the one hurtin', not me," Craig said in a voice raging with fury.

"I didn't do anything to deserve this. I sat on my ass every weekend listening to my stereo; watchin' everyone else do things and the one time I try to get involved a little bit, I get hurt. I'll never be the same. God didn't want me to be happy."

"You weren't hurt by God," Mrs. Meyers said angrily, joining her husband and son after putting away Craig's dinner tray, "you were hurt by an evil boy whose parents didn't have the time to teach him. If I had it my way, I'd throw Paul in jail for the rest of his life, so he couldn't do what he did to you to someone else," Mrs. Meyers declaimed.

With the tears in her eyes exceeding flood level, Mrs. Meyers hissed, "The system protects criminals like Paul and forgets the victims. If he's allowed to roam about the streets, Paul's going to drink and drive again. You haven't heard the last from Paul Michaels, that's for sure. Before he's through, he's going to kill someone, somehow. I know it!"

Rubbing her eyes which the tears of hatred ran from, Mrs. Meyers gasped, "I don't know if God can forgive me for this, but Paul could hold my soul 'ransom' and I'd never, ever forgive him for what he did to you. Never!!"

Changing the flow of the discussion from the negative and away from history which cannot be altered, Mr. Meyers interceded, "You're not gonna be in that wheelchair forever, boy. You've made too many gains too fast for that to happen. I'm not saying it's going to be easy, you *KNOW* that. You'll just have to keep bustin' your ass like you have and that ole brain'll do its thing. I'll be here with you to the end; until you get that brain of yours workin' again. Count on it."

Sensing his son's identification as an anathema needed resuscitated and wanting to smother the power this image had over Craig, Mr. Meyers encouraged, "It's just a matter of time and you'll be up and about. It's not a question of 'If' you get better, but 'When.' I know you, you don't quit. When you set your sights on something, nothing can stop you."

With his dad's pep talk, a rejuvenation of will and energy shot through Craig again and it was back to business as usual. Governed by the will to overcome that which has destroyed many, Craig started printing his letter to Valerie and, with his folks by his side, later showed them the route he takes when he does his laps in his wheelchair. The simple formula of listening to someone and showing that they're cared about can work wonders. Without it, rehabilitation is compromised.

On Wednesday the 21st, Craig's first attempt at standing in the morning Physical Therapy session was as successful as his initial attempt on Monday and as floppy as his tight rope walker impersonation on Tuesday.

Despite habitually spreading his fingers apart and placing his bad hand on his right knee to push down, Craig still could not get on his feet and stay there even with the support of Jan and Mary. Slowly ascending, about halfway up, Craig's knees would start shaking and—like a fawn that's just been born—became so unstable he'd end up landing back where he started. Thoroughly disgusted, Craig'd try again until—after countless trials—his frustration would just get the better of him, so he'd have to return home to his wheelchair to take a break. Cussing, Craig could not figure out what was going on.

Going up, Craig's heart would beat faster with the anxiety and excitement that goes with viewing the world from the angle it should be for him and not from the depths of a wheelchair. It would be, in essence, a tangible experience of the physical progress he'd made after being ridden in a bed for so long. There's naturally going to be fear when putting weight on a leg that exploded from being crushed, but it was more than that. A whole lot more.

Normally, when someone rises and stands, they instinctively know where they are in relation to the things about them. This perceptual ability is something the brain does without conscious effort. That is, if this control system is a healthy one. If it isn't and this autonomical function is not working as it should, the person literally cannot get their bearings. With Craig, his balance deficiency was due—in part—to the "position sense" function of his brain not doing its thing.

The only way Craig could stand tall over his disorientation and stop slip-sliding from Jan or Mary's clutches was to keep practicing in PT with supervision until his brain realized gravity was not a foe. By the end of the afternoon session today, gravitation would be Craig's ally.

Craig was hard on himself in the sense that he had a tough time seeing beyond what he can no longer do. Yesterday, a day which Craig was capsized by a wave of lost purpose, he took a memory test in Psychology. If Craig could have only known the results of his test score, he wouldn't have been so "down in the mouth" the day before. Some things were definitely starting to look up for Craig.

The Weschler Memory Scale, which Craig received the results of today, measure one's ability to immediately recall verbal and non-verbal material by utilizing several techniques including digit span (an oral memory counting exercise), verbal paired associate learning (matching exercise), general orientation questions, etc. The WMS showed Craig was now oriented times three and confirmed that his ability to learn new material of varying difficulty was intact.

Not surprisingly, this test showed Craig's visual memory (ability to mentally conceptualize images) was deficient. Anybody who had seen Craig struggle to remember what the different letters of the alphabet looked like, would hardly be shocked by this revelation. But that deficit pales in comparison to the encouraging results which show Craig could still attain and retain information.

Craig's uneasy parents were fearful that the portion of their son's brain which was darkened would render his capacity to learn forever dormant. As well as his own tireless efforts, the input from his family and staff developed passageways in Craig's brain which branched out and responded to stimuli. The brain processing external stimulation and storing it—not merely retrieving from the data banks material previously learned—gave the Meyers hope that the cognitive liabilities Craig shows now, such as his writing lapse, has the potential to be overcome. That Craig needn't be a prisoner of a mind ruptured of its knowledge and capacity to capture new understanding.

At Harmarville, while Craig was fighting the effects of his head injury, back in Washington, Mrs. Meyers was engaged in battle herself. Both Social Security and the Meyers' auto insurance wanted to volley back and forth their obligation to provide sufficient funding for Craig after he was hurt.

On January 1, 1982, Mr. Meyers was eligible for social security having turned sixty-two the month before. At this time, through his dad's social security, Craig was due to receive monthly payments according to a set pay scale. Through this benefit, which Mr. Meyers paid into for many, many years out of his paycheck, he applied for disability on Craig's behalf almost immediately after Craig was hurt knowing that Craig's regular social security probably will be jeopardized as soon as he had officially withdrawn from school. And it was.

Under the new Reaganomic plan (Omnibus Reconciliation Act), Craig is only eligible for regular social security payments until July 1982—or seven more months—while maintaining full-time student status. And this is where either the wool was trying to be pulled over Mrs. Meyers' eyes or the insurance company was not real keen about what Craig was due. In Webster's Dictionary, beside the words "thorough," "research," and "perseverant" is a picture of Mrs. Meyers.

Because Craig was a college student full-time, he was scheduled to receive a monthly stipend in excess of $275 from social security until this summer, following his freshman year at school. But, when Craig was hurt in February and no longer an active student, social security was then terminated.

Craig had received social security payments in January and February before he was forced to drop out of W.V.U. Now that he was no longer a student, social security stopped paying the stipend he was entitled for five more months under Reagan's July '82 cutoff.

According to the Pennsylvania No Fault Auto Insurance Law, when one has been disabled due to a traffic accident, lost income gets reimbursed from one's own automobile insurance regardless of who is at fault. Therefore, the Meyers' automobile insurance had to reimburse Craig for the five months' worth of social security benefits he would lose not being a full-time college student anymore.

The Medical Management Specialist unfortunate enough to be assigned Craig's case and tangle with Mrs. Meyers, didn't want to pay the boy who almost ended up in a body bag his June and July social security benefits. He believed Craig shouldn't receive both social security and the lost wages Craig would have earned in the greenhouse during those two summer months had he not been hurt, and sent Mrs. Meyers a nasty letter stating that Craig is only going to get the lost pay he would have earned working at the greenhouse and no more. Wrong move.

In response to this letter, to substantiate the edicts as they are written, Mrs. Meyers promptly sent documentation (Page 3 of the 1982 Social Security Administration Publication, No. 05-10048) stating that—yes indeed—Craig is to receive both social security and lost wages with no strings attached. Not at all happy being outwitted, the Medical Management Specialist sent Mrs. Meyers another tasteless letter stating that if Craig is to receive these payments, federal taxes are going to be taken out. Not so fast.

Mrs. Meyers pointed out that under No Fault, it stipulates that one has to earn in excess of $4,440 before they can be taxed by the Feds. With both the social security and the lost wages income, Craig falls way below this limit. En garde!

Mrs. Meyers' business college-training, as well as her experience as a secretary for the rationing board and a colonel during World War II, served her well during this never-ending demand for documentation. Besides having to keep track of the hundreds and thousands of miles they traveled on Craig's behalf, this mother/unpaid clerical slave undertook the unenviable duty of requesting, waiting for, and copying all of Craig's medical records and sending them to the different sources that needed to see them.

Just doing their job, the auto insurance needed confirmation of everything before they would afford Craig any money. They wanted copies of what exactly the primary insurer would and would not pay for, that social security did indeed stop their stipend to Craig, written proof from doctors stating what Craig's condition was and their prognosis for employment, who Craig's employer was last summer, how many hours a week he worked, how long he had worked at the greenhouse, duties at the greenhouse, etc., etc., etc. This always turned out to be a bureaucratic hassle.

By day's end, Mrs. Meyers would be exhausted. Her mind ragged from fighting for what she knows her boy deserves and her heart ached knowing that—under the old social security provision—Craig would have received these payments from the time he started college until age twenty-two.

Mrs. Meyers would not allow her son to be cheated in any way. When someone's been hurt as severely as Craig, there's no telling how many of those pennies will be needed in the future. At war with the symptoms which attacked him, neither was Craig going to cheat himself out of everything he could get.

In the short-term, Craig's efforts to get on his feet and maintain this standing position may not have provided him with much in the way of immediate gratification, but Craig would be cashing in on the long-term payoff. After Jan finished up with another patient, she walked over to Craig and said, "Well, are you ready to give getting on your feet another go?" Craig was more than willing, as the break did him good.

The morning's stalled attempts at trying to stand gave Craig some invaluable experience of the sensation he's to encounter when trying to get on his feet. This helped immensely. Not only because it was not a foreign experience for him trying to stand now—giving Craig some ammunition about the attitude he needs to have taking on this task—but because his central nervous system could capitalize on these building blocks which had previously only been stumbling blocks.

With Mary by Craig's left side and Jan kneeling along the mat to his right, this anxious patient not having been on his feet for sixty-seven days, Craig told these waiting patriots/gluttons for punishment he was ready. Her hand on Craig's back for leverage and support—in a voice sounding as if she was in a mission control center—Jan steadily rocked Craig forward, saying in a tone painted with encouragement and confidence, "One."

Quickly pushing Craig down and up almost as if getting back at him for yesterday, Jan then said in her firm commanding way, "Two." And then, holding her breath with wishful anticipation, Jan grunted while sternly rocking Craig forward, "Three!!"

Positioned under his pits again and their arms bracing his posterior side in case Craig decides to do a backflip, Jan and Mary pushed and hoisted themselves skyward, hoping this Harmarville gymnasium would be a Cape Caneveral for Craig and he'd take off his launching pad. With the rocket boosters blazing and the look of determination in his eyes, Craig's hindquarters catapulted off the mat. His head getting higher and higher after taking a nose-dive dip so his back would lunge forward, helping him straighten up, Craig wouldn't be denied. Craig's hands pushed down on his knees with a quick force before they could buckle. Straining, Craig fought the impulse his tattered brain was telling him to retreat.

Chest pounding, occupied only with the thought of beating the odds, Craig would not allow himself to be failures' conquest. There was only one way it was going to be, and that was going to be Craig's way. This time, the mission was not going to be aborted. The time had come to put this disabling condition of being bound to a wheelchair to rest. Rest in Peace.

Angry at what this injury had done to him, dipping his back going forward then holding his chest up, Craig pushed down, down, down on his knees with a prevailing force until they locked. "And we have lift off."

Standing on his feet for the first time in what seemed eons, Craig smiled so broadly the tiny space between his front teeth could be seen back home in Washington County. Feeling a joyous sense of accomplishment and pride in the work they do, Jan and Mary knew, however, the time to revel would have to wait.

With Craig standing, these two professionals were not about to waste this golden opportunity they could not say for sure would present itself again anytime soon, so they threw Craig's arms over their shoulders without delay to support him for the sequel to this attempt at doing some foot and legwork.

Under Craig's right arm to help him support his weight, Jan said, "Like I've shown you when you first started moving your wheelchair, when you take a step, you want to place the heel of your foot on the ground first, then your toes. Then you want to push off with your toes and roll on the ball of your foot, lifting your heel up. Now, let's move your left foot first. Remember what I said—heel down first."

Wary of putting any weight on his right leg, Craig leaned much of his 160 plus pounds on Mary's shoulders and quickly slapped his left foot a step in front of him. Craig's first step in a little over two months wasn't a pretty one, but he'd take it—at least it's a start. Now, for the real agonizing part—getting his paralytic right leg to do the same thing.

Not knowing how his right lower extremity was going to respond to the signals sent by a brain that has had to relearn everything, Craig leaned heavily on these two queens and—staring down—tried to pick his foot off the ground. Picturing his right leg snapping like a twig that's been bent too far if he put any weight on it coming down, Craig just stood there like a statue with his left leg a step in front of his right.

Sensing the tension, Jan said, "Go ahead, you can do it. You've done a super job getting this far. We want to take a couple of steps to the parallel bars, so you can do some work there." Encouraged by the confidence his therapist had shown in him, Craig did his Frankenstein's monster routine and dragged the top of his right foot up parallel to his left one.

Happy to see Craig take one step, albeit not a very smooth one, Jan was itchin' for more. "I know your right leg feels like it has no strength or control, but it does. Don't be afraid, your leg has healed; it can support any weight you put on it. Let's take another step. Go ahead and start with your left leg again. You can do it!"

Identical to what he did the first step, Craig leaned on the now red-shouldered Mary and stomped his left foot down immediately, so as to not put any weight on his once broken right leg. After his left foot slammed on the ground, registering 5.6 on the Richter Scale, Craig responded to Jan's claim in a voice shaking with panic, "I might be a little scared of putting weight on my right leg, but that leg can't pick my foot up!! It just sets there, not able to move!!"

Looking as if he was prepared to do a split positioned like he was, Jan hyperventilated in her calm voice to her patient in the ballerina pose, "You're able to move your foot and leg, you're not paralyzed. You have paralysis, there's a big difference. The only way we're going to be able to help you is to practice trying to get that brain to do what you want it to do. Now c'mon, you're heavy! They're going to have to give me and Mary CPR if you don't stop talking and start concentrating on getting to those parallel bars. C'mon, let's go."

Quickly, Craig skidded his right foot to where his left one waited while explaining why he was moving like he was, "When I don't have both feet on the floor to secure me, I feel like I'm going to fall over. With only one leg on the ground, I feel so unstable; so shaky."

Sweat burning their eyes from hauling this load, Jan told Craig that's why they need to take three more steps to the parallel bars; so he can get used to standing while having some support at the same time. Her own feet dragging lugging Craig, Mary gasped, "I can tell you've been eating double portions. Me and Jan are going to have a talk with the cooks in the kitchen, we don't get paid enough for this!"

After another quick move, banging his left foot in front of him, Craig then leaned on Jan's back as she bent over to pick his right leg off the ground, so that he could get the "feel" of what to do when he tries this on his own. Setting his one-time fractured limb back on the ground—still supporting Craig as he made himself comfortable on her backbone—Jan said, "You're leg's not broken anymore, it can hold you. You don't have to worry, it might feel tight at first, but your break isn't going to hurt anymore."

Knowing what he's feeling wasn't his imagination, Craig shot back, "When I lean to the right or roll over in bed, Jan, I can feel somethin' clicking in my upper thigh. I might be 'head injured,' but I'm not crazy. I think it's that fuckin' rod that's tearin' my leg up."

Telling Craig to watch his raw sewage language, sporting an elbow mark on her spine, Jan told Craig to first place the heel of his left foot down when taking his next step and concentrate on bending his right knee when trying to lift up his right foot. Strained and agitated, Craig's final two steps were as ugly as his first ones, as he held onto the parallel bar like it was a life preserver.

As Craig stood at the parallel bars, clinging on for dear life, several therapists and the intern—Andy—commended him for his efforts and some of the patients, who had seen Craig when he came in, told this proud patient how good it was to see him up. Before taking a much needed respite from Craig to work with some of her other patients, Jan told Mary the motions which Craig was to practice at the parallel bars.

Standing tall, viewing the gymnasium from an angle Craig wasn't sure he'd ever see again, Mary kept bending his right knee slowly telling him that this was what he was going to have to do when he wants to take a step. At this time, the emphasis was for Craig to be able to lift his right foot off the ground; the first step needed if he was to begin walking correctly.

Mary then stopped this modeling and told Craig to give it a try. Looking down at his right tennis shoe—visualizing it coming off the floor—Craig tried to pick up his foot, but all he was able to do was stare at this motionless mass. Somewhere between Craig's brain and his hoof, the message wasn't getting through.

Telling Craig to let her know when he was getting tired, Mary started manipulating his knee again. "Concentrate, not so much on raising your foot, but bending your knee;" Mary reminded Craig, "maybe that will help."

After several minutes of intense concentration, all that did was transfer the frustration of not being able to lift his foot, to the frustration of not being able to bend his knee.

Craig was getting mad that he wasn't able to lift his foot despite this thorough concentration and when Mary suggested that she get his wheelchair and for him to take a break, Craig said he didn't want that and insisted he was okay. Craig told Mary that if she needed to attend to someone else, then go ahead and just leave the wheelchair at the end of the parallel bars where he could get to it. Mary's main priority this afternoon was working with Craig, so she wasn't going anywhere. Instead, she kept lifting Craig's leg at the knee over and over with the hopes that his brain would get the signal from the Patella and Co. what it needs to do in order to get that foot skyward. However, all that was going up at this time was Craig's blood pressure.

Keeping an eye on her patient, Jan saw a guy who was just standing there hanging his head, looking at his leg which wasn't moving. Head bowed, Craig tried so damn hard, but it was to no avail, as he was shocked that he couldn't get his leg to move. The dissolution of Craig's ability to make his foot and leg abide by the brain's command was yet another passage in the horror tale which is a brain injury.

When someone has had a head injury, physical therapy is physical misery. If any gains are to be made when a patient takes on this most degrading and debilitating of physical experiences, they need to be almost obsessed with beating the odds and be focused for the hand-to-hand combat that's going to occur when going to war with the effects of a brain injury.

While Craig was wheeling himself down Harmarville's main hallway to his last program, Occupational Therapy, he had mixed emotions about what happened today in PT. Craig was ecstatic that he stood because it showed his brain was responding to his efforts and was proud of this accomplishment, for it wouldn't be paying dividends if he hadn't put forth the work/determination he had. However, Craig was in no mood to celebrate, for it scared him to death being unable to move his right lower extremities when he tried in vain.

As with his cognitive writing lapse, Craig's inability to physically lift up his foot showed him just how dependent a person is on the brain working as it should. Its functions taken for granted, until they've been taken away. The wicked tricks a mind wrought with lost capacity plays on those stricken can garnish the soul and challenge one's fortitude.

In OT, Craig had a tough time concealing the joy he felt about standing for that first time today, as he told his hand therapists of his achievement in the previous therapy. With her unmistakable, "Way to go"/"Go get 'em" demeanor, Wendy congratulated her patient who was "cheesing it up" from ear to ear, beaming from the thoughts of his magnificent accomplishment. Since she caught Craig in a mood other than the foul one that usually had a grip on him this time of day, Wendy thought she'd work with him on some exercises that usually made Craig hot under the collar with frustration. Oh well, so much for being in a good mood, but that's rehab.

Knocking plastic bowling pins down with a kickball, squeezing a rubber Snoopy dog, and putting different shaped pegs in its matching hole would be for another day. Today, Craig would be manipulating some color-coded Play-Doh-like substance with his right hand and fingers. Oh boy!

This therapy putty varied in its consistency from soft to firm. In order of resistance from the least degree of firmness to the most, the colors of the putty were yellow, red, green, pink, and blue. The purpose of this putty is to work on the different operations of the hand and to get a measurement the effectiveness the hand is able to undertake these functions.

The different hand motions Craig works on are Opposition (the act of resistance), Flexion (the act of bending), Extension (the act of straightening a bent limb), Abduction (the act of drawing away from a center or median line), Intrinsic (the act of isolating movements inherent of the hand), Deviation (the act of turning away from), Pronation (the act of turning the palm backward or downward), and Supination (the act of turning the palm upward).

Different exercises are employed in order to enhance these movements of the hand. Because this work requires great care and delicacy, the time involved to make any progress and to just go through with these exercises was significant. Hand just floundering in this dough-like cement, Craig's anger/frustration would percolate when gains weren't evident.

In one exercise known as Gross Opposition, Craig would flatten the putty into a pancake and lightly place his fingers and thumb on the edge of this flapjack before trying to draw them together. If it wasn't for his mouth moving, machine-gunning expletives, one would think a snapshot of Craig was taken doing this test of futility—for he wasn't moving otherwise.

Another Opposition exercise Craig tried was when he made the putty into the shape of a cone placing his thumb and fingers lightly at the top of this pyramid, pulling it up. While doing this, Craig would slowly bring his thumb and fingers together. Because the resistance was less than the Pancake Opposition exercise, Craig did a little better. Because the dexterity of his fingers was non-existent, Craig would not be asked to do the more difficult Pinch Opposition exercise where he would have to squeeze putty between his thumb and fingers or between two fingers.

Another putty exercise, Gross Finger Flexion, Craig put a cylindrical roll of putty in his right palm and made a fist. Craig didn't have a whole lot of trouble with this, all he had to do was think of the terror he was going to be put through in the Individual Finger Flexion exercise.

In this torture, Craig wrapped a sheet of putty around a designated right finger and—placing his wrapped finger in his good left hand—tried to bend the finger through the putty to his right palm. When one of the occupational therapists would enthusiastically beam, "Good Craig!," upon his isolating the movement of one finger—barely jiggling it—Craig knew they were only doing their job providing him with encouragement. But still, it gnawed at him inside knowing that he should feel gratitude for doing nothing.

The Thumb Flexion agitation test was one where Craig held the putty shaped in a cylinder with his right fingers and tried to dig his thumb as deep as he could into it and then would yank it out slowly (extension). For Craig, this was like trying to burrow a hole in concrete with his bare hands, as his knuckle wanted to snap from the pressure.

During the Wrist Flexion excursion, Craig's tendons just wanted to shut down. Here, Craig's right wrist hung over the table with the putty firmly snug in his palm. With Craig's palm up and the cylindrical tube of putty dangling between the middle and ring fingers, Craig held the putty with his left hand while he tried pushing it up with his right wrist. Talk about a mismatch.

With the opposition and flexion exercises mercifully over with, Craig was set to begin the extension misery exercises. Out of habit, Craig would start by picking his right arm up with his left hand and placing his paralytic wing on the table where he was going to be tortured. That is, until Wendy would tell Craig to try lifting his right arm on its own and attempt to spread his fingers without using his good hand, so that he can get used to moving independently of his left side. Therefore, the torture actually would begin even before Craig got his hand on the table. It was that bad.

Also, when Wendy asked Craig to move his side affected with hemiparesis, she wanted to see how much—if any—improvement had occurred with Craig's right side. Wendy's cold silence after one of Craig's tenacious and futile struggles to get his right fingers/hand/arm to respond some way, any way, was a barometer to how well Craig's brain was making those right upper body parts listen to what it was told to do.

With one Gross Finger Extension exercise, Craig would simply roll the putty into a tube and wrap this around his right fingers and the thumb. Stretching the fingers outward with the thumb serving as a base, this strengthens the digits and supposedly retrains the brain to open the hand up.

The resistance on Craig's fingers was such that opening his hand for a handshake was a formidable venture. In another Gross Finger Extension test of durability, strength, flexibility, and nerves, Craig would place his palm down in the putty with his fingers in a curled position. Slowly pushing away the putty, Craig's fingertips pressed into this clay-like substance, uncurling his fingers. Like the other finger exercise, when Craig wrestled with this conditioning task, it looked like he was going in slow motion.

The Individual Finger Extension was not an easy task for Craig either. This unavailing enterprise was one where a tiny doughnut was wrapped around the thumb and the unfortunate finger chosen to be tested. With the thumb stabilized, the finger stretches outward pressing against the putty and expanding this coil.

A wrist extension exercise which also incorporates the finger in a gross motor skill activity involves Craig gently rolling putty back and forth while he keeps his fingers and wrist straight. Pulling out putty and then rolling it back and forth, back and forth, back and forth would be a stabbing reminder for Craig just how far he's regressed in such a short time. This right hand which once picked some heavy duty riffs on electric guitar now can't even pinch a clothes pin.

Although a lot better since working out in the hallway every night, this right arm that once could fire fastballs past most hitters can no longer be stretched straight. Craig would have tested his right hand's coordination by coloring between the lines, if he could only hold a crayon.

Like the Wrist Flexion practice, in the Wrist Extension punishment, Craig's paralytic hand would hang over the edge of the torture table with his left hand beneath this tabletop, holding the putty. But this time, the palm of his bad hand faces down when pulling the putty up. This was another trying exercise for Craig, not only because the flexibility of his wrist was as tight as his right heel cord, but because he knew that if his right wrist does not respond to treatment, his days as a guitar picker are over.

The Finger Abduction challenge is utilized to help the person with a bad hand learn to spread their fingers apart again. With the fingers together and a coil of putty around them, Craig would struggle to spread his fingers sideways. If Craig's ever going to try to pick up a pencil again with his right hand, he'll need to develop this motion.

The Thumb and Finger Abduction drill, where Craig is to squeeze some putty between his right thumb and index finger or between any two fingers of his right hand, works on the skill Craig would need to hold a pencil or a guitar pick. And, if Craig is to emulate the "thumbs up" Wendy gives him for his effort everyday, he will have to master the movements practiced in the Thumb Radial and Thumb Palmar Abduction indoctrinations.

In the first one, Craig stretches his right thumb to the left away from the four tightly closed fingers and against the putty. In the latter, the four fingers are held tightly straight together again, but this time, instead of bending horizontally away from his fingers, Craig bends his thumb away parallel to the palm. Once again, Craig's fingers and thumb wanted to do their own thing, being insubordinate to the brain's command.

The left hemisphere of Craig's brain must be a real mess, for the ball his right fingers were curled up in weren't going anywhere—anytime soon—and his arm was going just as far. When asked to put either his right hand, fingers, or arm into motion, the emotional demolition which tore at Craig was profound. On the surface, it might have looked like Craig wasn't doing much of anything, but he was.

Like the gross motor skill of standing, the fine motor skills Craig practiced, but found impossible to do, required complete concentration. Concentration stimulates the brain to learn the movements needed to undertake an operation. Unlike getting on his feet and standing erect, because the movements he was trying to achieve with his right hand and fingers in Occupational Therapy were so slight, Craig would get markedly agitated not getting that brain to make things work as they should.

Identical to his right foot when he tried to lift it in PT, Craig's right hand and fingers would not move despite his undying efforts to make some kind of a connection between his brain and that which would not make the reception complete. When such relentless work is required to get so little, Craig would burn. Burn in the sense he would get angry, not "burn out" as if he was going to surrender. As a matter of fact, the anger sparked Craig to look for or develop a current which would make his right upper extremities adhere to the brain's signal to shake, rattle, and roll.

If he keeps working as he has, maybe one day Craig will be able to bend his wrist up as his arm lays on a table!!! Or raise a finger a few millimeters with his palm flat!!! Or bend a knuckle!!! After one's had a head injury, so little can mean so much.

In Physical Therapy earlier, Craig's right LOWER extremities wouldn't listen to his brain's command to get going, and in Occupational Therapy, his right UPPER extremities were doing the same thing. Craig's really getting a taste of the joys of head injury rehabilitation today. And the work ain't over yet.

When the last program of the day ended with Craig putting so much into it and receiving what seemed so little, this exhausted soul wheeled the short distance back to his room where his new roommate was sleeping. Finishing up his letter to Valerie, a process which took Craig twenty minutes for him to write five words because printing the wrong one seven or eight times before getting it right is time-consuming, Craig then started writing Jan Goga her letter. These two nurses being attractive had nothing to do with Craig's ending up writing them, uh, that was just coincidence.

A few weeks after Jan "saved" Craig from that old lady who wanted to lodge a fork in his forehead when he had to eat in the nurses' station, Craig had a choking episode just drinking some water and Jan came to the rescue again clearing Craig's pipes. Copying the letters, "D-E-A-R J-A-N," Craig wanted to begin writing a thank you letter to his Lone Ranger now that he can write a little better. Ahh, sweet guy, that Craig Meyers.

Not wanting to offend his cognitive therapists, afraid this could have a bearing on his date of discharge, Craig'd be liable to tell these "mind professionals" various flowery techniques they employed with him were working great. Theorizing that the tactile sensations of different letters would help his memory as to their form, anything worth a try to get this agraphic former journalism student writing spontaneously again, Craig was to rub his fingers over letters made of sandpaper. Quickly realizing that this outrageous method had no utility, Craig abandoned this quirky approach for a more traditional route.

In reality, what was really helping Craig in this process of relearning how to write was the multitudes of letters he wrote his nurse buddies. There's no substitute for hard work.

Being a meat and potatoes type of guy, Craig would have just as soon burned those Freudian "Short-Cuts to Overcoming Agraphia" books, than to feel the scratchy surface of a letter. Overall, however, the work these therapists were doing was spectacular. After having his visual memory stripped of all recognition, for Craig to even be able to write a little bit represented phenomenal progress.

The reemergence of functions in a brain once shaken can improve provided the warring person does what they can to facilitate this process. Because the restraints of permanent disability were not something Craig could accept, his fight to overcome his afflictions would not be an idle one.

With the right leg rest of his wheelchair gone, when Craig would wheel his riding partner, he would have to take tiny, deliberate steps. This didn't do much for the speed which Craig traveled from place to place, but it was getting that right foot to respond to the signals the brain was shooting to lift and make some semblance of a step forward. Bit by bit, with his right foot barely lifting off the ground, Craig's brain was being stimulated to relearn the action needed to take a step.

As he did when the footplate was taken off his wheelchair, Craig was going to go out to the hallway and practice. This time, however, making his right lower body parts abide by his brain's command being that he was leg rest-less. Or was it have his brain abide by his body's command to get a "move on?" Whatever it was, Craig knew he had a lot of work to do.

When Craig painstakingly wheeled himself towards the hallway to do his laps, he'd pass guys sitting on their ass at the tables in the nurses' station who'd be smoking, playing cards, and bitching about how life had been so unfair to them since they've been hurt. Without tackling the problem head-on, moaning and groaning would be their favorite pastime. Although talking about the many obstacles encountered when enduring a head injury is vital, when little is done to overcome these obstructions, the purpose of rehabilitation is defeated.

After he finished telling his parents over the phone of his milestone this afternoon, Craig was whisked into the shower where he had the stink of his wheelchair laps/ping-pong match with Valerie washed off and went right to bed. Craig had better get a good night's sleep, for tomorrow would be another sprawling with adventure.

In Communication Skills, the morning of April 22nd, Craig struggled to control what direction his left writing hand went when he tried to make a lower case "r," instead, Craig made an upper case "L." And, when Diane wanted Craig to put on his paper an upper case "A," he'd squiggle a lower case "q." Wanting to make an upper case "B," Craig would print an upper case "S." On this last try, at least Craig got the cases right.

While trying to get a few letters down on a tablet this new day, when the pen Craig was holding would touch that paper, he would hesitate before his hand would shoot off somewhere purposelessly. When he would do this, Craig would immediately stop, knowing this wasn't accomplishing anything. After identifying the letter or jumble of letters he mistakenly printed, Diane would tell Craig to break down what he intends to write into steps. First, TRY to get a mental image of the letter, know what direction the hand needs to move in order to copy this mental picture, and finally, force the hand to go where it's supposed to, not on some wild goose chase.

Slumped in his wheelchair battling the erroneous representations of his mind, Craig had no idea how to write spontaneously. Diane would tell Craig to stop and try picturing what he wants to put on paper, one letter at a time. Diane would say to Craig that while his visual memory is in this blank state it's in, he won't be able to cram letters automatically. Told to be patient with his brain for it needs more time to work properly since it's been disturbed, Craig's growing intellect realized the brain had been physically disturbed, but his emotions didn't want to accept any excuses.

Under normal circumstances, when a person whose brain is working decides to write, mentally forming an image of a word poses no trouble because picturing clusters of letters in their mind comes without hesitation. Like a word or words on a flash card, without effort, the cognitively intact person simply can see the symbol and transmit down to the hand what it wants replicated.

Somewhere during this process, a "disconnection" in Craig's brain either erased what was on the flash card or put so many symbols on the card it became an unintelligible, confusing sludge of nothing. And this usually caused Craig to print anything, usually a wrong letter.

In order to learn and have letters imprinted in his memory again, Craig would have to continue practicing and abandon his pursuit to just "take off" and write. Whether he likes it or not, Craig's just going to have to dissect each word into its individual letters, if he is to make any progress. And because of what he achieved yesterday, continued progress was all that was on his mind for his next therapy.

Although significantly quicker than yesterday when he first tried to propel his right leg and foot, the glacial pace with which Craig chugged down the hallway to PT in his wheelchair was a time used to envision the success he was going to experience in a few moments' time when attempting to take that first good step while standing, not seated in a wheelchair. Failure would not be considered. All Craig could see was his hopping out of that wheelchair and standing at those parallel bars, lifting that right foot up and taking step after step after step.

Wheeling around the corner to the entrance of the gymnasium, Jan must have been thinking along those same lines as she greeted her patient with a, "Are we going to take a couple of steps at those parallel bars today or what?"

Responding, "Damn right, we are!," Craig labored along in the wheelchair he was trying to say goodbye to and parked his means of getting around along the front wall where he always does.

Before she and Craig got started, Jan motioned for Theresa Gates to come over and told Craig that Theresa will be working with him for a few days until she comes back from her vacation. In addition to her high standard of professionalism, Theresa's, "Don't step out of line or you're history"/ "Tell it like it is," spunky personality would work well with Craig's own no-nonsense outlook on things. It was a good mix.

Seeing Craig work on different exercises in the gym everyday and having been filled in by Jan what he needs to practice, Theresa had a good idea of Craig's treatment plan and wasn't going to miss a beat. Before getting back to her own patients, Theresa was going to watch Craig up close, so she could get a "bird's eye view" of what Craig was having trouble with and needed to work on. The rambling Craig did yesterday down and up/up and down the hallway in his wheelchair got his brain primed and ready for what he was about to do in therapy.

Standing by his wheelchair, Jan told Craig to wheel up to the parallel bars. Motivated to get out of that wheelchair, Craig was much obliged. Telling her eager patient to slow down before he got ahead of himself, Jan instructed Craig that she needs to show him how to smoothly transfer out of his wheelchair first because it's slightly different from getting off a mat like he did yesterday.

The most vital requisite for prosperous rehabilitation to occur is a patient's incentive to get better. Without this, the person has nothing. By the same token, the person having sustained a head injury must be ready and prepared for the next seemingly impenetrable barrier, but not act on impulse. Not only does the inducement to crack the whip have to be present for recovery to occur, but it must be snapped wisely. One without the other, the patient isn't going to get out of rehab what they can. Haste making waste, they could even find themselves stagnating, regressing, or suffering a setback, if overly anxious. With Craig focused on conquering that which will not submit, the time had come to war with his mind's confusion.

Seated in his wheelchair at the end of the parallel bars, there was no doubt in Craig's mind that he was going to move along the continuum known as progress. Jan told Craig that what he's got to do first to transfer to the parallel bars is wheel his chair as closely as he can and lock the brakes. Then, Jan reminded Craig he needs to rock the three times down and up to get the momentum going before pushing with both hands on his knees to get up.

With a hearty, "Here we go!," Jan walked up to Craig's wheelchair and put one hand on his right shoulder and the other on the middle of his upper back. Decked out in her white physical therapy garb, Theresa was stationed to Craig's left in case she was needed to keep the ship from sinking or running aground.

In a matter-of-factly voice which sounded as if there was no doubt in her mind that Craig was capable of standing high and taking those first steps since walking out to Paul's car for the ride of his life which almost ended it, Jan reminded Craig again, "On the count of three, you're going to push down on your knees and stand up."

Sounding like the mother figure she had to be at times with Craig, Jan added without a trace of sarcasm, "And don't you even think about walking until me and Theresa are ready."

With the acid in his stomach shooting up his throat from the excitement of the big moment only seconds away and the faith his therapist had in him, Craig was revving up his engines when Jan led him down and said, "One." Myocardium pumping at warp speed, Jan had Craig up and down ripping out a, "Two," faster than he could say, "Jan, you're killing me."

And then, with the steam spewing from his exhaust pipes and the blood racing from his aorta, Jan rocked Craig and yiped, "Three!!!," as Craig pushed, pushed, pushed his palms against those knees that were shaking with excitement until—like fireworks shot on the Fourth of July—Craig was up, up, and away.

Seeing his therapists from the tops of their heads instead of staring straight at them from belly button level would be something most single guys wouldn't see as progress. But for Craig, nothing could have gotten his motor running more than having his feet support his frame. Now, if his brain can only get that transmission out of "Park" and into "Drive."

Standing, even with both hands clasping onto the parallel bars, Craig felt as stable as someone who's been on stilts for the first time. Despite viewing the world from this height for the better part of eighteen years, towering at an elevation of six-feet was like a new experience for Craig. Feeling as if his legs were just going to give out from under him, Craig felt a little unnerved waiting for Jan to position herself in front of him and Theresa in back. With the stage set, the show was about to begin. And what a gala it was going to be.

Looking at Craig's feet which hadn't supported much in the way of weight, Jan told Craig to concentrate on bending his right knee, so he can bring the front part of his foot up. The hours of practice Craig put in yesterday trying to get his right lower extremities to move his wheelchair paid off, for the message his bruised brain was telegraphing to his foot to get up from the floor was being dispatched.

Grasping the parallel bars so tightly the big blood vessels in Craig's hands were doubling in size, flat-footed, Craig raised his right foot a few inches and slapped it down a short distance in front of his left. Quickly, Craig took a step with his left foot completing his first step of the day. Hold onto those ribbons of paper, no need to get ready for that ticker-tape parade quite yet.

With his right knee bending just enough, Craig lifted his foot this second time and quickly smacked it on the ground as if he were trying to squash a fast-moving bug. The majority of his weight supported by his arms, not his right leg, Craig took a quick step with his left foot before plopping his right one. Craig could not, in any way, place his right heel down first. When Craig would waddle a step, he looked like Festus on "Gunsmoke," but Craig's spurs didn't click as fast.

Whipping his left foot forward a step and flinging his right, Craig repeated this pattern until he came to the end of the balance bar. What does he do now?

Jan explained that in order for him to turn around, Craig'd have to let go of the right parallel bar with his bad hand and grab a hold of the bar to his left. While always holding on with his good left hand, Craig was told he would have to shimmy his rear end ninety degrees, so that he'd be standing alongside the bar his left hand always had a grasp of. Then, grabbing with his left hand the bar that's now behind him which his right hand started off clutching, Craig's going to have to wiggle some more until he had completed his one-hundred-eighty degree turn. Riddled by sequencing difficulties and perseveration, Craig did not fully understand, but he knew better than to ask Jan to go through that again.

Anyhow, after looking like someone that's fallen out of a life raft while attempting to do this turnaround, Craig was now positioned to take some steps the other way. Craig started off plunking down his right foot and stepping his left foot out front so quickly one would think he was getting off hot coals. Occasionally sliding his right foot up to his left and always tilting his shoulders like a pendulum, Craig's next couple of steps would be ones where he would reach forward grabbing hold of a parallel bar before barely clearing the floor with his right foot while attempting to move.

Craig was slow, but he was getting the motion down. Prepared to do a turnaround when he got to the end of the parallel bar, despite his feeling he just got started, Jan told Craig to stop and take a little break while she shows him how to transfer back to his wheelchair.

After Jan demonstrated how to do this, Craig followed her lead and sat in the wheelchair he was getting closer and closer to leaving behind. Craig felt absolutely stupendous that he was able to rise above the mayhem of his mind and get his leg to do what he ordered it to. Never in his young life did Craig ever think that taking a few steps could make him so happy. Nor could he have ever imagined that so much work would be required to do something he, just a little over two months ago, could do without batting a wink or would spend two seconds thinking about. After his brief break, Jan had him back up ready to do an encore.

Excited over what Craig did taking step after step after paralytic step, Jan praised her patient for his efforts, pushing him at the same time. "I thought you did great earlier," Jan said wearing her proud smile, "but let's try to polish it up a tad. Concentrate on placing your heel down first before the other parts of your foot. I don't want to hear your foot slap when you walk."

The word, "walk," when used to describe what Craig was attempting to do sent chills of anticipation through his body. Only a month before last, Craig was in a decerebrate posturing position where the body sets in a grossly unnatural way, void of any messages coming from the brain how the body should be posed. Now, Craig was attempting to refine something few who had seen him lying comatose at Allegheny General thought he'd ever be able to do again in his life, let alone within three months' time.

But there he was, training that brain to stand and walk again. If Craig does as well in this next series of attempted steps as he did earlier, maybe commencing a ticker-tape parade wouldn't be such a bad idea, after all. At least toss some confetti in the air for the guy.

After Jan said, "Three!," in her quick, short startling way, Craig was up standing at the end of the parallel bar. This getting on his feet and standing was starting to become less of a challenge for Craig, as Mary—having returned to her lifeguard duty—barely had to guide Craig as he was shooting up.

Spreading the spastic fingers of his right hand, Craig put his palm on the bar. Looking down at his right knee, Craig bent this joint slightly and pulled up the lower part of his leg, lifting his foot three inches off the floor before slamming it down in front of him about ten inches. Leaning his weight on his left arm, Craig then dragged his left foot up to the right.

At this point, Jan told Craig to try bending the top part of his foot up, exposing the heel for a smoother landing. That might not have been so bad if getting the heel cord to bend a little bit was all that Craig had to bring into focus. Instead of following through when he took his step, Craig's right knee would lock and then bend back, rather than the natural progression of flexing forward. Balancing himself on a leg that crackled with pain and a brain that had no sense of where he was in relation to the things about him, also complicated matters. With so much not working, it's no wonder Craig's right foot went crashing down repeatedly when he would try to take a step.

Realizing this wasn't how it should be done, Craig said to Jan, "My ankle doesn't want to bend my foot up; it feels like there's an anvil on the top of it."

Disgruntled by the lack of progress, Craig complained, "Y'know, I wear that damn leg splint when I go to bed and it keeps me up all night because it hurts so bad."

Wondering what the purpose is of this cast, Craig asked again, "Why do I have to wear that damn thing, if it isn't going to do me any good? At least they could shorten it so I can bend my knee at night and get some sleep for a change." For the twentieth time, at least, Jan explained how this brace prevents drop foot and that he needs to be patient—that a brain injury takes time before things can work out.

Patience. Brain injury. Time. Craig's heard these words used together so many times he could get sick.

"Forget about all that stuff right now," Jan said, "and concentrate on what you're doing." Getting huffy, Jan prodded, "We need to get to the end of the parallel bars."

Knowing Craig needs a little booster, this physical therapist turned psychotherapist said, "You're doing really well. If you keep progressing like you have today, you'll be up and moving around before you know it. You've just got to keep on trying."

In a few hours, the afternoon PT session would come and go, with Craig continuing to throw his right leg outward in a semi-circular fashion when he took a step because this was the only way his brain would allow him to move, no matter how hard he tried. With the right side of his body, stiff and rigid from hemiparesis, Craig would attempt to take a step directly forward, placing the heel down first, but he simply could not. Moving along, hanging onto the parallel bars flapping his right foot in the process may not have looked like much in the way of stellar improvement, but it was.

While Craig was concentrating on putting that heel down first and bending the top of his foot up, his brain was being stimulated what it's like being in an upright position again. Distracted from being situated differently, while Craig wasn't making much progress in the way of placing his heel properly, he *was* getting a sense of what it was like to stand again. Sneaky gal, that Jan Alba.

About his being up and moving around, Craig could only pray that what Jan said would come to fruition and not be a faint hope which he could only "dream on."

Bar none, Craig is THE biggest Aerosmith fan east of the Mississippi, if not the western hemisphere. Joe Perry and Brad Whitford were the major influences in his decision to learn guitar. It was Craig's adoration of this hard rock band's music that gave Mrs. Meyers an idea for a cognitive exercise which could help her son get "back in the saddle." This turned out to be a taste of Reality Therapy for Craig as well, because it showed just how a brain injury—like a tornado—can wipe out anything that's in its trail.

Craig spent the days after school playing ball of some sort with his neighbor friends and, during the evenings, he spent most of his time practicing guitar and listening to his Aerosmith albums. The fifteen minutes between listening to the "Toys in the Attic" and "Rocks" albums was the time Craig devoted to homework. Until they burned out in 1979, Aerosmith was really the only band Craig ever listened to. Because of this, Mrs. Meyers brought Craig's "Aerosmith Complete" songbook on April 22nd hoping that the lyrics to the different songs would spark some memory.

Because these tunes reverberated throughout the Meyers' household from 3:00 P.M.—when Craig got home from school—until 11:00 P.M., when things had to be quiet so what was said on the evening news could be relayed without the use of closed caption, Craig's mom knew how the melody went to many of these songs. Playing "Name that Tune," with the exception of songs such as "Lick and a Promise" and "Big Ten Inch Record," Mrs. Meyers would either sing the different songs she knew the beat to or read the lyrics hoping somewhere in the shadow that was Craig's bruised brain something would come alive and make a connection.

To Mr. and Mrs. Meyers' delight, Craig was able to identify each song. The downfall occurred when Craig was not able to remember the words to a lot of the songs he had once lip-synced to a billion times and was, for example, unable to say the lyrics in the opening verse of "Walk this Way" because he couldn't form the words fast enough. Craig could not mouth the words Steven Tyler belted out because his brain simply could not keep up anymore.

Despite his parents' and brother's insistence that the sound of his voice and the words coming from his lips were now drastically different, Craig could not tell and thought they must be mistaken. For Craig, the mumble jumble characteristic of his voice that he was told about, had him thinking that maybe there was some truth to what they were saying now that he recognized he couldn't bellow out some words he once was able to croon without an effort. Not being able to lip-sync his band's tunes anymore, now *that* WAS catastrophic. Oh well, at least Craig can still jam some heavy duty riffs on his air guitar.

Friday, April 23 arrived as did every other day with the daylight shift coming in and the graveyard shift saying goodbye. Fran and Diane—two nurses' aides—would make their early morning rounds, waking up everybody on the unit with their terroristic tactics and getting the patients ready for meds, breakfast, and program.

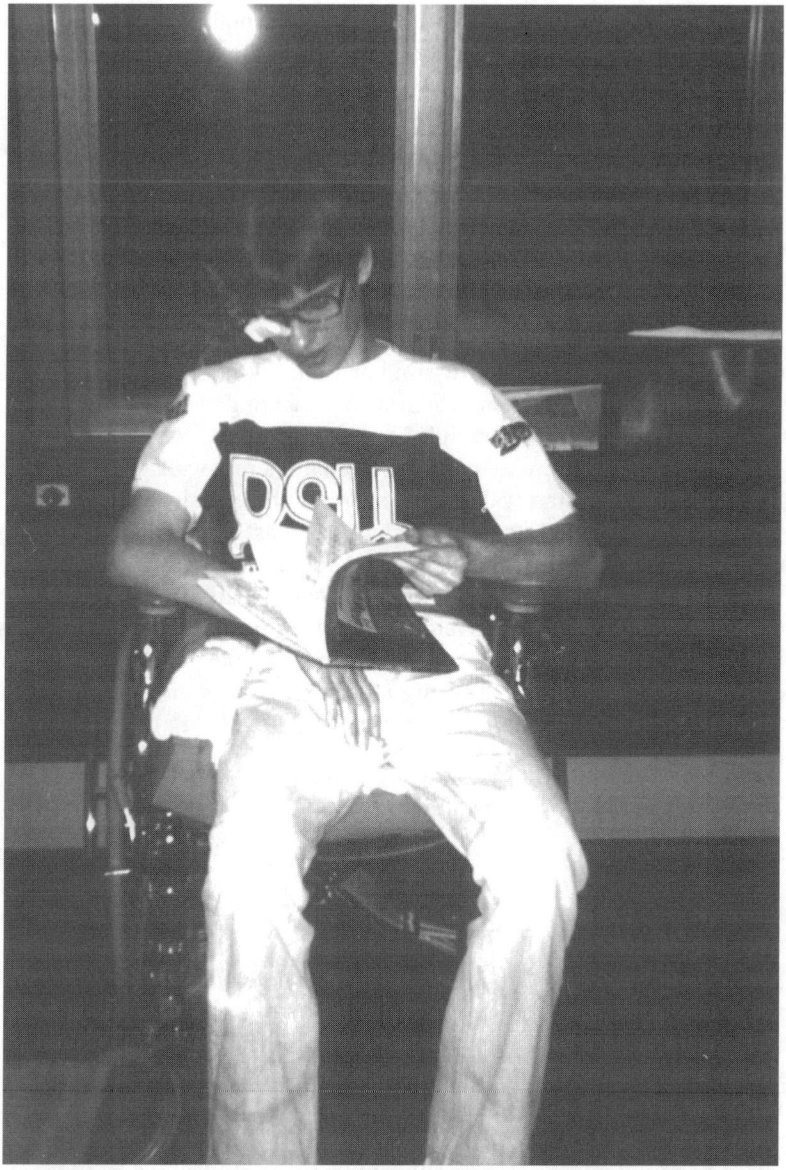

Having lost so much of his memory and intellect, Craig reviews a songbook from his favorite band, Aerosmith, in order to rekindle some kind of vision from his past. Note useless paralytic right hand and patch on right eye for double vision while sitting in wheelchair.

Craig's first therapy, Communication Skills, was nothing out of the ordinary. Sitting in his wheelchair, wearing his eye patch over the left eye, Craig continued to mistakenly print one letter when he was asked to make another. Nothing new, "same old song and dance."

Wheeling that left arm around and flapping that right foot like a fish out of water, Craig wasn't exactly galloping his wheelchair down the hallway on his way to physical therapy, but he was getting there. When offered to have his wheelchair pushed for him, Craig politely refused, saying he needs to practice. In PT today, Craig would continue to practice using his wheelchair—but in a different way.

In the Physical Therapy gymnasium, Craig sat in his wheelchair patiently waiting for Theresa to finish the twisting and turning range of motion exercises she was engaged in with a patient. Hearing the crackling of bones and scraping of joints, Craig wasn't so sure he was glad to be next in line.

But the fear was overcome by surprise when Theresa walked up to Craig and said, "Jan wants you to start walking behind your wheelchair today."

Shocked, Craig thought he'd be spending at least a few more days dangling from those parallel bars. But if his therapist thought he could graduate from hanging onto steel for balance to clinging onto his wheelchair for stability, while trying to motor around the gym, then motoring he would go. Pushy gal, that Jan Alba.

After Theresa told Craig what he'd have to do to transfer out of sitting in his wheelchair to standing behind it, Craig locked the brakes of his wheelchair and went about rocking and pushing his way up. Standing, Craig had his wheelchair maneuvered in front of him by Theresa and he was all set to go.

Theresa told Craig to move slowly and use his wheelchair for support, that if he felt shaky, then he was to stop and get his bearings. Theresa told this patient, who wasn't sure what to expect of this walking venture, to do what he did at the parallel bars yesterday and he'd be fine. And not to worry, that she'll be there in case he would need help.

Pausing for a moment, thinking of how he got his right leg up and moving forward yesterday, Craig gazed down at his right knee. Several seconds went by—nothing. Standing behind his wheelchair, squeezing the handlebars so tightly his sweaty hands were turning red, thoughts of the wheelchair slipping from his grip and rolling away from him as he stood helpless with no support, rushed his conscious. Just when Theresa began to say, "Why don't you try. . . . .," a surge of trust, strength, and confidence tingled throughout Craig.

Lifting his lower right leg straight up, Craig picked his foot off the floor a little and threw it out front about ten inches, slapping it down with a "thud." Then, clinging onto the chair's guide-bars as if his life depended on it, Craig took the step with his left. Presto!! Craig took his first step while standing behind the wheelchair. Because he needed his chair to get moving, the official scorer might not credit Craig with walking, but he couldn't care less, for this was the start of something big.

Because he lived close to his high school in Washington, Craig walked to and from Trinity every schoolday and never gave it a thought what he was doing during these hikes up and over the hill to his home. If someone would have told Craig his senior year that—within a few months—he would forget how to do something as automatic as getting his legs to move and taking some steps, he would have told them they were crazy because people just don't lose their memory how to walk. What Craig didn't know then.

Tossing his right foot out again, then kicking out his left, Craig proceeded to take his second wheelchair-assisted step. Repeating this sequence, Craig surprised even himself that he could advance the wheelchair without landing on his face. Those wheelchair wheels were rollin' now, spinning slowly, but surely.

Little by little, Craig walked the wheelchair to the doorway between the two gymnasiums while Theresa had her arms spread like an outfielder in case she had to make a catch. Trying unsuccessfully to place his heel down then rolling on the ball of his foot, Craig's upper body would shake when his right leg would slam on the ground and then his knee would bend awkwardly. Happy with the confidence he had snared, Theresa said little while trudging alongside Craig, except to remind him not to bang his right foot down so hard when following through with his step. Heel schmeel, Craig couldn't care less about the details of his walking at that moment because he was so incredibly relieved his brain still had the capacity to make the right part of his body move and take some steps.

Craig was on top of the world that he could control where he was going without being totally reliant on the wheels of a chair to get him there. Not having authority over what his body was doing or the movements it could undertake was a torment of unbearable proportions. Taking charge now, Craig was going to train his brain how to walk again.

Ecstatic about what he was doing, Craig lumbered around the gymnasium feeling positive about how he'd come out of this mess of a disability. Slowly limping around the PT gym, Craig never felt so good walking in his life. Craig knew that taking these steps was the first step to his regaining some of the independence that was taken from him. Smiling from what she saw Craig do, Theresa stopped Craig for a second and modeled what he had to do in order to smooth out his step. Turning the corner, Craig would be off again.

From the area of the gymnasium where she stretched a patient's arm to a point where no man has gone before, Mary congratulated Craig on his walking when he went by. Having spent much time under his arm pits yanking him up off his duff, Mary was one of the big reasons Craig was on his feet and stomping around. Circling 'round the gym, trotting down the home stretch, those endorphins were really flying now.

Little did Craig know, when he clipped the brakes on his wheelchair upon arriving for PT in the morning, it would be the last time he would do so from a sitting position. Because Craig had shown he was capable of getting around pushing his wheelchair without posing a threat either to himself or others, he was given the go-ahead to continue doing this throughout the day. And, if things go well, Craig's to walk throughout the weekend and report on Monday how things went.

After the morning PT session wrapped up, Craig pushed his chair out to the hallway where he normally would be heading for the cafeteria to eat lunch, but instead, walked to the unit where there was a pay phone. Bubbling with glee, Craig wanted to share with his parents his spectacular achievement of walking again. Craig knew collect calls made long-distance during the afternoon were outrageously expensive, but he knew his mom and dad wouldn't be too upset considering what he had to tell them.

When it was time for lunch, one would think Harmarville's staff hadn't had a bite to eat for weeks, as they all fly out of their offices and make a "B-line" straight for the dining room. Making his way down Harmarville's hallway which resembled Wall Street this time of day, Craig first passed the Psychology Department where—already armed with napkin in hand—Mrs. Joy enthusiastically greeted the patient she was due to see in an hour with a, "Lookin' good Craig."

Several slams with his right foot later, Craig came upon the Communication Skills offices and felt the floor beneath him rumble as if patients were stampeding from the PT gym fleeing Mary's range of motion exercises. It wasn't Mary that was responsible for this sensoround effect because she was already standing in the lunch line after having made a mad dash from the gym to claim a spot. Rather, the grumbling was Diane's, Bob's, and Vicki's stomachs anticipating the mid-day feast. Craig could not hear precisely what these Communication Skills pros were saying over this gurgling, but based on the expressions on their faces, he could tell they were overjoyed to see that he was up and about.

Approaching Unit 3, a white flash whipped around the corner. But Craig didn't have to fear for his safety unless he got in the way, for this lightning bolt was his Occupational Therapist trying to catch up with the cohorts in her department. Seeing Craig standing behind his wheelchair walking, Wendy extended her thumb and said, "Way to go, Craig! Go get 'em!"

Thumping along, Craig came to the lunchtime battlefield of the nurses' station where less-functional patients and nurses clamor. When June Golem, RN, looked up from her seemingly fixated position of looking at her watch while taking someone's pulse and Fran stopped singing, Craig knew that the site of him walking was something to behold.

Narrowly escaping this hubbub of activity, Craig went down the hallway past his room where the pay phone was and made a call.

When the phone rang at the Meyers' house, a lump would still get caught in Craig's parents' throats, not knowing if the person on the other line would be delivering dreaded news of some sort. After Mrs. Meyers picked up the phone and heard who it was, she yelled down to the basement where her husband was drilling a hole in one of the two steel bars he had gotten. Informed Craig was on the other end, throwing his tools on his workbench and letting the metal rods fall to the floor, Mr. Meyers ran up the stairs as fast as his sixty-two-year-old legs could take him. Heart racing that his son would call in the middle of the day, Mr. Meyers dove for the phone.

Paranoid, fearing Craig might have fallen or had that first seizure, Mr. Meyers answered the phone, "What is it buddy? Everything okay?"

Hearing those words, "I walked today!," coming from Craig's mouth, a shocked Mrs. Meyers said in a tone pasted with excitement and disbelief, "What!!?"

"Today in PT," Craig said with exuberance, "I got up and walked behind my wheelchair."

Huffing and puffing, Mr. Meyers cried out, "Ahhhh, that's great buddy, that's great." Stunned with elation, Mr. Meyers could feel a tear wanting to slip down his face.

Nerves wracked, Mrs. Meyers asked, "Did you have any trouble?"

Eyes red and face tear-soaked now, Mr. Meyers said after clearing his throat, "How far did you go? A couple of steps?"

"No, no, no," Craig said excited about the news of his day's performance, "I walked clear down the hallway from the. . . ."

"Clear down the hallway!!?," Mrs. Meyers said with surprise and a trace of horror before Craig could finish, "You walked all the way down that long hallway by yourself?"

"Was there anyone with you?," Mr. Meyers asked, fearing his son might have taken a spill, "Did you feel like you might fall down?"

"At first, Theresa—the therapist I told you yesterday that would be working with me today—was right there when I started," Craig said after his parents cooled their engines and gave him a chance to speak, "but after I started gettin' the hang of things, I didn't need too much help."

"You didn't fall did you?," Mrs. Meyers repeated, worried what Craig might say.

"No," Craig answered, "the only trouble I had was getting started and then it was off to the races. I feel great!"

Not wanting to jump the gun, but knowing his mom and dad have been starved of good news since Paul hurt him, Craig felt compelled to tell them, "If all goes well in therapy this afternoon, I was told that I can walk—pushing my wheelchair—all weekend. When you get here tonight. . . . ."

"What!!?," Mrs. Meyers said with even greater surprise the second time she blurted this out not letting Craig complete his sentence, "You can walk by yourself all weekend? Do they think you're ready for that?"

"Damn it Gwen," Mr. Meyers said with more than a twinge of disgust, "if you let the boy talk maybe we can learn something."

"Yep," Craig said when he finally got a chance to respond, "there won't be anyone with me. The team feels all the support I need is my wheelchair. Considering how well I do today, I agree; that's the only way I'll get my confidence back. And get better!"

"Confidence" could not possibly describe how the Meyers felt about their boy's prospects for recovery, because it would not be a strong enough word. Having lost track the number of times they had been "raked through the coals" since the accident, when Craig's parents hung up the phone in the afternoon, they were finally being swept by a sense of euphoria, figuring it would only be a matter of time until their son "got back into the game of life."

Seated next to each other, Mr. and Mrs. Meyers could only shake their heads in disbelief the alarming rate with which Craig was improving since he'd been at Harmarville. To think that in only a matter of several weeks, Craig went from being unaware of the world about him, to independently moving about it.

Mr. Meyers thought to himself that it wasn't all that long ago that his boy was dependent on an oxygen mask and intravenous tubes burrowed in his arms, just to ensure he didn't die an excruciating death. Now, independence can be something more than a cutting reminder of what Craig no longer commands, but a dream retrieved.

Because each hour crawls and so much had happened within this period, these two-and-one-half months since Craig had been hurt are weighted by the minute. February, when Mrs. Meyers was eternally grateful Craig opened his eyes a quarter of an inch and didn't succumb to a fiery demise when he was burning with fever, seemed like another lifetime ago. As if it just happened, Mrs. Meyers would always have branded in her conscious the image of her son comatose on that bedding in the hospital, moaning from pain and emotional distress. Mrs. Meyers said a silent prayer to the Lord Almighty thanking Him for the strength delivered to the family and Craig during a time when more than a few would have jettisoned all hope.

To avoid any problems, Theresa wanted to be sure Craig understood how to transfer in and out of his wheelchair since he'd be on his own this weekend; provided things work well in the PT session. Reviewing these steps again during the afternoon, Theresa told her week-long patient that when he walks to his destination and wants to sit down, Craig's to first bend down and lock his left wheelchair brake and then—tightly holding onto the wheelchair's right handlebar with his left hand—clip the right wheelchair brake with his right hand.

Holding onto the side rails with his good left hand, Craig's to shuffle in front of the chair and place his left hand on the left arm rest and his bad one on the other. Then jiggling his derriere in place a few inches above the seat, Craig's to gently—and under control—lower himself into his chair. Because of his deficient "position sense," this was not easy for Craig, as he would frequently "plop" down when he would sit.

Theresa stressed that Craig needs to use his right hand when he transfers because if he uses his left one for everything, his right will not relearn how to do things again and won't get better. She also told Craig to remember to place his heel down first when he takes steps, and to concentrate on not letting that right knee snap back when he lands on his leg. Demanding gal, that Theresa Gates.

Knowing that a wheelchair-free weekend (at least from a "not having to sit in it" standpoint) was dependent on this afternoon's performance, Craig stood behind his chariot ready to impress. Standing to the side of her confident patient, Theresa said in her encouraging way, "Alright Craig, show me what you got. Remember—take it slow and concentrate on smoothing out that step with your right leg."

After Craig told Theresa taking it slow was the only way he knew how, he came out of the starting gate like he had every other time he'd taken a step—whacking his right foot on the ground.

Craig strained around the gymnasium concentrating on picking up his right foot, placing the heel on the floor just before the anterior of his foot, pushing off his toes, rolling on the ball of his foot while trying to bend his knee naturally during his follow-through, and repeating. So much to think of and so much to do. Hardly appreciating the time when he did this automatically, what Craig wouldn't give to get a little bit of that back.

Craig tried to master what Theresa told him to do, but what he actually was doing and attempting were two different things. Being a University of Pittsburgh alumnus, Theresa was doing her best Johnny Majors' impersonation when she yelled across the gym.

"Watch that knee, watch that knee," she hollered, "you don't want it to bend back like that. If you can touch the ground with your heel first, instead of your heel and toes hitting at the same time, your knee will bend better." Craig sauntered about trying to get his right foot to obey, but he was still doing the flat-footed sashay.

"Lean to the left a little," Theresa instructed, "stay on your right leg longer." The only peace Craig would get this afternoon would be when Theresa had to inhale for more air for the next series of commands.

"Pick the front of your right foot up, Craig. Straighten your back; keep a good posture." Waiting for Tony Dorsett to sprint out of the back gym any minute, Craig couldn't believe all that he had to remember just to walk.

Hobbling around the gym, Craig sounded like a grandfather clock that had some glitches in its pendulum somewhere, as he would take a decent step with his left foot followed with a plunk of his right. However, considering all that had happened to Craig, this wasn't bad at all. To smooth out his walking, what Craig needed to do was practice. Like a man possessed, that would be exactly what Craig set out to do.

When they arrived for their weekend visit, the Meyers were speechless when they saw their smiling son standing behind his wheelchair, pushing it towards them.

Glowing, Mr. Meyers then whooped as he approached his son, "Hey, look at you! You look great buddy up on your feet like that! Talk about looking sharp."

Asphyxiated by emotion, Mr. Meyers said, "I told you it would be only a matter of time that you'd be up. Jus' listen to your old man."

Then sporting a shitty grin, Mr. Meyers said, "Those nurses better look out now. Heh, heh, heh."

Her eye shadow now setting on her cheekbone and her makeup running down her face with the tears of bliss, Mrs. Meyers tried unsuccessfully to contain the shock of seeing her son on his feet. Voice rattling, this mother joyous for everything Harmarville had helped her son to accomplish asked, “How’s it feel being up on your feet after so long? Does your leg feel okay?”

“Without the wheelchair here for support,” Craig said, “I’d lose my balance and fall down, but since I’ve been practicin’, I feel a little more comfortable. I’m getting used to standing up again, anyhow.”

“And my leg,” Craig continued, “every step I take, I can feel that damn rod clicking. I know it never has to come out, but if it’s going to ache like this, I’d rather have it yanked out.”

Reflecting on the nightmare he has even before he goes to sleep, Craig says, “I can’t even roll over in bed at night because it hurts so bad. I think that rod’s just a little too long.”

“Yeah, but the doctors who worked on your leg,” Mr. Meyers interjected, “had to work fast and there was just so much wrong with your leg, you’re lucky you have a leg.”

Without taking into consideration the magic performed by the orthopedic surgical team at Allegheny General, Mr. Meyers tucked in his shirt and straightened up his pants before announcing, “If it wasn’t for me, you wouldn’t have that leg.”

Explaining what he meant by this, Mr. Meyers told Craig, “I wasn’t about to sign any paper giving the doctors an easy way out, if surgery got tough. I told them to save that leg because you’re a ballplayer and you need your legs.”

Trying to make Craig’s physical discomfort a little more acceptable, Mrs. Meyers finished with, “Just be glad you got a leg that’s bothering you.”

Thinking of the horror she sees during their visits with Craig, Mrs. Meyers added, “I see lots of young people about your age who have plastic legs and arms. What they wouldn’t give being in your shoes right now.”

“You might have some things wrong with your thinking that they don’t,” Mr. Meyers said, “but you’ll overcome that in time. They’ll ALWAYS be missing their arm, leg, whatever. Be thankful you don’t need a prosthesis.”

“Without a doubt,” Craig told his parents, “I know I have a lot to be thankful for. I could’ve been blinded, burned, paralyzed, or in chronic pain.”

Not real comfortable with the direction this conversation was going, Mr. Meyers quickly interrupted, “Enough bullshittin’, show us how you walk.”

Slowly shifting his stiff body 180 degrees, taking tiny, meticulous steps so his wheelchair was pointed down the hallway where he wanted to go, Craig asked his parents who were gleaming with anticipation, “I know you’re not physical therapists, but give me some feedback what I need to do to improve my walking.”

Tick-tocking past the unit on their way to the dining room, Craig and his parents were stormed upon by Valerie and Jan Goga, “Daylight was telling us your were walking,” Craig’s ping-pong partner said beaming, “you look great!”

With a happy smile, Jan kidded Craig, “I didn’t know you were so tall.”

Unaware of his success history, Craig’s blond bombshell nurse/buddy said, “Before you know it, you’ll be picking up girls and dancing like John Travolta. Hee hee hee hee.”

Craig was a good example of how Harmarville staff pulls for their patients. From medical personnel to the therapists to nursing staff, the disciplines may vary, but the one thing universal about Harmarville is the caring these professionals have for those that they serve. God bless Harmarville.

Like every other weekend, Craig devoted his time to working on the various physical and aphasic difficulties which a brain riddled with disconnections will levy on one. And the furlough from this week's programs would be no different except that—instead of sitting in his wheelchair, putting it into motion out in the hallway—Craig would be making it roll by taking step, after step, after step, after step, after step. Standing behind his wheeled carriage, holding on for support, Craig would be energized by an unstoppable inspiration.

Since he'd had his head injury, Craig has had a whole slew of experiences and met an abundance of people. When Monday would make its appearance after the weekend's many miles of walking practice in the hallway, Craig would meet yet another key player in his rehabilitation. In the midst of being tested, Craig would have several experiences that would catalog itself somewhere in the cluster which was his long-term memory.

The person with a head injury is going to be forever changed from what they were before. Craig as he once appeared, was no more. A consultant was brought in to determine how much of the haze which was Craig's thought processes would forever linger and what, if anything, could be done to penetrate the mist of confusion.

The Front Page Assessment is an informal psychological test devised by Harmarville and got its name because it's usually the first page of a patient's Harmarville file. It is simply a series of brief, informal, writing and drawing tasks from which several preliminary assessments can be made.

In this test, Craig first would be asked to write his name and address (tells the level of his agraphia, if Craig can spell, knows where he lives). Then Craig's to write a sentence (reveals response time, if an ideomotor apraxia exists, gross spelling). Third, Craig is to put down the numbers, 27-458-1001, and add them up (divulges whether or not Craig can write numbers, do simple arithmetic, if perseveration exists). Fourth, a clock is to be drawn (indicates spatial relation capability, ability to plan and organize). Finally, Craig was to copy an abstract design (ascertains the existence of rotational errors, unilateral neglect, constructional apraxia).

As Craig struggled to harness that which he no longer can master, two probing eyes peered at the pencil he was holding, as this investigator could only wonder what it would produce next. Every motion, every gesture, every reflex was being mentally catalogued with detailed precision. While different impressions would abound, the personable, but distinguished English gentleman observing Craig would stroke his thick moustache one minute, rubbing his chin the next.

Anytime an error was produced, one hypothesis would formulate. If a delay in response time would occur, another related premise materialized. When a psychomotor lapse surfaced, another assertion or two developed.

With so much deductive reasoning and brainpower pervading these cramped quarters, when the heavy British accent permeated from this Psychology office, one may have thought Sherlock Holmes was inside doing his detective work. Instead, it was Harmarville's consulting neuropsychologist, Graham Ratcliff, Ph.D., trying to "crack the case." The brain is a mystery, but one that leaves clues. Craig's different aphasias left fingerprints as to what may be going on with his brain.

Eyes never leaving his patient, Dr. Ratcliff watched Craig as he slowly printed his full name. Because Craig has written "C-R-A-I-G M-E-Y-E-R-S" so many times since he lost his ability to write spontaneously, he was well-practiced putting this string of letters together and didn't have any trouble getting this down on paper. Printing his address was another story, however.

Holding Craig's chart for confirmation, Dr. Ratcliff asked the examinee what his address was. After Craig correctly responded, the good doctor asked him to write this without a cue. Sweat dripping from the end of his nose knowing a doctor of philosophy was sitting just a few feet from him—monitoring every move he made—Craig drew a squiggly diagonal line from the upper-left to the lower-right, apparently his version of a "one." Not feeling like the most intelligent of blokes at this point, Craig really felt the pressure when he couldn't remember how to write the other numbers or his street.

Because he didn't know the formation of numbers and couldn't picture what a clock looked like, for his back was turned to the one on the wall, Craig skipped to the last portion of this test. And here it was discovered that Craig could only perceive half his world.

Asked to copy a design that had a cross, triangle, rectangle, crisscrossing lines—as well as several other patterns—Craig focused on the abstractions located to the right part of the design, but did not attend to the patterns on the left. Craig could see everything to his left, but acted as if they weren't even there. Looking at his patient, Dr. Ratcliff noted Craig's gaze was deviated to the right which likely was related to this unilateral neglect, somehow. This left-sided neglect was first revealed when Craig took the Motor-Free Visual Perceptual Test (MVPT) in Occupational Therapy a few weeks ago.

The MVPT has five geometric, sailboat-like designs lined up horizontally with a target sample—either identical or similar to the others—set aside, and Craig's to match which of the five closet resembles the target pattern. Because of his right-sided focus, Craig would not notice the designs located to the left of the plane.

Also, Craig showed a definite response bias to the right when administered the multiple-choice form of the Benton Visual Retention Test. Like the MVPT, this is a motor-free perceptual test where Craig had to verbalize the response he wanted. In this test, Dr. Ratcliff asked Craig what designs he saw on each card.

Sometimes the card had as many as three designs set horizontally and the patterns would vary in size.

For example, one card had a very tiny circle to the extreme left, a triangle of larger proportions in the middle, and an abstract design equal in size to the triangle on the right. Scanning the configuration before him, Craig would not pay any mind to the circle on the left. Another card had an average-sized envelope configuration to the left, an equally large square to the middle, and a minuscule triangle to the right. It would not register in Craig's mind that there was a design which resembled the back of an envelope.

Out of a total thirty-two responses, Craig named twenty-five items that were to his right without even taking into account the design(s) that would be to his left. Because of this inattention to his left side, a true measure of Craig's overall perceptual deficiencies would be difficult to assess.

If this neglect wasn't enough, the Benton and the MVPT also revealed evidence that Craig did actually have several significant perceptual deficits. For example, when the designs were hidden within other patterns or rotated to a different angle, Craig could not identify the sister pattern. One whose mind has been sifted of its senses drifts within a child's scope of understanding.

Because Craig could copy letters, numbers, and designs in their appropriate dimension, but could not do so upon command without a cue, this suggests a disconnection of some sort occurring within his brain rather than a visuo-spatial difficulty, Dr. Ratcliff theorized. This "disconnection syndrome" entailed more than the ideomotor apraxia where Craig's hand just went off and did its own thing (often referred to as "alien hand"), but also indicated damage had occurred to Craig's corpus collusum.

The corpus collusum is the middle of the brain which allows functions occurring predominantly in one hemisphere to be transmitted to the other side making the brain one unified, well-oiled, smoothly-operating piece of machinery. When this corpus collusum cog malfunctions, it disconnects one part of the brain from the other. In a sense, making one person—two.

Because of Craig's agraphia, Dr. Ratcliff hypothesized that damage occurred to the nerve fibers here between the left and right hemispheres. The left hemisphere is where the language systems are located, as well as higher level motor programming functions such as the motions required to write or draw. The right hemisphere "takes in" what's in the environment and processes it.

In the left hemisphere, there is a receptor-like portion of the brain which receives messages from the "all-knowing" perceptual right hemisphere. After snagging the right hemisphere's telegraph, the receptor then sends a signal to another liaison sub-system in the left hemisphere which is headquarters for the Department of Handwriting Motions. With Craig being left-handed since the accident, this message needed to be volleyed back over to the right hemisphere of Craig's brain, so he could physically move his left hand in the direction it was supposed to in order to make the desired letters. When the corpus collusum freeway has so many potholes to be filled/oil spills to be sopped up, traffic's going to get bottled up somewhere and Federal Express delivering the message isn't going to get through.

Somewhere in this entanglement, the Dept. of Handwriting Motions never got the signal as to what the letters of the alphabet looked like. Therefore, didn't know what in hell to fax to Craig's writing hand. So the left hemisphere just guessed, doing whatever, without consulting the dictionary in Craig's perceptual right hemisphere. Not that this consultation would be of any use, for when Craig's head went through the side window of Paul's Volkswagen and collided with that pole, most of the pages of his dictionary were torn loose or indelibly smeared. Neurobehavioral terminology at its best.

Dr. Ratcliff conducted an informal test with Craig to see if his "disconnection syndrome" hypothesis was accurate. Because of Craig's agraphia, there was definite brain to hand interference and—if indeed the corpus collusm had been affected—there would be hand to brain deficits appearing as well in this object-holding test known as steriognosis. And appear they would.

With his eyes closed, Craig was given a pencil to hold with his left hand and was asked to name this object. Rolling the pencil around and feeling the eraser at the end, Craig correctly identified the writing utensil in his hand. Then, Dr. Ratcliff put a pair of scissors in Craig's hand, and with eyes still closed, Craig fiddled around with this for a little while before saying "pencil" again. Dr. Ratcliff then gave his closed-eyed patient a cigarette and Craig felt this for but a few brief moments before saying, "pencil," yet one more time.

Twirling his pipe in the front pocket of his dress shirt, Dr. Ratcliff's brain was hard at work after seeing this fascinating demonstration. Believing Craig's "pencil" response to everything he holds was due to his left hemisphere's perseverative speaking malfunction and not his right hemisphere's perceptual function, Dr. Ratcliff then put the pipe he was playing with in Craig's left hand and asked him what it was.

Eyes closed shut, Craig proceeded to feel the bowl and the damp mouthpiece. Then, wrapping his fingers around the bowl holding the pipe in its proper position for smoking, Craig told Dr. Ratcliff, "That's a pencil."

Noting how Craig was holding the pipe in the correct posture when one takes a few puffs, Dr. Ratcliff quickly told Craig not to open his eyes yet and to show him what one does with the object he was holding. Without delay, Craig brought what he identified as a "pencil" moments ago up to his mouth like it was a pipe!

When Dr. Ratcliff told Craig to open his eyes and Craig saw it was a pipe he was holding and not the pencil he said it was, an icy chill trickled down Craig's spine to his legs. Craig was fearful seeing, inches from his eyes, a tangible object which showed just how confused his thought processes had become.

Interestingly, Craig immediately said these correct demonstrations of use were in error—"See it's a pencil, but I put it in my mouth." It appeared Craig's left hemisphere was still trying to tell Dr. Ratcliff that what he was holding was indeed a pencil despite his right hemisphere already demonstrating that it was a pipe. It is true, as the old adage goes, "A mind is a terrible thing to waste," but having two of them can also be a problem.

Further testing of Dr. Ratcliff's hypothesis showed that Craig's left hemisphere would perseveratively blurt out any response which would come to mind while his right hemisphere knew what was going on. Craig correctly named two out of six common objects held with his left hand and identified four out of six with his right. As was the case with the pipe demonstration, out of the four incorrect verbal responses Craig made trying to identify that which was in his left hand, three demonstrations of use were right on the money. The results of these steriognosis tests reveal that Craig's upper-left limb (right hemisphere) is disconnected from the part of the brain responsible for language (left hemisphere). Simply put, when he tried to write, for example, Craig's left hand was out of his control.

This apraxia also manifested itself when Craig tried to draw. Craig copied letters without a whole lot of trouble because these are simple, concrete patterns that even Craig's twisted mind recognized as seeing before. But with complicated geometric designs that had never been previously processed, Craig's ability to spontaneously replicate these patterns was practically non-existent.

True, Craig's unilateral neglect did contribute to his inability to make accurate reproductions, overall however, Craig's trouble with drawing was due to his hand not doing what it was supposed to rather than not attending to the structure of the drawing. This difficulty copying drawings (constructional apraxia) was evident in Craig's attempts to copy the Rey Complex Figure, as the name implies, a design of difficult proportions.

For Craig to draw accurately from memory with any kind of spontaneity would have been nothing short of a miracle. Like his writing, if Craig were asked to draw a representation of an object, his right hemisphere would be able to project an image on *its* screen. But to have the projector relay this same image on the left hemisphere's screen—where the Dept. of Handwriting Motions could fax to the hand what it needs to do—would be impossible because of Craig's mid-brain freeway in need of those repairs. More neuro-behavioral scientific language.

The last test Craig was subjected to this day was actually two subtests (Trails A and B) called the Trail Making Test from the Halstead-Reitan Neuropsychological Battery. In this battery, Craig was first administered the simple component of this test where—without lifting his pencil off the paper—he was merely to make a continuous line (trail) connecting, in numerical order, a series of numbers scattered about the paper as quickly as he could (Trails A).

For example, if all went well, Craig would have his pencil at the number "1" to begin the test and—after searching the paper with the different numbers scattered about and locating the number "2"—he'd send his pencil in that direction before zeroing in where the "3" was hidden and launching his pencil for the third number and so on. Normally, a person who hasn't had a neurological impairment can finish this test in approximately twenty to thirty seconds.

Trails B is a test where, connecting alternately, Craig must make a line through a series of first, numbers then letters (i.e. 1-A-2-B-3-C-4-D). From the number "1," Craig was to make a connection to the letter "A" and from here, draw a line to the number "2" before heading for the letter "B" and then the number "3" and so on. This test takes people two or three times longer to complete than the easier Trails A. However, Craig wouldn't be so lucky.

These trails tests are sensitive to deficits in visual scanning, psychomotor speed, and one's ability to attend to the task at hand. However, the most useful information that can be gained from these tests is by looking at the difference between Craig's Trails A and Trails B performance.

Assessing the disparity, Dr. Ratcliff could approximate what some of the difficulties Craig experienced in relation to alternating between two sets of information, as a result of impaired working memory. In other words, the additional time that had elapsed doing Trails B would tell Dr. Ratcliff how well Craig could switch his mode of thinking from one type to another. This shuffling information in one's mind is a complex process, for the person not only has to learn and retain what they're asked to do during the subsequent task, but also must not allow what they previously learned and undertook interfere with what currently is asked of them.

During any one day, interruptions of varying degrees will occur time after time, where a person must stop what they're doing and focus on the intrusion. Then, to get "back on track," they must reach into their short-term memory banks in order to recount what they were doing and proceed from there. If one is to progress, this skill is essential. In order to help Craig get out of "Neutral" and into a gear necessary for survival, Dr. Ratcliff and Co. have got a lot miles ahead of them to travel.

With a sample Trails A before him Craig was to use for practice, Dr. Ratcliff explained what Craig was to do before the timed trail would be laid out and the real testing was to begin. Instead of seeing scattered numbers on a piece of paper—which is all Trails A entails—Craig's mind perceived what it thought was a complicated computer print-out which resembled the Waterhouse Price Index after a day laden with heavy trading and selling.

Mind numb from misperception, Craig's pencil stood frozen on the "1." Perseveratively, Craig's pencil/torpedo was fired hitting a target. Unfortunately, it wasn't the number "2" he should have sunk.

Sensing he was in for a long afternoon, one more time, Dr. Ratcliff modeled for Craig what he needs to do in order to successfully finish the trail. In his unshaken way, Dr. Ratcliff instructed Craig to be as accurate as possible and, by George lad, get that pencil moving as quickly as possible after finding where it needs to go.

As soon as Craig moved his pencil off the "1," the starting gun had been fired and—without fanfare—Dr. Ratcliff looked down at his wrist watch. For Craig, this time piece could have just as well have been "Big Ben" marking high noon for the pressure would be on.

With his pencil on "2," Craig scanned the paper momentarily before spotting the "3" tucked off in a corner before making the line into its belly. Not seeing the "4" right away, Craig frantically shot his head left then right then down then up. Still not able to find his target, Craig ovalled his head in a circular pattern. Tick tick tick tick.

Moving his head down, Craig spotted that sneaky little "4" and, fighting the impulse to shoot his pencil up, eventually found a way to get his pencil where it needed to go. Eyes zooming in this game of timed "hide and seek," Craig didn't find the "5" right away. Tick tick tick tick.

Looking up, looking down. Scanning left, looking right. Tick tick tick tick. Craig couldn't find the "5" until he forced himself to consider that things actually *DO* exist in the left hemisphere of a plane.

Playing tug of war with his unilateral neglect, Craig pulled, yanked, strained, crackled, crumbled, bent trying to free his mind from only recognizing that which is to his right. Tick tick tick tick. What had once been beyond the bounds of possibility, Craig was finally able to snap his trance-like gaze to the right and actually focus for a second that which was to his left. And this is where Craig found his elusive digit.

Knowing where the "6" was, Craig hesitated for a second before moving his hand several millimeters to the left of this sixth number to the "7." Apparently, Craig's mind was fixated on the six and associated what comes before and after this digit and off his hand went to the associative number immediately following the six. Tick tick tick.

Stopping mid-stride—halfway to the "7"—Craig knew this was a mistake and pulled the reins, stopping. Taking some evasive action, Craig soon captured that nasty little "6." After seizing the six, off Craig went to snatch the "7" he wanted to hook up with so bad.

Periscope up. Scanning down, scanning up. Scanning right, scanning down. Scanning up, scanning right. Scanning left (but not really looking), scanning here, scanning there. Tick tick tick tick. Craig couldn't find the last number until his right hemisphere perceived the "8" as being the only number that does not have a pencil mark through it and reasoned this must be the lost treasure he couldn't find, so away his pencil went to the "8" mark in the corner pocket to end the game.

Trying to be as inconspicuous as possible, Dr. Ratcliff glanced down at his watch and quickly scribbled in his notebook the sixty-some seconds it took Craig to finish Trails A. Before Craig could ask how he did, Dr. Ratcliff was explaining to his patient what needs to be done in order to properly complete Trails B. Mouth open, Craig's density was intense.

To get a sense of the tragic consequences brain injury has on the intellect, all one really needs to recognize is that a year ago, Craig was instructed how to go about completing the college entrance exam and now, cannot seem to grasp how this connect-the-dot game is played. When asked if he understands what he needs to do for this new trails exercise, Craig's teenaged "No Sweat, Dr. R" demeanor shot forth. Because he wasn't exactly sure what was going on—inside—Craig felt like Benny Hill must after one of his failed attempts romancing the ladies.

Craig at least recognized that in this second timed trails exercise, he would need to jiggle, shuffle, and shift his train of thought not only from that which he had just completed (Trails A), but whether his next target would be a number or letter. Sensing the complexity of the task before him, Craig felt like he was about to run a relay race where he must pass the baton from the right hemisphere of his brain to the left and back again several times. Yet another example of neuromedical jargon.

Somebody should have told Craig he needed to tie his shoes for this race and collect his thoughts for—when he was told to begin this practice Trails B—Craig was dumb-struck, not having any idea where to begin sending his pencil. With his pencil on the "1," Craig spotted the "2" and whipped that baby through the number two's chest. Looking at the number he just speared, Craig got that feeling in his gut one gets when sensing things aren't quite right. After Dr. Ratcliff reminded Craig that he needs to alternate between numbers and letters, in this case making a line to the letter "A," the timed trail trial was set to begin.

Heart pumping now, Craig shot off the starting block from the "1" to the "2" and—while the APB for the "3" was being sent out—realized he had made the same mistake again and needed to make his line through the "A" instead. In his barbituate-induced slow motion, Craig immediately erased this mark. Tick tick tick tick.

Scanning the Trails B, Craig spotted the "A" and zipped his pencil stabbing the "3" before remembering the "all points bulletin" had been renounced. Tick tick tick tick. Erasing the erroneous line, Craig tried to recall what it was he needed to look for because doing all this other stuff, he forgot. Tick tick tick.

Seeing the "A" with no slash through it, Craig figured this would be as good as any to shoot for, so away his pencil went whistling past the "A" to the "2" again. Tick tick tick tick. Doing a statue impersonation, motionless, Craig sat dazed and confused.

By some act of God—in several moments time—Craig remembered that he wanted the letter "A," saw this letter camouflaged amongst the others, and maneuvered his pencil penetrating the "A." Glory, glory, hallelujah. Now, it's time to hunt down that "2."

Focusing on the right side of the paper, Craig looked up, down, down, up before his courtesy glance to the left. Staring right at the "2," Craig's eyes then went north, south, east, north, back to east, up to north, down to south, back to east. Tick tick tick tick. Then, ziggin' when he should have been zaggin', Craig made his line to the "B" figuring he might as well do something.

Sensing this wasn't exactly right, but knowing time wasn't on his side and that he shouldn't just be sitting there, Craig sent his bloodhounds for the "3." After finding the "3" and seeing it already had a line through it, Craig wiped this line from the slate. Tick tick tick tick tick tick tick.

Hop-scotchin' right when he should have been going left, Craig made incorrect mark after incorrect mark until the Trails B looked like an Etch-a-Sketch toy that a hyperactive child got his/her hands on. With his brain's right hemisphere surveying the paper, Craig located the "2" sitting by its lonesome and put his finger on it before it ran away.

Erasing the line from the "A" to the "B," Craig then correctly sent his reconnaissance pencil from the "A" down to the "2" then across into the "B." After Craig nailed this letter, he had alphabet on his mind and went out in search of a "C" to harpoon. And so the story goes.

Craig botching up the Trails B hook, line, and sinker revealed he had sustained damage to the front portion of his brain as well. People with frontal lobe injuries are easily distracted and, based on his Trails B performance, it was quite clear Craig had sustained damage here because of his inability to proceed with the more complex trail without the image of Trail A interfering.

Craig knew how to go about doing Trails B, drawing lines through 1-A-2-B-3-C-4-D etc., but the "utilization behavior" where one sees something and does it right away could not be controlled because the frontal lobe function which filters out unwanted variables that keeps people from messing up had short-circuited. This impulsive condition, known as "frontal pull," frequently causes the person with a head injury to do and say things that are not appropriate.

Not that guilt-free Craig ever tried this, but this frontal pull has been responsible for more than a few nurses and therapists being propositioned by patients who have had head injuries. Like his perseveration, Craig could have used this ailment to his advantage, if he was only smart enough. Craig could have made a subtle suggestion to one of the many gorgeous females working with him and after being slapped in the face, could have said, "Damn this frontal pull."

These past seventy-two days since Craig practically had his head ripped from his body, the embers which had been Craig's conscious have been sparked by the flames of continued stimulation and healing. The accumulation of work, treatment, caring, love, and God's supervision made it possible that on the seventy-third day, resurrected from the ashes that were once confusion's cloak, the searing glow of understanding would appear. The darkness clenching Craig's awareness will be penetrated.

Chapter 5

THE AWAKENING

April 27th was a day unlike any other. Lying in bed, trying to get a handle on this new dimension, a feeling foreign to experience since being hurt greeted the rising. Wading in the darkness of misunderstanding and incapability was no more, for the ability to recount and file through the catalog which is memory and awareness had appeared with dawn's arrival. Waking up that morning, I know my thinking had cleared.

I know where I'm at. I know that I was in a car accident and messed up my head pretty bad and forgot a lot of stuff. I know that I can't walk or write and that's part of the reason why I'm here at Harmarville. I know that I'm not thinking real good, but today is different than any other. There's still a lot of blanks, but now I understand what's going on. What once was a hollow void is now being filled with long-sought answers. The fog that blinded my awareness has risen.

I was told that me and Paul Michaels went to a party at Rodney Ilyacoff's and that Paul wrecked his car into a telephone pole because he was drunk; that he almost killed me. I don't remember anything about any party or being in a car accident.

I know that I was in Allegheny General Hospital in Pittsburgh, but I don't remember anything about ever being there. I don't remember a whole lot about my past or anything about anything, for that matter. The last thing I can sense is being at West Virginia University. God, where have I been?

Before today, what I did know was a rehearsed comprehension of what I had been told like an echo repelling off the walls of an empty canyon. It was a surface realization, nothing in depth.

I know I was in a car accident and had a severe head injury which is why I'm at this rehab center. I know this because I have been told over and over by everyone that's what happened to me, but I have no real understanding or sense of experiencing what has occurred. There was never any true identification of Who?, What?, Where?, or When? Nothing had meaning. Nothing had substance. Everything is nothing in this realm of lost recognition.

I realized I had different therapists working with me on basic things I can't do anymore because my head had been "bashed in," but now I can truly appreciate what they're trying to do and why I've been bustin' my ass. It was like part of me was on automatic pilot where I was programmed to listen and work hard, but had no real control or understanding of what I was doing or why.

Amidst the massive confusion which took hold of my brain, there was a part of my thought processes which sensed what I needed to do to emerge from the chaos. Thank God this autonomic transmitter still had some spark or else I'd have withered.

The moment I got up this morning, I knew, I absolutely knew that I had come to some turning point and that my thinking had reached a level where I could now rationalize and perceive my world as it is, and not some unknown sphere of misplaced comprehension. No doubt about it, I know now I'm going to be alright and beat this thing. No doubt about it.

It's like a jigsaw puzzle where the pieces, by themselves, do not have great significance until they're put together and start forming an image. The accumulation of everything that's been done to and with me has built up to this moment: these are the pieces. Sometime during the night, something must have just "clicked in" and decided it was time to make some sense out of things: this is the image.

Getting up on my feet and walking, trying to remember how to write and figure things out again must have been the key which allowed me to break free from the forgotten ozone and return to this planet. The message, "Earth to Craig, earth to Craig, come in Craig," has been answered because I'm well on the way to entering earth's atmosphere again. Therapies from here on out will take on a new appreciation, meaning, and understanding.

In my morning Communication Skills session, Diane asked me to write "Today is Tuesday, April 27, 1982." But instead of just following through like the obedient pupil, I now know why I am doing this. My enlightened perception/new understanding that I can't activate the right hemisphere's visuo-spatial function of forming letters or put into motion the left hemisphere's function of getting this down on paper, made practicing this deficit that much more important and relevant.

Walking down the hallway behind my wheelchair to PT, I announced to anyone who might listen of my cognitive discovery. Although definitely pleased with what I was saying, the therapists seemed to accept my disclosure with a guarded optimism, for there is no telling if a PATIENT'S revelation is indeed authentic or merely a product of a broken mind. Fueled by my joy capturing this new understanding, I felt as if I was doing a pirouette around the PT gym while pushing my wheelchair with my tanned therapist by my side. Because of my heightened awareness, these practice steps with Jan took on a newfound appreciation.

During the psychology session with Mrs. Joy after lunch, when she also asked me to write, "Today is Tuesday, April 27, 1982," I was still frustrated I couldn't retrieve from my brain's right hemisphere how to go about making the first letter to the first word or get that frontal lobe to organize the steps needed to begin making that damned "T," but the bitter flavor this inability left behind was more tolerable, for this practice had a purpose.

Following my second physical therapy session of this spectacular day, I headed for yet another emotionally-challenging therapy—-Occupational Therapy. OT really got the passions growling because I put so much into it, but received what seemed so little in return. Until I turned blue in the face, I'd concentrate and concentrate and concentrate on getting that right hand and its fingers to respond in some way, any way, usually to no avail. Whether it be my unsuccessful attempts to spread my fingers apart when trying to pick a quarter off the table or my inability to flick a paper football, it would not be unusual for me to let the agitation-induced filth spew from my lips rapid fire. Although far from being overjoyed, I didn't let these hand and finger incapabilities ruin my day like they had on so many others.

Normally, when Wendy would ask me to pick up some wooden blocks with my bum hand and I'd end up dropping them on the floor after spending what seemed an eternity trying to clasp onto them, I'd be boiling. Or, when Stephanie would demonstrate a new way I could tie my shoes or button my shirt, the devastation of how far I've regressed would cave in on me. But being scorched and avalanched by emotional destruction would be for another time, because today I had a renewed vigor and grasp of what it is I need to do in order to get better.

My newfound freedom of awareness allowed me to recognize why I was constantly reminded by therapists, nurses, and my family not to use my left hand for everything—because if my right hand is to improve, I must use if for everything I can. If it were only that simple.

Having paralysis of the fingers and wrist feels like one's hand would after a rubber cement coating has hardened over these joints. There is barely any elasticity of the fingers and the wrist has practically no flexibility whatsoever. The fingers of my right hand are stiff and rigid, as if a stick of hard plastic were tied to each, making them anything but limber and responsive.

The fingers of my bad hand feel as if they weigh at least one hundred times more than those of my good one. There is no independent control of any single finger; at least two will move when trying to isolate the movement of one. The pinky is now severely double-jointed, as it will snap back and forth each time the fingers are individually—or as a whole—put into motion.

When I'm not focusing on the positions of my fingers or hand, my right-upper extremities natural position now is for the fingers to curl into a ball and for my hand to rest on my chest, as my elbow is still mortared at a right angle. Sleeping at night, my right hand forms a fist with my arm contracted close to my body.

Presumably, after being informed of my continued bouts with hemiparesis and double vision at the most recent staffing, my physiatrist, Dr. Amayo, told me when he did rounds that I had to start practicing some things everyday. First, in order to loosen up my tight heel cord, I'm to tap my right foot on the floor as if I'm listening to some music. The repetitive tapping motion strengthens and wakens the muscles that wanted to atrophy when I was in my state of no cognizance. Also, it reminds the brain which direction the foot needs to go and what motion is needed to undertake a step.

Like everything since my cranium put a dent in that telephone pole, this was tough because the front of my foot feels like a ship's anchor is holding it down. My ankles just can't seem to lift the front of my foot up. But if this foot-bouncing is going to help me stop slapping my foot when I walk, then you better believe tapping I will attempt to do. I can't keep to the beat of Judas Priest anymore, but maybe somebody's got some tapes of the Carpenters laying around. Nah, I'll do it without the music, thank you.

To help improve my double vision, I'm to extend my left arm straight out in front of me and, with the index finger pointing, follow my forefinger as I bring it towards me, touching my nose. I'm to do this while I'm not wearing my patched glasses. The theory behind this exercise is to stimulate that paralytic muscle behind my right eye and retrain the brain, so my eyes relearn how to work in conjunction with one another, instead of the left one dropping off and floating downward. Needless to say, when one eye has sunk and the other is where it's supposed to be, the brain is getting two pictures it must decipher.

Before following my index finger to my nose, I first have to determine which of the pair of forefingers on my left hand is the real one and which is a creation of brain damage. The way I do this is by turning off one of my optical TV monitors. Because of the hemiparesis, I can't close my right eye without shutting the other, so down will go my left eyelid. Either that or somehow try to block the vision of one of my eyes with my near-useless right hand. With the occlusion of one eye, I see normally and can tell which of the two digits I see is my actual finger as opposed to the mythical one.

If anyone sees me sitting in my wheelchair tapping my foot to no music and rhythmically bringing my forefinger to my nose and out again, I'll be discharged from Harmarville alright—-and put in Mayview State Psychiatric Hospital. But if this is going to help me see better and walk without being heard a hundred yards away, then I'll take my chances.

Without the patch over one lens, my vision actually makes me nauseous now. Seeing blurred images twice what they arc really gets the emotions bleeding and the stomach churning.

When my head's perpendicular to the ground and I'm looking straight ahead, one object is two and these two figures are side by side with the right elevated slightly above the left. Because of this, whatever I'm looking at appears to have an overlapping transparent coating. When doing the finger to nose exercise, my eyes shoot sideways trying to discern which forefinger is the real one and which is a mirage.

Head tilted to the left, the object is actually the image to the left and its apparition to the right. Shutting my left eye when in this position, the higher elevated ghost skips downward to where the object truly is located and I see as I should. Head leaning to the right, the left image is still where the body of whatever I'm looking at is situated. But this time, the left image is above the right and when the vision of one of my eyes is blocked, the right form shoots upward and I see things normally. The further I tilt my head, my vision becomes increasingly more horrific because whatever it is I'm focusing on spreads further and further apart as my head tilts more.

Any object located to my extreme left or extreme right appears as if they are significantly spread far apart. Without my "Pirate Pete" glasses, not only far away but close, I'll see double. For example, writing my practice letter, I'll see two pencils when there's only one to be seen.

When I'm tired at night, my vision is at its worst. When I'm doing my optical exercise in the evening before I go to bed and am not wearing my adhesive tape coated glasses, I'll just as soon put my left hand over one of my eyes to see than to close my left eye, because it's easier this way after a long, long day of rehab. I don't know if it's the distorted view itself, the emotional trauma not knowing if my eyesight is always going to be this way, or a combination of the two, but I actually feel as if I'm going to puke seeing the world as I do now.

At the very least, I'll have to put up with this for a minimum of one year because surgery isn't recommended until the brain has had twelve months to heal. I can tolerate the ringing in my ears all the time, but the suffering I'm going through with this double vision is cruel.

I am not going to acknowledge defeat to this brain injury or dwell on why I was that one in a billion who gets hurt, rather, I'm going to try to capitalize on the abilities I do have and do something about the things that are giving me problems in order to progress as best I can. This will require all the strength, willpower, and support humanly possible, for this condition poses many hurdles.

My fingers tightening in a ball while I'm sleeping at night and curling during the day did not go over too well with Dr. Amayo either, so he had ordered that a splint be made for my right hand that I'm to wear around the clock when I'm not using my paralytic mitt. This hand splint, which I got measured for in OT, is designed to keep my fingers apart and prevent them from curling.

It extends from my hand to the middle of my forearm and a cloth-like fiber resembling masking tape keeps my fingers and thumb spread open. The hard plastic from which it is made prevents my fingers from bending into a fist.

A pair of spongy foam rubber straps with a flannel covering connect onto two Velcro strips at the base of the splint over my forearm for stabilization. Already bothered by a leg splint when trying to get to sleep, I'm going to look and feel like the "Tin Man" from the Wizard of Oz when I go to bed at night.

Like the physical therapists earlier, when mom and dad came for their Tuesday evening visit and I told them that I know where I'm at and what happened to me, they naturally had their reservations. After all, this wouldn't be the first time

I had made a claim that wasn't exactly right. One of the few specific memories I have is my complaining about a kneepad that wasn't there bothering me.

Although far from being crisp, my memory of late has been showing signs of regeneration. My social worker, Miss Matthews, confirmed this when she called my parents this morning telling them the specific results of the Weschler Memory Scale I took last week. Mom and dad were encouraged when first notified of the general outcome of this test several days ago, but were unaware of the numerical value of the scale and its significance.Particularly, my yielding a score of 90 points which is in the Dull/Normal range. Informed of the specifics of this test, mom and dad were quite pleased that I was able to apprehend some of the knowledge which had escaped my conscious.

They were told that the first segment of the test consisted of an exercise called "verbal paired associate learning" where I'm read eight pairs of words and I'm to remember which words go together. Some of the words have an association with one another (ie. metal/iron, baby/cries) and are easier to recall. Others, have no relation to each other whatsoever (ie. crush/dark, obey/inch) and—because of this—are naturally more difficult.

After the list of words is read, two at a time, the first word of each pair is read again and I must identify the second word that went with it. I'm first read the list in a specific order, but during the testing phase, the order is different in the subsequent trials. The list of words is read until they all have been paired correctly. If—after six readings—each word has not been properly matched, the test is discontinued and scored.

Like the WAIS-R, the Weschler Memory Scale can localize approximately where some of the brain damage has occurred. Material that is well-practiced is generally believed to be mostly in the brain's left hemisphere and new information that is just being "perceived" is thought to be in the right hemisphere of the brain. The WAIS-R I struggled with yesterday indicated that I had a lot wrong with the right hemisphere of my brain and the Weschler did likewise.

Because I didn't have trouble pairing the Weschler words that I have learned in the past as being associated (ie. metal/iron, rose/flower), this was indicative that this left hemisphere function was reasonably intact. However, my memory wasn't sharp at all when I had to learn and "perceive" new associations (ie. crush/dark, cabbage/pen) and this lapse indicated that there was some neurological turbulence occurring in my right hemisphere.

When made aware that I was able to ease through the first part of the Weschler's mental control subtest where I counted backwards from 20 to 1 in a fair amount of time, mom and dad were elated that I not only could still formulate numbers in their numerical order in my mind, but had the capacity to reverse them. When told that I had no trouble with the second portion of the Weschler which had me say the alphabet as fast as possible, this didn't come as a surprise because I had done this in my practice sessions with mom, dad, and Ug many times before. Neither did it shock them that I did okay with the last portion of this subtest where, starting with "1," I added and counted by "3's" as far as I could (ie. 1-4-7-10-13 etc.).

Mom and dad have learned that how they feel about things is dependent on what they focus on. If they were told last April 27th that they would be ecstatic that their eighteen-year-old son had PROGRESSED to the point he now has the ability to count from "20" backwards or quickly say his A-B-C's this time next year, they'd have been crushed. If told this same thing two months ago, they'd have been jumping for joy.

Living in the "Here and the Now" and not yesterday, taking each day as it comes and appreciating any signs of progress—ANY improvement—is how mom and dad survived through this period where no one knew where I was at—not even me. If one gazes westward to mourn the day's passing, dawn's bright awakening may be forever missed.

Watching the sliding glass doors close behind my parents as they left upon visiting hours ending this glorious day, another awakening had occurred to me. Being of their own flesh and blood coupled with their life-long caring and nurturing of me, there was never any doubt that I was loved. Their incredible sacrifice, commitment, and devotion since I was wedged between that telephone pole and the Volkswagen made me truly understand that quantification of their love is impossible, for it is of infinite proportions.

My parents being of an older stature than other kids' parents my age was beneficial in the sense that they taught me the old standard work ethic where the importance of effort and perseverance are stressed. When you've lived through a depression and a World War, you can better appreciate the value of things and the struggle required to attain some comfort. Dad would always tell me that, if you really want something, you've got to scratch and claw for it.

Really all I can do for myself and my parents since February 14th is what I have been doing—and that's "giving it all I've got" by digging my nails deep into what's ailing me. This 110% effort is a must for, when it comes to the symptoms of head injury, there is no demilitarized zone because it's an all-encompassing around the clock battle. Because it's easier for me to say what hasn't been affected by this head injury than what has, I need to get to work again.

Pushing my wheelchair down and up the hallway doing my laps, it feels and looks like there's two of me. The left side is like the Craig of old, as I take normal strides and swing my relaxed, pliant left-upper extremities in a fashion just like anyone else, but the right side—that's another story.

When I take a step with my right leg, I'm stiff and my stride is only as long as my foot. And when I take a step moving my left leg, it's abrupt because putting weight on my right leg makes me so disoriented and feels as if I'm going to go tumbling down. One side moving fluently and the other lacking grace results in a limp characterized by hesitation of my entire right side.

I've got to swing my right leg out just to get moving, usually sliding the top of my foot on the floor. When I do make some semblance of a step forward, my foot smacks the ground and knee bends back. Landing on my right leg in an aggressive fashion with my knee snapping back doesn't feel real good. When I hyperextend my knee in this manner, that rod bites at my ass and clicks inside my femur. The knee itself feels as if it's been ridden with bursitis.

When I'm relaxed and comfortable now while I'm walking, it seems this is when I do things wrong. When things feel like they are falling into place naturally and I perceive myself as situated properly behind my wheelchair, is when I am not oriented at all. When it feels as if I'm overcompensating, I'm actually doing things correctly.

Relying more on my right leg to hold me up, which is what I've been told I have got to do in order to stand up straight, I feel so off-balance and awkward. When sensing that I'm crooked and going to fall over, this is when I'm standing like I should. It seems like my upper-torso needs to do one thing (lean more to the left) while my lower-torso simultaneously needs to do something else (put more weight on my right leg). I'm glad I got my wheelchair to stabilize me because, without it, my brain's malfunctioning position sense would leave me stranded or else I'd find myself constantly trying to pick myself off the floor.

To bend that "cinder block" heel cord of mine and to keep my right leg from swiveling out, the motion I have to undertake feels like I am doing an European goose-step march. The sensation I have is one where I feel as if I were doing some kind of high-step, but in reality, when I do get my foot off the floor, it's barely lifting off the ground.

In order to get my right arm to swing as naturally as possible along my side, I'd push the wheelchair with my good left hand and do what I sensed was an exaggerated swing of my right arm. With my elbow having the dexterity and resiliency of a cement slab, it would ache with tremendous pain while my right/upper extremities barely moved.

During this walking/arm swinging training, I'd be giving my designer hand splint a ride on my wheelchair because I would try to relax my paralytic fingers on their own and, if I would lose my easily-lost balance, I could break my fall better. My right arm trying to lock at a 90 degree angle and my hand trying to assume a shape resembling the head of a judge's gavel was just too much to deal with tonight, so I put on my splint and went back to my room to practice some writing. Court adjourned.

Stamina dehydrated, but fortitude reining, I forged ahead to write Valerie her letter. Writing Valerie a couple of letters a week is what has improved my ability to write from pre-schooler to second grader.

With the pencil in my left hand, I wanted to write her a letter telling her about how my thinking had cleared this morning and how much I need and appreciate her friendship. During the many hours and days that my family aren't here, I don't know how I'd keep from losing my mind without Valerie to talk to and spend some time with.

Just knowing someone can like me for who I am after what's happened to me means so much. And being an attractive female makes it that much more tremendous. With so many physical and intellectual scars, it's a concern whether I'm going to appeal to anyone, even as a friend.

With my alphabet board in front of me, but trying to be increasingly less reliant on it, I wanted to start the letter with "Dear Valerie." Because I started each of my letters to whomever printing the word "Dear," I had a lot of practice getting this word on paper and don't have too much in the way of trouble printing this now. Despite the majority of my letters being written to my #1 nurse/savior, often writing the name "Valerie" posed problems.

Pencil on paper all set to go, ready to make that "V," my hand quickly shot down then up, down then up making a "W" instead. Seeing the mistaken letter staring me straight in the face, I quickly scratched it out.

Knowing full well the mistake I just made, again my hand pulled the pencil down and—after a brief hesitation—pushed up, pulled down, pushed up, making another "W." I can't control what my hand does, it has a mind of its own.

A lot of the time, I don't intend for it to go in the direction it does, it just goes. Like in the case just now where I made a "W" when I intended to make a "V," my hand won't stop until it's damn well ready, void of any conscious neurological input.

After I've made the mistake, I know what I've printed is wrong and can identify the error that I've made on the paper, but I simply can't do anything about it. I can only wish that I could produce what I sense is right, because I have no mental picture of what the letters' shapes are.

Not only will my hand get manic being unable to stop, but will get going without having any idea of what it needs to do first in order to make a particular letter. My hand has no strategy of where to go or what to do, but away it will go anyhow. Even with the utmost effort and concentration, there's no guarantee it's going to abide by anything but its own accord. It just does what it damn well pleases and the control system guiding the hand— my brain—has no tapes of past experience it can refer to because they all have been erased.

For example, in time when a "V" does eventually flicker on my brain's television monitor and I am able to capture it and can get this letter down on paper, I'll want to make an "a," but images of an assortment of different letters simultaneously flash in my mind, making it virtually impossible to pinpoint the symbol I want because of the clutter. Detailing how the letters are laid out is not possible either because these images move around and fade quickly, so I just put down anything I know is a letter—provided my hand listens to me.

Recognizing these forms that flash before my mind's eye—when they stay still long enough or don't disappear right away—off my hand will fly reproducing the first figure on my mind's teleprompter without checking it out first. Being that the odds are 26 to 1 against me that the letter I print will be the correct one, or the low percentage my hand will stop when I want it to, chances aren't in my favor that I can keep from putting a tail on my "a" making a "q" or prevent my hand from circumnavigating producing an "o." One thing I can be thankful for is that my bruised "noggin" is allowing me to practice lower-case letters a little more. Survival is frequently dependent on whether things are seen as half-full, as opposed to half-empty.

Making a lowercase "l" seems like a simple enough letter to make—-just send your pencil straight down. If I could only get my schizophrenic hand to do this, I wouldn't have any problem. Whoever might say "just" send it down, has no idea what it's like having a brain that doesn't work.

"Inhibited" is not a word you could use to describe what my hand does when it attempts to make a symbol from the alphabet, for it will travel every which way, any which way. Without a lot of contemplation and restraint, the likelihood that I would jot down a simple vertical line to make that "l" are remote. It would be just as likely that I would make two crossing, diagonal lines forming an "X" or a horizontal line with a vertical line underneath it forming a "T" or some other confabulation, than it would for me to do the correct thing.

After failing to nab what this letter looked like, I referred to my alphabet cue. Saying my A-B-C's and pointing to each letter as I go along, when I said "ell" and distinguished the letter my left index finger was on as being the bugger I couldn't find in the void of no return which is my thought processes, down it went on the paper.

Not having control of your mind is terrifying. Things once done automatically without effort have now vanished. I don't know what the hell's going on. I'm scared.

Searching for this mystery letter and struggling against the forces which prevent my hand from going where it needs to, I finally was able to print that "l", as I whipped that pencil down and forced myself to pick that lead up off the paper before I gave it a little loop making a "b" or a hump forming an "h." Or stemming two horizontal lines of different size to the right constructing an "F" or three lines manufacturing an "E." Or sandwiching this "l" between two horizontal lines making an "I" or erecting another "l" while I'm at it and connecting them with a horizontal slash producing an "H."

I know all these configurations I just made without putting much in the way of thought into it are letters, but I don't know for sure which ones they are until I've put them down on paper and look at them because my mental notepad is missing. Being of a skeptical nature, if this wasn't happening to me, there's no way I could believe that someone could ever forget how to do something as automatic as writing. Unbelievable, it's absolutely unbelievable what a person can no longer do after their head's been "conked."

I looked down at the "DEaR Val" that took me five minutes to write and—recognizing the next two letters I need to put in her name are already there—I copied them, quickly scribbling these down. I wish I'd have thought of this when putting the "a" in Valerie. Because the "i" hadn't been printed yet, this was going to be a tough one.

Forcing myself not to look at my alphabet board, I tried to think of what an "i" looked like. I knew this was the letter that I had to use a dot somewhere. Let's see now, I think a dot is shaped like a circle, so that's what I'll make.

After luckily forcing my mind to remember what a "circle" looked like, I made this oval and impulsively stabbed a period in the middle of it creating an "eye," but not the letter. My gaze was gravitating towards the alphabet cardboard cue until I fought this powerful temptation with all the brute force I could. Head tilted, staring at the "DEaR ValER," I have no idea how to make that "i."

It seems all the letters of the alphabet are flashing before me except the one I want, that damned little "i." It takes all the strength I can gather to prevent that left hand from going ballistic and putting down what it wants to. It's weird, much of the time I don't have any control of what my left hand does when I write. As if it has it's own brain, my hand won't stop when I want it to. And if I want my hand to go in a particular direction that it has no interest in traveling, that's too bad for me because I can't do a damn thing about it, usually.

Even if my mind was able to provide my hand with distinct impressions of what each individual letter looked like, there would be no guarantee I could reproduce it. With a brain that can't distinguish one letter from another or develop their forms, what I have to do is try to tap some reservoir of past understanding in hopes that a gusher of recognition spews forth. Because of this lost ability to write spontaneously, I need to slow down and dissect each letter, so I can picture in my mind how it looks. Now, I'm going to try and snag that "i" that I'm positive is in my head someplace.

I know somehow it resembles the "l" I've put down and there is a dot, so I'll make a "l" and put a dot to the right of it. Looking down at my creation, I immediately know this is not right. Maybe the dot goes underneath the line.

Making another "l" and jabbing a dot beneath it, I know this was as bad as my first ugly attempt at printing that letter that comes between "h" and "j." Scribbling over this, I quickly sent my pencil from left to right making a horizontal line and then drew a circle under this. But this looks like a seesaw, not an "i," so away my pencil went and wiped this out.

With "might and mean," I yanked my pencil down making a vertical line and thoughtlessly dotted my letter to the left of my mark. I'm making a mess of this paper now, and if I scratch out anymore of these symbols I've made trying to rediscover what an "i" resembles, I'll tear a hole in the tablet.

Just getting this name down is a nightmare and I've practiced printing "Valerie" countless times now. Helpless, I'm just going to sit here for a little while staring at the word-and-a-half that required the thought and effort most authors put into a book-and-a-half, and try to regroup. Squeezing the pencil I wanted to snap in half out of frustration, I just kept thinking, "C'mon brain, do your thing."

Fired up and itchin' to make that "i," my hand went straight down, diagonally up and to the right, and back down again forming a backwards uppercase "N." Weakened, bitter, and brittle, I looked at the lowercase "l" I had printed and my hand just went and put a dot above the "l" making the "i" that I've been searching for. Somewhere in the torn battlefield which is the surface of my brain, my hand got a signal from the neurological command post and instinctively dotted the "i" where it was supposed to go. Hip, hip, hooray.

Damn it, I could've avoided all this trouble if I would have only thought of printing my first name and copying the "i" from "Craig." I was so wrapped up in trying to mentally visualize what this letter looked like, I didn't think clearly. Since my hypothalamus has been laying on Beau Street, what else is new?

Before wrestling with myself in order to find what an "e" looks like, I'm going to stop and think things through. Because I know the last letter in Valerie's name ends with the second letter in the word "Dear" I started this note with, I'll just copy this down. Hey, hey.

Now, I'd like to open this letter with "Thank you for being such a good friend," but where do I cross the "T" in the first word?

Having forgotten so much and being physically unable to do the most automatic of movements has stricken me with terror. Hearing about my non-stop efforts to overcome the aphasias with which I have been afflicted, Betty Stewart, RN, the Rehabilitation Specialist from our automobile insurance, said she wished she could bottle the fire that was burning inside of me and put it on market; that she could become rich off of it and retire.

I don't see what I am doing is anything special, however. I know I have a mess of problems and the only way I'm going to get rid of them is by practicing. It's like what I've learned playing guitar—the more you practice, the better you get. When you first start to take on this musical challenge, it ain't fun and it ain't easy, but it's something you got to go through if you want to be good someday. The more you put into it, the more you'll get out of it. I'll just have to keep my fingers crossed the same applies to this rehab challenge. But with brain damage, nothing is a guarantee.

I'm flattered Ms. Stewart thinks she could make a fortune off me, particularly because of her extensive experience with rehabilitation and seeing the multitude of patients she does being a nurse, but the thing that motivates me to work as hard as I do is not something that requires a patent. It's the simple formula of trying not to allow the various disabilities I'm experiencing now overtake me in the future and the overwhelming fear of what my life would be like if they did. And it's this fear that is the spark which makes me work so hard.

I couldn't live with myself knowing I didn't give it my all during this crucial period where the brain can be so responsive and receptive to training. My spirit would be sliced if I would have to live a life thinking, "If I would have only done more, I wouldn't be experiencing. . . . . " I need to take advantage of the ability I have knowing what needs done in order to get better and rise above the murk which many having brain injuries never have the opportunity to do.

A gashing, unbearable horror would tear inside of me if blank pages would be a document to my future because I didn't do what I could to prevail over what being squashed against a telephone pole did to me. If alarm lingers, disenchantment rules, and inability is to persist in the days forthcoming, I at least want the serenity knowing I did everything physically and psychologically possible to pull out of this. There's enough wrong with me, I don't want the chemical in the brain that is thought to provide one with a sense of calm and peacefulness—serotonin—to quit on me.

If the perdify of one that I trusted has taken away that which will never be regained, so be it. I'll just have to turn the page and go on and just be thankful a funeral procession wasn't played in my honor. But if there's a chance that tomorrow's happiness can be more than a figment of my imagination or I have something more to look forward to than the passing of the hour, I'm going to go for it. Call it being naive, stupidity, courageous, whatever, but I don't believe the script to my life has already been written and there are no more dreams to be snared. If I can do anything about it, there's no way I'm going to let my past be the epilogue to a life forsaken of its prosperity and robbed of the fulfillment it can offer.

I've always basically considered myself to be a fairly good person. I could never claim to be one who totes a bible around reciting scripture, however, I do definitely feel God's presence and that he's looking over me. With the ingredients for motivation in place, coupled with this powerful guiding force, I don't think my chances are so bad. Clicheish or not, I just may be here for a reason.

A life where I cannot walk without a wheelchair in front of me is one I would have a hard time picturing and in no way could I subscribe to. Being restricted as to where I could go and moving at a sundial's pace is something that I simply could not tolerate.

Like the bullet shot from a sniper's gun, no one can say with any certainty the direction my hand will end up when I try to write. Sitting there, mystified about what I need to do, I couldn't even begin to fathom the degrading thoughts directed towards me if I wasn't able to sign my welfare check or an application for unemployment. This inability to express myself via the written word is a situation I simply could not live with.

I can almost feel the agitation and disgust being unable to bathe myself, for I couldn't roll a bar of soap in a wash cloth or open a bottle of shampoo because my dominant hand and its fingers are no good. Modesty would be a thing of the past, as I would have to bare all in front of whomever, if I didn't want to reek.

It's an absolute given that I couldn't carry on with my eyesight as it is now. Having cloudy vision where things are seen twice what they are is something I'd have a hard time wishing on my worst enemy—except for the heinous foe that I was led to believe was a friend.

Imagine, if you can, a clump of mud slowly dissolving in your stomach. Acid rips into the walls of this brown mass melting off bits and pieces as the falling chunks splash gastro-intestinal fluid on the lining of your growling gut. This gel-like paste oozes down the side of your belly coating it with a putrid stench. This is how my vision makes me feel without having the vision of one eye blocked, and in no way could I endure this hell. Being the subject of burning stares when wearing my eye covering will not sit well with me, but it beats the alternative.

For the most part, being someone that always just wanted to be one of a crowd and not stick out, this foot slapping and rock hard stiffness of my right side would make me the object of too many curious minds for my comfort. When my right leg hammering the ground with my foot subsequently slapping down isn't the focus of unwanted glares, then my right arm dangling by my side will get the spotlight after enough has been seen of my patched glasses. Receiving uninvited attention goes with the territory when you're different and, as difficult as this might be, I just might have to accept the fact that I may not be the same as most others. You can bet your bottom dollar, however, that I'm going to work like a fool, so that I don't have to live through a life of these scenarios.

Because I'm not a fool, I also know that as critically as I was hurt and with the severity of my symptoms, I realize I'm physically never going to be the same as I was. But in the back of my mind, there's an egotistical part of me that's thinking maybe I will be the exception in order to set some kind of example. Denial? Possibly. Survival? Definitely.

It's this hope and the aforementioned fear of a life void of happiness which keeps me working like a dog. I thank God for the strength I do have to keep going and to work on what I can. Still, there are so many unknowns and pursuits not within my control.

I have been told that, because I have injured my brain, I will always be at risk for having a seizure. For the rest of my life, my head will be like a time bomb and, with the exception of avoiding excessive stress, sleep deprivation, and beverages containing alcohol and caffeine, there's little I can do to prevent one of these attacks on the body from occurring where a person either is physically shaking and/or becomes profoundly confused. These convulsions arise because brain waves have been disturbed and there isn't much one can do about the rhythmic, undulating flow of these neurological signals.

There are different kinds of seizures. A focal seizure is one involving only a specific area of the body. For example, a person might find their arm or leg twitching/shaking uncontrollably.

The word, "mal," in French means bad and, as the name implies, a grand mal seizure is the grandest/worst of all seizures and a petit mal seizure not nearly so excessive. Hence, the word "petit" meaning small, as in a little seizure.

A petit mal seizure primarily occurs with kids under the age of thirteen and is characterized by periods of inattentiveness and a shaking where muscles opposite each other tighten and relax alternately, causing rhythmic movements to occur (clonic convulsion). The grand daddy of all seizures involves a violent shaking of the entire body where all the muscles tighten and the person becomes a rigid, shaking spectacle (tonic convulsion). When this grand mal seizure hits, arms, legs, head, and everything else fly into a wild spasm and it may last from a couple of seconds to a few minutes. Naturally, the longer the seizure, the more potential for damage and this is why doctors want to know how long a seizure has lasted, so they can get a general idea of what additional damage there may be.

A psychomotor seizure is one where the person becomes mentally confused and physically compromised, as their movements lack coordination and are coarse. Seizures of this type don't necessarily involve involuntary spasms and contraction of muscles.

Nocturnal seizures are those that occur at night while the person is sleeping. If the seizure is a mild one (petit mal) or is localized in a small enough area where only a slight twitching may occur (focal), the person may not even realize they had a seizure. Often, seizures will begin in a certain area of the body, frequently starting with a twitching of a certain muscle group, and then expand until the whole body is involved. This type of convulsion is common with some forms of epilepsy.

My parents have been instructed that, in the event I would have a seizure, all they can really do is safeguard against me getting hurt. This includes, not only keeping me from falling where I could give my head another whack and/or break something, but to have a tongue depressor handy, so I don't bite into my tongue. They were told that if I do have this fit, at the very least I'll be utterly exhausted and confused afterward.

Since my head took the shellacking that it did, all we can hope for is that my anti-convulsant keeps doing its thing. So far, so good. But what will the next minute bring?

What did I ever do to deserve this? Will there ever be any enjoyment in my future or will it be one that I never stop asking myself, "What if?" Will I have to live life knowing all my pursuits are to be doomed? Will restriction and limitation be my lot in life? Is my fate one where I find myself never ceasing to submit? Has fortune become something I will never capture? Will success and accomplishment only be something I witness others attaining and not anything I'm to ever experience? Are the days gone where I can withdraw from the talent and wisdom I've deposited?

The things that I've always excelled at and brought me happiness were those that were physical in nature. Now, I can't even hold a pencil with my dominant hand, straighten my right arm without it shooting with a fiery ache, or take a half-assed step unless I bring my mind to bear upon each motion I'll have to labor through.

The stinging inferno of loss would blaze deep within me, if I were not able to throw a baseball or participate in sports again. This pain could only be topped by the tortuous ache which blazes from my elbow when trying to straighten my right pitching arm, or the misery I go through when the rod in my right leg decides it's time to shift. Being unable to toss a football or even jog around my neighborhood would be an agony of the cruelest proportions.

A hideous sting would plunge my heart, if I can't pinch a guitar pick. The countless hours I put into learning my instrument would be for naught and would have a hard time coping if I had to abandon something I loved with all my heart and has become such an integral part of who I am. The foregoing of a past makes for a life without meaning.

To sit back and dwell on how life might have been while watching the world go by is dangerous. For me to sit on my ass in my wheelchair wondering how things could have been otherwise is a sob story that's not going to do me any good. I've always been one that, when my back's against the wall, I'll fight like hell. And because of the symptoms my malfunctioning brain has levied against me, I'm in, not only the fight of my life, but a fight of all fights.

I might as well die if I approach things in a helpless/hopeless manner. The attitude I approach things with is one where, if I work hard, I'm not going to be stopped. I'm no idiot, I know that rehabbing and exercising with the goal of being how I was before is not going to happen, but I will attempt to get as close as I can. Hopefully, that can be a reality.

For me, this rehabilitation is like a slot machine where the coins are my effort and the jackpot is my health. I approach this rehab venture like the crazed gambler who jams quarter after quarter after quarter after quarter into their one-armed bandit hoping that the next coin will deliver those three cherries, apples, or strawberries and s/he can go home a new person. However, if my rejuvenation is to occur, it won't be from giving my money away. Rather, I need to attack it thinking that if I write one more letter of the alphabet, one more word, one more sentence, one more letter to Valerie, something in my brain is going to take hold and I'll be cranking out those words like you wouldn't believe. If I do one more lap, pinch one more ball of putty, tap my foot one more time, stretch my arm one more minute, or follow my finger to my nose one more trial, I just have to believe those fruits are going to come up somewhere down the road. Rehabilitation is a lot like gambling because, no matter how well you play the game, there's no way you can completely control what's going to turn up next and if Lady Luck is going to shine your way.

Because I know what's going on now, it has become more than an obsession for me to get better, it's now an addiction to work. The only way I'm going to get this "fix," this need to regain what has been taken from me, is to put forth an effort that I didn't know was within me. When the chips are down and I've got to play my hand in this not-so-forgiving game of rehab, I have got to play the best I can and play it smart, because if I fold, there's never any turning back. Never.

I not only can't remember what happened to me the weeks immediately prior and after I was injured, but most everything of what's happened to me in the past has been erased from my memory. It's one big blank what's happened to me, where I've been at these last few months, and, even more disturbing, I can't retrieve from my data banks any specific occurrence from my years in school, playing sports/guitar, living in my neighborhood, etc. Everything about me and how I came to be is now gone. Poof! In a matter of seconds, my life as I knew and experienced it has vanished.

I can say easy enough that I live in Washington, Pennsylvania, give my address and neighborhood, name who some of my friends are, tell you I was going to West Virginia University and went to Trinity High School, but I have no concrete event I can draw from my memory as proof that I can actually recall ever being at these places or associating with these people.

This is similar to the problem I have when trying to print a letter. I can say that a capital "A" looks like a tent with a line in the middle of it, tell you that the letter "o" looks like a ball, or that an "s" looks like a snake, but there's no way I could reproduce in my mind what a tent, ball, or snake look like, so these objects are merely words and don't represent images. Therefore, I might indeed be able to describe what the letters' configurations are, but I still have no idea how these letters look. Because language formation, such as speaking, is said to be a left hemisphere function and the formation of structure (perception) is a right, this is further evidence that my brain's right hemisphere got beaten up pretty bad.

I can recognize people and places—if shown a picture of them—but I can't go about telling you why I recognize the house in the photo as being mine, how I know the hairy stud playing guitar in the picture is Kevin Brezinski, or that Dave "Cobra" Parker patrols right field for the Pirates. My brain's recognition function seems to be working much better than its ability to retrieve new information asked of it. Once again, this is indicative of right hemisphere brain damage, for the left side is believed to be the storage compartment for material previously learned and the right is where the mechanism for new learning is thought to be. Then again, it might not all be my right hemisphere's fault I can't detail various happenings, it could have something to do with my mid-brain being whipped around. Whatever the case may be, I cannot remember any specific experiences during my life and bring it to my conscious.

For example, I can't remember any Christmases, holidays, get-togethers of any type, dinners, friends or relatives visiting, or spending any time there, but I know that's where I live when shown a picture of our house. I can't recall ever going any place with him, being in any of his high school or college classes, doing anything with him, or playing guitar around Kevin, but I know that we have a lot in common and are friends/Trinity '81 alumni and were roommates at W.V.U. I know baseball has always been a major part of my life and that Parker was my favorite player, but I have no hint that I've ever experienced him play despite somehow knowing that I've seen or heard hundreds, if not a thousand, Bucco games. Memory—-come out, come out, wherever you are.

It's incredible and frightening when there's a large segment of your life that you don't know where you were at and can't remember too much of anything. When my parents and Ug told me some of the things I did at Allegheny General and my early weeks at Harmarville, it shocked and alarmed me because it showed just how much my damaged brain altered my personality, for these dreadful acts were just the opposite of my character.

When mom told me I struck her both at the hospital and at the rehab a few weeks ago, my heart could have collapsed because that's something the "real me" could never, ever do, or would think of. When dad told me I've gotten out of hand in some of my therapies and tried to nail whoever was working with me at the time, I couldn't believe it.

I was informed that I took a swipe at Jan Alba, gave some PT intern a miserable time, and had gotten testy more than a few times in OT when the therapists would move my forearm or spread my fingers. Mom and dad both said I stretched and ripped articles of their clothing so badly when I was in Wonderland that some are ruined and others they wouldn't wear outside of the privacy of the house. I have absolutely no recollection/memory of ever doing any of these things.

Dad said I was so uncooperative at Allegheny General that I couldn't stay put in a bed and personnel at the hospital had to line my room with mattresses because I was so agitated and uncontrollable. He said I'd aggressively thrash my arm for no apparent reason and that I'd strangle him by the tie and yank him down towards me. Mom told me I grabbed hold of a couple of her blouses and pulled on them until they became what seemed to be two sizes bigger than they were.

She said that my respiratory therapst at the hospital dreaded working with me because I wouldn't let him put the oxygen mask on my face and when he did get it on, I'd just rip it off and throw it on the floor because it appeared that I didn't like anything touching me—not even clothing.

I could crawl in a hole and die when mom and dad told me of my stripping exploits during this stage where I didn't show too much in the way of reserve. They said all the nurses and therapists at Allegheny General saw me in the buff and quite a few at Harmarville saw "Goliath." They told me regardless of who was around, old ladies and little kids notwithstanding, off would come my gown covering me and I would bare all, as if I wanted to show off.

I was told it wouldn't take much to set me off. One minute, I'd be calm, pleasant, and serene, the next, away I'd bark the vulgarities and start swinging and swaying in my wheelchair as I tried to rip off whatever rock 'n' roll shirt I was wearing.

I can't believe the way I acted towards some of these kind-hearted nurses. I know it wasn't really me that kicked Fran, spit on Diane, called Rosemary "Crow face," or knocked my medications out of June's hands and I realize they knew this wasn't really Craig, but still, it's embarrassing when told some of the stuff you did when you weren't conscious of what you were doing. If a patient tried any of these things with me, whether s/he was aware of what they were doing or not, I don't think I could be as nice to him or her as these rehabilitation nurses are to me. Then again, few have the fabulous dispositions these Harmarville nurses have. God bless 'em.

If there's one occurrence I wouldn't mind remembering, it would be urinating on Ug a couple of weeks ago. To see him wrestle with my not-so-private privates, getting sprayed in the process while mom and dad stood there is a site I regret I can only imagine. However, as I understand it, my brother has been tremendously supportive and impeccably helpful during this whole ordeal. As much as I hate to admit this, there are times when even Ug isn't so bad.

The reason some memories have dissipated with the eye of the storm and others survived can only be left to speculation. It could be my brain had healed to the point where the memory center was capable of seizing events of consequence and storing them for future reference. Possibly, my brain was still in no shape to process and catalog what I had seen, rather, the significance of these events are why they stuck with me. Or simply, it could be a combination of the two.

There's a chance my hippocampus, which many in the neuroscientific community believe to be the location where memory becomes processed after new information has been absorbed by the brain, could have had a bruise on it as well that shrunk and this centrally-located seahorse-shaped organ of the brain healing some, allowed for neurons to transmit electrical signals to its neighbor nerve cells. Consequently, these connections enabled CMN (Cable Memory Network) to broadcast various images on the brain's television screen where I could retrieve figures from the past. Maybe my "think tank" sprung a leak, allowing this sea horse organ to get loose these past two-and-a-half months, until it healed shut a little. Regardless, there are several events that I definitely do have a vivid, distinct memory as occurring and not something my mind has allowed to go in one lobe and out another. Stellar usage of neuro-medical linguistics.

The very first thing I can remember since being crushed in that Volkswagen is an old lady firing her silverware at me in the nurses' station and hollering at the top of her voice, "Christ's son, Christ's son," and pointing at me. I know my one nurse, Jan Goga, came running over before I bought a fork between my eyes, and took this lady away. One can only guess why I cataloged this in my memory file and didn't do so with an assortment of other prominent events. Maybe the shock value and potential violence of the situation is why this didn't slip from my conscious.

Looking back, I can see my one roommate late one night lying awake smiling at me as I tried to lower my bed rail so I could escape, but didn't get too far. Thank God I got caught in this not-so-bright move. One could surmise that the reason this didn't become yet another episode that had been lost and forgotten, never to return, is the catastrophic consequences that would have occurred if I had managed to get out of bed.

I can think back to one afternoon when my family was all there and I asked this patient from Wheeling, W.Va. if he wanted to start up a rock group with me. That shows how good I was thinking; I can't even hold a pick anymore. I suppose I could recall this because I remember anything pertaining to guitar and music, brain damaged or not.

Carrying my thoughts back, I can picture Claire, Don, and Little Scotty visiting one time and Don sucked in all the oxygen out of the room when I told him, "I see two Dons, one's bad enough." More than likely, I grasped this memory because of the excitement in the air with my sister's family being there that I don't see but once or twice a year, and the relief this comment meant to everyone—for it showed a beacon of hope did exist.

Coming down the hallway, I can still see mom and dad walking towards me as I was stretching my arm in the hallway, disgusted with rehabilitation and how

Harmarville does not offer any formal counseling for its patients going through with this recovery process which requires much soul-searching. Feeling desolate about what was to become of me and seeing the two people who could provide me with relief probably is the reason this image didn't filter out of awareness.

Because this is an ongoing, recurring torment, it's no wonder I've always had tucked away somewhere in my mind's review, images of me ringing into my room a battery of nurses/aides then trying to talk them into taking that damned splint off my right leg. Flashes of me lying awake at night unable to sleep, feeling absolutely miserable, and moaning about how this no-compromising, hard plastic brace from Hell causes so much pain and discomfort has been a nightly occurrence and not just yesterday's passage.

Recognizing my newfound conceptualization of the world and orientation to that which occurs within it, my psychologist correctly assumed that I not only would be able to handle viewing the videotape her and I did together which depicts me severely compromised approximately two weeks after arriving at Harmarville, but that I would benefit seeing how I was a lost soul at one time. Knowing that the tape shows me in a state where I was profoundly confused, agitated, and physically inept, Mrs. Joy wanted to check with me one more time to see if I was prepared to see myself during a time where I have absolutely no recollection and barely knew who I was. Roll that tape.

Slumped forward, pushing the wheelchair back then struggling to sit up, I glanced at the photo of my brother-in-law Mrs. Joy was holding after she asked me to identify the person she was pointing to. No doubt agitated being in a sitting position, I couldn't stay still. Rocking my wheelchair back and forth and kicking the footrest, surely disturbed about my predicament, I reeled off some words in a language not of the Homo sapiens species. Babbling indiscernibly and playing with the microphone cord around my collar, before falling forward in submission, I was finally able to gather enough wind and approximate a sound. In a voice barely audible, I made a noise which resembled, "Daahn."

Right arm contracted, my head then went down in my left arm which lie curled on the wheelchair's table. When I would lift my head slightly, coming up for air, I'd rub either my left eye or touch the end of my nose as if I wanted to reach in and pick out a "goober." Intermittently sitting back and leaning forward, I took a longer look at the photo when Mrs. Joy asked if it was "Don?," but this time, I put a little more effort in my speech when I said, "Yeah."

Thrilled about this scintillating exercise, I then yawned and pushed my messed up hair behind my ear before Mrs. Joy asked me after reviewing the notes in her hand, "Where did you go to school?" Preoccupied with the mike cord around my neck, I went back a decade and told her where I went to elementary school. When Mrs. Joy asked me again where I went to school, once more I responded, "North Franklin."

Holding the folder which contained a profile of my past, Mrs. Joy asked me specifically, "Where did you go to high school?"

Preparing to slump forward, obviously disinterested in this test of question and answer, I once again said, "North Franklin."

Head now down in my arm like a grade schooler who's being punished, Mrs. Joy said, "Trinity," as I then immediately repeated "Trinity" and rocked my wheelchair back in such a way that I was letting my psychologist know I wasn't having a whole lot of fun playing this game, and really couldn't care less if I knew where I attended school.

In need of confirmation I knew where I went to school, the dedicated professional asked, "Trinity High School?" where I answered her with an "Ahh," which she interpreted to be a "Yes."

Camera angle shifting from a close-up of me to my left to a little further back to my right and getting a full frontal view, Mrs. Joy then asked me, "And what year did you graduate?" which was answered right away with a brief, succinct "'81."

When Mrs. Joy reflected what I just said, "In '81?," I was kicking my wheelchair and rolling it around ever so slightly when I let an "Ahh" roll from my lips and mumbled something which resembled, "Uh huh."

Looking excruciatingly uncomfortable, as if I were in pain and nauseous, it appeared I would have wheeled on out of Mrs. Joy's office if I only knew how. Also, my interrogator bracing the side of my wheelchair with her right hand as I was weaving back and forth would have prevented me from getting too far.

Head bowed, shadowing my eyes with my left hand on my forehead and giving my footrest the boot with my left leg, Mrs. Joy asked me if I was going to the "University of West Virginia."

Never hearing the school referred to in that way, I still must have known what she meant and responded with a, "Uhm huhm."

Still very much unsettled, pushing my hair back and behind my ear, I was then asked what I was studying there, with this inquiry being answered with a yawn. As if she asked me what my G.P.A. was my first semester at W.V.U., I then lowered my head into my bent left arm which was resting on my wheelchair tray.

When Mrs. Joy repeated, "Do you remember what you were studying there?," with back rigid and staring blankly into the face of confusion and straight in the eye of the video camera, I started playing with one of two strips of masking tape on my wheelchair tray.

With my attention now focusing on picking this tan tape off the tray, Mrs. Joy asked, "Journalism?," which I elaborated by saying, "Yeah"—but with no yawn this time.

Rocking my wheelchair back after briefly being out front, I put my left foot back on the footrest. Seeing that my attention was still undivided on the masking tape, Mrs. Joy asked while pointing at my new toy it seemed like I was possessed to keep loosening from the table top, "What's this on here?"

As if the difficulty of these questions had sifted me of my strength, I put my hand on my forehead, covering my eyes and lowered my head almost as if pleading with her to stop. However, this wasn't being considered.

"What do we call this, Craig?," the unrelenting professional in search of answers asked, hoping her patient could file through his brain's contusion-ridden left hemisphere and give her the correct answer.

Fussing with the microphone cord that was around my neck and wiping the side of my face probably wishing the camera wasn't rolling so I could go digging for some more "gold," I replied to this brainteaser in the tone of a whisper, "Masking tape."

Looking straight into the camera's lens with my dead stare and gazing at Mrs. Joy, she asked me to repeat myself because my hand being over my mouth and the slight pitch with which I gave my answer prevented her from hearing me clearly. Making eye contact with my examiner as if wanting affirmation to my correct answer and then after she prodded me with an "Hmm?," I repeated in a distinct—yet strained voice—"Masking tape," as the camera angle switched back to where it started.

Beaming like a proud mother, the intensity in Mrs. Joy's voice doubled when she excitedly exclaimed, "Masking tape!!!" Then, immediately reverting back to her desired persona as an emotion-free psychologist before anybody noticed, responded stoically, "Very good."

Anything within my field of vision or range of touch seemed to be fair game for investigation. Looking down, playing with the right side of my purple and yellow flannel shirt, the far-from-worn psychology trooper asked—referring to the mike—"What do we call this around your neck, here?" Looking down to where Mrs. Joy pointed, I said nothing, as I was too preoccupied with twirling my shirt.

When Mrs. Joy continued this inquiry with, "What does that look like?," it was obvious that I was worn, so I just let this P.I. know through my fussiness that I had had enough of this questioning. Not able to tolerate anymore, my aggravation had reached intolerable proportions.

With my lumbar straight up against the pillowed back support of the wheelchair, I started rambling incoherently, as the noise which gurgled from my mouth must have been what mom and dad meant when they said I spoke "Martian" at Allegheny General. Moments after I started this nonsensical jabbering, I exhibited what I thought to be the horrific wide-eyed stare mom told me about when I was in the hospital. As if in utter distress about what had become of my life, my head then fell into my left hand before I sunk into my wheelchair.

Agitated, I tried to find words amidst the haze which blanketed my thinking and the maze which drained me of my tolerance. However, anymore expression would have to come another day, for the video image of me bent back in my wheelchair faded away along with my ability to focus and concentrate.

Amazing. It's unbelievable the figure that should have died from blunt force trauma to the head depicted in the video is me. Because of what I had been told by my family and the medical/rehabilitation personnel who have worked with me since my life was almost sacrificed so a boy of privilege could have fun at a party,

I knew I was in sorry shape not all that long ago. Still, it's incredible actually seeing yourself on a television screen, incapable of doing anything and being light years away from coherence.

The mass confusion which pelted me put me in a state of oblivion. It looked like I just needed to escape out of the throes of whatever had me. I'm sure I didn't know precisely what it was, I just knew I had to get out from underneath the pain and disarray with which I was smothered.

When Mrs. Joy first told me about the existence of this video, I was stunned because I had no idea that one was taken of me. But now that I know that a depiction of me during a time when I was trapped by confusion, agitation, and physical contortion exists, I couldn't be happier because this is something I can build from.

I know that I still have a lot of things yet to work on, but seeing how I was only two months ago compared to how I am now, I feel great about my chances to come out on top of this disability. Seeing that I have made such immense strides in such a short period of time, an excitement that things will work out has emerged.

Although I can't remember a whole heck of a lot about this effort early on, I must've worked my tail off to get to the point I am now. To say I'm proud of the way I carry myself now, several weeks later, as opposed to when that film was shot would be an understatement. Thrilled, ecstatic, and jubilant would be more accurate. Viewing myself on video this first time and witnessing the astounding improvements I've made in a relatively short time, Mrs. Joy surely anticipated this favorable reaction would have a positive effect on my attitude about things. Remarkable prognosticator, that Mrs. Joy.

When someone's in rehab, they frequently don't appreciate the magnitude of the gains they're making, only seeing what they can no longer do. "Wanting more" is a natural reaction and a beneficial response, if it pushes one to achieve. However, it's also essential to "pat oneself on the back" once in a while in order to make the most of a recovery. No matter how nice, professional, caring, and understanding the people working with the patient are, head injury rehabilitation is an experience of misery. Deep-cutting physical and emotional pain is with the survivor from sunup to sundown when taking on this most vicious of wars. There isn't any escaping the struggle, but how one approaches it can dictate if battle fatigue will effect the warrior in the long run.

My all too frequent vulgar responses and bouts with agitation to the many inabilities I now have are a sign of the emotional turmoil which cooks inside me. Going through this restoration process, one needs infusions of hope along the way because the patient soon learns there's multitudes of anguish around every corner.

The video I just saw was filmed about two weeks after I arrived at Harmarville, following four weeks at Allegheny General where I was generally not responsive to anything. I not only saw myself horribly compromised cognitively during this short film portrayal of me, but also as a "physical wasteland."

In the video, I literally am experiencing torture from the abundance of physical ailments which this accident has left me to deal with. In addition to the mental incapabilities my bruised brain has caused me to struggle with, the various physical afflictions with which I am at war scream for attention as well.

Not only was my inability to remain situated in one place for more than a few seconds at a time caused by a brain that was tricked into believing every position I assumed was not a suitable one, but being physically confined and restricted in my wheelchair was a torment that even my perceptual malfunctioning brain must have been able to sense. This uneasiness is noted from the very beginning, as the wails of discomfort this lack of serenity creates blackens the audio portion of this taped biography.

As I watched myself endlessly trying to become situated, I could feel the infelicity with which I was plagued. Head down, head up, hand through my hair, then dropping to the side, then up covering my eyes, back down on the wheelchair tray, pushing the wheelchair back, then forward, foot off the foot rest, foot on the foot rest. Whatever direction I went or however I placed myself, I was going to be one disturbed mess.

Seeing my battered face on the TV screen, I can just imagine the powerful force my head went smashing through the side glass and ripping into that telephone pole, for it would result in my face still being black and blue six weeks after being sacrificed. Although healed significantly during this month-and-a-half's time, resembling the shadowy darkness of a closed casket, my face was still a haunting shade of gray.

Protruding from my sore forehead was a large, grotesque, lump where a shunt had been deeply planted. Seeing the size of this bump, I can only guess what having a monitor inside my skull felt like. Mom and Ug, who both have sensitive tummies, weren't kidding when they both described this marking as "gross."

When the camera angle shifted, I got a frontal view of my right paralytic side. Just a few feet from the camera's eye was my stiff, right leg which was a leaking artery away from being chopped off. With my right heel planted in the foot rest, my leg stuck straight out. I don't know if I didn't move it because it ached being mauled only a few weeks before or the bruised contents of my shattered skull prevented this limb from doing anything. Whatever the case, that rod slicing into me and my peculiar walk are a reminder that things are nowhere near to working as they should.

My contracted right arm wasn't doing much either except lying passively in the background, not far from my body. Like my leg, it was motionless, doing nothing but taking up spacc. It was like the left half of me was animated and the right, stillborn. Looking at the video as I appeared shortly after the accident, I don't see that much difference in the condition of my rigid right arm, curled fingers, and spastic hand despite going through continual physical agony and heart-wrenching disappointment in my therapies these past several weeks.

It could be that I am expecting too much, too soon, and I should lighten up some. I want to be 100% back the way I was—right now, right away. If I've got to wait for that messed up brain of mine to heal, they'll have to fashion another catheter onto my leg like the one I had in the hospital. It goes without saying, I've never been known to be one that exhibits exceptional patience. But that's all going to have to change, for a disability of this nature is one where time is all that's going to heal some of my afflictions. However, after viewing that video, it looks like time is on my side.

Although admittedly it's tough to see sometimes, I have made such progress since that video was taken of me, I am basically a different person now, as I am preparing to enter my third month at Harmarville. I know I still have many rigorous miles to travel and barren plains yet to cross, but the only thing I concern myself with is what's happening now with me. If I'm to improve and have better days in my future, I just have to put aside what's already happened and focus on what needs done today to get out of this dark stage of my life. If I look too far ahead, I just might be so overwhelmed with what I need to do in the days forthcoming, I wouldn't know where to start.

The expression of anger aside, I am fairly confident that if one-hundred patients viewed a videotape of themselves so intellectually and physically lacking, no two reactions would be exactly alike. Because of people's varying backgrounds, no response would be universal, with the exception of the one which would spawn an undying, deep-seated hatred.

Some may never want to see a video of themselves because it would be too disturbing and degrading watching him or herself so mentally "wacked out" and physically warped. Others may be embarrassed seeing how they were once needing for everything, from a wheelchair to ambulate to being so psychologically despondent they needed cued repeatedly just to identify a family member.

A few might be scared, fearing that some unforeseen trauma will occur because of an unsubstantiated belief that as severely as they were once hurt, the next logical step in the progression will be one where they suffer some kind of tragic setback. Maybe more than a minority of people might find it repulsive taking a look back to a time when they were anything but themselves, instead, vying to look ahead and try the best they can, so they have some control where their chips may fall. If someone who had never become well-versed about the steps a person goes through following a traumatic brain injury and the general condition during these phases, disbelief may evolve that the melancholic figure on that TV screen is them.

Immediately upon seeing myself in such horrid shape just a couple of weeks ago, I experienced two feelings. First, I was grateful my brain didn't succumb to a skull caving in around it. Not only COULD I have died from my head colliding with such a solid mass as a telephone pole at God knows how many intoxicated miles per hour, but I SHOULD have died. It's nice to think that maybe I didn't "cash in my chips" before their time because I didn't have too many marks against me.

Second, and this may be viewed as rather odd by some, quite natural to others, or a little bit of both for many, but I feel an overwhelming sense of pride. Seeing myself once tormented by lost awareness and terrified by the ills which I was imprisoned, I knew that it took an immaculate effort on my part to escape this suffering. No doubt, luck played a significant role overcoming the horror which I was being strangled, but if I didn't do what I could climbing this rehabilitation mountain, I'd be floating "belly up" right now.

I was thankful not only to God that I didn't pass on, but for the skills of the medical/rehabilitation professionals who had worked and are working with me, the strength and efforts of my family, and for the ability to recognize I have to "give it my all" physically, emotionally, and cognitively in order to advance to the next level. I also thank God that He gave me the strength not to shrivel up and approach things with a, "I'll never be able to. . . . .again, so why bother?" attitude.

Last, but definitely far from being least, I am grateful that my parents instilled in me a work ethic where there's no use crying over spilled milk; that if you want something bad enough, you've got to roll up your sleeves and fight for it. With this new enlightenment I have, the slugging has just begun.

To think my family saw me everyday in the condition that video depicts—and substantially worse, for this film shows me after I've had six weeks to heal—makes me wonder how they ever kept from collapsing. There's no way I could ever fully appreciate, understand, or empathize what it's like being a parent coming into a hospital everyday, wondering if your child had died during the night or not.

The pain they were subjected to and the fear which could have destroyed them evoked an emotion within me that could never be extinguished. And it goes without saying that my life being one where I will be debilitated in the days, weeks, months, and years ahead by someone I thought was a friend will fan the raging flames of fury within me for all eternity. I know that harbored feelings of wrath can turn one's heart to stone, but I'd rot in Hell before I could ever acquit Paul and his family of what they did to me and mine.

I thought me and Paul had become pretty good friends. We got along well and both liked the outdoors and sports. We were able to talk and just seemed to genuinely "click" pretty good. I mistakenly thought he was smart enough and cared enough about others he got along with that he wouldn't take a chance and do anything that might hurt them. By the looks of things, this couldn't have been any further from the truth.

When mom and dad were in the dark about the circumstances leading up to the accident and asked that son of a bitch Paul over the phone where we had gone, he lied saying we went to Canonsburg at someone's house he didn't know. As far as I knew, Paul didn't know Ilyacoff that well and here he was refusing to help the parents of a classmate he practically killed and supposedly became friends with at college, in order to protect an acquaintance. Good friend.

The damage has already been done and it's obviously too late to do anything about it—one can't change history or rewind the hands of time—but it's now all too apparent I put my trust in one's hands who must have had mentors that failed to teach the principle of consideration to their youngest. Looking back on it now, a little over two months after the crime, this artificial front was a facade of deception which I was fooled into believing was bona fide friendship. Was the person who showed no regard for me or my well-being the same guy who came across as such a good friend at school? Misreading this mask as authentic will forever leave me wanting.

If Paul had a conscience about what he had done to me, he'd have told my parents everything: where the party was at, who was there, what alcohol was consumed, where it was bought, or anything else they wanted to know. Instead, he didn't even have the balls to tell these suffering elder statesmen who were longing for answers where the location of the party was. Rather, he tried to steer them away from resolve. I wonder who role-modeled for Paul that this was proper behavior/moral etiquette?

Taking into account the therapeutic benefit of such a move and my need to return to my sanctuary of comfort, heading into the fourth month of my being disabled, staff made a decision not without its risks—they believed that it would be in my best interests, if I went home for the weekend.

Convinced the pros of returning to Washington for two days and two nights far outweighed any cons, staff pondered several factors. First, they attributed my slowly increasing frustration and moodiness to, not only my heightened awareness that tireless effort does not necessarily translate into improvement when one's had a head injury, but being constantly exposed to an environment of sickness and disability. Fresh out of high school, these couple of months have been the longest period of time I've been away from home.

Figuring that being around familiar faces and the place I've always referred to as "home" would do me a world of good, the therapy team had a hunch that I'd come back in better spirits and with a renewed vigor to bust ass in my therapies. They thought I'd have an enhanced outlook on things, a refresher course of what I'm shooting for/what my goals are, if I could spend a couple of days away from this aggravating rehabilitation setting. In addition to this notion of rediscovering what I'm working for and why I'm here, letting me go home for a break will show me that returning home is not far-fetched in the future and that—because I've been homesick from the "get-go"—I do have some control of what happens to me.

When someone's been away from normalcy, they can lose sight the importance of what this rehabilitation torture is all about and for what they're striving to attain. With the exception of counseling, Harmarville does not and would not skip a step in the rejuvenation process known as rehabilitation by leaving a stone unturned. On May 2nd when mom and dad would be here for their visit, the first step to my return home would occur. My docked ship, which has been my life since I was hurt, would be christened for yet another maiden voyage.

If I'm to spend my first weekend away from a facility which offers medical and/or rehabilitation services and be at a place where the surroundings are not foreign, I first have to demonstrate that I can tolerate being in a moving car again. Needless to say, I can't spend the weekend at home in Washington, if I can't get there because I'd be too terrified being in a car. My memory of ever having been in a car accident withdrawn from my recollection depository, I possess no recall about any mishap occurring in any vehicle, so I have no experience to "pull up" which would make me fearful about traveling. However, one person on this dinnertime practice run wouldn't be so fortunate.

As I pushed my wheelchair towards the Citation, I could tell mom was being eaten alive, thinking about the adventure on the ambulance she told me about when I was admitted to Harmarville. The sight of mom in the back seat, eyes bulged, mouth open, sweat oozing from her pores, back bent forward, arms spread wide, hands stationed parallel to her hips, palms sticky with perspiration, knee keeping the front passenger seat down as if ready to dart into action, was more terrifying than any thought I could have had of being in a car again.

Jiggling into the passenger seat using the transfer skill I practice in PT, after dad buckled me in and slid the wheelchair into the trunk, he started-up this two-door coupe, and we were on our way to Burger King. Making the short jaunt down Guys Run Road, the brown juice in dad's make-shift spittoon he kept in his right hand while he drove splished and splashed as he tried the best he could to miss the abundance of mini-craters scattered about this "Roadway from Hell." Because of who his passenger was this day, dad would take it excruciatingly slow and cautious down this road the Pennsylvania Department of Transportation (PennDot) must have forgotten about. Dad was at his classic best, slowly chugging along past houses, trees, mailboxes, driveways, "Winding Road" signs, and guard rails at a snail's pace because of his concentration being divided by driving and his need for a nicotine fix. Busy chomping, spitting, and wiping the tobacco juice from his chin, trying to put his spit can in the console, dad was able to manage spilling a little tar-colored saliva on his white shirt mom just washed. If there's one memory I wouldn't have minded remaining forgotten, it would be the enjoyable experience of riding in a car with my dad somewhere.

Thank God it's only a short drive to the bottom of the hill to the town of Harmarville's small business district where we made a left to Burger King. Taking a spot in the parking lot, dad got out, took my wheelchair out of the trunk, opened my door, helped me to my wheeled companion, where we proceeded to wait what seemed twenty minutes for mom to wedge herself out of the back seat of the car.

I don't think mom's getting her rear end stuck between the car's frame and the front seat was why everyone in the restaurant was looking at us, rather, we were the object of all those stares because of my needing assistance in order to make my way over to my wheelchair. As I was pushing my wheelchair to the front door of the "Have it Your Way" place with dad by my side and mom behind me with her arms outstretched, I know I was being looked at. Before I got half-way to the entrance, the door flew open and a man in his fifties held the door open for us; the smile on his face couldn't hide the sorrow in his eyes. Two seconds later, a teen-aged male employee sporting a mustard-stained "Hold the pickle, hold the lettuce, special orders don't upset us" ball cap flung open the other door moments before I got there.

It feels good that people are so compassionate—and I've met a bunch of them since I've been laid up—but I'd much rather be a "fly on the wall" then receive goodwill. Because of what this head injury has done to me and possibly, will always do, my days of being inconspicuous could be over. Enough's enough, where's my two regular hamburgers, large order of fries, and large Coke. I've been waiting a long time for this!

That was not only the best hamburger I've ever eaten, but the best meal I've ever had in my life. Although I can't remember any of them, I'm sure mom's Thanksgiving extravaganzas were great, but nothing could top what the taste of that hamburger and fries meant. Besides tasting fabulous, that quickie meal brought back a part of the old Craig which I wasn't sure would ever ascend from the darkness.

This represented progress. Chomping on that burger and chewing them fries took me from the hospitalization and rehabilitation horror—which is all that I can really remember about my life—and put me back to a time before I knew what paralysis, brain contusions, and comminuted fractures were. Not knowing how good you got it until it's gone, munching on fast food that you've sunk your teeth into hundreds of times before can be so special when you think how close it was to being something you'd never do again. If they have almost been taken away, the simple things in life can mean so much. Besides, it beats being fed intraveneously.

That short drive from the rehab to the restaurant was no big deal. For those that thought I'd get sick, have a seizure, or experience flashbacks to the night I kissed a utility pole, they worried for nothing. Because I have absolutely no recollection of the accident, the events leading up to it, or too much of anything about my past for that matter, I have nothing to be fearful of for I have no prior experience to draw from. However, the trip was just starting. Not knowing the outskirts of Harmar Township very well, dad didn't go out too far—he didn't have to.

Bordering Harmarville is the affluent community of Fox Chapel, and as we drove around looking at all the rich stiff's mansions, swimming pools, tennis courts, and Porsches, the three of us lied saying we wouldn't trade in our lifestyle to be in these rich prisses shoes for anything. Yeah, I'd be devastated if I got to miss out on shoveling Fritz's droppings out of our backyard because the butler already got to it.

Traveling through Blawnox, we were heading down to the Allegheny River checking out the Hulton Bridge before my brain took in what was going on and fired off a message to my gut that it was movement such as the one I'm experiencing now which preceded different parts of my body being splattered on Beau Street. "Bullshit," dad gurgled the best he could over the pool of tobacco juice which settled at the base of his mouth when I told him I was feeling "woozy." Turning around when he could, dad was heading back about five miles to the rehab griping—not because he was angry at me for having an upset stomach—but fearful that, and disappointed, I might not be able to go home.

Looking forward to his boy's return with all his heart, dad wouldn't be in the best of moods. Window rolled down, my dad's wind-swirled hair getting whiter by the half-mile and mom's petrified expression on her face caused my stomach to churn that much more.

Almost going the speed limit, dad was backtracking as quickly as possible. Accustomed to pausing at stop signs for at least ten seconds, dad barely stopped, as I was leaning on the passenger side door, sick as a dog. Whistling past Cadillacs, Lincolns, and Rolls Royces, dad wanted to get me out of Fox Chapel and to the rehab, not only because stretching out in my bed would likely make me feel better, but he didn't want me to open the car door and start cacking in some millionaire's yard.

We weren't successful in our attempt to slip by the nurses' station without being seen and the nurses working the weekend evening shift anxiously wanted a report on how I did. Clearing her throat, mom said, "He did just fine, except towards the tail-end of the trip, the excitement got to him a little bit," and that I want to lay down now.

"Nothing to worry about," dad said without hesitation, trying to ease any thoughts that I'm not ready for the weekend vacation yet, "he did as well as could be expected. He's a good boy, y'know."

As green as Unit three's walls, I just smiled the best I could and headed straight for bed before I left any burger and fry remnants on the floor. I'm not about to let a little motion sickness keep me from seeing my friends, sleeping in my own house, eatin' mom's food, and petting Fritz. One more week in this pen, then I'm going home!!! I'm going home!!!

Putting in a double shift of walking, writing, hand, eye, and heel exercises hasn't been as grueling this week as my previous overtime sessions floundering with my incapabilities because there's a light at the end of tunnel this time. There's going to be a big reward coming my way about four o' clock Friday.

It has been a little more tolerable these past couple of days when I write Valerie her letters and I don't know when to end one word, sentence, or paragraph and start the next. Or try so damn hard to get that right heel to land before the rest of my foot goes slamming down and the outcome is always a "banging" disappointment. Or concentrate on getting those right fingers to do something other than just setting there idle and not responding. Or want to pick up my glass case off the dresser, but instead reach for my Sporting News, a cup, pencil, watch, or God knows what else. Or attempt to keep that right knee from snapping back when I take a step, but away she'll go flying behind me anyway. Or struggle to bend that wrist without moving my entire forearm, with the result being less-than-profitable. Or focus on following my finger to my nose, but my eye will still drop off no matter how much effort I put into it to keep the bottom from falling out. Or. . . . . . .

Well, you get the idea.

I think the reason I'm not crushed by dismay is I don't give myself time to think, I'm always doing something to keep occupied. If I'm not walking behind my wheelchair in the main corridor, then I'm writing every opportunity I can, abusing the hell out of some putty with my right hand, stretching my right arm, or tapping my right foot to loosen up that damned heel cord. Idle time does not exist when you're rehabilitating—that is, if you want to get better. And this is one reason why my writing practice has been paying off.

Out of the twenty-six letters in the alphabet, about sixteen don't pose too much difficulty for me now. Specifically, when I try to print the letters, H-J-K-N-U-V-P-W-X-Y, either the upper or lowercase, I don't do so well. Requiring a good bit of thought, when I come across a word with one of these letters in it—if I'm not totally stumped—then it takes me forever for my mind to develop these letters' patterns on its teleprompter. Getting a glimpse of what these tricky letters look like, I can then send a signal to my now left writing-hand what to put down. However, most of the time, this teleprompter is blank. Because of these particular letters posing me with problems, I can't even abbreviate I was going to college at W.V.U. Thank goodness I can't make a "P" very well either, I wouldn't want to have to and write that I once attended Pitt or Penn State.

In addition to working with me on improving the dexterity of my fingers, hand, and wrist, Occupational Therapy has helped me find compensatory ways to undertake my activities of daily living (ADL). From brushing my teeth to buttoning a shirt, they've tried to teach me to be as independent as possible; many times not without its moments. For a guy not even in his twenties, it can be particularly devastating being reliant on others to assure you get clean and dressed.

There's this one really pretty nurses' aide in Unit Three, Renee, who's the same age as I am who came in one time about two weeks ago when I rang the call button for someone to help me take a crap. I could have cried when I saw she was the one who was going to hear my turds splashing in the toilet water, taking a whiff of their aroma, and sinking her beautiful hand in my hairy crack for the clean sweep. Situations like this one are why I was motivated to learn, as quickly as possible, alternate ways of taking care of myself hygienically. You don't really care as much if it's an older, motherly-type nurse that's going to be doing the wiping because you figure she's done this a million times before with her own kids and it's not really a big deal. But when it's someone you would have died for to take to the prom, that's another story. Not only is sickness, disability, and anguish around every corner when one's in rehab, but humiliation abounds as well.

Embarrassment from getting dressed in front of someone is a feeling I don't have to worry about or contend with anymore because my Occupational Therapists have taught me how to dress independently. Something as simple as tying your shoes is taken for granted until it's gone. I am lucky in the sense that I've developed barely enough dexterity in my right thumb and forefinger to pinch my shoestrings after I cross and tuck them, pull them tight, make the loop, and yank them tight again. This usually takes me a couple of tries and a few minutes, but I eventually get it done. You wouldn't believe how many vulgarities I spewed out in O.T. before I learned how to do this again.

On those rare occasions when I'm not wearing jeans and a rock 'n' roll T-shirt, I'm wearing jeans, a rock 'n' roll T-shirt, and a flannel shirt because it's cold. Because of this and my need to "spiff up" once in a great while, I have to learn how to button a shirt again. This is a lot of fun when you only have one good hand to do it with and your perseveration prevents you from grabbing the right button, but it can be done after a lot of irritation.

Many of my O.T. (Occupational Therapy) sessions have become AT (Aggravation Therapy) trials practicing reputedly simple things such as washing my face, cutting my nails, and buttoning a shirt. Like the shoestring ordeal, I was lucky I could push a button through a hole with my right thumb, as I manipulated everything else with my left fingers. Because everything you seem to do in O.T. requires the mastering of fine motor skills, this therapy can be particularly trying on the nerves when you're eighteen and can't even twist some "Play-Doh."

Because I can bear slightly more weight on my right leg now, I transfer out of my wheelchair better. When I get up and sit down, I require minimal assistance of one person for control, so I don't lose my balance. One who hasn't been in a prolonged state of dependence couldn't possibly understand how stupendous being able to get out of a sitting position and moving someplace by yourself is.

I not only can go to bed at night without ringing in a nurse to "tuck me in" like a little kid, but because there's thick, steel, looped handrails on both sides of the commode for those of us who are not that graceful, I can plop myself down on the toilet now without a Homecoming Queen type watching, hearing, and smelling me cut loose. Having your modesty taken away from you doesn't exactly promote good self-esteem. Damn it, now who used up all the toilet paper?

I've been responsible for more than my share of paint being scraped off walls. Dad told me about two custodians at Allegheny General who had their share of trouble avoiding walls and door trim hauling mattresses into my room for my Ranchos #4 sleeping pleasure. When they came in for their Thursday night visit, dad told me he and mom can understand what those janitors must have went through because they had done this very thing early this afternoon. Not at the hospital, obviously, but at home preparing the house for my return this weekend.

Because I forgot how to climb steps, mom and dad brought a bedroom down to me. From the living room, which is the main level, there's a flight of steps going up to the three bedrooms and a flight going down to the T.V. room. A few more steps lead down to the basement.

Dad assembled the frame for a single bed down in the T.V. room and then he and mom brought a pair of mattresses down two flights of stairs from the spare room, taking plenty of paint chips with them. I can almost picture the scenario when they told me what they did.

While mom would be making my bed, dad would proceed to detach and bring the shower curtain from my bathroom upstairs and drape it from the ceiling tile in a corner of the T.V. room, cussing all the while when things didn't go exactly as planned. With my brand spankin' new porta-potty mom just bought at the home health care supply store situated far off in the corner for my initiation, I've got me a bathroom. And alongside my bed is a rust-colored card table serving as my dining room. With the T.V. room/converted bedroombathroom-dining room next to the garage, it's only a short distance to the driveway where I could sit outside in my wheelchair, if I wanted. This mini apartment within the house provides me with everything I might need. Because her piano is already out of tune, I don't think mom will mind too much if I put a spare roll of toilet paper on her ivory keys.

For the first time since I was in Allegheny General's Intensive Care Unit, I'll have a private nurse. Dad will be sleeping along the side of my bed in a flip chair which will elevate him about six inches above the cold "rec" room floor. Three Christmases ago, when mom and dad bought me this pullout sleeper for my use when I lay on the floor to watch television, there's no way they could have ever been convinced that one day it would be used while one of them takes the night shift to safeguard against me having some kind of life-threatening nocturnal trauma. After one of its members has had a severe head injury, the family's life immediately takes on a transformation from what it was to a mystery where the clues are masked by the darkness of the unknown.

Not leaving anything to chance, Harmarville made sure mom and dad were instructed and understood what they needed to do to prevent some kind of setback and what steps need taken in the event something would go wrong. Through our social worker, Laura, instructions were given to my parents about the dosage and frequency I should take my medication and Colace, how I need to be transferred into and out of my wheelchair, the accommodations I'll need, there being absolutely no way I should attempt going up or down steps, and the time I should be at the rehab Sunday night.

Because they have been with me every moment they could since that tragic night before Valentine's, mom and dad were well aware of the "do's and don'ts" as they pertain to my care. They also knew Harmarville needed to double-check because, if there's one word that any medical/rehabilitation setting is terrified of, it's "liability." If a circumstance presents itself that my parents weren't prepared for, but should have been were it not for the negligence of its staff, that could spell trouble for the facility.

I can just imagine how mom and dad feel. On the one hand, they want to safeguard against me hurting myself somehow, and on the other, they want to see me continue to progress and therefore don't want to "baby" me. Whatever the weekend has in store for me, I'm just glad to be going home. There was a time not all that long ago when few thought this would ever be possible. But I fooled 'em.

After my last therapy of the week ended today, May 7, 1982, I limped out of the OT workroom pushing my wheelchair to the nurses' station where mom and dad were waiting. When they saw me coming out, their smiles could be seen clear from the Oakmont Country Club. "Well buddy," choking on the emotion of what he was about to say, "are you about ready to saddle up and go home?"

Looking at the nurses around him who never saw a man bubbling with such genuine happiness, dad finished with, "Or do you want to stay here with these pretty nurses?"

Although the scenery around here can definitely stimulate those hormones, that question was a "no-brainer" and isn't worthy of an answer. After what's happened to me, going home for the first time in eighty-three tormenting days could not be topped.

Being her methodical self, mom did some double-checking of her own. Looking down at her little notepad she jots pertinent information on, mom ran by the nurses—for the third or fourth time—the type of medication, their milligrams, and frequency which they are to be taken just to be sure. "He's to take one Phenobarbitol capsule in the morning, lunch, and bed time?," mom said to herself around the nurses knowing they'd interrupt her, if she was mistaken.

Glancing up from her handy reminder, mom said to the RN's huddled around her in a voice blackened with worry, "And if we should have any problems—God forbid—we're to call you at Seven—Eight—One—fifty-seven hundred?"

Eyes gazed at the nurses hoping they'd add an hour or two, mom said in a tone with a trace of sorrow, "And we should have him back here Sunday night, no later than eight o'clock?"

Hands in his pockets jiggling his keys and rolling back and forth on his heels, dad said in a voice filled with anxiety, "Now c'mon, the weekend will have ended and we'll still be in the unit."

Wanting to see me back home ASAP, dad told us, "Let's go back to your room and get your stuff. Fritz misses his buddy!"

I don't think there's a word in the English language which could possibly describe how I feel about going home. I guess "fantastic," "awesome," "stupendous," and "spectacular" are about the closest. And I know mom and dad are equally ecstatic and wouldn't miss a step preparing for my return. Although they would be hard-pressed to concede this, I know there was a time when my parents were skeptical that I'd ever call anyplace "home" other than a hospital, personal care boarding home, or some kind of dormitory where the residents need some kind of supervised living arrangement.

Taunted by the possibility that my capacity to learn has forever disappeared in a crevice of lost opportunity, mom and dad were psychologically preparing themselves just in case their golden years were spent taxiing me to aftercare or partial hospitalization programs. If I would take up residence at the house somehow, they probably figured it would be a stay where I depended on them to provide me with the essentials such as brushing my teeth, giving me sponge baths, making sure I ate my Gerber's, changing my catheter and/or diaper, and stuffing suppositories in my anal canal to dissolve.

Being in their twilight years, mom would make sure that after her and dad passed on or could no longer care for me, I would be taken care of in a CRR (Community Residential Rehabilitation) program where remedial classes would be offered and basic skill training courses provided. Sadly, I could advance to the intermediate curriculum level once I've proven I can build a popsicle stick house without supervision. After day program, if I'm to spend the evenings at home, nurses would come to ensure that my belly was full, bottom wiped, urinal was within reach, meds were taken properly, and that I wasn't in agony or unconscious from having a seizure. Nice way to spend your retirement years.

Because things have rarely gone their way these past three months and because we haven't felt this good during that time, I wasn't about to say anything that would spoil the moment. Specifically, me not remembering ever being at the house. I know that would tear at mom and dad's heart.

With my visual-memory not working, I have trouble picturing what the inside of our house looks like. I know roughly how it's laid out because mom and dad have described it to me many times since my memory has been taken from me, but I have no personal recollection of ever being there despite being at these dwellings fourteen years. When mom, dad, Ug, and my lovely sister-in-law would work on memory tasks with me at the hospital and the rehab here, they'd show me different pictures of people and places which I was familiar. One of these snapshots being a frontal, outside view of our house, I couldn't remember ever being there.

Recognizing the house when shown a picture of it was simple, but before seeing this picture, there's no way I could set up in my mind what it looked like. I couldn't tell you that the aluminum siding was white, the shingles black, or that we had a front porch with big, green bushes in the front of it. If mom and dad didn't inform me of this, I couldn't tell you there was a patio out back that dad built or that there's a big hill in our backyard.

Because I can't recall seeing any pictures taken inside of the house, I have no idea how the interior design is arranged precisely, beyond the description my parents gave me. If I have to rely on a mental picture of an experience within the house, forget it, it just isn't there. Not being able to pull out from the memory banks what the house looks like indoors, but can identify the house when shown a picture of it, is further evidence that the recognition function of my brain is working much better than the recall function. Being unable to picture in my mind what our house looks like has stricken me with a fear that I'll never be able to remember ever being there. In about an hour and a half, that will all change.

Once we approached the first exit in Washington County off Interstate 79, Exit 10 in Canonsburg, things started to look familiar. When I told mom and dad that's where Claire used to live a couple of years ago, you'd have thought we won the lottery, for their hoot and holler could probably be heard outside of the Citation which was burning rubber at 50 m.p.h. Pitter-pattering past the "Meadowlands Exit," I said that's where the horse racing track is.

There's no way a winner of one of the harness races that take place here could cheer any louder than my parents when I recalled this. It didn't hurt my memory any that underneath this exit sign is a smaller sign that reads "Race Track." Because things are coming back with such ease and falling into place surprisingly well, I needn't need to mention this, for I didn't want to spoil the mood.

Pulling onto Route 70 West off of 79 South underneath the sign that reads "Wheeling," I felt absolutely no ill-effects from being in a moving car. The excitement of going home and recognizing these various landmarks distracted me from believing I was in some kind of danger. Being that we were on the highway and not some two-lane backroad like we were on when I got "woozy" the other day, dad thought that this had a lot to do with me not getting sick. He thought that seeing all those telephone poles through Fox Chapel, Blawnox, and the other small communities we went through might have alerted some sensory passageway in my brain that I was in trouble somehow. Whatever, when we passed Exit 6/"Jefferson Avenue," we were approaching the last leg of the trip.

After we got off our exit on "Chestnut Street," I was right on the money when I told my thrilled parents that the Franklin Mall is right here after the bend. Going past the mall, we made the right onto Franklin Farms Road where we took it out to Park Avenue where I correctly identified the tiny corner market store, Gabby Heights, as being the place where I used to buy baseball cards when I was little. My parents couldn't have been happier that I was able to rewind my memory about fifteen years and tell them something I did when I was a little kid.

Approaching my elementary school a block up to the left, Mrs. Joy would have been proud when I told mom and dad pointing, "Up there's where I went to grade school—North Franklin. That's where Mr. Gough was my favorite teacher in the fifth grade and where Trinity plays its home baseball games in the field there."

With his now customary enthusiasm and optimism, dad said, "Attaboy Craig, you're absolutely right—that's where you guys lost all your high school games."

Climbing the grade up along the cemetery which I also identified—maintaining my recognition average at a perfect 1.000—we then made our way towards Trinity where I lamented, "To the left here is where I didn't learn too much in high school."

After mom told me that was my own fault, dad asked, timing his question to avoid a debate, "Do you know what we're coming up to now?"

Looking over my shoulder, I saw the mountain I climbed everyday after school which never looked so inviting before and, a second later, I then saw the majestic grade leading up to home sweet home. Sending shock waves through my parents' systems, when I told dad what lie on the other side, he and mom both yelled out in deafening proportions. Not knowing this was the yellow brick road leading to the neighborhood I've lived in so many years would have pulverized my parents.

Going up the embankment, I could feel my heart pounding with anticipation and excitement. Reaching the top of the hill, brain damaged and all—without any trouble—I recognized the houses situated in a circular pattern down in the valley as being the place I've spent most of my life.

As topping on the cake, while we were veering to our street, I identified who lived in some of the houses. "The Moore's are the first house here to the right. My good buddy, Dave McClellan, lives down the hill a house here to the left. 'Sam' lives a couple of houses down on the same side. My first friend I got to know here in Washington when I was five—when we moved here—Jeff Little, used to live in this house to the left." My parents were being flooded with joy, not only because I remembered who currently lives in these homes, but that I could recount something from 1968.

Starting to make our descent, I didn't bother to say the Sprowls lived up the cul-de-sac to the right because a beautiful site I was so close to never seeing again appeared before me. Before dad could finish asking me what was in front of us, pointing in the direction of our castle, I said with exuberance, "There's our house!!! It never looked so good to me before!"

A few rotations of the tires later, dad flicked on his turn signal and pulled in the driveway. "Home at last!," I said, "I'm back where I ought to be."

Sitting there in the driveway, it was like I never left. I can't say everything is just the way I would have pictured it because I couldn't formulate an image in my mind what our house looked like. But now that I'm home, it's no big deal because being here has been enough to bring it all back. All my fears that I wouldn't remember ever being here or had forgotten how everything looked were unfounded. Our next door neighbors, the Ruffner's to the left and the McNamara's to the right, their houses look the same and didn't magically lift off their foundations and go anywhere.

When dad helped me out of the car to my wheelchair, I hung on staring down to the foot of the hill where a lot of my friends live and it was a scene which registered in my mind as one I've seen a billion times before. The Day's, Kerr's, Johnson's, they're all still there. Their homes, as well as all the other nice houses in the development, look like palaces to me now.

After mom eventually got out of the back seat, giving the shock absorbers the jolt of their life, dad whipped open the garage door and there at the end of the garage was our old "Model T" white Whirlpool refrigerator, clanging as loudly as ever. Shooting a line drive wad of tobacco spit into his can, dad then disconnected the springs which pull the screen door shut and flung open the door to the altered "rec" room. My haven for the next few days and hopefully in the weeks to come, with all the compensatory modifications made preparing for my return, this den now looks like a "wreck" room.

Walking into my transformed efficiency apartment and chomping into his "Workhorse Tobacco," dad opened the door leading to the upstairs. On the other side, Fritz waited to pounce on whoever it was that came in. As the portal cracked, Fritz jammed his head in this tiny opening and nudged the door open. Anticipating our schnauzer to greet me with a licking "Welcome back," dad was more than a little disappointed when Fritz darted in towards me, but only so he could smell my wheelchair. After affectionately nibbling at dad's feet, our loyal watchdog ran upstairs because his curiosity had been satisfied.

I don't know how long my absence translates into "doggie years," but being away at the hospital and Harmarville for approximately three months, I thought I'd at least get a courtesy sniff. Wearing my patched glasses and hand splint like I was, I guess I ought to be thankful that he didn't sink his teeth into me thinking I'm a stranger. It's all how you look at things.

Thick index finger as stiff as the wooden spoon mom used to threaten to crack me with during one of those rare occasions I wasn't an absolute angel, dad said, "You are not—under any circumstances—to try climbing these steps. If I don't kick your ass, then I'll send you back to Harmarville in the blink of an eye, if you even think about it."

I can barely pick my right foot off the ground when I walk and there ain't no way I'm going to do anything stupid like trying to elevate it onto a step. I'd end up on the carpet, if I would try to go up the stairs because I drag my right foot as it is when I push my wheelchair.

Getting a mole's-eye view of the living room, I was seven steps down from the main floor. Where I was straddling behind my wheelchair, I could see the couch, two chairs, the wall clock, some pictures, and the flight of steps leading to the bedrooms. Like the neighborhood coming in, I was pleasantly surprised all these things were very familiar and clicked into my right perceptual hemisphere as something I've seen countless times. One could say that I'd only be gone three months and things should be recognizable, but until I arrived here a few moments ago, I had no idea what the house looked like. However, three months to a person whose visual-memory tape player has all but disappeared seems like an eternity, especially if three millenniums worth of experiences has occurred within these three months.

If I wouldn't have recognized the "rec" room, it wouldn't have been because of my head injury. Mom and dad disposed of the hot, sticky, brown leather couch nobody liked that was against the wall, and put a bed where this bouncy sofa that I broke was. With my make-shift latrine propped up prepared for when I let loose with some heavy duty relief, bed set up for plenty of relaxing pleasure, and card table ready for my dining cuisine, I was all set for my first weekend home.

Maybe it was because we never went anywhere—including out for dinner—but every opportunity we got, I wanted to stop at either Burger King or McDonald's now. Maybe my memory got knocked into my taste buds and they could remember how much I used to like eating at McDonald's when I lived in the Towers at W.V.U. Timing their visits for suppertime like they always seem to do, Ug and his lovely wife missed out this time because we were just finishing our burgers dad got.

Seeing me in the house again was something Ug was not sure would ever happen again, so he showed a little compassion by not ragging on me immediately—he waited two minutes. Having just eaten and seeing my brother, I had to try out my new potty.

Inevitably, after I got my belt buckled and smelled up the room pretty bad, I got my first "real" visitor. My nextdoor neighbor and childhood friend I enjoyed dominating in sports when we were little, Frank McNamara, came over. Either he got word I was home or the wind took the scent of my presence to his house—prematurely ending his mom's birthday party.

Me and Frank have been the best of friends since I was eight and because of this, we have more-than-a-few shared delinquency experiences together. The therapeutic benefits of the events Frank told me about were worth their weight in gold because occurrences of my past are something that Harmarville knows nothing about and obviously can't help me with. After telling Frank that I practically have no recollection of my past, he shifted into high gear and started firing off different situations I should know about.

When Frank said that me, him, the two Hobbs, four Hunts, Craig Johnson, Dave McClellan, John Woods, "Sam," and "Claude" would play two baseball games a day behind Johnson's, I could mentally see the field and picture everyone there. Then, after Frank told me we outgrew that field and started playing softball and football behind the Legion everyday, I could see the pasture that was the outfield/end zone, the tree behind first base/marking the 50 yard line, and the creek along the third base line in foul territory. I could still hear them griping when Frank told me our mothers would burn upon bringing our filthy, mudcaked clothes home after one of our swampy sandlot football games.

Frank asked me if I remembered when Claude broke his leg during one of these games, when we would have one of our daily debates whether Dave Parker or Al Oliver were the better player for the Pirates and whether Franco Harris or Rocky Bleier the best in football for the Steelers. When his nature-loving brother, Dennis, got an irritation that looked like diaper rash on his arms/hands trying to catch frogs in the bacteria-infested pond before they built Oakley's house on the lot and the time he tried to pet a squirrel and got bit. When Eric and Danny would have one of their classic brotherly-love fist fights, when the two of us and Danny would compete against each other to see who would complete the entire Topps' baseball card series first every year, when we would team up and beat up Timmy Johnson and Eric Kerr because they were too little to defend themselves, when we would get together and watch the Major League Baseball All-Star game every year, when we would make fun of the guy down the street for being skinny, etc., etc., etc.

Everything Frank talked about, I could remember and it really felt spectacular that I had pieces to my history which has formed an image of who I am and came to be. I have a clearer sense of belonging; that my life had a little bit of substance to it and my index of the past is still there, but that I need some help being able to make a reference through it.

Like an essay vs. multiple choice test, if I'm given a list of possible answers, I can usually recognize the correct one, but if I'm to file through and retrieve something out of my memory without any hints, I can't do it. Appreciating that there are systems within our brain that catalog various events over the years and stores it for future retrieval is not easy. What's even more difficult to get a handle on is how accessing this information can be impossible when a tiny bruise makes one's history forgotten

After giving Frank a synopsis of my physical condition, he went on to tell me about how he heard about the accident and how a lot of people in the neighborhood and school thought I was going to die shortly. Hearing an assortment of versions about exactly what happened and what I was like, being the first on the scene, Frank wanted to hear from the horse's mouth what the story was.

Needing to get this inside scoop before anyone else, Frank asked me how I ever got to know Paul—for he couldn't ever recall us associating together, where the party was at, who I went to the party with, who was at the party, if I had been drinking, if Paul had been drinking, if I remember the accident was anyone else hurt, if I had heard from anybody that were in the car with me, what took place at the party, if I remember anything about being in a coma, etc., etc., etc., etc., etc., etc.

Were they. . . . . ? Was there. . . . . ? Who was. . . . . ? What kind. . . . . ? Are you. . . . . ? How long. . . . . ? Did anyone. . . . . ? Which way. . . . . ? Questions, questions, questions. That boy Frank should be an attorney someday for he sure likes to talk. Because of this, I'm sure I don't have to remind him to let everyone know that I'm not on my death bed. After counsel lcft, it got inexplicably quiet. But by tomorrow, this peacefulness will have ended.

Prior to his bunking down alongside my bed in that uncomfortable three-piece urethane foam cushion, dad did something I never saw him do before and wasn't sure how to handle. With just me and him in the room—for mom went upstairs to go to bed—my dad cried. The only time I could ever really remember dad showing emotion was when his mother died. And here he was, barely able to say three words without pausing to clear his throat of the sentiment which made what he wanted to say difficult to understand.

"It's good to have you home buddy," dad pouted, wiping his eyes. "You don't know how good it is to see you under this roof again. With me, your mother, and Ug—the family didn't seem complete without you. You being home, the family seems more like a unit again. Welcome back Craig, it's good to have you home."

Breaking down, sobbing over what he just heard himself say, dad continued in a voice weary from this emotion, "I never lost hope, but still I couldn't be sure I'd ever see you home again. But now, here you are. You don't know how good it is to see you."

Face now soaked and jaw trembling, dad said in a fired-up and encouraging tone, "I know you're going to come back, I can just feel it. You're going to make it."

Stopping for just a moment to capture his breath, the thought of an epicedium almost being played on my behalf made the tears come crashing through the flood gates. "When you were in the hospital," dad said whimpering, "and no one knew for certain if you were going to make it, I kept telling everyone that you're a fighter; that it's gonna take more than a drunken bastard to keep you down. That my boy's gotta lot of life to live and that you're gonna beat this thing. If anyone would have told me your condition was terminal, I wouldn't have believed them. And God help the person who would even think of asking me to donate your organs because that would have been the last of them. Now look at you, here at home!"

Putting his arm on my shoulder and his head in my chest, dad repeated, "You'll never know how great it is to have you home again. I told them you'd be back. I told 'em so. I missed you, buddy."

After reflecting on what he just said and processing its meaning, dad's voice then turned back to the way I'm used to hearing it, "Now get to bed, mom's making us apple pie tomorrow."

After dad flicked off the light, I lay in bed thinking just how badly people get their priorities confused. My pleas with my dad to let me drive, play baseball, and buy me a guitar, all pale in comparison now to what's really vital. Getting an education of some sort, preparing one for a job, so that a person can get some dollars to buy the necessities in life is important, but there are many other things more pressing. Frequently, too much emphasis is placed on acquiring material things and not enough on what really matters. One's health and how much they're cared about are things which cannot be rung out with a cash register, but their value cannot be quantified because it is of infinite proportions.

People can lose focus of what's truly important, like having someone care so much, they'd give up everything for you. When you got someone that likes you so incredibly, like the guy that'll be snoring unbearably loud alongside my bed here any minute, you got more than you could ever imagine. When a human being would give everything they've got and ever had to assure you're safe and happy, that's priceless.

Love has no price tag and cannot be put on market. It's invaluable because its impact on lives is immeasurable. When one receives love unconditionally, there isn't a greater gift. When love is a given, not something that has to be earned or deserved, this is the single most important guiding force influencing a person's life. Just ask someone who feels their life has been void of this compassion and affection.

To my dad, discipline was something where one "toed the line"/didn't question, and was one way he expressed his fondness for someone. His mother being a brigadier general of sorts instilled in him this strict sense of obedience. To give you an idea of how faithfully dad abided by the principle of conditioning oneself to adhere to authority, when he was in the service during World War II, his superiors knew that he had the "no frills" character to advance far beyond his tech sergeant ranking and recruited dad to begin Officer's Training School. Dad never attained Lieutenant status because the war ended six weeks after he started the program and there was not the urgent need for ranking officers anymore, so instruction discontinued and the candidates were told to go home with everyone else. I'm sure proud this guy likes me so much.

Often, we don't relish what we've got until something happens. You realize the beauty life has to offer is not of unending proportions. Once the irreplaceable has left us, it can be an absence you wished you could have only appreciated more. Dad, stick around for a while, I don't know what I'd do without you.

Waking up to the smell of mom's classic french toast, my brain knew that it had been aroused by this fragrance many times before. Like the burger and fries I had at Burger King that first time, mom's home-cooked breakfast brought back a sensory memory no mnemonics technique could ever come close to matching. Being in an environment that I've come to know as home has raised my spirits incredibly because I now know that what I've had taken away from me memory-wise can be restored. Only remembering a rehab center as being my past, I could not say for sure that my childhood hadn't dissolved into an amnesia which could never be withdrawn from my malfunctioning neurological processes. I haven't even been home a full day yet, but coming back to Washington has been an immaculate step towards recovery because it gives me a flavor of what my lifestyle was like and the surroundings which have been a part of me. I don't have a real clear image of my history yet, but returning home is turning out to be an experience of "lost and found."

Finishing off that morning feast doctored up with the Gwen Meyers' touch was nothing short of fabulous. Harmarville's food is tasty, but those taste buds can tell the difference between "almost there" and perfection. This being the food I've been used to eating for eighteen years and not having it in such a long time, one could say I'm a tad biased. Because it stirred up a sense that was a part of my slowly resurrecting past, this petit dejeuner was the piece de resistance. I know those two semesters of French mom told me I took in high school would come in handy someday.

No sooner had I got done eating and cleaned up, that the doorbell and phone started ringing. I'm sure glad I slept soundly last night because the visitors would be coming today non-stop. I knew Frank McNamara and dad could talk, but I never fully realized how much until now.

I'm glad coal was never dug for under our house, because if it was, with all the people on our driveway the afternoon of the 8th, we would have definitely caused mine subsidence. Knowing that there was a demand to see me and knowing this was an opportunity to put his socialite skills into practice, dad wheeled me outside for all the neighbors to see. Of course, this was after he already had notified them I was coming home today.

Within no time, Mr. and Mrs. Ruffner and their three girls stopped taking a morning dip in their beautiful underground pool and made their way over. Mr. and Mrs. Day and Brian came across the street to see how I was doing, wanting to give their best. The McNamara's, Johnson's, Hobbs', Kerr's, Hunt's, Jack Switzer, Delsignore's, and others all came over to wish me well and a few, I suppose, wanted to see for themselves if it was true that I had one foot in the grave. There was more people congregated in our front yard than a lot of the Pittsburgh Pirates' home games.

It's nice that the neighbors are so supportive and offering any help they could. And I must admit, realizing I was the reason for this gathering, I enjoyed the attention. It goes without saying, however, the cost of being the focus of everyone's concern was not quite worth the price.

The multitude of questions Frank asked me yesterday were the same ones being thrown at me by the neighbors. I'm sorry if I disappointed any of them not knowing the answers to a lot of their inquiries, but that couldn't be helped. However, before I knew it, I was face-to-face with the neighbor who could help me with some of these answers. But, for some odd reason, that wasn't going to happen.

I don't know if Sam were sweating because the May sun was only beating down on him this warm afternoon, or if he was getting hot under the collar because he'd just as soon skirt this visit. Knowing each other since kindergarten and being that we attended the same party which created all this havoc, it would not only look strange if he wouldn't have stopped by, but a little on the suspicious side because it possibly could lead one to believe that Sam played some kind of a contributing role towards my getting hurt.

Wanting to ascertain who was at fault for this accident, representatives from the Michaels' insurance company conducted interviews with various people who attended the party. With a shrug of his shoulders, Sam was stricken with such a bad case of amnesia when asked some of the particulars of this house party, one could have easily thought he had sustained the head injury. Well-liked, Sam didn't want a smudge on his popularity by implicating someone.

My parents had very little idea of what happened to me when I was barely alive at the hospital and neither Sam nor his family came forth with any details of the night in question which would have at least given my exhausted folks some light of understanding in their time of darkness. When asked by investigators some of the circumstances of the night, this guy who was my blood brother when we were little, couldn't offer any assistance. All this Eddie Haskell clone knew was that he went to the party with me and Paul, left with some girl, but had no idea what happened in-between.

As tight as a noose wrapped around a hung man's neck when we were kids, Sam would rather see me dangling from this rope than to give specifics of the party now that we're older and have grown apart. When these reps wanted details such as where the alcohol was bought, all my long-time "friend" contributed was, "Duh, I dunno anything."

While he was standing in our driveway with his P.R. smile, I asked Sam if I had been drinking at the party and he shook his head "no," but there's no telling what he told the insurance people. Thanks buddy.

Saved by the bell, it was during this time that "The Man" came to see me. Everyone scattered and dove for cover as the light blue Chevy Nova rumbled into the driveway. Recognizing the car and its driver as his non-consensual love making partner, our schnauzer ran over to greet this visitor. Once the driver's side door opened, one could almost hear the theme song to "Love Story" being played. After Fritz was peeled off Kevin's leg, I sat in my wheelchair gazing at my friend whose 5' 7", 235 pound frame never looked better.

Either he or his family getting daily accounts of my progress, I would imagine Kevin wasn't too surprised to see what kind of shape I was in. I think Kevin had to struggle to put some spring in his voice when he said, "Hey Craig, how you doing!!?" upon seeing his battered roommate sitting in a wheelchair.

I have known Kevin since our infamous tenth-grade French class we took together. It's been a little over three years since I met Kevin and you couldn't have a better friend. Since I've known him, we have been around each other practically every week and have a surplus of experiences together. Kevin is incredible in the sense that he is like flypaper when it comes to snatching experience and never losing it. And was I ever going to benefit from this.

After the crowd broke up, Kevin and I had a chance to talk by ourselves. Like Frank the day before, I told Kevin about my disappearing memory, but it was no act. Being the magician of sustained recollection that he is, Kevin pulled some rabbits that were lost experience out of the black hat which was my memory gap.

If there was one time I wished my brain's recognition function wasn't working so well it was when Kevin told me some of the things I had done at W.V.U. that first semester. Because of their relative recency, I remembered each of the antics I engaged in after Kevin told me about them. However, I needed these specifics because they were the essential pieces to the puzzle which had previously been consigned to oblivion. I had to know what occurred leading up to February 14th in order to make some sense out of this tragedy.

This lapse of memory regarding the precursors to what happened leading up to being bounced off that pole has been torture. For instance, I had no idea of who, what, where, when, or how I was invited to that party in the first place until Kevin informed me Paul had asked on the way up to Washington from Morgantown in Mrs. Bostko's car. Knowing that I'm in a condition where I'll always be lacking, but not knowing why, was a torment that's spell cannot be broken until some clues are brought forth. Now, I have some answers which shed some light on this sealed melodrama. "Well, what can I say?," is how "The Man" would respond if I told him, "Merci beaucoup Kev, you're a genius."

Forming some kind of image how I got the way I am now wasn't all Kevin resurrected in my memory. Handing me his most recent engineering innovation, dad could only hope a repeat of March 19th could be avoided. This was the day my guitar was brought to Harmarville, but I couldn't play it because I couldn't pinch a pick and forgot how to finger it with my left fretting hand. But the scene couldn't have been better for me to start that long road back towards regaining the hobby that had been my obsession.

Because I can barely pinch, dad took one of my flat picks and cut an arch into it with a lathe. Being that I can curl my fingers enough to hold a ball, dad put "2 and 2" together and reasoned that if a pick were connected to a ball somehow, the sum of all parts would equate into me being able to hold a pick. So, what he did was solder one of my picks into a wiffle ball. Voila! I now have the means to pick and/or strum, if I only knew what to do with my other hand. But that's where Kevin comes in.

Hearing me play AC/DC and Judas Priest riffs galore before I was hurt, Kevin was speechless when he realized that my damaged brain caused me to forget everything about guitar. I didn't know where different notes were located on the fretboard, how to form the most basic barre chords, or how to go about playing the different tricks characteristic of rock guitar.

Playing "Girls Got Rhythm" and "Living After Midnight," I knew these songs and recognized the power chords Kevin was grinding out. Kevin told me I should be familiar with these songs because I'm the one who showed them to him. My recall of this is zilch.

When Kevin told me I had just learned by ear an AC/DC song entitled, "Beatin' Around the Bush" right before I was hurt, a feeling of disbelief and sadness overwhelmed me. Disbelief because I have absolutely no memory whatsoever of ever trying to learn this song, and sadness because it sparked my awareness just how much ability I had that eroded away, for this tune is a fast one that only a player with some talent could possibly pick out and play.

After Kevin showed me how rhythm chords are positioned on the neck, in no time my left hand comfortably went right where it needed to go as if I had done this a million times before. In fact, I had done it a million times before, I just didn't remember until Kevin went about showing me what my left-handed fingers needed to do. While I concentrated on what the fingers of my left hand were doing, Kevin acted as my right hand doing the strumming. Now, if I could only take Kevin to the rehab center with me, I'll be able to practice. Muchos gracias, Kev. And he didn't think I studied in French class.

His family owning a business in town, Kevin hears a lot of talk through the grapevine. When stories get passed from one person to another, certain things can get deleted and others added, with no basis for this editing or embellishment. Getting the play-by-play since I was hurt, Kevin tried to put to rest some of the false rumors which were spreading about my condition and the circumstances leading up to the accident.

Kevin sounded as if he were annoyed when he heard people say such things as I'll never walk again, I lost a leg, I had brain surgery, I lost my right arm, I'm permanently mentally retarded, I've lost an eye, I'll never be able to talk again, I'm deaf, etc. It's funny how things get twisted when people have a need to fill in blanks, but don't have their facts straight. Speaking of straight, I didn't hear anything about me supposedly having phimosis. Now that would be terrible.

Knowing the truth, Kevin was non-committal when we informed him of the propaganda tactics utilized by the Michaels where Paul was supposedly too late in his courageous attempt to swerve—avoiding a glaze of ice—when he smashed into the pole. That the blind curve on Beau Street and the hazardous weather conditions of that February night kept Paul from seeing any forthcoming danger. I wonder who fanned the flames to that story.

I woke up laughing Sunday morning—May 9, 1982—seeing my dad in his classic nocturnal pose before he fell off his improvised bunking arrangement, breaking a sound sleep. Imagining the spectacle of himself rolling off the flip chair, dad cracked more than a smile too before he crawled back into "bed."

For me, the mood quickly changed from a light-hearted one to the somber feeling of guilt. Seeing my 62-year-old dad practically lying on that cold asphalt floor with just an afghan thrown over him, I was getting a first-hand taste of what kind of sacrifice my father was making and had made since Paul had almost killed me.

What right did I have blowing the money he worked so hard for when I was at W.V.U.? Did he labor tirelessly as the Director of the Western Area Vo-Tech School so I could give a minimal effort in college? Could the tears that have poured on my behalf been avoided if I weren't so naive? Did my striving for more and supposedly better create a situation where I didn't see what I already had? Was I so hurt and inexperienced in the ways of life that, in my attempts to attain these pursuits, prevention of the inevitable could not have been within my realm of understanding? Did I not have the strength to prevent being seduced by what I perceived as promise?

A combination of this introspection, what dad said to me my first evening back home, and Kevin reminding me of what I did precisely, my conscience was telling me I have to fill in some pieces of the puzzle for my dad. Telling dad of my marijuana use, I didn't know how he was going to react. God be with me.

Underestimating my dad, I wouldn't have blamed him if he "blew his top" like I've never seen it blown before. However, instead of waving his fist, his face turning that terrifying shade of red, jaws locking, and calling me every vulgarity under the sun and then some, dad's eyes watered when I told him my feelings of confinement were just too much to take and I started smoking pot as a means to escape the reality of me being dismal. When I told him being isolated from everything and everybody like I was at home transferred over to college, dad was shocked because I had always let on things were fine.

I said that, because I was never given access to go anywhere or do anything, I never developed the social skills I could have and didn't learn how to socialize beyond the friends in the neighborhood. In essence, I didn't know how to have fun unless I was tackling someone or catching a fly ball. And I told dad—like anything else—if one wants to be proficient at something and be their best, practice must occur once in a while. I said that I was thrust into the situation of going to college and building a future for myself when there wasn't much of a foundation to stabilize this hoped-for development.

When I told dad I was absolutely miserable retreating into isolation away from others because the means to be involved simply weren't available to me and that I was utterly dejected missing out on so many things, he was at a loss for words. Eyes saturated with commiseration—not burning into me with ferocity—when dad first started talking, his voice was one of compassion before taking on a much-less understanding tone, "Do not tell your mother what you just told me; she's been hurt enough."

When dad said that, I knew that stare as being one where he meant business. If I didn't listen to these orders and said a peep about anything that occurred that initial semester at school, being in a wheelchair or not, I couldn't be sure that the compassion wouldn't evaporate.

Voice returning to its original state of concern, dad immediately wanted to know if I started using any other, more potent drugs. When I told him that I hadn't, his relief lasted only until I told him the frequency and quantity of my marijuana usage.

Then, there was a silence which felt like it was going to last forever. After dad took a deep breath, I thought for sure that this was the end. But he only did this to get enough wind so he could ask me if Kevin was the one I got high with. When I told dad that Kevin was as pure as a virgin's bottom, I got the impression he was relieved that his trust in Kevin was well-placed and judge of character right on target.

When I told dad that the "Bossman" was the one I mostly elevated with, he was surprised, but not shocked. I think dad shifting the focus off of me and expressing concern for "Boss" was his way of letting me know that he had heard enough for one day and didn't want to hear anymore.

Feeling sick, I told dad that I was afraid our relationship was over now and would never be the same because I know what he thinks about drugs and those who use them. He told me not to worry, that we'll get back to the way we were; that the most important thing now is for me to concentrate on my therapies and to learn from this experience. By the expression on his face and the tone which his voice changed, I think dad was both happy in a way that I confided in him something so difficult, and remorseful because I think he sensed the complexity of factors leading up to my stepping out of character.

It was here that the thump, thump, thump of mom coming down the steps cued dad to put his index finger over his lips to stop this conversation and to be quiet. "Things'll be allright," he whispered, "mom's bringin' down our pancakes."

Parents—sometimes they're not given enough credit.

The lines were crooked and so ugly one could have thought someone from a kindergarten class made these letters, but I know mom couldn't care less. Having me home for Mother's Day to give her the card I bought in Harmarville's tiny gift shop was enough to make this the best Mother's Day ever for her. Sure, it would have been nice to print "MOM" on the envelope without soliciting the help of dad, but sometimes you can't have everything. But if there was one thing mom would have plenty of on her day, it would be visitors. I guess some of these people came to see me too.

In addition to Ug and his lovely wife making a return visit my second afternoon home, taking the time away from their own families to spend some greatly appreciated time with me were "The Man" Kevin, Frank, Danny Hobbs, and Brian Day. The crowd dwindled quantity-wise, but not quality-wise.

Hearing in the wind I was home for the weekend, my longtime baseball buddy I've been friends with since kindergarten, Angelo "Sonny" Alberta, made his visiting debut this afternoon. Unless an umpire makes a bad call against him, this guy simply never gets flustered. Describing "Ange" as mellow or laid-back might still be too abrupt because the majority of the time it looks like he's been breathing in an anesthetic all day. I'm sure it's this demeanor which makes him such an exceptional athlete and I know this non-threatening, non-judgmental persona is why he's so widely-liked by those who really know him. Similar interests and his easy-going predisposition aside, I think we've always gotten along great because I'm one of those people who can make Angelo laugh without saying anything; not only "with" me, but "at" me. And this is where he brought back a baseball memory I would have always "cherished" had I not had my head crushed of its memory.

With a devilish grin while saying, "Do you remember the time when you. . . . . .?," Angelo unfortunately went on to tell me about a play I was involved in during a high school game where the batter hit a fly ball out to me in center field and after I caught it, the runner on third tagged up. Having a real good arm, I decided this would be an ideal time to show off my cannon, so I rifled the ball all the way into home, ignoring the cut-off man. Angelo, who was pitching, stood in front of home plate and watched the ball that I "gunned" soar—not only over his head—but over the mile-high backstop behind home.

Wanting to crawl under second base, I then could remember Coach Hughes putting his hands on his hips in disgust and kicking the dirt as Assistant Coach, Mr. Stanish yelled, "Keep your throws down, Craig!" No kidding. Next game, I found myself in left field. Not only was that the position I manned the rest of the year, but where I was at mentally too.

Before I was hurt, I had always had the memory of an elephant when it came to anything that happened in one of my baseball games. But there's no way I would've recalled this unforgettable play, if I wasn't reminded of it. I guess I should have kept my mouth shut instead of asking Sonny to help me with my memory. Why couldn't he have told me about some of the good plays I had to have made. Play ball.

While Angelo and I were reminiscing about our high school baseball days, my brother must have been thinking back to the time he tried to play. Hearing the crack of bats and balls whistling over the outfield fence as he delivered another pitch, one could almost tell Ug was visualizing the two-thirds of an inning he was on the mound during his high school pitching career. These memories of greatness fresh in his mind, Ug picked up the green sponge Nerf ball and started throwing it around the horn. The three of us tossing this toy in a circle wasn't going to make anyone forget the double-play combo of "Tinkers to Evers to Chance," but it was a way for me to engage in a therapy for my arm that I'd enjoy. I guess my brother isn't always intolerable.

Tossing the ball around the room trying not to break anything, somebody came running down the steps and flung the door open. It was my turd nephew, Little Scotty. My sister Claire and her family made it over on this holiday from Ohio including my niece, Donna, this time.

Seeing this as an opportunity not only to reacquaint me with how the rest of the neighborhood looks, but to attract any neighbors who might be able to light a memory, dad decided it would be a good idea if I were wheeled around the neighborhood to take a look at things before I had to go back to the rehab later. Being put on display would probably draw some familiar faces who otherwise might not have spoken to me either because I didn't know them well enough for them to feel comfortable coming into my home, or they'd be fearful I was some deranged heretic now that I've bumped my head. Whatever the motivation, this exhibition would provide dad with ample opportunity to "flap his jaws" to the neighbors. I didn't feel real comfortable being the object of show and tell to say the least, even with assorted friends and family by my side, so let's get this over with.

I know dad's been through more trauma these past few months than he has his entire life, and troubles shared are troubles lessened, but I wish he would have taken into consideration a little bit the humiliation I would be going through being looked at. I don't want to be remembered like I am now by my peers who I've known since I was little. What made this even more unbearable is dad seemed to be enjoying the attention once those wheels got rolling. I can't wait until I'm given permission to get out of my wheelchair and push it on my own during these weekend visits home because dad's moving too damned slow. I guess I should start waving to everyone and smiling because it feels like I'm in the Macy's Day Parade.

If ten steps were taken without one of the neighbors I had never spoken to in my life stopping us, it wasn't too often. Embarrassed beyond belief, after catching all the neighbors on this, the initial descending leg of the trip, I was pushed up the hill where, if any of the brigade of Hunts missed the opportunity to gawk at me yesterday, they'd get another chance here in a second.

Not wanting to see me hit my head again because of a failed attempt at trying to do a wheelie, dad wasn't about to let Ug push my wheelchair. "Hey dad, I'll push for a while," Ug said with his sparkling wit, "When I'm through with him, Craig won't think riding in a car again is that bad, after all. Ha Ha Ha Ha Ha Ha Ha Ha Ha Ha Ha Ha Ha Ha Ha Ha Ha Ha Ha Ha Ha Ha Ha Ha Ha Ha Ha Ha Ha Ha Ha Ha Ha Ha Ha Ha Ha Ha Ha Ha Ha Ha Ha Ha Ha Ha Ha Ha Ha Ha Ha Ha Ha Ha Ha Ha Ha Ha Ha Ha Ha Ha Ha Ha Ha Ha." As terrible as this experience is, I must admit one thing, however, and that is it's really nice that even neighbors I don't know too well are claiming to be thinking about me and saying I'm in their prayers.

Coming up to the end of our street, John Woods' family all rushed out to see me. John and I played on the same Colt League baseball team three summers ago and I would just as soon his folks view me as a former teammate than to see me now in a wheelchair. In a way, it's no doubt nice seeing all these people again and everyone I was running into—rather wheeling into—seemed to be glad to be catching up with me as well, but the sympathy I see in their eyes is not easy to handle.

Whipping around two corners and going up the hill past Sam's empty house, we came to McClellan's, but they weren't around, so we just kept on going. I wish Dave was outside working on his car like he always does because I'd really like to see him. Age-wise, Dave's got about five years on me, but you can't tell that he's older because he's got such a young-hearted personality. Dave's a real nice, friendly guy who would do most anything for anyone. He's one of those guys who always has a smile on his face and you'd be hard-pressed to find anyone who didn't like him because he treats people with respect and greets people in such a way that they know they're accepted. He might call someone "dickhead" once in a while, but that's only his way of saying you're okay.

If you want to find Dave, just listen to wherever there's commotion on a ballfield and you'll find him in the middle of things. Dave's been a really good friend who I've played football, softball, and volleyball with an average of a couple of times a week for the past couple of years.

On the adrogynous side, Dave has a good balance of what it takes to be the elite stud without turning off the kind-heartedness and sensitivity we've all come to know him for. Dave craves sports for survival, but doesn't let this get in the way of his innate tendency to be affable. Dave's a great guy; I know I'll catch him next weekend, if he's home.

Hiking to the top of this steep slope, the end of the marathon was within sight. By the time we started walking this last lap—like society in general—my nephew, Little Scotty (9) loosened up from the first time he saw me after he realized that I wasn't a head injury-induced serial killer, but still wasn't exactly sure how I was, so he just kind of played it cool—opting to keep his distance. Scotty was very tentative and apprehensive around me, almost as if he were waiting for some kind of Charles Manson in me to come out. Boo!!

Donna, 13, was like society in general too in the sense that, after she could be assured 100% that there would not be any risk involved whatsoever and wouldn't be put out of her way too much, she relented and tried to approach me without letting on she was the least bit skeptical of me. When my sister's family minus Donna came to Harmarville March 28th to express their concern and caring, my niece's absence didn't sit too well with dad. Personally, I couldn't blame her one bit because being around someone you can't be sure if they're a mentally disturbed "kook" or not isn't exactly comforting. Why deal with something when you don't have to?

Donna's apparent viewpoint was identical to that of society's as a whole for, if you can avoid involving yourself with one that's had a head injury, by all means stay away until you're obligated somehow. Donna and Scotty are very young and the acceptance of those with head injuries by society is also in the adolescent/pre-adolescent stage as well. Until more is known about the brain and we can step outside the shadow of ignorance, it's going to stay that way for a while.

I think dad planned for us to take the difficult way around the neighborhood, for he wanted to save the best for last. Approaching the cul-de-sac, the two brothers I've played a lot of ball with in the past—T.D. and Brad Sprowls—yelled down, wishing me luck and waved at me which was cool. But when their gorgeous sister—who would be a "10" on anyone's attractiveness scale—cheered me on and said, "Hi Craig! I hope you're feeling better," I started having second thoughts that being pushed around the park wasn't such a bad idea, come to think of it now. We've been neighbors for years, but I couldn't say with any confidence that Darci even knew my name until now. It's nice to know—and even flattering—she knows what I go by when people address me, but I wish I could have discovered an easier way to find this out other than to be splattered on the east side of town.

All good things must come to an end. If that statement were to be used to describe this weekend, this would be a gross understatement then. This weekend was probably the greatest two-and-one-half days of my young life and this was the main reason I was way "down in the dumps" about returning to Harmarville. Traveling the one-and-one-half hour trip back to the rehabilitation center, it was so quiet in the car, you could almost hear my heart drop.

Thinking about the cognitive and physical agony that I'm going to be experiencing this week really clutched ahold of my conscious now that I know how life should be. Working to find ways to walk and write are not how an eighteen-year-old should spend their days. I ought to be going to school, working, playing my guitar, and being around friends, not doing first grade homework or learning how to walk again. Because of the rebirth of my memory, I can now at least look forward to weekends without having to worry whether or not I have dementia.

The events of this weekend put me on seventh heaven and I can use this as a springboard to help me through the week's hardships in program. Things looking familiar to me, Frank filling me in about different things when we were growing up, Kevin answering many of the questions leading up to my being hurt/ helping me with guitar, getting some things off my chest that were bothering my conscience, dad still liking me despite the things that have happened, Angelo reviving some baseball memories, and Darci knowing my name were all memorable occurrences which should help me through the week.

Within a two-week period, from April 5th to April 19th, four tests were conducted to assess my hearing and these test results reveal normal peripheral hearing sensitivity. The outcome of this test did not surprise me because, beyond a low-intensity ringing, I fortunately hear just as good as I ever have. Despite my insistence I was phonetically balanced and hearing just fine, that probe still went in one ear and a headphone on the other. I guess the audiology staff supervised by Dr. Amayo figured anybody whose ear looks like ground beef like my right ear does and had their lobes twirled around smacking a skull has got to have something wrong with their ability to pick up sound.

My ability to discriminate speech patterns in both ears was good (96% right, 92% left). The vibrating of my ear drums, tympanometry, was within normal limits bilaterally as well. Testing of the membranes within the ear showed that the involuntary response to a stimulus on the same side of the ear, ipsilateral reflex, was absent on the right ear and slightly elevated on the left. Opposite side reflexes, contralateral, were present bilaterally although slightly elevated when the left ear was stimulated.

I thank God that my peripheral hearing sensitivity is normal, for this indicates that nothing outside of the central nervous system which influences hearing has been affected. If, for example, the spiral cavity of the inner ear (cochlea) had been damaged, which is quite possible when one has sustained a severe head injury, I would have irreversible hearing loss. As much as I love her, I wouldn't want to know firsthand how my hearing-impaired Grandma Barnhart experiences the world.

Because of my perceptual aphasias and agraphia, Dr. Ratcliff hypothesized that there had been damage to my brain's right hemisphere and the corpus collusum. An audiology test which was conducted on me (Auditory Brain Stem Response) seems to support the doctor's theory. The audiologist conducting the evaluation, Barbara Vento, M.S., CCC, wrote in her progress note dated 5-10-82: "ABR test results were consistent with a lesion in the right brainstem at the level of the mid-brain."

When I must decipher amongst a multitude of stimulation, there will frequently be an abnormally long pause until I process in my mind how things are and what I want to do. The damage to the tissue of my brain which causes this decision-making hesitation may also be partially responsible for the delay in response time of my hearing. In audiological terms, "latency" refers to the time a noise is produced until it gets processed/identified in the brain stem, and my hearing examination showed the slightest abnormality existed. Maybe a trillionth of a second.

Stimulation of the left ear showed all waves present at normal latencies. In my right ear, test results indicated waves I through III were present at normal latencies, but wave V was not identified. This is evidence that somewhere between what my right ear is picking up and my parietal lobe is sensing, things are going awry ever-so-slightly.

If I can overcome the paralysis of my right hand and the spasticity of its fingers and be a musician again, trying to learn songs by ear while having tinnitus won't be fun, but it beats what I could have been like. It's spectacular I hear normally because Judas Priest is coming out with a new album and I understand there's a rockin' single called, "You've Got Another Thing Comin'," off this LP I wouldn't mind learning someday. Music being such an integral part of my life, I don't know how I could exist without it. If this infatuation was taken from me, you definitely would find me "screaming for vengeance."

What is it about the month of May? Preparing to leave for Morgantown in the fall, I had just finished up my high school finals about this time last year. It's now 1982, one year later, but the exam this time around isn't so much to measure what I've learned through reading and studying, rather, who I am as a person. On the week of May 10th, Mrs. Joy administered the subtests of the Weschler Adult Intelligence Scale-Revised (WAIS-R).

The WAIS-R measures a person's intelligence within a verbal and performance realm. The Verbal subtests are those where the examinee must use their expressive language capabilities (a left hemisphere function) and orally present to the examiner the correct answer. The Performance subtests are ones where the examinee must utilize their perceptual abilities (a right hemisphere function) and, with the exception of one of the modes, physically construct the correct response.

Analysis of my relative Verbal and Performance subtest scores should reveal approximately where some of the damage to my brain is located. With this road map, an educated assumption can be made what some of my current and future deficits/weaknesses may be. And because of this information, remedial interventions can thus be planned.

Specifically, in order of increasing difficulty, the six Verbal subtests are: Information, Digit Span, Vocabulary, Arithmetic, Comprehension, and Similarities. With the least difficult listed first, the five Performance subtests are: Picture Completion, Picture Arrangement, Block Design, Object Assembly, and Digit Symbol.

In order of their administration, the different subtests are described. First, the Information subtest is one where I'm asked twenty-nine questions of general information. No specialized knowledge or academic prowess is necessary, for this Verbal subtest measures basic intellectual functioning. Picture Completion is a Performance subtest despite being one where I am to respond to verbally. The reason for this classification is because I must be able to "perceive" what is missing from the picture before responding.

Digit Span is where I would be read a list of three to nine numbers and I'm to reproduce what I've just heard. And then, in the second half of this test, backwards from what was said, I must reproduce the list. In Picture Arrangement, out of order, I am presented cards that have drawings on them and I'm to put these in sequence so that, when completed, the arrangement tells a logical story.

In the Picture Arrangement, I am presented three cards that show a man building a house. One card, the man has just begun getting his brick wall started and is carrying planks towards the wall. Another has the brick wall and a wooden frame. The third has the man painting the house. This sounds like a simple enough exercise, but when one's sequential ability has been swollen against the skull, it's almost impossible to make logical sense out of things.

Looking at the three cards, I had no idea how they should be situated from what comes first to what goes last. Perseveratively, I'd shuffle the cards as if wanting to deal them, only to put them down again before picking them up once more. Gazing at each card, I could not formulate an image of what was occurring in the picture.

Coaching me to think to myself what story the combination of pictures could tell did not help right away. Sure, I could say that the drawings tell a story of a man building a house without too much difficulty, but my experiential memory file could not be retrieved. I could say what was going on in the pictures, but could not take from my visual data banks an experience where I would know Step A comes before Step B followed by Step C. This was too complicated a sequence for a mind scorched of its ability to mentally construct images.

Upon Mrs. Joy's instruction, after I slowed down and took it one painfully slow step at a time, I was able to find the deductive thinking which had been scrambled somewhere in my brain's right hemisphere. And when I was able to find this lost reasoning, I could determine what was going on—-maybe. If nothing else, I wish I could be back in college, for the testing is easier.

Vocabulary is where—one at a time—thirty-five cards with a simple word on it are shown to me, while Mrs. Joy says the word out loud. At first, the definitions were easier and I could spit out their meaning without too much trouble, but as Mrs. Joy and I went along, the words became increasingly more difficult. Because English was one of the few academic subjects I put an effort into, I would get annoyed when I couldn't remember the meanings of some of these words I once knew.

I had a lot of fun with Block Design where I'm shown a red and white design on a card and given a one-inch cube with six different configurations, one on each side. Choosing which of the six designs to use, I'm to assemble the abstract design on the card. To choose one of the patterns on the block or to omit others, I must first try to form a mental picture of what I need to have in order to replicate the design on the sample card. When I'd try to construct the images on the blocks in my mind to form a cohesive whole, they'd disappear or just wouldn't stay in one place for any length of time before scattering.

When my brain was alright, I was not really that great at math in the first place. Now that my brain isn't alright, I'm absolutely horrendous.

In the Arithmetic Verbal subtest, I'm read fourteen problems that a kid in grade school could answer. Without using paper and pencil (not that this would help me, anyhow) I'm to figure out these basic addition, subtraction, multiplication, and division problems in my head. I might be able to do this if I only knew what the different numbers looked like and the numbers would stay still long enough for me to align them. Like when I would try to read and the sentences would move, I couldn't keep the numbers from jumping around

The subtest that gave me the most difficulty was Object Assembly. Here, paper cutouts are to be put together in order to make a flat picture of a common object. Seeing only fragments of a whole, I could not fish out of my memory what these familiar items looked like in their entirety, therefore, I could not construct this puzzle. I could easily tell Mrs. Joy the deterioration of my spatial relation is no day at the park—she just better not ask me to draw or construct an image of this recreational area. Unless, of course, she has no one else scheduled for today and she's not in a hurry.

The Comprehension Verbal subtest was the next to be administered. The format of this exercise is one where I'm asked sixteen practical questions in order to get an idea of my judgment and common sense. These do's and don'ts, right and wrong, questions also measure my ability to dig in my left hemisphere and find the correct words to express an idea, thought, or question. The final Performance subtest I had a ball with was Digit Symbol where its key has nine symbols paired with the nine digits. Given a minute and a half, with the key before me, I'm to fill in as many symbols as I can under the numbers on an answer sheet. My inability to transfer one set of information to another indicates my ability to take in material and processing it in the memory over time is suspect. Similarities is the eleventh and final subtest presented where I'm shown fourteen items and have to say how two things are alike. If Mrs. Joy says, "Peach-Apple," I'm to say, "Fruit." Or, if she were to say, "Einstein-Craig," the correct response would be "Opposites," etc.

The results of my WAIS-R showed a Verbal score equal to 45 with a Verbal IQ of 90. My Performance score was a paltry 22 and my Performance IQ was 66. These results gathered the second week of May 1982 indicate my Verbal functioning was in the average range while my Performance capabilities were in the mentally retarded range. It's tragic when a few too many drinks can wipe out twelve-and-one-half years of education in a matter of seconds.

My exceptionally low scores on the Object Assembly and Digit Symbol Performance subtests revealed that I had sustained damage to my brain's right hemisphere because these exercises measure spatial relations and this function is believed to be primarily one of the right hemisphere. That brain of mine sure took a beating, for my right hemiparesis and communicative deficiencies show significant left hemisphere bruising as well.

In her Communication Skills therapy session with me, Diane Rosato had me verbally identify four common objects laid out on a table in front of me (key, comb, toothbrush, cigarette) which I had no problem doing. Nor did I have any trouble spelling these objects—-orally. However, when Diane had me write on paper with a pen these same items, that's when I had trouble and couldn't do it. This inability to write spontaneously wasn't out of the ordinary for me now; the fact that this particular cognitive therapy session was being videotaped is what made this day anything but typical. I don't know if the buzzing of the two video cameras which are aimed at me will distract me while I'm taking this test, a form of the Porch Index of Communi cative Abilities (PICA), but here goes nothing. Lights! Camera! Action!!!

One video camera was positioned over my right shoulder and pointed down on a piece of paper with the numbers, 1-8-75-6, in one horizontal line and the letters, F-G-L-J-K, in another. Underneath these sample numbers/letters, I copied these symbols without any difficulty.

Portraying a frontal image, the second camera will be showing me sitting in my wheelchair with the patch covering my right eye, my right arm lying on my knee out of the way not rendering assistance like it always does, my uncoordinated left hand doing the writing while Diane holds the notebook down on the table, and me stylishly sporting my Van Halen '81 Worldwide Tour T-shirt.

After naming the objects placed before me, Diane asked me to write the names of each one of these. Following this stumper of a question, I looked down at the four objects I just identified, but didn't know how to follow through with what Diane had just asked me.

In my mind, I could look at these items collectively naming them all, but could not break down each as a separate entity, think what the single object is called, formulate the images of the letters making up their name, and reproducing it on paper within a reasonable amount of time. This "sequence" of steps is still too difficult for me.

Attacked by mass confusion having to pick one of these items to begin this exercise, I felt absolutely helpless and dumb-struck not knowing where or how to start, as the only noise being heard was the drowning hum of the video camera. Just sitting there holding the black felt pen above the paper, I was also drowning, but with disorganization not knowing which of the four I should attempt to print first. My inability to map out a plan and break down the steps needed to undertake Diane's instruction is indicative of frontal lobe damage amongst a host of other possible unknown reasons.

Knowing there were only so many minutes of video film, Diane anxiously prodded me on when she asked, "Which one do you want to write?" Instead of picking the easiest object which I would have only had to write three letters to identify it—key—I picked the most difficult—cigarette. That's right hemisphere damage for you.

Slurred, in a voice I've been told is difficult to understand, I wearily forced, "C-I-G-A-R-E-T-T-E," after Diane told me to spell the object I had just chosen to write. After Diane said, "Okay," indicating I was correct, clearing the runway for me to start writing, it looked as if I was going to have a clean takeoff.

Immediately and with no hesitation, I made an uppercase "C" and dotted an "i," with this dot miraculously being where it was supposed to go instead of being poked somewhere it should not be. However, that turned out to be a fluke because, before I hit cruising altitude, my brain ran into some turbulence.

With that "Ci" on my paper looking so pretty, I was ready to rock now and fling down that third letter and all the rest of them after that. But this is where my damaged neurological teleprompter started scrambling. Before my mind was able to file through its alphabet index, my left hand went about writing the letter "Z" with a slash through it. I can only guess why I wrote this letter which is in so few words. Possibly, it might be because the motor skill of printing this letter is easy, for you don't have to lift your hand off the paper. Whatever, once I recognized the letter I put on the paper as being the last one in the alphabet and not the "g/G" I wanted, I scratched it out and correctly said what I produced, "C," "i,"—"z."

Without saying anything, I looked at Diane wanting rescued with some kind of hint what I should do next. Realizing she wasn't going to help me cheat—once again—I looked down at the paper I was supposed to be writing on, not having a clue as to the shape I should make. Different letters, numbers, and symbols may flash in my mind, but until they're put on paper in front of me, I can't identify what their shapes represent.

My brain's monitors blank, not saying a word, I made an oval somewhat similar to the one in a lowercase "g." Was this the big moment we've all been waiting for? Was it time to cut loose the confetti and celebrate the dawn of a revived beginning? Was it time to hail the coming of a new era of enlightenment and conceptualization? Was this the breath of cognizance I needed to sustain my awareness? Were these the building blocks needed in order to develop a renaissance of understanding? Had the time arrived where I was to capitalize on my search for knowledge? Was I now to bear the fruit of my labor and disband from an identity where all I grasp is struggle and disappointment? Will this be a christening where a rebirth of sense and idea abound?

No. Instead of correctly printing a tail underneath this circular configuration, I put a straight line slanted from the upper-left to the lower-right making an uppercase "Q." Maybe somewhere in the process that was once my thinking, I knew that a lowercase "q" resembles a lowercase "g," but instead I made its uppercase brother. More than likely however, because this would require some deductive thought and I no longer have this reasoning ability, I just put down whatever my hand once knew was the direction to produce a letter. Only God knows and I'm fairly confident He doesn't know what's going on the majority of the time with my writing, either.

"What letter do you want to make?," Diane asked while I scratched out the "Q." I told her, "g," but that doesn't make a damn bit of difference because I still can't formulate in my mind what this symbol of the alphabet looks like.

Hearing the camera lens shifting on the second camera, the next image on the video must be a frontal close-up of me lost, trying to picture how this "g" is formed. Expression surely blank, trying to capture the proper image in my mind, Diane threw me a life preserver when she finally asked, "How about if you try another word?"

Like the "i" I dotted a few minutes ago, immediately and with no hesitation, I gladly said, "Okay." Sounding like Foster Brooks when he does his drunkard impersonation, I brilliantly asked Diane if she wanted me to choose from the same four objects and when she told me she did, I utilized the common sense I still have remaining which is why I chose the next to the hardest object to spell—toothbrush. I'm sure Diane was thrilled about this selection for, not only is perseveration always a constant when I try to print one letter and end up making another, but I might be here all day making that letter "o" over and over again.

After Diane asked me and I told her how the word "toothbrush" is spelled, I proceeded to make—you guessed it—another "z" before scribbling it out. Trying to get that damned "T" down, my left hand didn't want to lift the pen off the paper, so it impulsively decided to make an "s." After scratching out the "s," I didn't know what the hell my left writing hand was going to do next. I don't feel as if I have any say what it does. Ideas abandoned, I know nothing of writing the symbols of the English language.

Time is ticking, but my hand still doesn't have any idea how to go about making that "T." Sensing my frustration as I sit there with the pen hovering over the paper, but not writing anything, Diane suggested we call it quits. That's the best thing I've heard all day, as I'm sure the camera's image of me is going to fade out just like the forms of letters has in my visual memory

Having my deficits put on tape is something I don't feel real comfortable with, but if it's going to help me in the long run or some patient down the line, I might as well "go for it" and make the best of things. I sure hope something good comes out of this taping because I'm making an incredible sacrifice allowing Mrs. Joy and Co. plop my ass down in front of a camera to film me. Sometimes I feel as if I'm being mistaken for an actor and not a patient. I'm getting a little bit pissed off that I'm missing so much program in order that my aphasias and physical limitations can get captured on video tape.

For example, this latest video segment where my agraphia gets taped, I missed a physical therapy session. When one has had a brain injury, in order for optimum recovery to occur, it's vital that the patient attends all their programs and puts forth a solid effort. If the day should ever come where I would want access to these tapes which I am the object, I'm sure Harmarville would be professional about this request and make these tapes readily available to me. Scene #7, take 4.

I guess there could be a day when I look back to the way I was and be thankful this time was captured, so I can appreciate any improvement I've made. Until then, I still have a "ways to go" yet. I just hope there's a pot of gold with my name on it at the end of the rainbow. If I'm to put my name on this treasure chest without making it a research project every time, I'm just going to have to continue working like a dog.

I'm scared to death not knowing when I'll be able to write spontaneously again without taking forever to print one word. Because of the subtle improvement I see in my letters to Valerie, I know I will be able to write again someday, it's just a question of how long is it going to take to regain this ability. I mean if I write like a second grader now, will it be ten years before I'm able to write like a high school senior again? If that's the case, I'll be twenty-eight-years-old before I could take college freshman courses again. If that scenario occurs, this head injury will have taken ten precious years from my life.

What if my writing will always be limited and never advance beyond, say, a sixth-grade level? What kind of future am I going to have? Will I be kept out of society's view and stuck in the stock room of a department store piling cardboard boxes atop one another because that's all I'm intellectually capable of doing? What kind of life am I going to have? God, help me. Please help me.

Hearing that tone in Jan Alba's voice before and seeing that look on Mary Smith's face during times of transition, I know something's up. It's more like what I don't hear and don't see that tells me there's going to be some serious business going down in Denmark. Jan not "ragging on me" about my ever-increasing waistline and Mary not laughing at the clothes I've selected to wear to program today, I began worrying.

I can recall hearing Jan's voice like it is now when she wasn't sure how I would respond to pushing myself up from a sitting position after being down so long. I can still picture the look on Mary's face the first time I stood at the parallel bars when she was by my side to brace me, and that's the expression she has on this very moment. When Jan instructed me how to go about standing behind my wheelchair, her voice currently sounds like it did then. The look of concentration in Mary's eyes is similar to when she guided me along those first steps I walked behind my wheelchair.

When my physical therapist smiled and asked me how I was feeling today, I knew I was in trouble. If there's one thing I've learned while being at Harmarville, it's when a physical therapist smiles, pain, terror, and/or unbearable frustration are just around the corner. And this time was no different than the others.

Jan told me that after I lock my brakes on my wheelchair and push myself up, to just stand there because she and Mary are going to throw my arms over their shoulders and we're going to take some steps together without using the wheelchair for balance. I hope Jan and Mary had a relaxing weekend and are well-rested, because I have a feeling they're going to think they are U-Hauls here in a second, lugging my dead weight body.

Shaking from being physically unstable and maybe more than a little from fear, I wasn't used to being in an upright position without something being in front of me to break a potential fall. Noting my body was twitching, Jan nonchalantly told me to take a step forward with my right foot first like I have been doing all along while I push my wheelchair. A lot shorter than myself, and not quite as filled out as I am either, I was definitely concerned whether Jan or Mary could support me should my brain decide it's time to lose sense of where I'm at, causing me to wipe out. Jan under my right pit and Mary joyfully positioned under the other, I picked my right foot off the ground and quickly slammed it down in front of me about twelve inches.

Yes!!! My first "wheelchairless" step!!! Now it's time for the second therapist/therapist's aide-assisted step, with my left foot this time.

Trying to support my weight and balance me at the same time, Jan and Mary resembled a weight lifter who tries to dead lift an incredible amount of weight. Not exactly making anyone forget about the grace of Fred Astaire, I tried to balance myself the best I could on my right leg as my left foot slapped down so hard one could have thought the two Ginger Rogers guiding me had left those barbells drop on top of my foot.

Like a captain whose ship's taking on water, Jan alerted her shipmate Mary to be prepared because I'll be lunging my right foot out and putting my anchor's weight on her. But before they could "batten down the hatches" and "unhitch the life rafts", my right foot ovaled in front of me, as I took another step without too much trouble. I guess Jan knew what she was doing having me push my wheelchair all this time.

With less difficulty than my right foot, when I step with my left one, I'm able to place my heel down first a lot easier. Concentrating on what my feet and legs were doing, Jan and Mary took it slow with me. Resembling a soldier that's been wounded during battle with two medics by his side when we started, by the time we approached the middle of the gym and they saw I was doing okay, Jan and Mary allowed me to be slightly less dependent on them. Not much, but a trace more on my own.

Wanting me to walk as naturally and independently as possible, but still letting me know that they were within arms' reach if my balance function in my brain decided to act up, Jan and Mary removed my arms from their shoulders and placed their hands on my back and side as I stomped along. When it was time to turn around and head back to my wheelchair, Jan told me to take it easy because I knew she didn't feel like ringing the alarm "All hands on deck" in case I took this U-turn too fast and went down.

Coaching me along, telling me how to go about making this 180 degree turn, Jan and Mary had me going back to my wheelchair, slowly but surely. Doing my "Hop-a-Long Cassidy" during this final stretch, I was cruisin' now. Not wanting to see the ship go down—with them on board especially—Jan and Mary made sure caution prevailed.

It is a little unnerving moving along without any support available to me should something go wrong, but I just have to put that out of my mind the best I can and tell myself, "Everything's going to be fine." Because of the multitude of people they work with, therapists have a good idea of what's going through a patient's mind. When they tell a patient to relax and "remain calm," these rehabilitation tradespeople know what they're talking about because I know that if I would get too flustered, I couldn't think rationally about what I have to do to get better. It wasn't easy, but once I put my trust and confidence in the professionals working with me, some real good things started happening. Although I'm worlds away yet from where I want to be, the combination of my efforts and the knowledge of my therapists is why I've progressed as I have.

From an attitude standpoint, what works best for me is to block those things out of my mind which aren't going to help me. Instead, I try to focus on what I need to do today in order to improve tomorrow. And I know I probably won't see much in the way of progress at first, but I realize if I keep battling, I've got a better chance of succeeding in the long run than if I just sit on my ass bitching about how unfair life is. If I'm to overcome the many physical disabilities and aphasias I have, I need to set aside the negative thoughts which want to overtake me, and put some faith into the people working with me. Letting them go to work, these miracle workers have been trained how to get patients back into the "swing of things."

I can do my part by practicing the exercises and doing the things they think are best for me. Too many times, I've seen patients being combative which doesn't do them a damn bit of good. People do this for a multitude of reasons.

Like myself at one time, a lot of these folks are simply not aware of what the hell's going on around them. Most of the time, patients who have had some type of neurological impairment have no idea what in God's name has happened to them or what's being done with them. They know their world is full of pain and confusion, and when things don't feel too good, the natural reaction for the person is to try to stop what's being done to them.

A lot of patients, like myself now, do know what's going on and become scared and frustrated by their various incapabilities/slow progress. The inabilities caused by an injured brain are terrifying because the most basic functions are usually affected and there's no telling if these afflictions will be permanent. This isn't something I've learned because I've read a "Disability 101" textbook, rather, it's a horror I have lived everyday these past couple of months and quite possibly will have to endure for the rest of my life. The pain one experiences after a head injury is not only physical, but emotional as well. All I can do is work hard, have faith in God's will, and hope for the best.

The vast majority of therapists try to understand the psychological trauma a patient is going through and when a patient does things—or more accurately—doesn't do things because they feel that they know best, sometimes it's tough getting them on track. The longer one remains derailed, however, the worse they'll be because the time that they're not listening and not working is time wasted. With head injury, this can be particularly devastating because time is of the essence. It's like the Olympic trials in the sense that if one doesn't qualify, they don't get to compete in the various sporting events. However, with my head injury, if I come up short, I don't get to participate in life.

In one way, I've just got to have tunnel vision and tell myself that there's no way I'm going to let this disability keep me down and beat me despite its many obstacles. I'm just going to have to give myself that little extra kick in the ass and fight another round. On the same hand, I can't get too carried away and expect things that just aren't going to happen. I need to keep some sort of a healthy balance, if that's possible. If I reach for the stars fully expecting to touch them and don't succeed, I'm in for one helluva fall. But then again, who's to say I'm not going to be successful.

Being told that yet another one of my cognitive therapies was to be taped and I was to take some steps in PT without a wheelchair wouldn't be the only surprises I would be delivered this week. When they came in for their Thursday evening visit, mom and dad told me that they were scheduled to come in tomorrow morning—Friday, May 14th—for a conference with all my therapists, to review how I am doing and go over the treatment plan.

Not only were my parents coming in to check on my progress at the meeting, but they are going to attend my therapies all day tomorrow. Because they weren't allowed to attend any of my formal therapies while I was in Allegheny General, this was going to be a new experience for them.

I'm sure they're going to have some mixed emotions about the whole thing depending on the frame of reference they happen to be operating from at any given moment when they view their "brain injured" son. If they see me thumping along with Jan and Mary in PT and think that it wasn't all that long ago that they couldn't be sure if I'd ever regain consciousness, mom and dad would definitely be counting their blessings. Viewing me from the vantage point of being a good athlete not that long ago either, would fill their minds with fury and/or a raging remorse.

Having me fling down on paper with a pen anything my hand has a mind to, will not make their day when they see me do this tomorrow in Mrs. Joy's and Diane's sessions. But if mom and dad look at it with the attitude that there was a time when I didn't even know what a pen and paper were, they won't be struck down so hard.

If they see only from the perspective of how I am now compared to what I was like this time last year—preparing to graduate from high school—they would definitely have a harder time coping with my struggles to get words down on a piece of paper. Tough as nails, only concerned with how I withstand this trauma, I know mom and dad are going to do what's best. They better, or it could be them that's in for a surprise tomorrow.

Professionals will say that people who have had a head injury will go through a transition in their personality. They do not mean this to be taken in an encouraging or positive manner, rather, as another symptom which could have a lasting negative impact on the person and their family. I have seen quite a few who have digressed and become demented. However, like a few other things about my head injury, this is not the case with me. Without sounding egotistical or as if I now have a narcissitic personality disorder, I now feel as if I have some worth and that I am special in my own little way.

You learn a lot about yourself when the chips are down. Being that I have a little difficulty smoothly adjusting with transition, my adolescence has not been an easy one. I have spent too much time on the defensive and never had the opportunity to see what was really inside of me. Feeling as though I never quite measured up, I never had much in the way of a healthy self-concept. Self-esteem was something others had and an elusive dream I could never seem to corner. But tackling my problems head-on—like I have since I was hurt—not vying for the path of least resistance, has given me an "awakening" as to who I really am.

My effort has opened my eyes to what I have always been and always will be. Even if no more gains are to be made, I am proud of the productive way I have faced this adversity. I can hold my head up high knowing that I've been reaching deep within me and "giving it my all."

Not seeing myself as worthwhile, unfounded criticism has been something I have been too readily willing to accept as the truth. Because of what I've achieved in my rehabilitation thus far, I can now see the misguided cynicism for what it is. It is not the fabric of my character, as I was led to believe, rather, a weapon used by those who had no idea of its lasting impact. This tool of ignorance used so skillfully by these cynics prevents them from finding true meaning. Perhaps they have discovered their own misgivings and absorbed themselves in their artificial facade where belittlement keeps the focus off who they truly are.

No longer do I feel as if my fiber is anything less than what it should be at this stage of the ball game. Everything that happened to me in the accident and what I'm doing in the face of this tragedy, has paradoxically provided me with a different kind of strength.

With a brain injury, there's no room for complacency and no easy way out. For those who are capable, one gets what they put into it. Unfortunately with this disability, only those lucky and strong enough withstand the barrage of pain/question and come out on top. Luck and fortune have a profound effect on one's recovery, but I also know that if one doesn't put in the effort, good things aren't going to come their way. I'm just happy as all hell with the way I've played the cards I've been dealt. Being told how bad I was at Allegheny General and Harmarville those first couple of weeks, and seeing that first video of me where I could barely talk, made me believe that I could rise above all my afflictions.

Beauty, money, power, and material objects are, without a doubt, great if you have them, but these aren't the most important possessions one can own. If these are the things that make a person happy, perhaps the one looking back at them in the mirror has had a life of fortune. What's really precious is one's health. It's so invaluable. As far as having a realization, an "awakening" of who I am and what I represent, this accident has provided me with a foundation with which I can start to build my character. That's how this head injury and almost being killed has changed my personality.

I should have told on them. With mom and dad standing in the PT gym, Jan and Mary were at their best behavior. Mary didn't make one crack about how she likes my other black Judas Priest T-shirt better and Jan didn't say a word that the sweat pants I'm wearing must have shrunk a size from last week. While walking alongside of me, with courtesy and congeniality, these angels instructed me how to go about taking these steps. Within a short time, however, they couldn't resist any longer and the masquerade ended.

While I was taking a short breather, Jan walked over to my parents. "Mr. and Mrs. Meyers," Jan said within earshot sporting her devilish grin, "Y'know, Craig's a real delight to work with."

"Yeah," a smirking Mary said when it was her turn, "we really like him a lot."

Smacking me on the shoulder—all kidding aside—Jan and Mary went on to tell my folks how hard I've been working, what they are trying to do with me, and would like to see me accomplish. For a second there at first, I wasn't sure these were the same two people I've been working with in PT all this time.

Mom and dad were ecstatic with the way I've been progressing within the physical realm of my rehabilitation. Fearful I might be confined to a wheelchair for the rest of my life, mom and dad were thankful from the bottom of their hearts that I not only had such knowledgeable professionals working with me, but ones I got along with well. It makes for an easier ride when one's going through the bumps of rehabilitation.

In a short time, the fun and games will be over because I'll be off to Psychology next. Well, I don't know about the games, but I do know the fun is over.

Looking down at the worksheet which depicted different geometric figures, I was wrestling with my brain's right hemisphere perceptual deficit to remember what went where. Giving my parents a quickie "Neuropsychology 101" lecture before I started, Mrs. Joy explained how the various damage to my brain will translate into behavior/responses on the various tests I'll be taking in their presence. Without getting too elaborate about their names, the tests Mrs. Joy will be administering will be the Benton Visual Retention Test, the Motor-Free Visual Perception Test (MVPT), and the WAIS-R (Picture Arrangement).

Not being able to discern differences in the various displays of figures, not noticing designs located to the left, and my inability to put in order how a comic strip should be set up, I gave my parents a disheartening exhibition of my brain's right hemisphere perceptual difficulty, unilateral neglect, and sequential deficit. After making one of my mistaken responses on the Benton, apparently Mrs. Joy noted the look of sheer terror on mom's face and winked at her as if to say this wasn't a surprise and this is something that's being worked on.

Loving to read the comics on Sunday, dad stood there and watched in disbelief as I couldn't do something as simple as figure out the logical order of events when asked to piece together some pictures which would tell a story. Covering how he really felt about this, dad tried to laugh this off as a joke. But the trembling jaw told another story.

Oh, I wouldn't just sit there and do nothing. I'd put the middle picture where the first one belonged, the last where the middle was supposed to be, and the first where the last one should have been placed. What was amusing was that I tried to make sense of how I set these pictures up. You want to talk about one strange story.

My pen going down and over when it should have been going up and across was something mom and dad had seen many times, but when I started doing this in Diane's therapy session, it brought home for them that this aphasia was something that wasn't going to be fixed easily. Knowing the concerted efforts by the therapists and my diligently working to overcome this agraphia has not reaped the rewards as they had hoped, mom and dad could only watch and pray something would "snap" upstairs, making this writing ability automatic again. The sooner, the better.

Back to the unit for my last therapy of the week before I make a much-anticipated return trip home for the weekend, it was my turn to try and be on my best behavior. I can only keep my fingers crossed the Occupational Therapists won't tell my parents how disagreeable I can be at the end of a long day of rehabilitation. I'll even try to cross the fingers of my right hand without using my left to help, if they don't say too much about how shitty I can be.

Having a brick for a hand that used to bullet a football and shred guitar strings is a transition that could make an angel scowl. Sugarcoating things, Wendy merely told my parents that my "mood will fluctuate from time to time" because I'm so motivated to get better, and that the minimal improvement being experienced upsets me. Way to go Wendy, you came through once again. Now get out of my way, I'm going home for the weekend.

On the trip back to Washington, dad told me he built a little wooden ramp leading from the back patio to the dining room allowing me to have access to the upstairs now. Going from the sideyard to the back, I can have my wheelchair pushed to this upper level where I can take a look at the living room, dining room, and the top hallway where the bedrooms are. Last weekend when I could only get a glimpse of these from downstairs, the images of how these areas of the house looked started coming back, but I still couldn't be completely sure how these were laid out until I saw them with my very own eyes. But now I know.

I no sooner got pushed to this upstairs haven when a few of the neighbors started coming over and the phone began ringing. For the most part though, like last Friday when I came home, this evening would be a quiet one where I was given the opportunity to spend time with family. Like last Saturday however, a flock of friends and neighbors phoned, saying they'd be over when they could, which was great.

Thanks to these folks, I have an understanding of myself and that which has been a part of me. Before last weekend, I didn't remember being healthy and I had no recollection of my childhood. Nor did I know how I was going to be received, or if I would be accepted. I guess tomorrow will tell me a lot about that.

Just because I'm home for a few days doesn't mean that gives me license to "goof off;" not that my parents would permit this or I would want that. The time in between talking with friends and getting reacquainted with things, which wasn't a whole heck of a lot, I spent my minutes practicing my printing or worked on hand exercises.

Talking with my psychologist earlier this afternoon, Mrs. Joy gave mom and dad some ideas of board and card games they may want to invest in which could help with some of my cognitive difficulties/aphasias. It's been a long time since mom gave "Mattel" any business on my behalf and she isn't going to feel real happy about getting her college freshman son toys to play with—but if it's going to help me—she'll put aside the personal discomfort, as long as it brings me out of the dark cloud which I've been trapped. If it helps me regain some semblance of my former self, she and dad will play different games with me "until the cows come home." Being that I can think of better ways I'd rather spend my time too, I hope we're not milked of our sanity.

The impetus behind my drive and willingness to work is the knowledge that if I don't take full advantage of my strengths now to help me overcome my weaknesses, then a fulfilling life down the road may be out of touch. Unless I was reading sheet music for guitar or watching some sporting event on T.V., I wouldn't spend much time sitting, which is one reason I never really had gotten into board games all that much. Loaded with a mess of these brain twisters, when mom came home resembling Santa Claus, I knew I was in for some serious "downtime" and right hemisphere testing.

To help with my spatial difficulties and compromised eye/hand coordination, mom bought the game "Perfection." For my memory, she got the hand-held game, "Pocket Repeat" and to address my spatial and concentration lapses, "Word Master Mind" was purchased. "Snake Puzzle" was also in this pile of goodies which could stimulate the right half of my brain. And she shelled out some cash for the Chinese Tangram puzzle game, Changram, which would also tickle the right side of my brain. For the purpose of eye/hand coordination, sequencing, and memory addition, the card game "Uno" was another cognitive gift I'd be playing with. In order to help clear up some of my spatial inabilities, mom got the geometric puzzle, "Pythagoras." Since the card game, "O'NO 99" would help me with my memory, addition, and direction, mom couldn't resist getting her hands on this and brought this home.

Like I said before, I dont' get too caught up in games like these, but if it's going to help my brain's right hemisphere function any better, then shuffle those cards and let's get going. When am I due to return to Harmarville?

Majors, minors, thirds, sevenths, fifths, suspended fourths,Kevin was at it again showing me different chords on guitar and Frank came over to tell me about more stuff we did as kids. Using the tank and armored car models we would build, Danny Hobbs told me how we would play World War II on my 4 X 8 board plywood board down in the basement where the Americans would always kick the Nazi's ass. And Craig Johnson asked me if I remember the many cabins and tree houses we used to build in the cemetery. It was little stuff like this that I was informed of that meant so much in reconstructing my days of years past. I didn't have all that long to bask in the glory of my childhood, however, because something weird started happening to me.

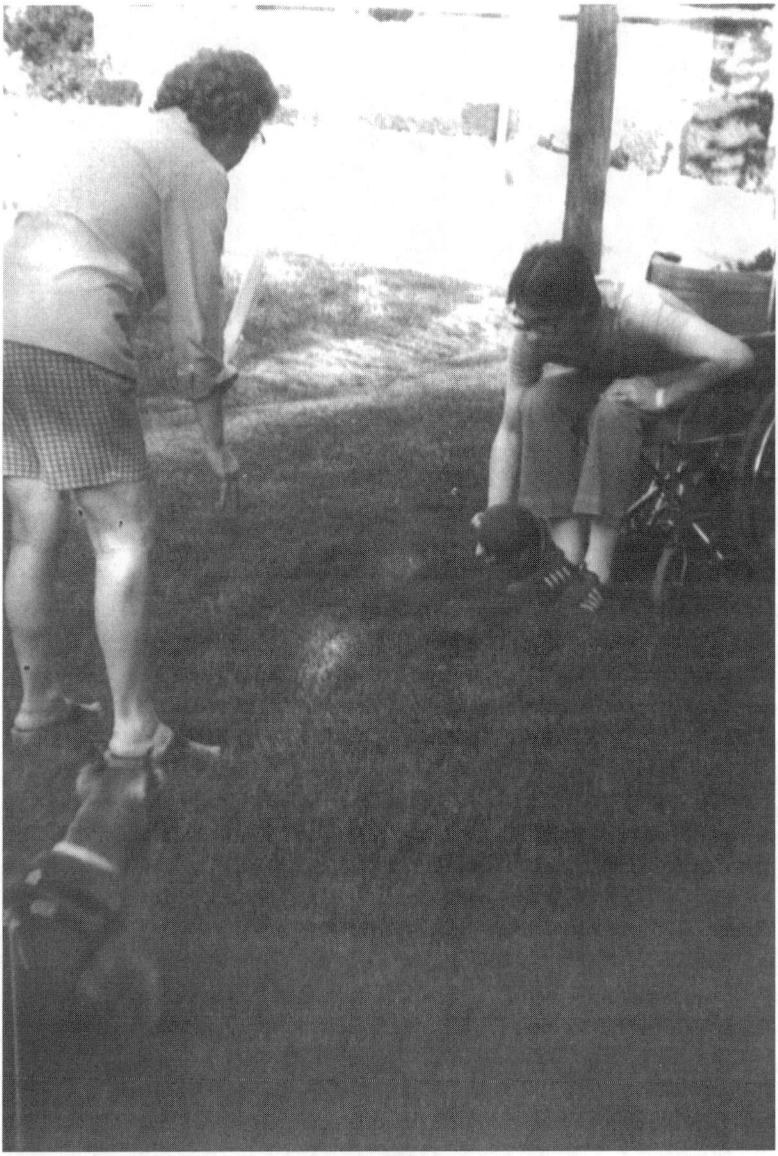

Going from aspiring W.V.U. baseball player to tossing a Nerf Ball to his mother, as the Meyers' schnauzer looks on, is but one barometer as to how far Craig had regressed following his traumatic brain injury.

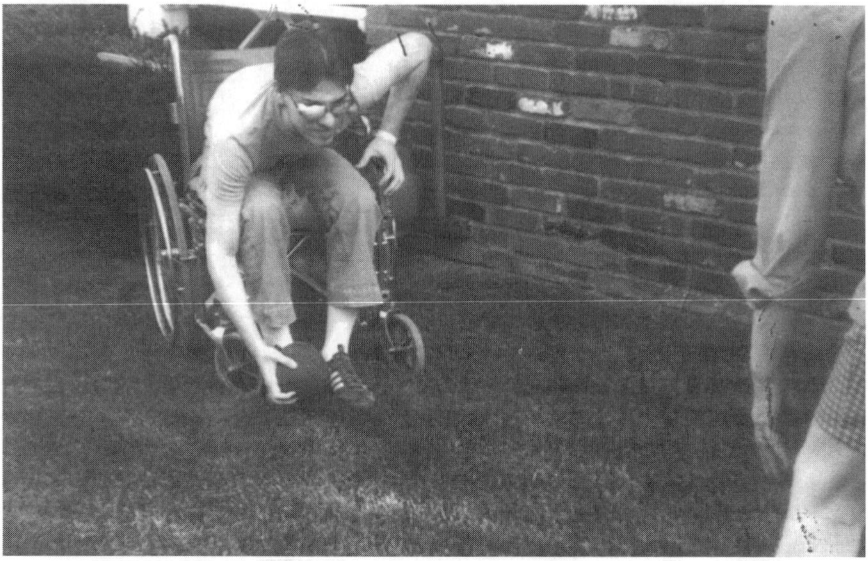

Unable to walk or use his dominant right hand very well, Craig attempts an underhand toss from his wheelchair to his mom in their side yard.

For some strange reason, on this Saturday afternoon, my right foot started to swell. Fearful the passageway in my leg for blood circulating was closing up, mom and dad got on the phone and gave Harmarville a desperation call reporting this swelling.

Wanting some instruction as to what they should do, they were told that when someone hasn't used one side of their body too much and starts working it again, parts of the inoperative side can sometimes respond in strange ways. Harmarville said that because I've started moving my leg to walk and I slap my right foot every step I take, that this is the body's reaction to being "awakened" after such a long time in a dormant state.

But to avoid any further problems, Harmarville informed my parents that if this condition gets worse, take me to a doctor and have my foot looked at. And when I get back to the rehab Monday, the doctor will check my foot. Overall, Harmarville said it wasn't anything to fret about.

Normally, I'm a right-handed hitter in baseball, but because my right side isn't getting the job done, I have to bat lefthanded now. But that didn't make any difference when I went to bat against my brother this final day of the weekend, May 16th. Even sitting in a wheelchair, batting the opposite way that I'm used to, I was stinging the tennis ball. As Ug delivered another one of his customary fat pitches twenty-five feet away, spraying every one of his thrown balls to all fields with the wiffle ball bat, I "stuck" his hanging curveball like Pirates' legend, Willie Stargell would. I wasn't the greatest hitter of all time, but against my brother, I have always been able to slug the cover off the ball.

Whether it was his spinning knuckler, "It's outta here" rendition of a fastball, belt-high sinker, or hanging curve, I was cranking 'em. Having the heart that I do, however, when I saw the devastation on my brother's face after repeatedly "lighting him up," I'd miss every once in a while on purpose, so he wouldn't feel so bad. I think Ug appreciated my controlled display of dominance because he helped me with some of my cognitive deficits afterward. "Ha Ha Ha Ha Ha Ha Ha Ha Ha Ha Ha Ha Ha Ha Ha Ha Ha Ha Ha Ha Ha Ha Ha Ha Ha Ha Ha Ha Ha Ha Ha Ha Ha Ha Ha Ha Ha Ha Ha Ha Ha Ha Ha Ha Ha Ha Ha Ha Ha Ha Ha Ha Ha Ha Ha Ha Ha Ha Ha Ha Ha Ha Ha Ha Ha Ha Ha Ha Ha Ha Ha Ha Ha Ha Ha Ha Ha Ha Ha."

Apparently using me as his model following my exhibition of athletic superiority, Ug drew a smiley face beaming from ear to ear and asked me to draw a hat, tie, and moustache on this depiction of me. Like my swing after one of his throws, I was right on the mark when I drew these three things.

However, when a blank piece of paper was laid in front of me without any kind of facial cue, I could not make a hat, tie or moustache without this hint. Whenever something is written on paper, this serves as a substitute for my failed visual memory. When this foundation is not on paper, I can't go on, and my ability to identify/replicate these figures by writing them down collapses. Verbally, I can describe what a hat, tie, and moustache are and how they look, but just don't ask me to draw them because that's where I get lost. Strange, very strange.

There's a guy who lives in the neighborhood who thinks he's James Dean and is always working on his cars or motorcycles out in his driveway. Because Dave McClellan likes his hot rods and bikes too, he spends a lot of time now down at "James'" house tinkering under a hood or shining up his wheels. I'm absolutely positive Dave knows that I've been home these past two weeks because "James" saw me when dad put me on exhibit around the neighborhood last weekend, and it goes without saying that he told Dave I was home. I'm a little surprised Dave hasn't stopped to see me and I'm a little miffed. I know he's home because I saw his sports car thundering past the house yesterday.

I realize that people have other obligations and Dave has a lot of friends because he's so good-natured, but because we are pretty good friends, I thought for sure he'd at least alot a minute in his schedule and check to see how I'm doing after almost "checking out." I would really like to see Dave because he's such a nice guy who comes from a super family and, like Frank, could really help my memory with regards to neighborhood happenings. Oh well, as I sometimes do, maybe I'm reading too much into things. I'm sure he'll stop and say "Hi" next time I'm home.

Sometimes I only wish I wasn't so cognizant of what's going on around me because I'm now aware of the battle I am up against. I know the disability which I'm tangling is one where sparsely anything is known which makes it that much more powerful and threatening. But I try not to see it as omnipotent because then

I'd be beaten even before the battle lines have been drawn. I can't quit now and let this injury take everything from me. That would be like flushing eighteen years down the shitter and I'm not about to let that happen, if I can do anything about it.

I try to keep my head above water by what I tell myself, but sometimes this is hard. I don't want to lie to myself, yet, I can't give in to what's going on around me. I have to keep telling myself what David did to Goliath. I guess my will is my slingshot. But will I have enough rocks to fling?

For me, being in a brain injury rehabilitation program, the days last forever. Every waking moment I'm reminded of what's wrong with me and what I can no longer do. Keeping from caving in is a constant struggle. Working on basic things, doing them time after time after time, over and over again with no end in sight is enough to drive you crazy. This is when one starts to wonder if the pain will ever leave. Is time being wasted on a dream that will never be more than fantasy? Sometimes I just wonder if my fortune has been all used up and I just better start getting used to the way I am now because this is all the farther I'm going.

I know I've progressed and have progressed rapidly thus far, but I feel as if things are in slow motion now and I should be getting more in return for my efforts. I've been driving myself up a wall working like an idiot. Why aren't things happening as I want them? Damn it brain—heal!!!

The discouragement and frustration not being able to do the most basic things is enough to make anyone mad. Yet, I'm encouraged by others that it can be done, that I can do it. This helps me to stay afloat, but with a brain injury, you just don't know. Will I bust my tail in therapies only to have my brain not cooperate?

No matter how hard I practice my writing, walking, manipulating my right hand, trying to clear things up with my perceptions/thinking, there's a definite possibility this labor will be all for naught because these functions will have been permanently ruined by the damage to my brain. I can't control the etiologic factors responsible for my limitations, but how I approach this warfare is something I'm not going to let slip from my control. I need to have a fighting spirit, if I'm to regain what is no longer within my possession and triumph "against all odds."

Maybe thinking too much can be dangerous. But how can you help not to think? When one's life has been so drastically altered, there's no way you can help from having thoughts that have the potential to be defeating. It takes all the strength one can gather to keep from giving in, but you have to tap this resource of stamina—and then some—to keep from breaking down. But it ain't easy. Nothing with a brain injury is.

One can't help but ask themselves, "When's this all going to end?" The days are just so long now, you just want to rip out your hair. I try to keep from thinking that this struggle is one where I'm putting in so much effort for a hopeless cause. I just need to look deep inside myself and find the strength to overcome my fears and endure. Although I think I do one helluva job concealing this, I'm totally shocked, saddened, and worried beyond belief what's happened to me. But I have to put these negatives aside, if I'm going to advance to the next level.

This is the key for me and how I need to go about my business—putting negatives aside. I need to look at things from an angle where I recognize the many gains I've made and support I have, instead of allowing my continuous disabilities discourage me, because nobody knows for sure if any of the difficulties I'm having now will necessarily be permanent. I have to view my situation in the manner that—because so little is known about the brain and its capacity to heal—no one knows how far I can go, so nobody can tell me what I can and can't do definitively or what can and can't be achieved. This is one of the things that lights the fury in me to excel even when the odds appear not to be in my favor.

I know that attitude is such an important factor when approaching a situation, which is why I try to balance all the bad that goes with this type of disability with a "never say die" demeanor. The reality that so many lingering uncertainties exist with head injury cannot be denied, but all you can do is make the best of what you got and don't wave that white flag before your time. Good things can come to those who wait. And the passage of time is never fleeting when the mind has been anchored in disarray.

I need and want to improve, but it seems I'm just getting started. I know this isn't the case deep in my heart, but it feels as if the race hasn't even begun in this contest where I'm trying to outrun my afflictions and not let them overtake me. Unfortunately, with this disability, I don't think there's a finish line. I guess I'll just have to keep running, keep battling, keep running, keep battling, keep running, keep battling, keep running, keep battl. . . . .

Because this conflict is never-ending, it's tough to maintain a healthy, positive perspective because of all that's wrong with me. Often, I can't help but think that maybe getting on track again is something that just isn't going to happen because of this injury to my brain. I couldn't live with that or accept that I'll never enjoy life as I had hoped, so I just try to believe that things will work out for the best. I might be living an existence of fabrication, but if this keeps me working as hard as I have been, then fabricate I will do. I can make ignorance work for me. Maybe the reluctance to accept that which is not known for sure will open new doors. Necessity is the mother of invention. Without doing anything stupid, one wouldn't know limits until they've been tested. I don't have too much to lose.

I still can't walk without four wheels helping to take me where I want to go and I can't write yet. My thinking is one confused, muddled mess and my right hand is no damned good. What goes here? When's this torment going to end? It isn't fair that my life's been dealt such a devastating blow. Then again, who ever said life was fair?

Maybe this is reality's way of giving me a chilling slap in the face and telling me I'll never be right again, that I'll always be lacking and unsuccessfully searching for an existence where there is promise. I'll say to myself that this can't be happening, pinch me and tell me it's not so; that it's only a bad dream. I thought I was immune to tragedy and bad things were something that happened to other people, not me.

I know there's a time and a place for everything, and "now" isn't the time to be dwelling on all this because I've got too much work to do. I'll just have to bury all these thoughts and put them on the back burner. I just have to keep active and occupied. Since there's so many basic things I can't do anymore, I'll start working on these for the gazillionth time.

Where should I start? Manipulating putty with my bad hand? Practice printing the alphabet? Pushing my wheelchair out in the main corridor? Tapping my right foot to loosen my tight heel cord? Follow my finger to my nose to help my double vision? God please give me the strength. I'm too young to stop living.

I won't give up on myself. I can't have a "What's the Use?" mentality, I've got too much to live for and too many dreams to capture. I just hope there is a "next level" I can advance to. No, I know there is.

The work my cognitive therapists have done with me and the multitudes of letters I've written are starting to pay off. The piece of cardboard that has the letters of the alphabet printed on it is still by my side when I write my letters to Valerie or Jan in case I might need to refer to it, but I'm not as reliant on it as I used to be. Instead, I will now say the alphabet to myself and simultaneously print the letter I'm saying in the air before putting it down on paper. Since I've written so many letters to my two nurse darlings, I'm slowly starting to get an idea again what the different letters look like.

True, tracing each individual letter in the air for confirmation as to what they look like before putting them on paper isn't the ideal situation one wants to be in, but at least it shows my conceptualization of the shapes of letters is returning. Being able to skywrite each letter instead of being totally dependent on a cardboard cue to write is an absolutely spectacular gain.

My ability to do this is indicative that I'm developing images in my mind again how the different letters look. I know that even neuropsychologists can't say with any kind of certainty what is going on exactly with a brain that's been injured, but I guess it can be assumed that new passageways are being formed in my corpus collusum which allows me to picture in my mind the framework of each individual letter. Relaying the patterns to my left hand to write, these new transmitters have apparently taken over the writing function once operated by cells now unable to carry through with this operation because they're irreparably damaged.

With repetition, I've learned to put a harness on my writing hand, so it doesn't take off before I've captured each letter's image. The perseveration, coupled with my inability to identify letters, has been the "Tag team from Hell" I have been up against in my attempts to write again. But before this match is over, I know I'll beat this double threat. "When?," I can't say precisely, but it's coming.

Because of the repetition and practice, my mental monitor is starting to pick up strings of letters forming words as well, rather than grappling to find the configurations of different letters then joining them to form a word. Like when I now want to start my note to her with, "Dear Valerie," I'm gradually starting to see the word, "Dear," as one unit instead of trying to snare the four sub-units/letter symbols, "D"-"e"-"a"-"r." I'm also beginning to see the name, "Valerie," as one unit instead of seven elusive letters I can't remember how to print. On a good day, I'll even see the two words together forming the opening phrase to my letter. More often than not, my left hand will go in the proper direction to form these letters. I might occasionally forget to include the comma, but I don't think Valerie will mind too much.

I know that effort on the part of the patient is the main ingredient with any kind of recovery, but rapport one has with their therapists, nurses, and doctors is also a vital component to the mix. Since being at Harmarville, I've been in the fast lane towards recovery. It's been a one-way ticket towards progress since I've been at the rehab and there's no looking back.

Because I can finally see what this rehabilitation business is all about now, I've grown comfortable with the Harmarville surroundings and realize this environment promotes the utmost in care. There's nothing here that would prevent me from focusing 100% on what I need to do to overcome my various ailments.

In traditional psychotherapy, a patient's therapist cannot be involved with their client beyond a professional level and objectivity must prevail. Within this psychodynamic framework, when personal matters come into the picture, sacred ground is being treaded upon. Never inappropriate, the professional at Harmarville is seen not only as qualified and knowledgeable, but someone who cares as a friend would. They've definitely been one of the major factors that have helped me to look at life differently. Freud might not go for an approach that promotes such a union, but that's what has worked best with this patient and others who are progressing. Now, where's Valerie, I want to play some ping-pong and make that "Id" of mine happy.

Look mom, no hands!!! Nor was I hanging on to Jan or Mary around the neck either, holding their heads down as if I was about to give them a Dutch rub. I wasn't going to make people forget about any of the Olympiads at the last games, but the time I've spent on the rockpile trying to get my walking down is definitely worth honorable mention for some kind of medal.

As if I were handling nitroglycerine, I put one foot in front of the other with great care and concentration. I continued in this tortoise pace, trying to filter through my memory the multitude of things I need to do to take a step. Don't let that right knee snap back! Down slap your foot down so hard! Don't lean so far to the left! Don't let your arm dangle! Don't drag your right foot! So many "don'ts" I was still doing and so many "do's" I wasn't. I never knew all that walking independently entailed, until I forgot how.

Getting my neurological control center to physically move my body like I want is one thing, but now I have to psychologically prepare myself that there won't be any wheelchair for me now, if I lose sense of where I'm at and my brain dictates it's time to go down. Jan told me if I learn to walk using a cane, I could be discharged sooner. However, the combination of her not wanting to see someone as young as

I am forever dependent on a compensatory device to get around, and with the way I've been progressing to this point, Jan wasn't about to shoot for that as a goal. Am I ever glad Jan would not settle for anything less. While teaching me how to walk again, I just hope Jan and Mary don't go out with a bang. BOOM!!!!!!!!!

I really look forward to PT now because during this time I can discard my wheelchair and try to walk on my own, which gives me a taste of my old self and a renewed enthusiasm that things are getting better. After being bedridden and confined to a wheelchair for so long, it feels absolutely fantastic getting up and hobbling about without following my wheelchair-walker everywhere I go. I may not be real smooth when I walk around the PT gym—with Jan and Mary not too far off—but to think I've achieved so much independence after being hurt so bad, I feel pretty good about what I'm doing, no matter how loud my foot bangs. But there's always plenty of room for improvement, which is why I'm never satisfied. This can be good in a way because you're always pushing for more, but it can be of great harm if you don't stop for a moment and look at the many miles that have been traveled. You gotta smell them roses once in a while.

Around the unit and everywhere else I go, I have the wheelchair guiding my way, but like my cardboard cue when I print, I'm nowhere near as dependent on it as I once was because I'm finding that my stability/balance and comfort is improving as I walk more and more. The foot slapping, exaggerated leaning to one side, and lost sense of balance aren't good and are still there, but now I'd have to say the most disturbing thing about walking now doesn't have anything to do with my malfunctioning brain, rather, the severe bite that rod in my right femur is giving the top part of my leg. This pain and discomfort is barely tolerable. Each step I take, I'm reminded that my leg was broken. Like so many other things since this injury, I just have to learn to suck it up and make the best of what I got. "Ouch! That smarts!!!!!!"

Things that I once thought were important, now seem so trivial to me. After my brush with death, you kind of get a new perspective/an "awakening" as to what's of value and what isn't. Because of almost having my "chips cashed in" for me, I've matured and grown beyond my years.

I'm not intending to give the impression that I'm never going to enjoy things young people should like, it's just that other things take on a more significant role in the scope of importance. But then again, this new vantage point which things are seen may not be attributed totally to accelerated maturation or development, rather, a kind of bitterness.

Bitterness in the sense that I've been robbed of my chance to take delight in my growing years. With this, a sort of pessimism has emerged because my aspirations have been taken from me and I haven't finished being a kid. A lot of opportunities are not only deferred, but gone, never to return. Just because one's in college doesn't mean that they're grown up. I think I've proved that. If my maturity was ever lacking, this catastrophe has helped me to catch up—and then some.

This "awakening" as to what is of worth and that which lacks depth may not have anything to do with what happened to me at all, it merely concurred with the maturation process. But I wouldn't bet on that.

Without a doubt, things are definitely starting to come together in this rehabilitation excursion. I'm starting to see some dividends from my practice and repetition. Rehabilitation can be the ultimate in boredom, but when a patient starts showing the fruits of their labor, there isn't an excitement more immaculate.

By the time Friday, May 21st arrived, the straw broke the camel's back and I was printing without the use of that cardboard cue. It was still slow and sloppy, but I was printing letters straight out of my head now without having to take a peek at anything for a hint. If I get stumped as to how a particular letter is formed, I'm just going to have to get those chemicals in my brain to connect and figure it out on my own. This will be an exercise in futility, as I'm sure I'll be wrestling with my brain's fuzzy visual-memory as to how some letters look, but it's definitely going to enhance my independence. Besides, since my long-range plans at this juncture are to go back to school, realistic or not, it would look kind of funny if I would lug a cardboard cue to all my classes so I'd be able to print my name on my paper. "Let's go-oooooooo, Mountaineers!"

My hand still wanted to go every which way, but I wouldn't let it. Wanting to cross an "i" and dot a "t," I was able to force my hand to go where I wanted it to, instead of where it had every intention of going. The frustration, pain, and fear is incredible when my hand wanted to do one thing when I truly had a desire for it to do something else, and it wouldn't listen to my command because the impulse was just too strong. What was equally—if not more scary—was that I didn't know what I should order it to do. But now there's a corpus collusum hookup between my brain's right hemisphere perceptual monitor and the left hemisphere's language production system. If I could only jump, I'd be doing so for joy right now.

Perceptually and cognitively, my brain is beginning to make some sense of its world and I was making some equally remarkable headway physically as well. Jan wrote in her progress note dated this Friday, that I was showing significant improvement in all phases of my physical therapy program. With both sitting and standing, my posture was better and I was able to monitor just how well I was doing with these. Noting if my stance was how it should be, I knew what revisions needed done to make things better. This doesn't necessarily mean I made the right adjustment, I just knew how I should be adjusted.

Done with minimal cueing, I was independent with my weight shifting and my knee extension when I walk. With proper weight-shift forward and bearing on my right-lower extremities, I was able to stand without any trouble. However, when I got on my feet, my standing balance was only fair. But this should get better in time because my overall gait was improving, for the weight-bearing on my right side was increasing.

My right foot was still whacking away at the floor, but not as much, for there was increased heel to toe action. Keeping my hips forward was not easy for me, with Jan occasionally reminding me to, "Get up there" and straighten my backside.

When I'd slouch some, I always got a little nudge, as Jan's fist would go digging into my back. I think the smile on Jan's face indicated she enjoyed the pain she was inflicting because this was her way of getting back at me for all those times I tried to swat her when I was a Ranchos #4 terror upon admission. Jan didn't think I knew what I was doing. "Ha Ha Ha Ha Ha Ha Ha Ha Ha Ha Ha Ha Ha Ha Ha Ha Ha Ha Ha Ha Ha Ha Ha Ha Ha Ha Ha Ha Ha Ha Ha Ha Ha Ha Ha Ha. . . . ."

This third weekend home would be a continuation of PT, for I now have clearance to practice walking behind my wheelchair. Knowing how the contour of our neighborhood is, Harmarville said it would be okay if I practiced pushing my wheelchair, just not up and down hills because I haven't been prepared for manipulating hills yet. About the only level place near the house where I could get up and stroll around then would be our one-car garage and the very top of the driveway. Well, I guess you gotta do what you gotta do.

Dad looked funny twirling around the middle of our tiny garage as I kept circling him like the apaches do when they want to attack a wagon train. But my gruff dad didn't mind looking like a ballerina as long as this would help me. Used to going down Harmarville's infinite main corridor, I definitely felt cramped playing this ring around the rosie. But it beats just sitting in my wheelchair getting fat—ter.

The reviews on this wheelchair walking were mixed. When I was fresh and rested, I was able to place my heel first on the ground before my toes a fair amount of the time because I was clinging onto my wheelchair for support. However, being so dependent on my wheelchair to support me, I lifted my right foot too high. During this march step, the rod in my leg really dug into me, tearing into my ass.

With my "position sense" so off-base, I could not tell whether I was making strides as I should, or if they were awkward. The manner in which I walk could be described as both an "ataxic gait," where my foot is raised high and the sole comes crashing down suddenly, and a "spastic gait" which the legs move in a stiff manner and the toes of my right foot drag each step I take. In a way, I kind of resemble Frankenstein's monster when he roams about the castle. Not only is my walk similar to his, but we have about as many stitch scars. However, the emotional scars of having to be in a physically subordinate position to that of my peers will be something I soon will not have to contend with.

Having my friends standing alongside my wheelchair towering over me didn't make me feel real comfortable, so being able to get up and take a look at them in the eye should do me a lot of good. And I know dad would feel proud showing off how far I've come. Getting up out of my chair would be an ideal way I could show anyone who came to see me how well I've been progressing. I know my friends would be glad I'm doing so well too. Let's see now, we played board games last night, "Ring around the Rosie" in the garage this morning so we could "Show and Tell" this afternoon; I guess "Patty Cake" is next. Reverting to decades past is all too common with brain injury.

Not only would it be notable who I was playing "Show and Tell" with this weekend, but who I wouldn't be. Kevin made his weekend visit Saturday and was telling me of the various people we both know he runs into during the week and how they're wishing me well. A few of my better friends he has crossed paths with have said they would be stopping within a week or so to check up on me.

Kevin's really the best of friends with the valedictorian from our class and I'm a pretty good friend of Randy's as well. Not anywhere close to being in the same league of tightness that he and Kevin are in, but we get along good. Kevin was talking with Randy this week and Kevin informed me our brilliant classmate said he was going to come see me soon.

That's great, I'm looking forward to seeing friends who might be able to "click on" some recollection in the darkness which is my past and the void which is my memory. If I can't go back to W.V.U. right away, I wonder if Randy wouldn't mind sitting in for me during my absence; I need to get that G.P.A. up.

Brilliant. That's one thing that can't be said for Sam's memory. When he came to see me Saturday, he still had a mental block as to what the specifics were leading up to the party and what occurred during this outing. He just kind of shrugged his shoulders and had a blank expression on his face when asked what took place at and before the party. Not wanting to "fink" on anybody, could selective forgetting be the order of the day again?

I guess Sam was better friends with those that were at the party than me now, and didn't want to get any of them in trouble. We can assume this is why he's being so tight-lipped, but still I wonder who he's trying to protect. Because I don't remember anything about what occurred leading to and during the party, could it be Sam did something? With all the questions me and my parents drilled Sam with the first time he visited me on that first weekend I was home, it's a wonder he stopped by today. Feeling uneasy, you'd think Sam'd just want to stay away. But here he was—and he wasn't alone.

Accompanying Sam this afternoon was his right hand man, "Claude." Living in the same area of the neighborhood, these two guys saw each other a lot and were really good buddies. I've known Claude for about eight years and we have played a lot of ball together being neighbors. We'd get along fine enough, but we were not exactly bosom buddies because aspects of our individual personalities just wouldn't mesh. Demeanor tough to gauge, depending on who was around would largely dictate how one was approached by this lanky dude. Although not overly abundant due to Sam's disparaging influence, I suppose me and Claude had our moments where we'd "click" alright, however, and I guess that explains why he's here. Doing right by me now, realizing people change in time, I can only presume that my wariness towards Sam's pal is just my imagination. But still . . .

I can't figure it out; I don't know what the story is. I'm a little pissed off now. At first, I thought it was a case of him being pressed for time and not being able to stop, or not knowing I had been home. I know he's become pretty good friends with James the past year or so, but I wouldn't think that would change Dave's favorable attitude towards me. We've always gotten along so well and I don't think what anyone might say would change his opinion of me.

Playing football, softball, and church volleyball together, we always got along great. But now I don't know; maybe I didn't read our friendship as it truly was. I mean Dave likes his cars, bikes, beer, and females and I never had much experience with these. Over time, people change as can their interests, and maybe this has something to do with Dave not dropping by to see me.

The one thing that tied me and Dave together—sports—may not be so important to him anymore. Possibly, these other interests could have taken precedence over anything else when it comes to sustaining a friendship. Since I don't know too much about motorized vehicles or dating, I can only assume that I've been forgotten about because sports likely are a thing of the past for me and we wouldn't have so much in common anymore.

We always got along well because Dave always liked those who have excelled at sports and kind of let those that weren't too good fall by the wayside. I'm sure he has heard how physically bad off I am now and knows that sports are more than likely something that I can no longer participate in, so he just doesn't bother. Or, it could be because of his own short-lived attempt at giving this a try, Dave never really warmed up to those that went to college. Although I wasn't exactly a magnum caum laude, I was still enrolled as a college student at the time I was hurt, and this might've changed Dave's perspective of me.

Nah, Dave's a lot deeper than that. Maybe he thinks he'd be bothering me if he were to come by the house. If he has a vision of what I'm like based on the fictitious images depicted on T.V. of those that have had a brain injury—I know he didn't read any books about it—he could be a little leery of being within close proximity of me, thinking I might try to sink a knife into him. I guess I could give him a call and just talk to him over the phone, letting him know I'm not a brain injury-induced sociopath that has no sense about things. I think a person who has been injured contacting a friend for a potential visit is just something that isn't done and isn't exactly appropriate. No, Dave will come when he's good and ready. Chances are he'll be popping in here next weekend to tell me what the holdup has been.

Sundays are so depressing now. Leaving home and bidding farewell to my parents as Harmarville's visiting hours end is a not-so-subtle reminder of what has happened to me. Being alone at the rehab, miles away from my friends and the surroundings I've come to know as home made this Harmarville experience feel as if I have been indicted and convicted of a crime I did not commit and this is my sentence. It's when I start wishing I would have gotten the death penalty that I start doing my wheelchair laps out in the main corridor to distract me from this thinking.

Pushing my balance chair towards Unit 2, I started reflecting about the events of the weekend. People that really care are those that'll put their own lives aside to make someone who has had a kiss with tragedy feel a little more comfortable.

Ug and his lovely wife have been with me from the beginning and, without their support, things could not have fallen into place as they have to this point. Kevin and his family have been in my corner through this whole ordeal and without people like the Brezinski's rooting for me, this climb I'm making to attain some degree of normalcy would be steeper than it needs to be.

People like Frank McNamara, Craig Johnson, Angelo Alberta, Brian Day, and Danny Hobbs are my real friends and would do what they could to make things easier for me and my family. Despite the reservations, I know deep in my heart that Dave McClellan fits into the "true friend" category as well, which makes what's going on with him that much more confusing and hurtful.

This "awakening" has allowed me to see that those I partied with were people who really didn't give a shit about anything other than having a good time. Misery enjoys company and the more on board the party bandwagon, the merrier. I could be reasonably sure that the "party crowd" thought that it was a misfortune what happened to me, but sometimes shit happens when you're just trying to cut loose. I know nobody was glad when they heard I was hurt, but I don't think that's a definition of "friendship."

With this "awakening," I now see that they don't care. I was not the happiest of campers before the accident, but to get involved with who I did to find some joy is something I will suffer from for the rest of my life. People who love and/or care about me are also paying for this mistake. I never thought being wrong could be so costly or hurt so bad.

I still need an incredible amount of work on the basics, that goes without saying, but this Monday—May 24th—my therapists had their eyes on the future. To ensure the patient's program corresponds with their progress, Utilization Review meetings are held every two weeks on each patient —several people at a time— where the therapists of each discipline and various members of the medical personnel discuss progress and forthcoming interventions/treatments. Because of the advances in my ability to print these past few weeks and subtle improvement in my hand, Harmarville's staff didn't want the progress to stop there, so they decided at this conference to make some drastic revisions.

With the idea of me returning as a Journalism major, which is what I'm still hoping I can pursue, I took an Initial Vocational Evaluation aptitude test Friday in the Vocational Department upstairs to see just how feasible this might be someday. The results were in on Monday and they were, to say the least, less than ideal.

To ascertain the likelihood I could continue to pursue a writing career if I'd ever return to W.V.U., I was administered an information questionnaire which I would have to jot down my achievements and interests to see what careers I have a potential for. Because of my difficulty writing, I had to have my vocational evaluator fill this out for me. Good start. I guess my desire to be a journalist can be ruled out at this time. "Let's go-oooooooo, Mountaineers!"

Vocationally, along the same line of thought, Occupational Therapy started to work with me on the fine motor skills that will be involved, if I'm to pursue this journalism career aspiration. My long, skinny fingers are perfect, not only for playing guitar, but when I want to nail those typewriter keys. Excuse me if I brag, being that this was one of the only classes I did really well in during high school,

I'm going to elaborate on my typing class performance. Out of about thirty to thirty-five students in my typing class, I was THE best. Numero Uno. Head of the Class. Valedictorian of the home row keys.

I knew that being a productive, efficient journalist, one has to type effectively, so I really put forth the effort to be good at this. In OT, Wendy had me working on the typewriter because she knew I'd have to be proficient with this tool of the trade, if I were ever to return as a journalism student and I might as well get started pecking those keys. Like water dripping from a leaking faucet, a letter was being hammered on that paper about every ten seconds. Good grief.

When I first sat down, I was intimidated because I used to be so good at getting those letters and words stamped on paper, and now I can't even remember where the letters are. Why aren't they just in alphabetical order? I guess that would be too easy.

In time, however, after looking down at the keyboard, the arrangement of the letters started to look vaguely familiar. After initially being hazy in my memory, I soon realized that the home row keys were still where they had been before and I recognized the other letters hadn't gone anywhere since I first started learning how to type. But now, because of my bad right hand and my missing memory as to how the various keys should be fingered and struck, there was no way I could type other than to use my left index finger and scan the keys row by row to find where the different letters were. When I got going, those type bars weren't exactly fluttering.

After the OT session ended—with Wendy trying to cover several yawns—I typed between three to four readable sentences in thirty-five minutes with an abundance of errors, apparently caused by my uncoordination rather than my limb apraxia.

It's lost abilities such as this one which makes Occupational Therapy so difficult to handle at times and really gets the agitation brewing. If at all possible, OT is geared for righting wrongs, but sometimes this gets to be so trying on the emotions because the task being attempted is one any four-year-old can do with ease or something that was once done automatically. Being eighteen-years-old and not being able to tie your shoes quickly without help, for example, would make anyone with a little bit of pride boil.

With my typing like it is, I guess working for a newspaper isn't an option. I couldn't keep a deadline and it would take me a week to write a daily column. With a head injury, even skills once mastered are not immune from being deleted.

Chugging along in PT with either a therapist and/or an aide by my side and scratching out mistaken letter after mistaken letter as a cognitive therapist looked on, it was more of the same aggravation I've been dealing with for what seems a lifetime. Although Wendy and my other Occupational Therapists try to make the exercises as diverse as possible so I won't lose interest, there's only so many ways you can stretch a ball of putty.

In Communication Skills, if it wasn't the California Phonics Survey, it was some other test I'd be taking which would make me feel—well—like I've had a head injury. In Psych, if it wasn't putting blocks together or pairing funny shaped designs that I'll never see again in my life, I was asked to arrange some cartoon strips. It's a wonder I haven't had a recurring nightmare where a man-eating octagon or an axe-wielding Dennis the Menace has been running after me trying to "get me" since I've been seeing Mrs. Joy for Psychology.

Like a broken record, the three words I hear all the time in PT are "Don't," "Straighten," and "Lean." Many nights, I'm surprised that I haven't awakened from a sound sleep only to find myself in a pool of cold sweat, believing that I had just heard those very words barked at me. "You don't want to lean so far to the left, straighten up!" "Don't drag that foot! If you'd keep your hips forward, stop leaning, and straighten your back, you'd walk better. Now, I don't want to have to say it again." Never having been enlisted, I obviously couldn't say for sure, but PT can't be too much different than basic training.

I wonder if I'll ever wake up in the middle of the night thinking that I am being strangled or smothered. I can imagine a dream where the therapy putty I work with so much in OT had transformed into a boa constrictor which would wrap itself around me and choke me of my last breath. Or, a shirt I practice buttoning in my ADL training ends up getting tossed over my head by someone who wants to "do away with me" and gets squeezed tight, so I can't get any air.

Because I've done these therapeutic interventions over and over again in program, it's a wonder they're not part of my subconscious. Practice, repetition. Repetition and practice. That's what brain injury rehabilitation therapy is all about. I can't tell you how many times I've thought, "Oh no! Not this again," when told to undertake a particular movement or exercise. For the most part, being that the majority of the training is nothing new, I'll need the patience of Job to get through this. Been there, done that, here we go again.

If Thursdays get me down a little bit now because I'm alone, all I've got to do for a "pick-me-up" is tell myself why it's this way now. During the workweek, visitors are permitted in the rehab Tuesdays, Thursdays, and Fridays after program. Since I've started to go home on weekends, I told mom and dad not to bother coming on Thursdays anymore. Dad's put close to 10,000 miles on the Citation since I've been at Allegheny General and Harmarville, and I know they need a much deserved break from the rigors of travel.

Knowing how they think, I'm sure that they're both worried and relieved. I can just picture mom sitting in the living room biting her nails because she hasn't seen her boy for three whole days and wondering if I need anything. Because he usually finds something to repair when he comes in, dad's probably going to be concerned whether my wheelchair or bed need some adjustments only his trusty wrench can correct.

I know they're going to have their reservations about not seeing me every opportunity they can, but deep inside, I'm confident they're happy as can be that I've improved to the extent that I'm not so dependent on them for everything, everyday, and have shown that I can cope on my own a little bit. Besides, it'll give dad some extra time to work on the project he's started on my behalf, and mom the added opportunity to continue her correspondence to our insurance carrier.

I'm definitely missing them, but because I love them with all my heart, I owe it to them to do what I can, so they get a little break from all this. With the long Memorial Day weekend starting tomorrow, we'll have plenty of time to get at each other's throat.

Primarily, Memorial Day is reserved for those who have died and once defended our country in battle; soldiers are paid tribute and remembered for their heroics. Over the years, it has evolved into a day where family members recognize the passing of a loved one. Words alone could not possibly describe how my parents were feeling that their youngest was spared from being only a memory. And it is for this reason that Memorial Day 1982 will be remembered as the one that was not being acknowledged by honoring a family member who left before his time.

Because of the perfect way they have handled everything in the face of this adversity, I am convinced that—bar none—my parents are the greatest ones who ever lived. I guess this proclamation could be considered a bit biased, but one thing that is not subject to scrutiny is that a family can play such a vital role in a patient's recovery—or lack of. Dad has commented on several occasions how he feels bad that some patients are always by themselves, never getting any visitors, and always appearing to be so sad. Families who are involved with their loved one, or at least show some interest in their afflicted member's progress, can do so much to enhance the rejuvenation process. Maybe not physically, but a family can do more for the healing of the emotions than any kind of medication. In this regard, my family has been absolutely spectacular.

Mom and dad have given me support when support was what was needed, but what's more impressive is that—as difficult as this was for them—they've gotten out of they way and backed off when getting out of the way and backing off were needed. In my book, they're tops.

This "awakening" has allowed me to see that when things really counted, they came through in their customary fashion. Looking back, I am ashamed of some of the things that I thought and did before all this happened. When it truly mattered, they pulled through and gave me everything they had, everything humanly possible. I don't deserve them.

Feeling as if my diligent effort should reap equally productive rewards and my wanting this control, I got really agitated today—Saturday, May 29th—when I saw no improvement in my vision. Seeing two distinct fingers coming in towards my nose when only one should be seen, I really got steamed because I've done this finger to nose exercise at least a thousand times now and my vision is as bad as it was before I started doing this.

I feel for my parents because they're the ones who hear me bitch about things that have been bothering me all week. Because Harmarville doesn't have the expenditures to employ a Psychotherapist, so much stuff builds up inside of me I've just got to regurgitate to someone what's eating at me.

With some symptoms—depending on the location of the brain damage and the pathways disturbed—I know that no matter how much I put into it, no improvement is going to occur, for the area of the brain effected is just too extensive. I haven't had any improvement with my vision despite all that I've done. With a head injury, nothing is a guarantee, for one is frequently at the mercy of how much that brain decides to heal. Progress isn't a given, as luck deals the cards all too often. Maybe I'm not only working like a fool, but being one too, for I'm still playing for that Royal Flush. Go ahead and deal them cards, don't let me stop you; I've got some walking to do.

I suspect my assessent about him was off-target. After I got done walking out in the garage alongside dad—leaving my wheelchair behind like Harmarville said I could, and while I was practicing standing up from a sitting position—Sam's partner in crime, Claude, came over to spend some time with me. Apparently, I must not have read him accurately, for Claude was talking to me like a well-developed young man and kidding around with me like we've always been the best of pals. We just had a good ole time doing nothing but enjoying each other's company and enlightening one another with our diverse, unique qualities which developed us as individuals.

Claude strummed my guitar for me as I fingered the chords, and we reminisced about the neighborhood gang getting together for football and softball games all the time. Me and Claude had always gotten along well enough, but I never knew he was such a great guy. He showed me a compassionate and empathetic side of him I never saw before and didn't know he had. Always believing Claude wanted to be seen as someone a little rough around the edges, I feel guilty now that I never gave him much of a chance to prove just how genuine a fellow he could be.

Because a fair share of the people Claude was friends with could be on the hoodlum side, I wasn't exactly sure what to think of him. But people change and it looks like I almost missed out on getting to know such a kind and considerate guy such as Claude. I got me a good buddy now.

Claude will be graduating from high school shortly, and wanted to know what college was like, for he would be going to school up north in the fall to catch the academic world on fire and wanted to get an idea of what to expect. When I told him that I couldn't remember anything about my freshman year in college and that my memory was largely blank about everything, this seemed to open a can of worms.

When I asked him, Claude said he wasn't at the party, but he was mighty interested what I could remember about it, though. In a casual, non-chalant manner, my new chum quizzed me whether or not I remembered anything about the party or about any of the stuff that occurred surrounding this event. I told him I couldn't recall anything prior, during, or following this extravaganza. As smoothly as he introduced this topic, he slithered into another one.

Because this is something that doesn't get discussed outside of the family, I was more than a little surprised when Claude uttered the three-letter word which leaves a hollow kind of sensation in the pit of one's gut. When he asked me if we were going to "sue" anybody, I told him nothing was being planned at this moment; that any type of suit is not currently being considered. But since we've become such good friends and he's trying so hard to win over my confidence, I felt compelled to tell him I didn't know right now, but that this could be a possibility somewhere along the line.

Switching directions, taking an interest in my various symptoms and listening intently to anything I had to say, Claude then helped me with the writing exercise I was engaged in and was telling me how the different letters are formed. A swell guy whom I had no idea was so understanding, Claude looks like he wants to be a respected confidante.

I don't know if it's a kind of morbid curiosity where he was waiting to see if anything thrilling happens with someone who's injured their brain, but Claude stuck around for quite a while being pleasant as can be and taking an interest in me that was second to none. I saw Claude like I'd never seen him before. Not realizing the degree to which Claude was so humane, I feel bad. Maybe it's a case where I simply didn't appreciate how much he thought of me. Yet, I wonder. . . . .

Because you couldn't be sure from one minute to the next what his mood was going to be, I had always assumed it was tough being friends with Claude. Depending on who he was around at any given time, you were rolling the dice whether he was going to be affable or anything but. Maybe it's a case where I didn't realize how much he regarded me. Yet, I wonder. . . . .

I'm sure he went somewhere for the long weekend. Why else wouldn't he have stopped? Although the numbers have dwindled significantly since that first weekend I was home, there's still a pretty good flow of people dropping by to see how I'm doing. I mean it's a sure thing that Ug and his lovely wife are going to visit a couple hours everyday I'm home. After he's done working at the store, Kevin always makes it a point to come over. And Sunday, Kevin brought his parents and sister. Frank and Brian didn't come over because they were away, but my cabin-building pal, Craig, stopped for a few hours this holiday. And then there was Claude. . . . .

Dave didn't make it over again. I guess the time has come where I shouldn't be expecting him. I don't know what to make of his not seeing me. Could Dave be trying to tell me something? If he is, what point is he trying to get across?

I can't remember the last time I've seen Dave or talked to him, but I don't think we had any kind of argument or anything. Unless you call him out of bounds when he wasn't, or "out" at first base when he was safe, Dave's one of those guys who doesn't have a disagreeable bone in his body.

I'm probably just being paranoid; there's surely a very logical, understanding reason why he hasn't gotten around to seeing me. Next weekend, I'll probably see Dave's souped up car whipping in our driveway and him popping out apologizing for not coming sooner, but other things needed to be taken care of first. But I'm not counting on it.

Hand over hand, I was turning that steering wheel. Accelerating and touching the brake, the car was moving pretty good and slowing down. I was doing okay. At least the car never went off the road or went into another telephone pole. Then again, if we had changed places and I was the one driving and dad was doing the simulating, more than likely, Life Flight would be making a return trip to Washington. But instead of one Meyers aboard, there'd be three of us.

Feeling sorry for me, dad wanted me to start practicing the motions of driving a car in order that I can develop again the eye/hand coordination, concentration, and attention needed to drive. If I was going to drive before the age of forty, I might as well see if I can physically undertake the movements necessary when operating a vehicle.

Physically, I may have been barely capable to steer that phantom wheel and apply some mythical brakes, but with my current psychological state, it would be unlikely I could travel any distance—safely. Having perseveration and maneuvering an automobile is not a match made in heaven. I could picture a scene where I'm stopped at a red light—and for no reason—my brain tells my right foot to stomp on the accelerator to get going, no matter how many cars or people are in the intersection.

If dad thought he had it bad a little over two years ago when I was starting to drive, he's really got his hands full now. Not only can't he be sure what my brain is perceiving, but whether or not it will remain calm/seizure-free while I'm behind the wheel. If those brain waves decide it's time to act up and I have a convulsion while I'm driving, that car's going to lose control and end up wherever, into whomever. Because of my current physical limitations and various aphasias, obviously driving isn't even a remote possibility at this time. Shaking, preparing me for that day if and when I am ever given the "go ahead" to drive, dad had me operating these imaginary controls as we headed back to Harmarville.

Where did the weekend go? This extra day off was just what the doctor ordered. Being home an additional twenty-four hours fired me up to really give it my all in therapy this week. Normally, I'm really down in the mouth on these return trips back to Harmarville, but this time I'm itchin' to get down and dirty. If I knew what lie ahead, I may not have been so eager.

Imagine a chain saw grinding into your hip. The spinning metal rips into the top part of your leg with a thunderous fury, as bone chips and flesh spray within the bloody mass that was once a leg. Arteries and veins are being tugged, pulled, twisted, and torn beyond the threshold of tolerance. You grasp the leg because it feels as if it will detach itself from your body, if you don't. This is how my leg feels when I lift my right leg up any distance, and now I'm going to practice climbing the stairs off the main corridor in PT. Lord, please have mercy.

Trying to ignore the tremendous, severing pain in my right leg will be virtually impossible, for that rod stabs me with an incredible biting force. The agonizing pain of that titanium metal clawing at my leg is a reminder that the bone was once shredded into splintery fragments. Tearing at my emotions with an equally devastating stranglehold was that I actually had forgotten the motor movements required to go up a flight of stairs. It's bad enough that amnesia forces me to relearn almost everything, but on top of all this, when physical misery prohibits me from doing things, that's a double whammy I've got to contend with. And then there's the triple curse against me which is the psychological aspect that's part of the retraining process.

Preparing for the ascent, I clutched the handrail along the right side of this stairway with my bad hand. These steps, looking like a mountainside to me, were a menacing opponent. I could picture myself tumbling backwards down these flight of stairs because my sparse coordination had abandoned me. Neck bent, the weight of my body pushes my head into the hard, metal steps as I do backflip after backflip down the stairs. Mouths open, Jan and Mary descend the staircase as I was falling back, trying to stop this out-of-control backspin. I could feel my warm blood splashing onto my face as I see the ceiling, light fixture, my feet, ceiling, light fixture, my feet, flashing before me as I roll backwards. My distorted vision makes what I am perceiving that much more treacherous.

Twirling violently, my head crackles and snaps back like a branch that's been popped in half. Entire body aching, a sick surge goes ripping into and through my gut. Hearing the twisting of bone and snapping of tendon, my spine recoils from the crushing pressure of my lower torso.

"All right," Jan said breaking my trance, "here's what you got to do to get started." Having a vivid imagination isn't all that good when you're within the grasp of the perils of PT.

Watching Jan model what I needed to do to ascend these steps, one at a time, the anxiety built up within me. I could almost feel the rod knife into me seeing my therapist elevate her right foot on the step, putting all her weight on her right leg, as she hoisted her left leg up to that same step. Ready or not, it was my turn now.

Reaching over with my left hand, I spread the fingers of my spastic right paw and grabbed hold of the right handrail. Heart racing, I know the moment's here for me to tackle this challenge head-on. Looking up, I never thought a stairway could be so intimidating. Looking down, I knew I was in for some heartsickening pain, but I have to get that out of mind and concentrate on what I'm doing, for my brain needs to be taught again how to do this.

Inching my right foot up to the step, I was positioning myself to confront this threat. Putting out of my conscious the vision of me falling back uncontrollably, I replaced this with how I know I'm going to feel once I reach the landing and prevailed over this psychological barrier.

Getting that electrifying tingle in your chest when adrenalin spews throughout one's body, my stomach was churning and I could feel the hair on my back standing. Taking one last breath, I was ready to go when—- laughter filled the stairwell and a heavy door went clanging shut. It wasn't Jan beside me or Mary behind me doing the cackling, rather, some therapists from upstairs coming down. Talk about shitty timing, but Harmarville's a busy place.

After seeing what they interrupted, these workers apologized and went about their merry way. Trying to psyche myself out again, two films started playing interchangeably in my mind. One, after doing my backwards somersault down these flight of steps, my face and eyes had swollen like Rocky Balboa's after his title fight. And the other, I was hopping around like him after he won his bout. Feeling like a kamikaze pilot must before his fateful dive, I sucked it up knowing that rod would be digging into my leg through the bone that was sliced into pieces and bent my knee, lifting my lower leg up.

With that rod piercing into my thigh, the suffering was of intolerable proportions and the hurt was inhumane. Although I didn't do this, it felt like I broke my leg again. It was as if the femur was no longer a bone, but a bayonet which ripped into me, as if I were the enemy. Though there's nothing wrong with this, I wasn't about to let the tears roll from my eyes like they wanted in front of my physical terrorists. With my right foot on the step, I immediately pushed off with my left foot, so I'd be able to help my bad leg support my weight.

While I hoisted my left leg up onto the step, all my weight was supported by a right leg that was once held together only by a pin sunk deep within my femur. It was only a second at the most that I did this balancing act, but when it feels like a 16-penny nail is being hammered into your bone, the pain can't end quickly enough. Tick, tick, tick, tick, tick.

Bearing all my weight on this fragile limb, the pain exceeded being excruciating. The ache which exploded within my leg was intense, but my stubborn male pride prevented me from conceding how badly I was hurting. Noting the grimace on my face and my short deliberate breaths, Jan knew I was in misery and gave me a couple of much-needed seconds to collect myself, before I attempted the next hurdle. Jan, you're too kind.

I actually wish my leg had fallen off, so that I wouldn't have to endure the imminent torture when attempting the next step. When I'm standing solely on my right leg as I'm lifting my left, it feels as if someone has taken a sharp hook and jammed it in the side of my bum limb, ripping all that gets in its way.

Clinging onto the rail with my right hand and my left ready to spring into action, I bent the lower portion of my aching leg up again and—dragging my foot over the top of the step—put my hoof on the next tier up as quickly as my tormented mind would allow me. In-between steps when I'm putting all my pounds on the right leg that was fractured, it feels like the bone is being pulled out from my leg. I can actually feel that there is something in the bone of my leg, and when the rod clicks within the top of my hip, I sense that it has protruded outside of the bone.

This steel shaft helping to hold my leg together, it just sticks out enough to catch my thigh, making this one incredibly miserable sensation. Scraping the inner part of my leg, it feels like my hip is being devoured from the inside out. I know I need to be thankful I've got a leg, but when you're in the midst of agony, it's tough to be grateful for anything.

As I drag my right foot over top of the second step up, the area around the bone in my leg was throbbing. Sore from this mountain-climbing of one and one-half steps, I quickly pulled myself up with my left arm which was hanging on to the left rail for dear life. Sliding my foot atop the step, I was perched one level higher.

Scared to death, I never thought going up a few steps could be such an expedition of will, courage, and fear all wrapped into one. Afraid that it might just get in the way, I abandoned using my right hand for this stair climbing excursion and focused on utilizing the strength of my good left arm and hand to get me through the rest of this nightmare.

W.V.U. students aren't called "Mountaineers" for nothing. Because of where the different campuses are situated, there are many hillsides to climb in Morgantown just to get to class. And where there are hills, there are steps. To think I climbed thousands of these over the course of a semester and now I can't even go up one flight of stairs is representative of just how much a brain injury can take from someone.

Going back to school seems so impossible, but I can't worry about that right now because I've got to practice going down these steps. I've learned that, with a head injury, setting long-term goals is not realistically possible; that the short-term variety is all one can really go for. With the hope that the accumulation of these tiny triumphs will allow one to broaden their scope of aspirations, a patient having sustained a brain contusion will just have to dust themselves off until they get it right. This is symbolic of what I'm doing at this very moment: taking this rehabilitation one step at a time. "Let's go-ooooooo, Mountaineers!"

Like a potter at his wheel forming a vase, Jan and Mary twirled me around carefully, watching for any sign that their project may collapse. Spinning not quite the speed of a top, after one revolution, I was preparing to descend these babies. Hopefully, one step at a time and not in one fell swoop.

Clutching onto that left handrail with all my might, I felt as if I was dangling from the ledge of a window on the top floor of the U.S. Steel Building because the foot of these stairs seems so far down from where I was. I looked down at all those steel steps thinking how badly it would hurt, if I were to to tumble forward and catch my head on each one of these.

Eye ripping from its socket and the knee of my once broken leg hyperextending back, I could see my shoulders bouncing off one side of the wall to the other, as I try to break my stinging fall. Ricocheting off one wall towards the next, bruised and battered, my immobile right arm gets caught between my body and the titanium handrail. I finally stop when there is nowhere else to go and my head slams against the iron wall. Flipping forward, my shocked body penetrates this mass of metal with a puncturing force. Tension not forgiving, the pathos would be overwhelming.

"Take it slow," Jan cautioned freeing me from the image which I was choking, "me and Mary will be right here, if you need us."

Using the psychology which comes so naturally to her, Jan said, "You'll be doing just fine Craig, we'll probably just get in the way. Remember, right foot first." Well, here goes.

Knowing that this would mean I would be in for a not-too-gentle landing, I tried not to stoop too far forward. Applying pressure to my lumbar, Jan used the heel of her hand as a prod to remind me to keep my back straight. Flat-footed, I abruptly smacked my right foot down on the top step. Because I've learned to support the majority of my weight with my left arm, the twinge in my right leg wasn't quite as bad as when I went up, but it was still there. Lowering myself slowly, I got down to the next step when—you guessed it —someone needed to go upstairs.

Someone could have dropped killer bees at my feet and I wouldn't have let go of this safety rail. Clutching the handrail as tightly as I could with my left hand, head down carefully watching every tiny step I took along this narrow stair, I sort of towed my body towards the wall. Frozen from fear, I wasn't about to move so, inconveniencing her or not, that nurse with the firm buttocks is just going to have to change lanes and get out of my way 'cause I ain't going nowhere. Knowing what my view would be, where was she when I was heading "up" the stairs? Talk about incentive. At least my head being injured didn't do anything to those pubescent pleasure urges.

"C'mon Mr. Testosterone," Jan growled annoyingly, breaking me from yet another fantasy after this goddess had gotten out of the way and the door slammed behind her, "get your mind back on what you were doing. You don't want to spend all night here, do you?"

"Depends if she comes back," I answered.

Timing her placement perfectly, Jan poked me with her fist in my lower back again, so I wouldn't slouch and to get my mind out of lustland. Cut me a break, I'm only eighteen and I'm at my peak. I've never seen so many beautiful females gathered in one place before and this really hits home how much I've been deprived. I hope I don't slip in my saliva.

With my back now rigid too, I carefully placed my right hoof down as smoothly as I could. I rely a lot on my functional left arm to support and balance me while I'm going down the step, but I still can't make the placement of my right leg any smoother, as I kind of vibrate after I land. Admittedly, being scared plays a role in my not standing on one leg long enough, for I have a difficult time sensing where I'm at in relation to the things around me and the gravitational pull yanking me down just seems so powerful. It isn't very comforting when it feels as if you may lose your balance and go down for the count.

I kind of wish I wasn't told now that my femur was broken because, if it wasn't for that damn rod gnawing at my leg, I would not know anything happened to it. Realizing how badly my leg was broken and that I almost lost it, however, I'm very leery about having it support any of my weight. If I want to progress, that's a fear I'll just have to get over by telling myself that things'll work out for the best.

Because of trauma-induced decalcification, I imagine a scene where I place weight on my right leg, but it can't support me and the bone snaps again, protruding from my hemorrhaging hip. Twisted with terror and pain from what this compound fracture has done to me, I plead with God to stop the agony, as the fiery red blood streams down my leg.

However, realizing the importance of relearning how to ascend and descend steps, I have to block this horror flick from my mind and go about the business of getting down these steps. Although I know he'd do this without complaint, if it was his only recourse, I don't think dad would be real keen on the idea of buying a ranch house because I never learned how to do steps again. Showing his confidence in me, even before I started this step-climbing adventure, dad had started planning to install handrails along the two flights of stairs in our house and a metal banister down to the basement. With this encouragement and my not wanting to take a "handicap" elevator everywhere I go—if one's available, I'm just going to have to take what my leg's going to "dish out" and make the best of it.

Jan guiding me like an emergency medical technician and Mary below me with her arms out/preparing to cushion a fall, didn't do a lot to ease the stress I was feeling, but I'm definitely glad they're here, just in case. Rehabilitation—I just love it.

Going from point "A" to point "B" is not always a flat endeavor. Getting to point "B" usually has ditches to climb out of and hills to get over if one has a disability. My right leg didn't feel too good after this stair practice, but I felt a proud sense of accomplishment about what I just did. What this means for my future takes away some of this ache. Someone who's never been seriously hurt neurologically or physically probably would have trouble understanding what the big deal's about; just grab the rail and go up the steps. But my mind and body aren't quite ready to do that yet.

After Mary walked me out to the PT gym where I was resting in my wheelchair, someone from the Education Department approached me, telling me that I had to get going because the camera was ready to roll and that I was going to be in another video. When I said I hadn't practiced walking with my aide around the gym yet, apparently that wasn't as important as the cameraman's schedule, for I was told to leave at once. Last month, light bulbs flashed in my face for Harmarville's monthly newsletter while I was in Psych, now this again. It only takes one quick look at me to tell I'm not a model, but a patient. Oh well, I guess I don't have my priorities straight.

Revised treatment plan or bust, the emphasis this week in Communication Skills and Psychology has been on building my vocabulary, so that I may resume my educational pursuits someday. Surprise, surprise, in these therapies I worked on a variety of expressive language exercises. With remedial treatments designed to reprogram the brain, one too many times is still not enough.

Using the various "Apple Computer" programs to develop not only accuracy, but speed, I was engaged in several problem-solving activities again this week in Communication Skills. Far from a wunderkind, I was showing steady progress with my speech and writing. Also, Diane tested my reading comprehension to determine just how much I was improving with this facet of my program. To say that I wasn't ready to read "War and Peace" yet, would be an understatement.

Whoops! I didn't want to do that. Not nearly as often, but my hand still has a mind of its own sometimes when I try to print, as it will go this way when I should have made it go that way. Without any kind of cue, I was having a little tougher "go at it," but I was getting better at forcing my left hand to print what I had intended. And the mind which tells my hand where to go is getting clearer reception on its monitors how the letters are structured.

I don't know how they do it, but whoever came up with the saying "Patience is a virtue," must have had the cognitive therapists who work with me on my writing in mind. Surely, wanting to twittle their thumbs and/or pull out their hair on those occasions when my brain was being stubborn, those in the Communication Skills and Psychology departments not "giving in" has gratefully made this printing practice an experience of operant conditioning.

Chink——Chink——————Chink————Chink————Chink————Chink. In Occupational Therapy, away I was jabbing at those keys on the typewriter in preparation for a scholastic venture into the world of journalism, if my bruised brain ever permits. The effort I'm putting into my therapies now is extremely difficult for me emotionally because, like when I first entered college right out of high school, I have some reservations about pursuing this journalism career. One's heart really has to be in this profession to be proficient at it. From a professional and personal frame of reference, this can be a very rewarding career for some. However, even when I was intellectually and physically capable, I was far from being certain that this was what I really wanted to do. Now, it looks like I'll be working like a dog just to be barely efficient at something I can't say for sure is worth the blood and sweat I'll be putting into it. And it's very questionable whether or not I'll ever attain the physical and mental capacities again to pursue this vocational choice. Chink—Chink.

How one goes about approaching a rehabilitation dilemma can be the single most influential factor which determines how things will turn out. In many, if not most cases, attitude is everything. For some, it's not going to make the least bit of difference how things are looked at, for there are many afflictions which one doesn't have any control. Those who do have a say, however, but do nothing except give up and stick their tail between their legs, are not going to achieve anything. My outlook and desire about this journalism endeavor very much in flux, the prognosis for achievement within this realm does not hold much promise.

If it wasn't bad enough my existing therapies were gearing their interventions toward this "supposed" journalism aspiration, an additional program was being put in my schedule to help me achieve this goal that I have always had serious doubts about. With this new plan of treatment structured in such a way that I'm being pushed to select a career, I unfortunately can sense how I felt entering college again. This being an atom for my current predicament, the feeling I'm currently experiencing is one I'd rather remain lost in my brain's contused conscious.

I don't know, I guess I should be thankful. Only those who have shown some kind of potential get this far. I guess Harmarville wouldn't include this program, if they didn't think I would benefit from it. Maybe they see something I don't. I still think they're rushing things a little, though. But I trust that they know best. For the most part, they have so far.

Maybe this accident somehow was supposed to happen in order that I wake up and smell the coffee, so that I can make some realistic decisions as they pertain to my future. Most everything I've ever wanted to do career-wise and interest-wise has been physical in nature, but now it looks like I'm going to have to develop the academic potential that I've always seemed to have. The writing's on the wall that I'm going to have difficulty undertaking even the most routine of physical activities, let alone excel at something where the body must respond in some heightened fashion. I'm not exactly a diamond in the rough, but if luck continues to be good to me, someday I just may be able to shoot for "Joe Average" status. Considering what's happened to me, I suppose this is terrific and I should take a bow, if I'm ever able to attain this.

For a few things, it's been characteristic of me to buck at change, as I will occasionally oppose adjustment if I don't feel it's advantageous to modify things. I know they want their patients to go as far as they can, but I think Harmarville's getting a little carried away with this newest treatment approach with me. Hell, I can't write yet, I can barely move, and my brain still doesn't know what to make of things, and now they're trying to tell me I need to start thinking about a career.

"Vocational" is the component of one's rehabilitation program which attempts to prepare the patient for the work world. This program ascertains how the injured person's limitations may impede them from doing a productive job and what, if any, accommodations may be needed to assure a fruitful work performance. Not only are past achievements, abilities, and interests considered when taking into account what jobs may be appropriate for a person with a disability, but what they are no longer capable of doing efficiently. Whether it's white or blue collar, the training provided the one in this vocational track is individualized to meet their specific needs. But before services can be tailored for the patient, an assessment needs administered, so a baseline of these interests, aptitudes, and achievements can be drawn. After this general information is gathered, the evaluator can outline different training alternatives which should appeal to the patient. I think I know what's up the rehabilitation center's sleeve, they want me to do another video entitled, "From coma to college to career: The Harmarville Way!"

4+1=5. 7-3=4. 2 X 4 = 8. 15+. . . . .. Hey, no fair! That last problem has got a number with two digits in it. It isn't calculus, but it sure seems that way to me.

My Vocational Counselor, Donna Sebastian, Voc Ed., started me on some prevocational activities, so she could get an idea of what she was working with. Verbally completing the Interest Inventory wasn't tough because this is merely a personal preference survey/questionnaire which attempts to make a match between things that capture one's fancy and a job whose employees characteristically share the same interests. And based on these results, a list of work positions are provided which should correspond with the test-taker's personality.

The formula is a complicated one, taking into consideration different aspects of an individual's make-up by the choices they make. A question might be, for example, "What would you rather do on a Saturday afternoon? Go to an art museum and look at some paintings from the Baroque Period or listen to records on a stereo?" Duh, I'll stick to spinning Ted Nugent's "Cat Scratch Fever" album, thank you. Because of the timing of this inventory when limitations outnumber capabilities, I'm sure the results will show I'm either destined to ripping ticket stubs at a movie theater or be a roadie for a heavy metal band.

Nuclear Scientist? Mechanical Engineer? It would be a good idea if I could get out of my ten tables in Arithmetic before I'd consider these as a career option. Trying to figure out some basic problems (Classmate 88 Math) in Vocational, I was stinking up the place pretty good. The right side of my mind couldn't get a grasp of what numbers were supposed to represent and thought addition, subtraction, multiplication, and division were abstract concepts beyond the realm of understanding. At least this head injury didn't do anything to effect my ability to do mathematics.

Altogether now, "It's Howdy Doody time. It's Howdy Doody time. Let's give a rousing cheer. 'Cause Howdy Doody's here. It's Howdy Doody time. It's Howdy Doody time. It's time to start the show. So kids, let's go!!!!!!!" This last line was the cue for the little ones in the studio audience to go crazy with anticipation. I was going crazy too, but not from waiting for the show to begin.

Why am I wasting my time with this Recreational Therapy bullshit? This spittin' image of Howdy can sing alright, but she doesn't know how to play guitar. For some of the older folks who have had strokes or some of the recent admissions who have extensive damage to their brains yet, this might be some thing they'd enjoy. This should be an elective therapy, not something you're required to go to.

I must admit, I'm not putting much effort into trying to be jolly, but can I be blamed? This is the time I usually reserve for practicing my walking, writing, stretching, hand dexterity, eye exercise, foot tapping, etc. and I'm supposed to forgo these because I'm scheduled to attend a program where playing the card game, "Go Fish!" is of primary importance,

For me, this is time wasted just sitting here in the evening listening to this "professional" strum the acoustic guitar and croon to her heart's delight. How in God's name am I supposed to benefit from this? "RT" is the abbreviation for Recreational Therapy, but for me, it stands for Regression Therapy because it's taking time away from the things I need to work on. This must be the CEO's sister and she needs a job.

And I know this program has not been individualized because Howdy thought it would be fun if we all played with the crossword puzzle tonight. Only needing to glance at their medical records, I know someone who didn't do their homework.

If this "therapist" had done a little research on the people who were going to be throwing away their precious time with her, she'd have found out pretty damn quick that I have agraphia and can't fill out the blocks of a crossword puzzle because I can't write or print.

If this lady who looks like she just came off the set of a "Kukla, Fran, and Ollie" episode wasn't a member of the professional staff, thus not permitted access to the medical records, what the hell was Harmarville thinking, allowing someone like this work with patients who need the utmost in support/ care and don't need to have their already beaten psyches further trampled? I didn't want to come here in the first place; now this.

I've been through enough trauma these past couple of months, I don't need or deserve to be humiliated and laughed at having this aphasia exposed in front of all the other patients. My cognitive therapies are, for the most part, done on a one-on-one basis to preserve confidentiality. And this woman with too much rouge and the fakey, "Isn't life grand?" demeanor had me feeling shameful for something I couldn't help because she didn't prepare enough for her session.

The same ignorant patient who made an embarrassing ruckus when my wheelchair had been pushed in front of his in the lunch line my first day I was to eat in the cafeteria, was having a great time laughing at me as I sat there dumbfounded with pencil in hand, not able to print the letters I wanted. Because of the limited time staff has to eat before going back on duty, they have to cut in line during mealtime. Harmarville wanting to make this first experience not eating in the nurses' station as stress-free as possible, a nurse was assigned to accompany me in the dining room and didn't get at the end of the line because of these time constraints. Not seeing the nurse as the culprit of this "cutting in line" behavior, but the one who had no control over the situation—me—the vulgarities were flung my way by this West Virginian who was about my age and got his head whacked when the car he was in drove off an overpass following a wedding reception.

It doesn't feel real good when things outside of my control create an unpleasant situation, but you just have to keep in mind who it's coming from. A lot of these peoples' lives have been turned upside down and they have little sense how their actions affect others. Then again, there are some patients who were trash before being hurt and their particular disability has made them that much worse.

I know what the recreational "therapist" did wasn't intentional, but a patient has the right to expect such disgraceful accidents to be safeguarded against. I guess I just don't have my priorities straight again. Buffalo Bob wouldn't be proud.

Once again, no pain, no gain. Without a doubt, her outstanding efforts are definitely showing some dividends for me, but I still need to get away from her—the further, the better. Doing all that stair-climbing practice this week, my leg needed a weekend break from Jan.

I have improved so rapidly with my step-hiking that by the end of the week—Friday June 4th—I was going up and down those stairs with minimal assistance. Although I was using the rail to pull my weight down and up, Jan and Mary didn't have to trail me like a shadow anymore to keep me from going "down and out" because my balance/posture were improving and I was getting accustomed to the jabbing in my right leg.

I come to a standing position independently now and when I do get up, my orientation was getting better. Unsupported, my standing balance has improved significantly, as I am bearing a lot more weight on my right leg and my knee control/heel to toe action is increasing as well. Functionally, I roll, sit, and transfer on my own and—although my gait is improving—I still have to work on different areas of this, for my extension and stance are still not adequate. But hey, how much fun would rehab be then if there was nothing else to fix?

More of the same, same of the more. At it again, flexion, extension, abduction, supination, pronation, and every other exercise possible were the order of the week again in OT, as was what I was doing at the typewriter which could be classified as anything but typing. However, I was making some gains isolating motor control of my right arm/shoulder, as well as improving with my transfers, ability to stand, managing my wheelchair brakes with my paralytic hand, self-care activities, and elbow strength. But I need an incredible amount of work yet, before I could even hope to isolate the movements of my wrist or hand.

Right now, with the way my right-handed fingers feel and are responding, I'll just have to be happy with the small increments of improvement that may occur and any heightened performance of a fine motor skill which could develop. I do think my right-upper extremities are getting better, but the progress is so gradual, I could climb the walls.

Because one uses their hands for practically everything, any disturbance with its ability to function properly is torture, especially if the dominant hand is the one not working as it should. But to go from what it was a few months ago when my hand was in a fist contracted under my chin with the fingers curled in a tight ball, to what it is like now, is nothing short of amazing. I just have to remind myself of this next time I am feeling blue about not being able to stretch that putty like I want. Same of the more?

I'm feeling ecstatic because I can sense a lot of things are coming around—even mom and dad were around the corner. After someone's had a severe head injury, they're in a daze not knowing what's going on. Not certain whether or not this is how life is going to be from here on out, when functions return you couldn't be certain you'd ever see again and/or your thinking clears to the point where some sense of things can be made, no feeling could be more dynamic.

Rightfully so, some things are just taken for granted and are expected to work properly like one's physical and mental capacities. But if something happens and these abilities are taken away, devastation will want to overtake the person. An equally powerful feeling of exuberance occurs as well upon the reappearance of abilities and a new appreciation of basic motor skills/cognitive functioning develops because they've been missed so much. The four-day therapy week having just ended, I was overflowing with joy as it was, but watching my folks making their way down was topping on the cake.

It was literally awesome seeing my parents walking down the hallway this Friday because this was the first time I had seen them this week. My Grandma Barnhart is in a nursing home near Youngstown, Ohio now and my parents had to head off to Johnstown to get her some clothes, so they didn't have the opportunity to get down here this week for a visit. Because last weekend was a long one, they figured this extra time together would carry over into the week and we could carry on. They were right, we survived. And it might have even done us a little bit of good that we could separate for a time.

Before I met mom and dad for the weekend trip home, I was talking to two newer admissions who were having some troubles adjusting to this rehabilitation business and accepting all that's happened to them. Knowing that we approximate each other in age, are enduring many of the same types of symptoms, and I suppose because I've made some good progress and can express myself pretty well, nursing staff thought it would be beneficial for these guys and their families if I would talk to them about things. Being in the same fraternity of sorts, they really wanted to hear what I had to say.

Although there's still much therapeutic work to be done on my part, I can imagine the hope these patients and their loved ones must be feeling knowing how I once had similar difficulties as they do now and was able to overcome them. It can't be stressed enough how vital it is to talk with someone when things get to be too much. Rehabilitation professionals who learned their trade through the reading of books and witnessing other peoples' grief can be very knowledgeable about the impact disability has on a patient and those around them. Discovering someone who is not only intellectually competent, but has personal experience coping with the trauma and humility of disability/rehabilitation can be a commodity of invaluable proportions.

When I first started to become somewhat aware of my surroundings, speaking with some of the more astute patients helped me deal with some of my sadness. And seeing how the clerical staff, custodians, and volunteers Harmarville employs who have disabilities conduct themselves has provided me with solid role models I can pattern some of my behaviors after.

Ironically, one of the new admissions I was talking to is from Washington and graduated from Trinity. The other, an accomplished pianist, lives only about twenty miles or so up Route 19 in the South Hills and he too is only about a year younger than me. Both had sustained severe head injuries and needed someone who had "been through the ropes" to talk to because they believed they were at the end of theirs'. I felt for them being so young like me and because they're on a collision course with a disability that they will be tempted to let get the better of them. My recently married social worker, Laura Matthews-Beninati, wrote in her progress note about me regarding this situation: "He enjoys socializing and appears to enjoy helping other patients when he can." I'm just passing the torch and doing what I can to help.

Gliding over the strings between the two silver pickups, that wiffle ball pick was being directed by a loose and limber right hand that has produced music countless times before. On the fretboard, the chords A—G—E—E—E—G were being fingered much better and sounded almost okay together once I shook off the rust from not playing and got mom to move the pick to the rhythm of the simple AC/DC classic, "T.N.T." While I was doing the chord switching down on the fretboard, mom was thumping, whacking away at the strings over the body of the guitar. Angus wouldn't be real happy with the way we botched up the song, but I'm sure Bon Scott wouldn't have turned over in his grave, if he only knew the improvement I've made playing since Kevin showed me this song again last weekend. "It's dynamite."

At the base of the neck, over about the nineteenth fret, I then gave it a "go" trying to make my right picking hand do some strumming for me. I can't do this string sweeping up close to the bridge like it's supposed to be done because the fine motor skill entailed when doing this just isn't possible now. My wrist is barely able to go anywhere, as the wiffle ball pick seems to weigh fifty pounds. Making single notes impossible to pick, there's no way I can control the movements of my right hand, so I can isolate on any one string. Lucky when I can bend this joint enough to make it strike all six strings, my right wrist is just too rigid and stiff to make this motion.

When I attempt to make this carpus flex, it just doesn't move, so I've got to use my entire forearm in order to make a downstroke over the strings. Because of the tightness of my wrist, upstroking is impossible. With this limitation, I guess my hope of being the next Eric Clapton isn't going to materialize. If I'm lucky, someday maybe I can "jam" like Slim Whitman. Thanks to my two best friends, however, they're going to make sure I don't stay down in the dumps too long about this.

I'd know that rumble anywhere!!! Could it be!!? Looking out our front window, I saw Dave's sports car coming down towards the house!! Because he's such a good-hearted lad and my memory still very much draws more blanks than not, I'm really looking forward to speaking with Dave.

Pistons firing now, that Camaro was thundering down the road in all its glory. Wanting to throw their undergarments on the hood of his "babe mobile," the young neighborhood teenaged girls stared in awe at the 22-year-old driver, doing what they could to keep from letting out squeals of passion. Mag wheels rollin', I was a lot away from seeing my stud buddy.

Picturing Dave's "bad-ass" wheels roaring into the driveway and him hopping out telling me to hurry up and get better because he can't wait to kick my ass in football, I was feeling pretty good. Surely wanting to make a grand entrance that corresponds with his outgoing personality, Dave revved up his engine until the entire house vibrated. I wasn't about to roll out a red carpet for him, but I'd be more than happy to see him just the same.

But then a lump the size of a boulder got lodged in my throat and the butterflies which were swirling around in my stomach with anticipation only moments ago, died when the pounding of Dave's engine didn't let up any and he drove past the house. Accelerator then touching the floor, with a boom the sound of a cannon, Dave whistled up the hill out of sight. Stunned, I hung around the window a little bit longer thinking that was only a scouting lap and he'll be around in a second or so after he sees we're home.

I tell myself not to count on things because if they don't happen, I won't be disappointed then. I try to assume this attitude when it comes to Dave dropping by, but it's not easy. I have no idea what's going on with him.

Although this isn't the greatest of feelings, I do see a lot of improvement in how I'm handling this situation in the sense that I no longer feel resentment or bitter towards Dave, just let down. I couldn't have imagined a guy I had always gotten along with so well and spent so much time playing sports with these past few years not coming to see how I was faring, after almost being killed. Despite trying my best not to let it, this confusion still hurts. Suffice it to say, Dave didn't come back around.

That blue Nova has been a fixture in our driveway on weekends since I've been hurt, however. It would be difficult for someone to find a better friend than that hunk of hair playing my guitar. We've gone to battle together many times before and now that I need a medic to bandage my wounds, Kevin's efforts to help me pull through this attack are one reason my memory is coming around as it has. And before long, my newest great buddy would come by to see just what—if any—new things I could recall since last weekend when he was here.

"You can't remember anything about what happened to you the night you were hurt?," Claude asked subtlely, masterfully spacing the different times he inquired about this. Thinking nothing of it, listening closely, I told my curious pal that nothing's new from the last time he asked me this. Since my new friend is so vitally interested in me, once again, I went on to tell him about my recollection of things being gone.

Since Claude's been coming by, I haven't seen Sam. Not that I thought anything of this, I just figured Sam was working full-time somewhere this summer and that if he wanted to tell me something, he'd leave a message with Claude. I know that anything I would happen to say to Claude would get back to Sam. Without a doubt . . .

When I come home on weekends from Harmarville now, things are looking strikingly similar to how they were before I was "banged up," in the sense that boredom rules again. The only difference is that after my parents and I get done looking at each other, instead of me sleeping, eating, listening to my stereo, playing my guitar, and going outside, I sleep, eat, listen to my stereo, play my guitar, and retrain my brain.

This weekend, when I was reteaching my neurological systems how to print again, I gave it a new twist by attempting to do this with my dominant, spastic right hand. When I eventually did get something down on paper, it was awful. Frustration went into overdrive when I would lose grip of the pencil each time I applied a little bit of pressure on it. I wasn't about to let my physical limitations interfere with my attempts to overcome my cognitive ones, so I'd quickly put the pencil back in left hand. How 'bout that for excitement?

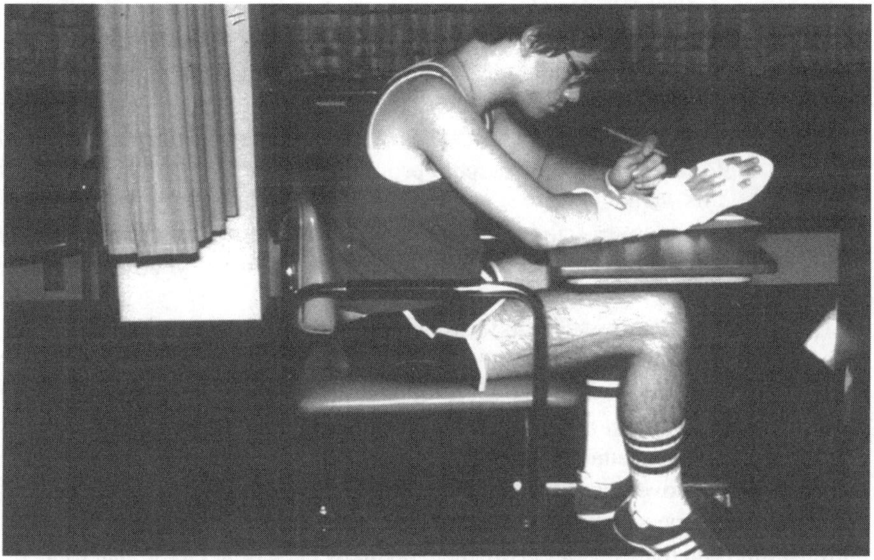

Literally forgetting how to write (agraphia), Craig trying to retrain his brain how to formulate letters was a common scene at Harmarville, as he would attempt to jot these elusive letters down with his non-dominant left hand. Nobody who treated Craig at this time would have ever predicted he was to one day author a book and earn a Master's Degree.

With my schedule of therapies as they are, lightning does strike the same place twice more times than not as far as diversity of interventions is concerned. Until the passageways in my brain pick up what they need to do, I'm just going to have to repeat these treatments over and over and over. Both physically and cognitively, repetition is the key for success with head injury rehabilitation. The week of June 7th would be another where I would be compensated handsomely for the duplication of therapeutic procedures.

When it comes to getting those letters down on paper, instead of all the lines being straight and squiggly, they're now also going to be rounded and squiggly because I'm starting to work on cursive writing. Because I require minimal cueing when I practice my printing now, away I'm going to leap into the world of continuous curved handwriting. Yippee, yes siree.

I must have known something no one else did. A few months back, when the first of many videos was shot of me where Mrs. Joy asked me where I went to high school and I kept on telling her my grade school, I possibly had a glimpse into the future, for the work I'm doing now is reminiscent of my days at North Franklin.

First, to get accustomed again to the physical motion entailed with writing, I made waves and ovals of varying size and direction. Unable to hold a pencil with my right hand, I copied these non-stop practice lines depicted on this writing-training pattern sheet with my non-dominant left hand. What I wrote on my paper was ugly, but the important thing was that my brain and hand were getting a sensation again of how to produce letters without lifting the pencil off the paper too much. With some of those professors at W.V.U. giving their lectures at the speed of light, I could see me trying to keep up printing my notes.

Alright boys and girls, today's lesson is learning new letter forms. And the first form we're going to be working on is overcurves. Can everybody say that for me? "Overcurves!"

Copying from a sample sheet, I was to reproduce the lowercase overcurve letters, "a" and "o", where the initial line is curved over the meat of the letter. Hey, I bet that's how they designated this type of writing, "over curve." I wonder if I'll get a sticker of a star put on my chart on the bulletin board for that good answer.

After I got these letters mastered in a few sessions, I was then to move on to the more difficult overcurve assignment of making a lowercase "n," then a lowercase "m." If my perseveration decides to act up, I might be sitting here all day putting humps on that "m" or making one too many each time I try to make an "n," finally producing that "m." So what I guess I've got to do if my perseveration clicks in when attempting to make an "m" is pretend I'm making an "n" and hope for the best. If I want to make an "n?" I haven't figured that one out yet.

Now for two "toughies," the lowercase overcurve letters "v" and "x." Having started so many letters to her with, "Dear Valerie," I've printed the uppercase "V" many times since I've been agraphic, so I wouldn't think this would be too different from writing the lowercase version. Just the same, I'm glad I've got a model in front of me which I can copy. I don't know if I'd be put in the corner or not if I'd just put some thin paper on this sample sheet and did some tracing. But I'm not going to chance it.

This small "x" looks like a doozy though. Because I haven't written letters to any "Xaviers" lately, I don't have the motions to produce this third-to-last letter of the alphabet down too well. There seems to be a lot entailed with writing this letter. Concentrating on the sample lowercase "x," slowly, I not only start this funny looking letter with an overcurve, but finish it off with a fancy looking tail. I crossed my "x" with a downstroke diagonal line when the instructions say I should've gone up. I wonder if I'm going to get my knuckles rapped by a ruler for this.

Undercurve letters are, obviously, just the opposite of overcurves in that the initial line dips slightly under the meat of the letter, and the first two letters of this type I'm going to work on are "i" and "e." I need to learn the proper motion involved with writing these letters because when I write the name, "Valerie," I want her to be able to read it. But I don't know how to join these two letters.

Oh boy, thank goodness there's a section which shows the beginning writer like me how to connect letters to form words. To connect these particular two letters, I have to "slide" between the "i" and "e." I'm going to have to copy the sample words, "is," "me," "car," and "was" to get accustomed to this sliding hand motion again. But before I reach the end of Valerie's name, I have to learn how to "swing" between the letters "a" and "l." To accomplish this movement, this high school graduate is going to practice the sample words "an," "on," "no," and a real tricky one that's going to give me some trouble, "ox."

When these letters are written, there's a roof on an "r," a hook in a "c," and a curve in a "s." A retrace in the lowercase "v," as well as a trace with such tall lowercase letters as "d," "t," and "p." The lowercase tall letters "b," "l," "h," and "k" all have looped tops which require my hand and brain to do something slightly different than the traced tops. And the stroke I have to learn when writing a "g," "y," "j," and "z" requires using a lower loop. I wouldn't want to skip these handwriting exercises and chance getting paddled because Diane and Mrs. Joy look like they could pack one helluva wallop.

Overcurves, undercurves, slides, swings, roofs, hooks, curves, traced tops, looped tops, lower loops, etc., I always thought writing was something people were just able to do automatically. Like walking, I never realized all that it entailed. There's so much with this writing business I need to get a handle on again. I know one thing: <u>I'm never going to be able to write a book!</u>

Mind over matter. I just got to keep trying, something good's gotta come of this. I can. . . . . Just one more time and I'll be another step closer to getting over this. I am going to improve and keep getting better. Nothing's going to stop me, I'm going to beat this thing. I'm going to come out on top. If I don't want to be like this for the rest of my life, I've just got to bust my tail and kick some ass. Just keep trying, it'll come.

These thoughts that I made sure I told myself were just a few that helped pull me through these next couple of weeks. Attitude is everything when it comes to rehabilitation because <u>you feel how you think</u>. When it comes to this self-talk, I guess in a few ways I've been a "Rock of Gibraltar" type. I don't see this mindset as anything unique or special, rather, a necessity a patient must incorporate, if they're not going to allow their disability ruin their lives.

If one approaches things in a helpless/hopeless manner, they're not going to have the energy to behave in such a way as to overcome the various ailments a debilitating injury levies on one. Nothing irritates me more than to see someone give a "half-assed" effort in therapy when they can do so much more. And it is usually this type of patient that bitches loudest about their condition. They talk one helluva story about how hard they work, but talk is cheap. When their back is against the wall, the true character of patients like this comes to the front and all they do is moan about how they've been victims all their life and that there's no use in trying because nothing good is going to come of it, anyway.

Nobody bargains for this disability or rehab business, but sulking only gets you so far before you have to tighten your chin straps and get down to business. If it weren't for the "shake it off and pick yourself up" property my parents instilled in me, I don't know what I would do. I guess they knew what they were talking about.

My intent is not to sound like a hard ass, this lolly-gagging behavior is just the way it is with some people. Maybe not the majority, but more than a few. It needs stressed that, more times than not, you get what you put into it. All patients will face a series of emotional hurdles.

Fundamentally, the steps both patients and families go through after one's been seriously disabled are, in order of progress from worst to better: Shock, Denial, Anger, Depression, and Acceptance. In certain circumstances, maybe one of these will get skipped, but generally this is what people experience when someone's hanging in the balance, teeter-tottering between psychological extremes after the onset of a severe disability.

Shock is the initial trauma one will face after an accident. Denial is when one is not accepting the extent of the affliction(s). Anger occurs when one comes to grips with the fact that their life has been forever altered and become enraged about the degree with which they've been hurt/how the injury will impact them the rest of their life. Depression evolves after the heightened emotion has subsided and a sadness envelopes the person after they've reflected how the mishap will have a permanent disabling effect on their life.

Acceptance is the healthy step of this progression where things are obviously not embraced, but tolerated. This is the stage where a person realizes all that has happened to them and what it means for their life. When this understanding occurs, the person not only finds ways to live with what has happened to them, but can move on in such a fashion that they find ways to limit the influence their condition has on them. It is difficult to reach this "acceptance" phase, but it is of crucial importance that it gets attained, for the implementation of compensatory strategies can then begin. Having limitations doesn't have to be prohibitive, the person with a disability is just going to have to find different ways to get around what they have trouble doing.

With the effort I put into my therapies day in and day out, as well as how hard I work on weekends when I'm home, maybe this is indicative of how I haven't reached this self-actualized level of acceptance yet, for I'm still vying for how I was before being hurt. Maybe shooting for the stars is my way of not letting go of a fantasy where I want recognized for excelling at something. If this is a form of denial, it appears to be working for me, however.

It is true that if one's goals are not realistic and outside the realm of possibility, they'll really be in for a fall that they might not get up from. But sometimes you don't know how things are going to turn out until you try. I know more than work is involved if one's going to make any achievements following a neurological impairment, for luck and good fortune are going to have a vital say in how one comes out of this. In the days and weeks ahead, the focus for me will be to continue refining abilities I've rediscovered, developing skills that have vanished—and as always—pushing limits. Same ole, same ole.

As time crawls on—with God on my side and fortune in my corner—a bridge was being built connecting me with a new beginning, a second chance I'm not so sure I'm worthy. Maybe there's a reason why I survived "against all odds" when it shouldn't have been this way. To dwell on the inconceivable serves no purpose and to spend precious moments pondering this equation with no apparent answer is not wise, for time is of the essence.

I don't know what the next day is going to bring, but I can feel that a foundation is being set for a prosperous passage into tomorrow. Each block for this entryway's frame and stone for its wall has had the perilous price of pain and suffering. The shrine which is my future is why I set off in this pilgrimage know as rehabilitation. And the signs seem to be leading me to this destination.

June 7th (Monday): On this day when I started to write cursively, Mrs. Joy made an observation and recorded in the progress note, "Emotionally, Craig's overall affect is appearing less flat and wider range of emotion noted."

June 8th (Tuesday): Check-up at Allegheny General Hospital with my neurosurgeon, Dr. Prostko.

The mild-mannered doctor was very pleased with the way things have been turning out with my recovery. Happy to see that I could straighten my right arm to about 75% of its normal range, this brain surgeon wasn't surprised the hyperactivity of my right muscle stretch reflexes remained from the last time he saw me, which I was told was April 6th. Scraping the sole of my right foot, a Babinski reflex was noted. When this toe-bending response exam is done with someone who hasn't had damage to their brain, the toes normally bend down, but my small ones fanned out and the big toe went up, which indicates abnormalities in the cerebral cortex's motor control pathways. These reactions were expected, given that I was hurt only a little while ago. However, with so much working in my favor, Dr. Prostko was encouraged by the progress I was making.

So much so, he said there's no reason I couldn't play baseball again someday. I have the highest regard and respect for this outstanding physician, but with all that's wrong with me and the way I'm feeling now, I don't see how this could be possible and have resigned myself that my ballplaying days are over.

Because he is a man of sincere compassion, I can't say for sure if Dr. Prostko has the heart to tell me athletics are a thing of the past, knowing how important this was to me. To give a precise prognosis to one that's had a brain injury is not humanly possible, but then again, I guess I've made some gains in a few areas which challenge the accepted logic of "what is" attainable and "what is not" after an injury of this sort has occurred. Maybe this and the fire in my eyes will indeed help me achieve desires that were once—not so long ago—only a foregone dream.

Although it's only been a little under four months, it seems a lot longer that I've been taking anti-convulsants. Despite never having a seizure or feeling as if a convulsion were coming on, the doctor wanted me to continue taking my Dilantin as prescribed. Saying that no assurances could be made whether or not the electrical impulses in my brain will remain calm, Dr. Prostko said I probably will be taking seizure medication of some type for the rest of my life, given how badly my head was pounded. As a matter of fact, Dr. Prostko wanted to check on how my brain was doing, so he scheduled for me to have a Cat Scan conducted which X-rays the interior and exterior of the brain. Better safe than sorry.

> June 11th (Friday): I got weighed at Harmarville and I'm only one-half pound below what I weighed at the time of the accident. Harmarville's tasty food and double portions are doing the trick. Oink, oink.

> June 12th (Saturday): I went to Washington Hospital for the CT Scan, then later left for the greenhouse where I worked last summer for what I hoped to be a memory-reviving visit.

With practically every part of my body having been X-rayed at least once since the night I was wrapped around that utility pole, it's a wonder that I don't glow now. Today, my head was subjected to thousands of volts, so a detailed picture of my brain's terrain and inner workings could be taken. This may be wishful thinking, but I just hope that being "zapped" by so much radiation doesn't have any kind of long-term detrimental effect. It's a wonder I don't get electrocuted now when I take my shower.

After I got my head probed, I was off to where I spent four months last summer getting down and dirty. Everybody I worked with was happy to see me. However, knowing them like I do and because we liked each other so well, I'm sure the acid was churning in each one of their guts seeing me in such a compromised position like I am now.

While I was hanging onto my father for balance, my boss, Mr. Aaron Stimmell, came out once he saw my dad's car to greet us. Cliff and Mrs. Casper also came out after they saw the Bobcat which transported me to and from work everyday pull into the Floral Hill driveway. Mr. Stimmell's youngest son and little daughter stopped too.

As I was looking at the familiar outside perimeter of the greenhouse, my buddy I had worked with and talked to quite a bit—Bill—walked up and said it was great to see me. Teary-eyed, Bill told me I better get to playing my guitar again soon because I had promised to play for him someday.

With mom looking on, I told those I had broken my back digging, hauling, and planting with about my failing memory and that I barely remember anything about this place or anything I did here. Immediately then, as I hung on to my dad for leverage while standing on the rough terrain, Mr. Stimmell proceeded to give me a tour of the greenhouses where I used to sweat, get dirty, and smell like a pig.

Eyes burning with a somber compassion, my boss was pointing out some of the areas where I had worked during my 3:00 P.M. to 11:00 P.M. night shift and told me what some of my duties were. As I was taking all this in, my mind was trying to form some images of being at these different places and doing these various tasks. Some of the areas we had walked through looked very familiar to me and a good bit of what my good-hearted boss said struck a chord with me.

However, there were also a lot of things that I was told and saw that I just didn't recognize. The huge water tower out back tipped over a couple of months ago and fell on the glass-framed mum house where Mr. Stimmell said I spent a lot of time laboring over the flower beds, but I couldn't remember ever being there.

Maybe if this spacious mum house hadn't been destroyed and I could've stepped in and taken a look around, some things might have come back to me. This seems to be another example of how my brain's recall function needs a recognizable stimulus before it can generate a memory response.

Shown the main houses, I could vaguely remember putting the black curtains over the flower beds here before I'd start piling boxes and arranging carts in the garage out front. And I can recall putting flowers in tubs of water on carts and packing others in cardboard boxes while I was out here. Some things looked very familiar to me and I could recollect, others were as if I had never been here in my life. Even things that sparked a memory, I couldn't have remembered without seeing first.

Going home, mom told me that while Mr. Stimmell, dad, and me were in the greenhouse looking around, Bill must have been taken back seeing me and started crying. I can only guess that Bill had an image of me lugging heavy buckets of dirt, carrying big boxes of flowers over my shoulders, and chopping away at the soil in those flower beds with a hoe like I was doing last summer and couldn't bear seeing how I am now, having to lean on my dad for stability, so I could just stand up.

People who have known me since before the accident see me differently than I see myself. Remembering how I was before my brain was torn to shreds, friends and acquaintances have a distinct picture of what I was like when I was healthy and know how much I've regressed. Because the images of me when I was physically intact are simply not there anymore, I have nothing to judge myself by, other than what I have been told. Because there's no concrete picture of me in my mind as ever being healthy, all I have to go by is what I'm like now, as opposed to how I was at Allegheny General. And that being the case, I don't think I'm doing so bad knowing what I could have been like. Maybe it's for the best, after all, that my history is someone else's. Someone I'll never be again.

> June 18th (Friday): I walked 7/10ths of a mile around our neighborhood—without my wheelchair.

To think that just a little over a month ago, I was being pushed around the park by my dad in a wheelchair and now I'm making these steps up and down hills on my own with dad beside me—not behind pushing—is a real tribute to everyone who has helped me come this far. When I started to get up out of my wheelchair and began to push it, it wasn't long after that the brain got a wake-up call how to do some strolling again. When it was safe to do so, Jan and Mary let me go and I've been off, off, and away ever since. Way to go ladies, thank you.

Four months ago, few at Allegheny General could be convinced that the comatose patient having rock 'n roll music blared in his ears would ever come out of the deep unconscious which he had sunk—let alone be walking without assistance—but here I am doing exactly that. Snapping out of a state where death almost had me, to where I'm at now is something I can't explain—-I'm just glad I'm here.

Making so many gains in such a relatively short period of time leaves me to wonder, "Why?" Why was I spared when so many people—good people — haven't had this fortune? I know how incredibly hard I've worked to overcome my various symptoms, but I've seen lot of patients work diligently with less-than-productive results. I think I've definitely been lucky in this game of life. I also realize that people make their own luck. I suppose there's a fine line between the two.

In any kind of game, there are rules and the game of life is no different. My Christian belief is, and always has been, that when God made the earth, there were laws of the universe the players have to abide by. If one steps outside the bounds of these laws/rules, then some unfortunate consequences could result. If the violation is too extreme, the game may end.

On February 14th, my game of life was almost over before it had much of a chance to begin because the basic law of the universe which states, "No two things can occupy the same place at the same time," was broken. "Why" I'm able to walk around the neighborhood when others who have had head injuries are forever unconscious, I don't know. Maybe if I was sitting an inch over to the right in the VW that fateful night, I too may not be aware of my world. Or, possibly if I were sitting an inch to my left, closer to the driver's seat, nothing would have happened to me. There may be an answer, there may not. I just know I don't fully understand what the reality of this situation is. And it's unlikely I ever will—at least not in this life.

Divine intervention? I'm sure God was looking down and He knew what was going on, but I could never say for sure if I was blessed somehow by a ray of light from Heaven or not. I definitely have the practical belief that God does work through the hands of others and that the doctors in the ER., nurses in the hospital/ Harmarville, and the therapists here all have themselves one efficient co-pilot. Whether the pieces in this game of life were arranged in some way where I would have some kind of an advantage or the rules had been stretched some, I'm in no position to understand because I'll never know.

It's nice to think that The Spirit touched me somehow, for some reason, and I experienced a sort of spontaneous remission. Why I was able to grasp the joy of awareness and given the opportunity to operate within my environment is a mystery that I may never solve or absorb the meaning of. However, if there's one thing that is crystal clear to me, it's that as I go walking around the neighborhood, I am grasping a happiness I couldn't be sure I'd ever experience again.

> June 21st (Monday): My ability to climb and go down stairs had improved to the point where I could now do this step over step with minimal assistance.

If one hurts their brain, it's unbelievable what they forget how to do. A wooden staircase model of about five steps is kept in the PT gym, so that patients who have lost their ability to go up and down stairs can get some practice. Possessing that incredible Alba foresight—apparently thinking the time spent working at this imitation staircase could be better spent elsewhere—Jan didn't bother utilizing this "dummy" stairwell and had me working on the "real thing."

As I went up the stairs off the main corridor, I tried my best to make sure I was balanced and positioned properly on each step. Now, my concentration doesn't have to be so intense and, at the same time, my speed is going to increase significantly because of this alternate-stepping action. That rod still stings and I need to continue using a rail for stability and posture as I go up and down, but I was happy as the day is long now that I was getting this down. I never thought I would appreciate hiking up and down some steps so much, for this is just one of those things that is taken for granted. Rather, "was" taken for granted.

> July 2nd/July 3rd (Friday and Saturday): Scheduled to see my opthalmologist, E. Ronald Salvitti, M.D., in Washington for an appointment about what I'm to do about my double vision. And practiced ascending/decending the steps at home.

Overjoyed, I wasn't only seeing fireworks because my independence was returning so incredibly fast, but because on this Independence Day weekend of all times, I was informed that there were a variety of options available to me to free me from this tortuous eyesight which I have been held captive. With the hopes of full recovery, Dr. Salvitti first talked about prisms being ground into the lenses of my glasses to correct the problem where I'm seeing pairs of everything when only one object is there.

Dad, firmly entrenched in his own form of denial, wasn't happy at all hearing about this form of correction because he didn't want me to rely on any type of compensatory device as a result of this accident. He wanted his little boy back 100% like he was before being crushed against that telephone pole. Usually though, with head injury, what one wants and what they get are two different things.

Dr. Salvitti said that, hopefully, this vertical diplopia will resolve itself without treatment. However, if this fourth cranial nerve palsy on the left doesn't heal on its own, then the need for surgical intervention becomes a distinct possibility, if not a probability.

Because she has glaucoma, mom sees Dr. Salvitti on a regular basis. On her most recent appointment with our family eye doctor, Dr. Salvitti surprised mom when he told her that he and his wife witnessed me being taken out of the VW the night of the wreck. Dr. Salvitti said that he had made himself available in case he was needed, but that the paramedics, fire departments, and the other medical emergency personnel on the scene did such an excellent job, his services weren't needed.

Years before, prior to his specializing in opthalmology, Dr. Salvitti was a neighbor of ours living on the other side of the park. Because he had two sons who approximate me in age who I used to play some ball with, Dr. Salvitti knew me personally when I was younger. The night of the accident, however, while he was on stand-by in the event his numerous medical skills needed utilized, he had no idea it was me that was being extracted from the car because I was a bloody, mangled mess.

When mom came in for the appointment to have her eye pressure measured, Dr. Salvitti told her that I had lost such an incredible amount of blood that my blood pressure was probably "zero." Whether I had died or was "just" in shock those forty-five minutes I was trapped in the car with no attention, there's no way I could ever know this. But I know that I couldn't have agreed anymore with this talented doctor when he said, "You're lucky you're here."

Energized by my regained capacity to make my way up some stairs and get back down, dad and I practiced this step-climbing in the house until about 12:30 at night, so I could polish up this step over step mountain climbing I have been working on in PT since June 21st. I could feel the rod stabbing at my right hip, but because I was so elated that I could do this step-skipping ascent smoother and what this will mean for my independence, I forgot I was hurting. I guess it's just a matter of living with the pain and not letting it control me. I just have to "bite the bullet" and try to ignore this extreme discomfort, if I'm to get around.

When me and dad were stomping up and down the staircase, the clock struck midnight and this marked the beginning of my parents' 39th Wedding Anniversary. You might think that going up and down some steps so your son learns how to do this quickly again is a helluva way to start a day of celebration, but since it has been practice such as this which I'm getting the feeling will allow me to sleep in my own bed pretty soon, I know dad won't mind too much. The night I'm able to sleep one room over from him will really be a cause for celebration, because this was oh-so close to never happening again. Happy Anniversary, mom and dad.

> July 6th (Tuesday): Remarkably, I continue to show significant gains within all facets of my rehabilitation program. But equally incredible, because of this, I was denied Social Security Disability.

Jan put in her progress note dated the 6th day of July that I'm showing various improvement in my ability to ambulate, transfer, and shift positions on the mat. Climbing the steps at home has really benefited me, for Jan dictates that by this date, I go up and down stairs skipping a step with minimal cueing and assistance. Still needing watched closely in case I stumble, I hold my trunk stiff during this and other activities.

Also, because of this difficulty doing steps, I need a visual cue as I head up or down. In other words, if I don't look down at the steps as I'm going, I can't judge the depth between steps confidently. I try to overcome this faulty sense of depth perception by taking a firm look at where I'm going. Looking straight ahead as most people do when they're climbing or going down steps would spell certain disaster for me. Unless you've had one, it's tough to fathom the "chills and thrills" one who has had a severe brain injury endures. I'm just going to keep my hand in close proximity to this left rail, so I don't take any spills.

Whether this is only fear which taunts my psyche or just plain common sense, I don't do stairs well or comfortably unless there's a rail on my good left side. If I would lose my balance on steps and would need to rely on my right arm or hand to bail me out of trouble, I'd be good as dead. But OT is trying their best to do something about this.

As always, Occupational Therapy's emphasis this first week of July has been on decreasing spasticity, so I can increase the isolated movements of my hand and wrist, as well as extend my fingers more. To help with this dexterity, I continue to wear the wrist/hand platform splint which has been effective in decreasing the tone in my fingers, but that isn't all it's decreased.

I know because my fingers are responding a little better to what I want them to do, I guess this splint has been worth the lost sleep and the overall discomfort I'm feeling wearing it. Try going to bed holding a bowling ball and see how much "shut-eye" you get. However, I'd much rather experience this loss of comfort for a time than to have the fingers on my right hand permanently curl in a ball, as if set in mortar. But it would be nice to get some sleep once in a while.

Someone must have pressed that rewind button because I'm at it again working on my memory, speech, and writing in CS and Psych. My Communications' therapist, Diane, wrote in her 7-6-82 progress note that, "Craig Meyers continues to attend program daily. His written language expression is at present fully functional. Speech and spontaneous verbal expression only rarely show word recall difficulties. Verbal associative tasks reveal good capabilities in this area." It looks like I'm getting back on track, thank you, Diane. I don't know what I would do, if I couldn't talk.

To assure that brain of mine continues to snap to attention, Mrs. Joy had me working various videos in Psychology again, so that my visual memory would further develop. The capacity to form images in my mind has improved tremendously because of the multitude of brain-stimulating cassettes my psychologist has jammed into her VCR. Because I've spent so much time in front of these, I could probably change my college major from Journalism to Computer Science and graduate in the fall. Having that kind of rapid progress with such a trying major isn't feasible, but I was swiftly showing significant gains overcoming my various aphasias to the point my program was becoming progressively more advanced. As Mrs. Joy recorded in her progress note on this 6th day of July:

"Patient continues to be seen 4X weekly for cognitive retraining with present emphasis on cursive writing and visual memory using Atari video cassettes and Apple computer."

"Patient's cursive writing ability neat and accurate, but his performance remains slow."

Mrs. Joy, your efforts have been greatly appreciated and beneficial, thank you, mam.

I guess I wasn't hurt bad enough. A combination of blue collar guidelines for white collar strivings and ignorance about what a head injury does to a person's intellect, led to the Social Security Administration rejecting the claim for disability benefits filed on my behalf.

Knowing the impact this brain injury could have on my ability to earn an income, mom wasted no time applying for SSD. A little over two weeks after having my skull fractured, March 1st to be exact, mom applied for disability for her comatose son.

Hoping that dad putting aside money out of his paycheck for social security all those decades would harvest an income for their "brain damaged" son when he needs it most, mom was devastated and shocked when she received the letter from the SSA stating that her claim for disability was being denied. SSA had determined that I was not entitled to benefits because I did not fall within the disability requirements/physical and mental limitations established by the law to receive payments at the time the application was filed.

In reaching this decision, SSA considered how much my condition will affect my ability to work for the next twelve months. SSA's guidelines state that the impairment, whether physical or mental, must be so severe that it prevents the person from performing any substantial work with the key word here being, "any." Also, provision of benefits is dependent on the condition having lasted or expected to last at least twelve months. Realizing this injury will cause me to experience hardships of varying degree not only for the next year, but for the rest of my life, mom and dad appealed this decision in writing to the Disability Determination Division of the SSA.

My case appeared to fall in a gray area of the law, for the Social Security Act stipulates that a disability must prevent a person with a disability from doing "any" significant work before they would receive cash previously set aside by a working family member. Because my brain stem being smacked against my head bone wouldn't prevent me from wiping feces off a toilet seat in a gas station or from cleaning up stalls at the Meadowlands horse racing track, the Social Security Administration came to the conclusion that I was employable then.

Without taking into consideration I'd still be in therapy for months to come following my discharge from Harmarville, or that I'd be pursuing an education which would allow me to attain a position more in line with my capabilities, SSA's denial response was almost as quick as mom filing a claim, for—on March 28th—my parents received word that no money was coming my way.

SSA wrote that they based their decision on reports from nine sources about my condition ranging from physicians, therapists, my psychologist, hospitals, Harmarville, and even my high school. In their explanation of the denial determination, SSA wrote that the medical evidence shows that I did suffer a head injury, but recent intelligence testing is not severe enough for disability purposes. The Explanation of Determination slip notes that my right leg and ear injuries were corrected surgically and that I am constantly improving with therapy. SSA stated that because I should be able to lift twenty pounds maximum, ten pounds frequently, and walk/stand up to six hours a day within the year, I'm not eligible for Social Security Disability. In this Social Security Notice which states all the reasons why I'm not eligible for Childhood Disability (Ages 18-22)—thereby rejecting our request for compensation—SSA concluded with, "While your son's impairment is severe at this time, it is not expected to last a continuous period of twelve months as required by law."

I know hindsight is 20/20, but this shows just how ignorant SSA is about the effects of a head injury. Talk about being between a rock and a hard place. You either don't work in therapy and experience physical/cognitive atrophy, but you get what's coming to you monetarily. Or, you work and progress, but because of this, you don't get what you are entitled from previous savings because you're in too good of a condition. You can't win for losing.

> July 9th (Friday): Tonight, on mom's 59th birthday, I slept in my room for the first time in five months.

So this is what my room looks like. When I'm home on the weekends, I work to improve on those things I have been reintroduced to in the rehab center during the week in therapies. Dad finished installing the last segment of railing along the stairs this week, so my weekend is going to consist of me doing some legwork on these steps. Cultivating the stair-climbing ability that I had forgotten how to do, I'm prepared to practice at home now.

Clutching onto the thick, ugly, black rails dad put alongside the stairs—a dozen times—I hauled myself up and down the thirteen steps leading from the rec room to upstairs where the bedrooms are. I didn't know if I'd ever be able to get up here again, but here I am.

Anticipating the ascent to my bedroom this weekend, during the week mom and dad joyfully moved all my stuff from the rec room back to where it was before I had left for college. The last time I was in my room was the night of February 12th and even then it didn't look or feel exactly right because my stereo, speakers, clothing, and clock were in Morgantown. Arranged exactly like it was during my high school years, I never thought I'd be so happy returning to the room where I spent the majority of my adolescence moping and never being satisfied. Compared to the way I am now, I didn't realize just how good I had it then.

My bed, stereo, dresser, clock, rocking chair, and amplifier are positioned precisely where my brain's recognition function last pictured them being. Without actually seeing them before me, however, I couldn't form a visual image in my mind of how these were placed in my room or even what was in here. Now that I am looking at them here in front of me, I know now this is where the closet and window have always been, but I couldn't have told you this five minutes ago, or until I was looking at them.

Being able to stand in my room is analogous to what I'm striving for in rehabilitation. Elevating up some stairs represents progress and reaching my room is symbolic of how goals can be attained, if one remains focused and puts forth the effort. Grasping a part of me I couldn't be certain I'd ever experience again, I was thankful from the bottom of my heart. I haven't reached my pinnacle yet, but I'm getting there as things are looking better and better. God helps those who help themselves. Happy birthday, mom.

> July 13th (Tuesday): Mom and dad appealed the SSA's ruling that my physical and cognitive conditions were not severe enough for me to collect disability, as they filled out a Request for Reconsideration questionnaire last night and got

it off in the mail this morning. In Vocational, I was readministered the Wide Range Achievement Test (WRAT).

July 16th (Friday): When dad was at the rehab center for the weekend pick-up, my social worker, Laura, informed him that all my therapists thought I was depressed.

Things are becoming all too clear now that, no matter how hard I try, my physical limitations and maybe even a few of the cognitive restrictions I'm currently experiencing are always going to be with me. Despite discarding my wheelchair a few weeks ago, which was an immaculate symbol of what I have achieved thus far, I am not cheery. The accomplishments I've made in the past few months are not something I savor because I am saddened knowing that any triumphs I may make in the future are going to be few and far between now, and of a far less magnitude.

I know that I've been told that after one has severely injured their brain, they are never going to be the same again, for an insult of this type always results in some permanent loss of function of varying degree. But that went in one ear and out the other when I was told this because I figured being eighteen-years-old, Superman, and invincible, that things will be different with me. I'm afraid not, junior.

This diagnosis might apply to everyone else who has had a severe head injury, but I'm Craig Meyers and I'm going to work my tail into the ground and prove everyone wrong. I'm not going to hear any different. Now, get the hell away from me before shit hits the fan.

I'm getting "teed off" that I can't twirl this little wooden cylinder between the fingers of my right hand, tell time very well, or read a damned sentence without it jumping all over the place. My heel cord isn't loosening up any, my right arm still agonizes me when I put weight on it, that rod in my leg bites my ass like a bitch when I raise it, I can't balance myself on this right leg, and my eyesight sucks. God, why'd you do this to me? You could've prevented all this from happening!!!

July 18th (Sunday): Being away from music which is so incredibly important to me hasn't done much to sparkle my mood any so—figuring this might pick up my trodden spirits some—I got permission from Harmarville that I could bring my guitar to the rehab, and that's exactly what I did when I returned back tonight. But the other patients needn't worry, I left my amplifier behind.

July 19th (Monday): With my claim that I want to pursue a journalism career in mind, Vocational solicited the help of a tutor who was going to help with my writing/English skills. This volunteer, Betty Schwartzberger, was a former school teacher and is going to help me relearn basic rules of grammar and punctuation.

July 20th (Tuesday): Despite so much still falling in my favor, it has become apparent that the extent which I have been hurt is going to have an impact on me my entire life and I'm starting to feel heart-broken.

The realization of this unfortunate consequence of my head injury is being translated into a souring mood when I attend therapies during the day, but I was still putting forth the effort needed to improve. In her progress note dated 7-20-82, Jan wrote: "Craig is now working on incorporation of proper weight shift and pelvic motion in ambulation to improve gait. Showing improved ability to self-monitor gait pattern. Pace has improved significantly along with increased control in stepping, initiating ambulation, and in negotiating turns. Gait still shows decreased weight bearing on the right."

Jan also dictated that because of stiffness, pain, and the clicking sensation near the pin insertion area in my right hip, I have been limited as to what I can do during elevation exercises of my right leg. She reported that I go up and down steps independently now using the left rail, but that I have difficulty doing this when someone's not right there with me.

To end it on a bright note, Jan writes that I am independent in all mat position changes, transfers, and ambulation. Also, my physical therapist wrote down that this patient "continues to be motivated." Jan's assessment about the fire which burns inside me is accurate, but to attain this drive now, I've got to tip-toe around some emotional land mines that have the potential of dismembering much of what I've worked so hard for.

Since being twisted with the metal in Paul's car, the days have always seemed to last longer than 24 hours, but now they are really dragging. When you work yourself like a slave with no end in sight or few substantial rewards being reaped from this effort, I can't think of too many things more discouraging. I know I'm not the easiest to satisfy, but that's me. And I know my distress is evident to everyone who has the chore now of working with me. But everyone pulled together to help guide me through this mine field.

Focusing on the positive has worked up to this point and I know I've got to keep on doing this if I'm to survive through the duration, but my ability to continue this functional self-talk is getting to be more difficult because after incapability after incapability after incapability slaps you in the face, it takes all the strength you can get ahold of to keep from just "hanging it up." And it's here when I just have to keep reminding myself just how bad off I could be, and that I wasn't spared so I could take the easy way out and quit.

Seeing me evolve into a Scrooge, Harmarville thought it best that I get involved with their new Wednesday morning group discussion with other patients who can relate to what I'm going through. Although you would never wish this on anybody, a patient can take a perverse sort of comfort knowing that others have had similar hardships, but were able to pull themselves up and maybe even grow from the experience, so future setbacks won't be so trying.

At least during this psychology rap session, Mrs. Joy won't be having me play with any "piss-ass" crossword puzzle because she knows my case too well. If done properly, group therapy can work like magic. If it's done in a bush league fashion, however, it doesn't do the trick which is why I'm not about to go to Howdy's recreation/waste therapy anymore.

I've been emotionally descending down into the pits for a while now; I don't know how much more psychological heartache I can take. My disintegration into an ogre state has been recorded in at least three "progress" notes by three people fortunate enough to work with me.

My Occupational therapist, for example, writes in her 7/20 progress note: "Frustration tolerance appears to be decreasing when doing upper extremity activities. Craig appears to be somewhat depressed and withdrawn." "Appears" nothing, I'm scratching bottom hook, line, and sinker.

You know my dejection has topped out when this commentary comes from Wendy, because she has heard me growl when others haven't and would know when I felt spinning the chamber of despondency would be one option of escape. This wasn't going to happen, however, because I always seem to be able to redirect this anger I'm feeling outward and make it work for me. Okay, so I'm not Superman.

In just a few words, my social worker captured the essence of my current demeanor, as she put in her 7/20 progress note: "Craig remains motivated, but is realizing fully his deficits and shows occasional discouragement." That's good Laura, but instead of using the word, "occasional" to describe my discouragement, "increasingly more" would be more accurate.

Using different words, but describing the same thing—this discouraged inpatient's temperament—the Vocational Educator sugarcoated my predisposition these last few days when she wrote in her note: "His energy level seems lower this past week." Seeing myself as a person who no longer posseses a future, I hope these healthy group leaders can relate to me because I really need some help handling all this.

Although it was difficult doing so, I tried not to let my not being upbeat interfere with what I ultimately had to do in my therapies. I was bummed, but I had enough rational thinking working for me not to let up. This will be a key if I'm to overcome this unforgiving disability.

For example, Donna wrote in her progress note that, despite my current downcast nature, I have been working with my tutor "concentrating on writing skills." And that I continue to work on Classmate 88 Mathematics and received a grade of 70% correct in Division, 84% multiplication, and 91% addition. I know that if you take two nickels from five, you have three nickels left over or fifteen cents when you started off with twenty-five cents before taking away those ten cents. See? I'm good now—damn good.

In Wendy's OT, although not in the greatest of spirits, I was attending program as scheduled and working independently. I was still limited as to what I could grasp and release spontaneously, as I would demonstrate sufficient control, if the object were not real small and could wrap my entire hand around it. But if I have to get each individual finger to work for me so that I could manipulate smaller things, forget it, because this just isn't going to happen for me—right now.

If I'm to climb out of the ashes of disgust, I just need to keep my head up and not allow my perception of things suck me into a hole where I see no escape. Little things can mean so much now when it comes to boosting my spirits like when Valerie makes it a point to track me down every night now, so that I can give her guitar lessons. Sometimes it's tough to keep my head above water, but my efforts and the personalities of staff are keeping me afloat. I know that paranoia can be one common symptom of head injury and is something I would like to think I don't have. Still, I can't help but think that the words, "Titanic" and "therapy" have the same number of letters in them. I wouldn't think that would have any meaning—would it?

Spring thaw. That was the last time I was tested so extensively. If I thought I was back at W.V.U. taking mid-terms when Mrs. Joy administered the WAIS-R and the Weschler Memory Scale baseline tests on the week of May 10th, I haven't seen nothing yet.

Not only was the week of July 26th going to be the time I'd be readministered these psychological tests, but I would also be getting my grade on the Wide Range Achievement Test (WRAT) I took in Vocational and the Gates-MacGinitie Reading Test—Form F, I was administered in Communication Skills. To say things were looking "up" might be understating things some.

Aptitude tests are designed to measure one's potential in a particular arena and achievement tests are used to assess how much a person knows or has learned. Baseline refers to the position a person or thing is at during the beginning of an assessment, and from this, a comparison or measurement can be made at a later juncture.

The Wide Range Achievement Test Donna gave me is a standardized test used to measure competency in basic abilities and assesses the elementary skills one needs to possess in order to manage their life in today's society. Specifically, this test was administered to assess my functional abilities within the speaking, writing, and arithmetic computation realms.

On 6-14-82, the first time I had taken the test, my baseline score was 8.2 grade level. This meant that during the middle of June 1982, I possessed approximately the same amount of knowledge as someone in the second month of their eighth grade year. That means I have lost about six years of knowledge because of this traumatic brain injury, for my second month in the 8th grade would have been October of 1976. God help me if I got to go back to the Trinity Middle School again to finish junior high. With the speed which I'm getting better, however, I won't have to concern myself with this.

As a matter of fact, on 7-13-82, I took the WRAT a second time so that an estimate could be gathered where I was operating a month later, and the score improved to a 10.0 grade level, or as if I were starting my sophomore year in high school. That's one heckuva jump, especially if one considers that only five months before that, I wasn't even functioning at the preschool level. Being a freshman in college—with an asterick before this classification—I know I'm three grade levels below where I should be, but I'm climbing up that ladder at an encouraging rate. Who knows? Since I took that test two weeks ago, it's a distinct possibility I've climbed another grade these past fourteen days to an 11.0 grade level.

My brain healing has allowed me to ascend these rungs at an amazing pace. The Gates-MacGinitie Reading Test I took in CS was evidence of this, for I scored in the 38%ile of 12.8 graders. In other words, 62% of students about my age are dumber than I am in my current state and I bet these seniors didn't have head injuries to contend with. That either says something about the healing power of the brain or about the deficiencies in our school systems.

The returns are in. The first time I took the WAIS-R on the week of May 10th, I received a Verbal IQ score of 90, a Performance IQ of 66, and a Full Scale IQ of 77. The second administration—done three months later—yielded a Verbal IQ score of 108, a Performance IQ score of 79, and a Full Scale IQ of 94.

In Mrs. Joy's progress note assessing my WAIS-R performance, she concludes: "All areas reveal improvement over baseline testing with lowest gains appearing in those subtests requiring visual spatial skills, re: block design and object assembly." Attention directed towards my low Performance IQ score on the WAIS-R, my psychologist dictated that I "continued to exhibit some mild deficiencies suggestive of continued right hemisphere involvement, namely in spatial relationships, visual memory, and complex visual perceptualization." In roughly ninety days time, my Verbal IQ score had improved by eighteen, my Performance IQ score by thirteen, and Full Scale IQ by seventeen. If I keep advancing at this pace, maybe I could be a Nuclear Scientist or a Mechanical Engineer, after all.

Right now, with the way I'm going, I'll just be happy if I ever get my freshman year out of the way. In the same report appraising my WAIS-R score, Mrs. Joy wrapped it up with: "It is yet premature to consider return to academic setting." So much for finishing on a positive note. "Let'go-oooo, Mountaineers!"

> July 27th (Tuesday): Because the pain that rod was inflicting on my hip wasn't subsiding any, I was scheduled to go to Allegheny General today for an appointment with the surgeon who operated on my fractured right leg. Apparently, because of the improvement I'm showing in most facets of my program, when Harmarville's Utilization Review meeting was staffed this morning, I was granted an extended stay at the rehab for only seven days, instead of the usual fourteen.

Dr. Imbriglia said that he never would have believed I'd be standing in his office talking to him given the near-fatal condition I was in that February 14th early morning when he inserted that thick, seventeen-inch titanium rod into my femur. This orthopedic surgeon said I'm very lucky to be alive and that he can't get over how well I'm doing.

When the good doctor told us he would surgically remove the rod after I told him how it was bothering me, me and my parents' initial reaction was one of dread, for we thought that I wouldn't have to be subjected to anymore operations. Originally, we had been informed the rod wouldn't ever have to be removed; that it would be sort of a souvenir permanently lodged in my leg. But since this steel bone-support has been acting up whenever I move my leg or put weight on it, this surgery proposition was something we had kept in the back of our minds as something that could very well happen. We weren't 100% sure being carved with a scalpel was the only option available to us towards relieving this severe discomfort I was barely tolerating, for we still held out hope that it would rectify itself somehow over time. Nice try, but I'm afraid it's not going to work that way.

Going under the knife isn't something people look forward to, but if it's going to alleviate the ripping sensation in my upper thigh, then it can't be done soon enough for me. Sensing a foreign body in one of your bones is not the most pleasurable of experiences and when it tears into you like it's going to penetrate your skin, the agony is both physical and psychological. Being informed that an operation is all that really can be done to stop the pain is not the most delightful news we've ever received, but if it takes away this unbearable ache, few things could top this.

Not wanting to do anything to disrupt the functioning of my newly transplanted artery by rushing things or cut into a leg that's been sliced open enough lately, Dr. Imbriglia said that he would remove the rod from my leg in March or April of next year, after he sees how things are going at that time. Instead of taking an attitude where I'm telling myself that this will mean I have to put up with the nagging twitch in my leg for eight or nine more months, I'll just have to look at it taking the view that at least something can be done about it. I know I'm not going to like it, but it's just something I've got to live with for now. At least the fear that nothing can be done has been alleviated, which had been weighing heavily on my mind.

My nurses and therapists couldn't possibly know how I am feeling because, if they did, I wouldn't be seeing those smiles on their faces. I am totally shocked, saddened, and worried beyond belief. This can't be! There's something wrong here, someone must have made a mistake. No way am I ready for this. Rehabilitation is supposed to be synonymous with restoration and I'm still broken. I never thought my condition was thought of as a hopeless cause by the professionals caring for me, until now.

I'm just starting to walk without two therapists helping to take me where I want to go and I still am sluggish when I write. I can't make my way up and down steps without clinging onto some side rails and having someone shadow me every step of the way. My thinking is still muddled and my right hand is no fuckin' good. What goes here?

I want to improve and it seems I'm just getting started. I know that I have had the blues as of late and wanted the hell out back a little while ago, but I've had a change of heart because I can see what this rehab's all about now. I hope this isn't a sign I'm being given up on by those with the sometimes unenviable task of having to work with me. I know I haven't given up on myself.

I get irritated because I try so damned hard and the gains aren't coming like I want them to. This agitation is not a reflection of what I think of the rehab center or the people that work here. I hope this didn't have anything to do with the decision that was ultimately made.

I know that in the past I've made references that it sometimes seems I'm just wasting time and so little is coming from my "back-breaking" effort, but I can see now that I'm in the right place, if something's gonna give and I'm going to get back to being healthy again. The determination that was made is leaving me in a state of flux.

I can try to look at it from the positive perspective that I don't need such extensive treatment anymore, but this isn't easy because of all that's still wrong with me. I know that effort on the part of the patient is the main ingredient with any kind of recovery, but rapport one has with their therapists is also a vital component to the mix. This can't be happening, there's still so many basic things I can't do.

Maybe this is reality's way of giving me a chilling slap in the face and telling me I'll never be right again; that I'll always be lacking and getting on track again is something that just isn't going to happen because of this injury to my brain. I can't live with that. Totally unexpected, Harmarville was planning to discharge me.

Basically, Harmarville is geared for those with the very worst of disabilities and I guess they figured that I'm "out of the woods" as far as possibly regressing and it's time to let me go now. Because I'm progressing so well, one would think that since I've got such a good thing going, to stick with it until conditions prove otherwise. If it ain't broke, don't fix it.

I guess Harmarville figures because I've missed home so much and really benefited from my visits back in Washington, that going back full-time now is the answer. I can only assume that they reasoned my walking, writing, hand, and perceptual lapses have progressed to the point where any outpatient therapy program would be able to provide me with the treatment I would need to improve. And because I can understand now what needs done to advance to the next level, I'm sure Harmarville feels that I can do—as I have done—a lot on my own without structured supervision.

Since being at Harmarville, I've been in the fast lane towards recovery. It's been a one-way ticket towards progress since I've been at the rehab and there's been no looking back. Now they want to take me from this environment where so much has been accomplished with me and I've finally grown comfortable. One can't be at their best if they are within surroundings which don't promote the utmost in care. And this was the trump card that was going to be played.

Because of where the discharge plan had me going for my continued therapy at home, peering eyes would have made optimal recovery difficult. The stress and tension of having Paul's worldly parents staring at me while I would be working in my therapies would prevent me from focusing 100% on what I would need to do to overcome what their son had done to me. Ready or not, it would have been too easy for Paul to be "just passing through" and dropping by for a visit with his well-rounded parents and taking a long, prying look at me which would have been uncomfortable to say the least.

A patient's therapist can't be involved with them beyond a professional level and objectivity must prevail. When personal matters come into the picture, sacred ground is being treaded upon. Being a co-worker with Paul's parents, therapists would have a natural loyalty to their fellow employee, thus the patient in need of having primary care established, would get second consideration. When a patient has had a head injury, anything other than undisturbed focus on the part of the patient and therapists can be catastrophic. During the course of the next week, Harmarville will have the opportunity to contemplate our position.

Our social worker's progress note of 7/27 summarizes me and my parents' feelings about being released at this time. Laura writes, "Craig states he is very disappointed that he may be discharged. His family is very supportive and also hope that Craig can stay at HRC longer to receive intensive therapy."

There's not much I can do about this, but to ride out the storm and keep my fingers crossed that things will work for the best. In the meantime, I'm just going to concentrate in therapy on what I need to do, if I'm to go this week and apply the finishing touches on my inpatient rehab.

One last time or will there be more to come? I was conscious of the fact that this might be my last dance, but I couldn't let this get in the way of what I have to do during treatment.

In PT this week, I was improving with the advanced exercises of backward walking, fast walking, as well as running. Also, I was going up and down stairs now by myself and walking a distance in excess of 500 feet. When ambulating, I was showing an increased ability to shift my weight and perform the proper pelvic motion.

In my cognitive therapies, Psych and CS, I was swinging that left hand of mine writing those cursive letters with increasingly more fluency. This wasn't exactly being done at the speed of light, but that corpus collusum of mine had healed to the point where I was now reproducing letters without any kind of a hitch. My typing, although not done with a blur, could now be measured in increments of words per minute (WPM) rather than words per week (WPW). Because my reading comprehension was in the 38%ile when the standard is the 46%ile, improving upon this will be a focal area the next five days in Communications. With those low WAIS-R Performance scores etched in her mind, my psychologist outlined her program this week to address these right hemisphere residual cognitive deficits.

Since my career pursuit is one where a mastery of English concepts is required, my Vocational program this week continued to supplement those areas which work on language skills. With my tutor, I continued to work on rules of grammar, punctuation, and writing.

There has to be a major short-circuit somewhere in the switchboard that controls my right hand. The lack of progress I see in my right fingers and wrist has always been trying for me, but now that I'm bringing my guitar to hand therapy to work on my picking, this therapy is now devastating for me. And embarrassing.

Because I learned how to play the instrument well in a short amount of time, I never thought I'd be ashamed with the way that I pick the guitar—until now. My left fretting hand would switch chords smoothly, but I had to slow down until my right hand caught up. With any kind of musical instrument, if the two body parts playing are not synchronized and working together as a team, the wail produced is a disturbing noise, not music.

In front of my therapists and the other patients, I sounded like shit. I know they understood my disability prevents me from playing up to my past capabilities, but I still felt like a louse because my playing ability was something I was so proud of and talked about quite a bit. And for everyone to hear just how bad I sound now was tough to handle. After Kevin showed me what to do, at least I'm able to press the strings down against the frets at the proper position with my good hand. That's a start and you gotta start somewhere, I suppose.

Because of the fingering my left hand was doing, my therapist could tell that I once could play pretty well when my right hand could move. Realizing the trouble I was having holding onto my pick with my paralytic right hand, Wendy thought dipping those slippery little buggers in a blue liquid which becomes a sticky rubbery coating when it dries might help. I'll give it a shot if she thinks it'll work. I know that if I want to have a quick picking hand again, that wiffle ball pick will have to go one of these days. Besides, the sooner I can get back to normal, the better I'll feel about things. This blue stuff on the pick isn't exactly natural, but I'm definitely going to give it a shot, if it's going to get me back to playing again.

Guitar wasn't only a part of my life these past three years, it had BECOME my life. From a general frame of reference, the number of years I have been playing were not many, but because of my desire to learn and be proficient on the six-string, I practiced many, many hours each and every day with the result being I was better than or just as good as a lot of players that had been picking two and three times longer than I have. Now, it's 1979 all over again when I first picked the instrument up and all that time and torture learning this obsession is wasted because now it takes all the concentration and effort I've got just to make sure I don't drop my pick. Damn you, Paul, you spoiled, drunk-ass, rich bastard.

Processing this discharge situation from our vantage point—while keeping in mind that there is probably a certain degree of separation anxiety on my part about leaving the only environment which I have a vivid recollection—on Wednesday, August the 3rd, Harmarville met us halfway and extended my inpatient care two weeks. This grace period of fourteen days will give me some time to emotionally adjust and psychologically prepare myself better for the return to the outside world than to be "thrown to the wolves" without much in the way of advanced warning. Thrust into surroundings which I should take comfort, but where little is known and any understanding will be a new beginning, is a nightmare which could never be one I fully become acclimated. Being a circumstance I will need to learn to accept in time, embracing life as it will be for now on shall be a torment I shouldn't have to endure, but one that I must if I'm to coexist with the inabilities that will test my endurance and willpower to overcome. Hopefully, this added period of adjustment at the rehab will help me cope with the conversion to my "new" environment of being home.

This extended frame of time would, just as importantly, provide my parents with some breathing room where they could make all the necessary arrangements for my return home full-time. For them, this additional block of time will be used to secure the services I will need to keep in pace with my goal of getting back to where I was before Paul left me for dead that Valentine's night. Rather, as close as I can get to the way I was.

Seeing me in the rehab twice a week and on weekends in my compromised condition was torture for my parents, but to see me at home everyday struggling will be a state that will take some time getting used to. But like everything else since I tangled with that utility pole on 672 E. Beau Street, they'll do whatever is needed, so that things can work in my favor.

By now, you'd think I'd have learned something. As usual, Harmarville was right. My lobbying for this extended stay and being stubborn about how this was going to benefit me hasn't worked like I thought it would, for all I'm doing now is spinning my wheels. I'm becoming bogged down into the dark pit of realization that, as Harmarville foresaw, hasn't done a whole lot to glisten my outlook of things. The premise behind this awareness is one where, what I see now, might be basically all that I'm going to get.

During this two-week prolonged agony, it has become increasingly more apparent that no matter where I'm at, whether it's Harmarville or someplace else, I'm at the point where much of the magic could be over. Time to build from what little I feel I've got, I must start putting together the pieces of a life which—for all intents and purposes—should not be. Hopefully, what becomes assembled will be a puzzle which shows a passage into a tomorrow which glimmers with hope and prosperity.

I thought this encore of intensive therapy at Harmarville I insisted upon would be fourteen days of continued stellar progress, however, it has been anything but encouraging. If there is a gain from this experience, it would be that I know now that I have to find someway to learn to appreciate the achievements I have made and accept what I've got now is more than I could have ever hoped for. I'm just going to have to revise my thinking of things and learn to live with my shortcomings, if I'm to proceed in a healthy fashion. But it's impossible to completely satisfy a person who keeps needing more.

This drive definitely has helped in my rehab effort, but could prolong unneeded turmoil, if it interferes with my ability to see my condition as is and how my disability will play in my future. When trying to walk this rainbow, believing it's a bridge to a brighter horizon, it is soon discovered that this path of hoped for prosperity is one that cannot be traveled because it does not have the firm foundation of reality. With God's will, the only way for me to reach that radiant star which is tomorrow's triumphs is to confront my denial and overcome the fears which I sometimes feel I have been trapped.

Almost having my head knocked off actually has put it on straight. My eyes have been opened as to what truly is important. Being in the midst of tragedy, I have learned more about myself and my family these past several months than my previous eighteen years combined. When one's back is against the wall and you've got to come together to pull through, this is when you find what you're made of.

What's really vital is the strength in your heart and the support one has to develop. Often, many teenagers who are lacking have to play a game, so they're seen as strong and of value when they are really hurting and not full because the majority of their time is spent covering up how they really feel, instead of doing something productive about it. These adolescents are extremely intelligent in the sense that they can make this front that has no meaning appear to be a foundation of maturity and development. Unfortunately, my grasping onto a person who exuded these false qualities for acceptance, almost led to my undoing.

Kids of this nature frequently do not receive the discipline and caring from their parents/primary caregivers that they are deserving, so they must preserve this facade. For those who live this existence which lacks any kind of authenticity, this artificial appearance needs maintained so that they can continue to be perceived as feeling worthwhile about themselves when, in fact, their life is one which lacks substance. Mistakenly believing this masquerade to be how life was for most, I was never satisfied and continually craving which made me one lost, vulnerable soul with no direction.

Being in this state where I perceived myself as deprived, I only could see that which I didn't have, but wanted. Because of it almost being taken from me, I now have a grasp of the many precious things that are in my possession. My character as a person and the love of my parents are two invaluable entities that no amount of money could ever buy. My efforts at Harmarville and the people here guiding me along the way made this "awakening" possible. This knowledge and understanding I have finally captured will help me persevere when the days are overcast and seems as if the sun will never pierce the darkness. This fresh conception has provided me with the freedom to look at the world from an angle blossoming with promise, rather than one where all is bleak.

This new outlook I never want to surrender has molded my personality into one where I now have purpose and an optimistic view of what I'm to achieve. Because of this, the potential which always seemed to be in lasting hibernation can now bask in the warmth of production's arrival. This changing season where I've experienced this inner blooming has enhanced my interactions with others 1000%. Most everyone I've been in contact with at Harmarville have been special and many have been exceptional which, I'm sure, will have some impact on me for the rest of my life. There's one person, however, I've met here at Harmarville who will forever have a place in my heart.

She doesn't have a slew of initials after her name, but that's not important to me. Having a smile that warms my heart and a laugh which puts me at ease that everything will be okay, my friend came at a time of my life when it was so important to have someone show they care from both a professional and personal level.

What Valerie showed me was, despite my physical and cognitive limitations, I was still whole and someone that mattered. Valerie accepted me for who I am now, not for the person I was when I was healthy. This was extremely important to me because I know deep inside that the Craig Meyers who was in physically mint condition will forever be a memory. I needed to receive this message that I was of some value, for I couldn't be sure this was possible given the way I am currently.

Having so many doubts about myself could have stranded me at a dead end, but when I needed to be shown a passage around this emotional blockade, Valerie's friendship and caring helped me get out of the "blahs" and erase some of the negativity I too often create for myself. Because I can be my toughest critic, if I really want something, sometimes I'm impossible to please.

Valerie wanting to spend a little bit of her time with me and involving herself with some activities we could enjoy together made me feel good about myself and that my appealing to someone of the opposite sex someday doesn't have to be impossible. If it weren't for Valerie playing a little ping-pong with me and allowing me to give her guitar lessons during the week, I would really feel repulsive about myself, I'm afraid.

I never met anyone like Valerie. Because of my past experience, I always thought a friendly female was something you only read about in a fiction novel, but now I know better. Valerie was also understanding in the sense that she wouldn't let me get too discouraged about what I had forgotten, always highlighting my improvements. And one thing she noted was that the mist hazing the images of my past was clearing.

It didn't hit me at first because a lot of what I knew and remembered about W.V.U. when she told me this was not clear at the time. Valerie had said her and her husband lived a short distance from the rehab center, in a community called Penn Hills.

I didn't think anything of this until the associative function in my brain eventually healed enough a short time later where I could match people with places. Putting some thought into it, I knew I had heard of "Penn Hills" before, but I could not remember where. But then it came back to me.

Ironically, the only other attractive female who ever seemed to take an interest in me premorbidly was also from Valerie's hometown as well. The music major goddess who sat next to me in English class at college seemingly several milenniums ago and who I'm almost positive came to my dorm room when I wasn't there was also from Penn Hills. Even more astounding is that Valerie knew of this Mountaineer vixen.

There must be something in the water there which makes females from that area think I'm appealing. I've got to bottle me some of that and take it back to Washington with me. Either that or splash that nurse with the sensual buttocks who was going up the stairwell when I was practicing steps in PT and hope, she too, is from this eastern suburb of Pittsburgh.

This "D minor" chord never sounded so sad. The guitar lesson I was giving Valerie this Tuesday night was bittersweet. One of the things I've always been striving for since being at Harmarville is almost here, but the goodbye I will need to give to my special friend in a few hours will not be easy.

There's usually a positive that comes from any tragedy. If I hadn't been "banged up," there's no way I would've ever met my dear buddy Valerie, who has impacted how I will think of myself for many days ahead. All I had to do so she'd like me was for me to be myself, which she taught me was just fine and that I didn't need any major revisions personality-wise. I now know that wearing different hats just to please everyone else is not the answer, for I'm sacrificing who I really am. And when this happens, you sell yourself short.

Because of Valerie's influence, I learned that I can be appreciated for the qualities I possess. Because of this "awakening," I can comprehend that the traits I do have can take me a long way. Valerie could see the intricacies of my character as they were and her insight/subsequent approach with me allowed me to express the part of my inner workings I had always been afraid to, but for which I longed. Always having been conditioned to avoid that which instinctively a person needs to be happy, Valerie's friendship showed me that there's nothing wrong with being open and that it's quite natural to want a sharing union with someone. And the most significant aspect of all this is that I learned I don't have to be anybody but myself to attain this.

Writing an occasional letter to someone who has left such a profound impression on me seems like so little, but that's about the only way we're going to be able to keep in touch now because by the time she comes to work her shift tomorrow, I'll be gone. Thank you Valerie for everything you've done, you're an incredible friend. I'll never forget you.

August 18th (Wednesday): I was discharged from Harmarville Rehabilitation Center.

Looking into a mirror, before I came to Harmarville, the person I would be looking at had a deep-seated inferiority about himself. Lacking confidence in most of my abilities, I retreated into a horror which I felt condemned. I'm not saying this was necessarily the case, but the image gazing back at me felt as if his word was disregarded and actions never good enough. Feeling as if I never measured up, I buried myself in a harrowing discord that I knew I couldn't get out of. Self-mutilating perceptions of myself continuously harassed me and these masochistic thoughts which I struggled with were the core of my feeling comfort only when I was in isolation and insulated from damaging disparagement. I did not see these editorials of me as the misdirected fabrications that they were, rather, as the backbone of my character.

Needing to find the solace which comes with accepting oneself, I reached out to whomever I believed might help me discover this elusive serenity. Unfortunately, those I latched onto for approval did not have the foundation of character they were so cleverly able to falsify and wanted others to think they had.

Formulating a healthy image of how I felt about myself was dependent on how others perceived me and whether or not they gave me a passing grade. When one thinks in this manner, they are surrendering control of their life to everyone but themselves. This is extremely volatile and dangerous if the person you've assigned this authority to is one you may have reservations about because what they portray might not be who they are. Being a prisoner of a war that I conjured in my mind was a battle I could not win because I would be the only casualty in this confrontation, for I was my enemy.

However, my efforts following my accident and all that I've accomplished "against all odds" has given me an "awakening" as to who I really am. For all that I've had to endure physically and psychologically, I now see myself as a person with incredible emotional fortitude and strength. I know there are still many mountains to climb yet, but to do what I've done in the face of destruction is nothing short of amazing. And any person who has been through the hell I've been and comes as far as I have, can't be too bad.

Obviously, this new awareness could not have been achieved were it not for the prowess of those medical professionals at Allegheny General who worked with me, and for this, I owe them my life. Because I don't remember ever being at AGH, it goes without saying then, that my character enhancement had to have occurred while I was at Harmarville. The way the professionals here were with me allowed me to feel good about myself which was something that I didn't experience all that often.

I know they reciprocated how I was with them and I'm sure my effort, overall attitude, and regard had something to do with the way I was approached, but Harmarville's amicable interactions with me went well beyond the call of duty. I may have had a head injury, but I'm not dumb; I know that with any patient/caregiver alliance, unconditional positive regard must occur. However, it's not too hard to sense when a relationship between these two parties exceeds mere courtesy and duty into something with a little more depth. The personalities and dispositions of the professionals working at Harmarville made me feel worthy, respected, and liked. Harmarville staff's ingrained good nature was the key which helped me to unlock the vault where my assertiveness and self-esteem had been lost.

Because those who hold such a high opinion of me are authentically good, quality people, not fakes whose sole purpose is a self-serving one, then I must be okay too. I had to go through a lot to see this. God works in mysterious ways.

Welp, this is it. Considering how I was coming in five months ago and the way I am now, I don't think I'd be mincing words much if I'd say this Harmarville experience has been magnificent. Not only from a cognitive and physical restoration standpoint, but from a self-acceptance one as well.

If one looks hard enough, often there's some good to be found in a bad situation. The growth I've experienced since I was hurt has propelled me into a new beginning where my outlook on things has risen, so that I now have a clearer image as to my place on this earth and for what I stand. Out of the darkness which blinded me from understanding my purpose, I now can say with confidence that my role in life is one which is inclusionary, not a tragedy where I should take comfort in being excluded and alone. I always thought I had the makings of someone who could be of significance, but I could never seem to tear down the self-demeaning barriers which penned me in and kept me from attaining what I wanted.

Making the wondrous achievements few thought possible since I was almost killed, had provided me with a confidence that I can master whatever I set my mind to. With some of the people I have the misfortune of knowing, I know words will be used as a wrecking ball in an attempt to demolish my pillar of strength, but it will take more than a verbal assault now to reek havoc on my structure because I've been fortified with this new power of understanding.

Submissiveness is no longer inherent of me, for I can now see the motives of those who tried to forever imprison me in this unwanted position. Since being at Harmarville, my sentence has ended. In that sense, this accident was the best thing that ever happened to me.

This past Friday was the 13th and marked the six month anniversary I went out to the party which led to all this. On this Friday the 13th, the tutor mom and dad contracted with to work on my cognitive deficits at home, Mrs. Joni Russell,

M.Ed., came to Harmarville and sat in on my cognitive therapies to get an idea of what she could do to address my limitations. To see and hear from my rehabilitation therapists firsthand what it was I would need to continue progressing, my home-based cognitive retrainer got a flavor of what I would have to work on in order to prepare for college again. However, for good reason, not all were optimistic about this desired return to W.V.U. "Let's go-oooooo, Mountaineers!"

In CS and Psych, Joni (pronounced like the male name "Johnny") caught a glimpse of my existing right hemisphere spatial and perceptual aphasias, as I continue to have problems of varying degree with certain exercises. While observing what my brain being injured did to my ability to conceive my world, Joni was given some recommendations what remedial treatments might benefit me. Along with her own bag of tricks, Joni was mentally mapping out how she would be going about making some cognitive repairs, so I'd be able to go back to Wild, Wonderful, West Virginia. "Let's go-ooooooo, Mountaineers!"

Based on my previous college performance and continuing cognitive afflictions, while I was out of the Psychology room talking to my soon-to-be private instructor, my parents were told not to be surprised if my college performance is a less-than-passing one. Given the intellectual deficiencies I currently have that may always affect me, my parents were informed that attaining my Bachelor's Degree seems far-fetched at this time. This dim prognosis likely an authentic opinion given what is generally acknowledged/ accepted about head injury, I can only surmise that I'll never possess the capabilities necessary to attain a Master's Degree.

However, what this accident has done is allow me to see the proverbial "light," and my needing to prove to myself that I'm back—emotionally better than ever—is all the motivation I will need. Because of my "awakening," without a doubt, I'll find the stamina to reach my summit.

On this last day I would be at Harmarville as an inpatient, there was also no doubt I was confused about the revision in my schedule. Patients fortunate enough to be discharged from Harmarville have their schedule altered on the last day at the rehab center, so that any loose ends can be tied up before they leave and so that they can get out of here by mid-afternoon. With this frontal lobe damage I've sustained, it's confusing for me to decipher the adjustment that has been made in my program on this day where I'm finally cut loose. I guess Mrs. Joy's reservations about me going back to college are pretty well-founded.

Feeling like I did when I took the Trails A and B Test a few months back, after having mixed emotions about finishing up my final abbreviated Communication Skills session with my gem of a therapist, Diane Rosato, I asked her and Laura if they'd point me in the right direction for my next therapy. At that moment, trailing me to all my therapies this last day with his camera embarrassing me, my corny dad whipped out his Keystone Everflash 20 and snapped a picture of me fashionably decked out wearing my hand splint and patched glasses with these two beauties who would make Hugh Heffner pant. To tell you the truth, this is one picture I wouldn't mind having enlarged.

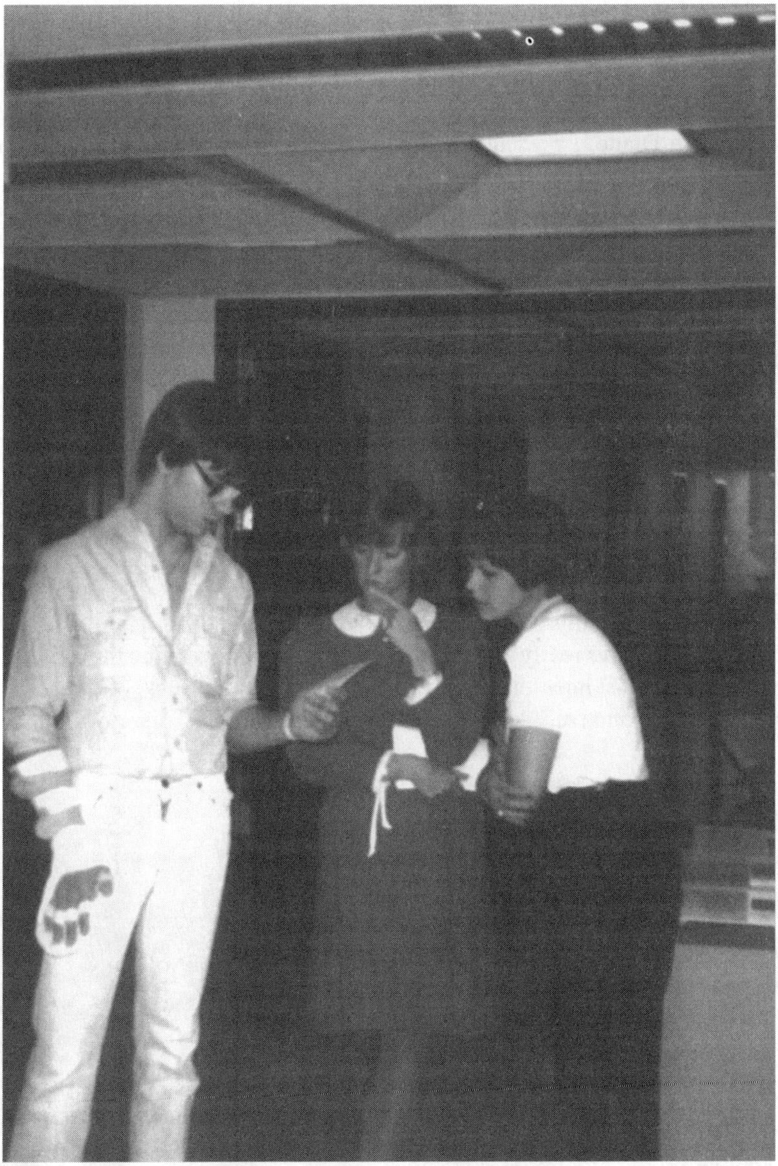

Laura Matthews-Beninati, M.S.W. and Diane Rosato, M.A. looking at Craig's revised program schedule on the day he was discharged from Harmarville.

Waddling down the hallway one last time towards the PT gym, I said my goodbyes to the lady who pulled off a miracle getting me back on my feet and walking again, Jan, and another skilled therapist with a million-dollar personality who worked with me periodically, John. As a small token of our undying appreciation, like I did with Diane, I presented Jan with a gift wrapped box of candies mom bought. We figured that these Sarris chocolates would give Jan a little extra energy boost the next time she encounters another agitated Ranchos 4 admission like I was. As I made one last inpatient crack about things, dad would flick another picture. This photo might have been worthy of framing too had John shaved this morning.

Next on the agenda was saying farewell to my Vocational Counselor. Feeling somewhat sprightly, Donna had the fortune of running into me as I was getting into a fired-up mood being that my last day at Harmarville was coming to a close. Far from being consensual, I snatched Donna up, threw my arm over her shoulder, posed for dad this time, and had a picture taken with my shocked counselor standing in the main corridor where I used to do my practice laps. Engaged, I don't know how thrilled Donna was, as that smile on her face she was wearing for the camera looked as if it took a lot of effort. Having had a head injury and this being my last afternoon at the rehab, I figured I could get away with this without getting hit. Besides, I knew my dad would be there to protect me just in case Donna decided it was time to put me in my place.

The adrenalin was really gushing through my body now being that this OT session would be my last inpatient therapy program at Harmarville, but I was still able to down that cake and fruit drink spread these Occupational Therapy darlings laid

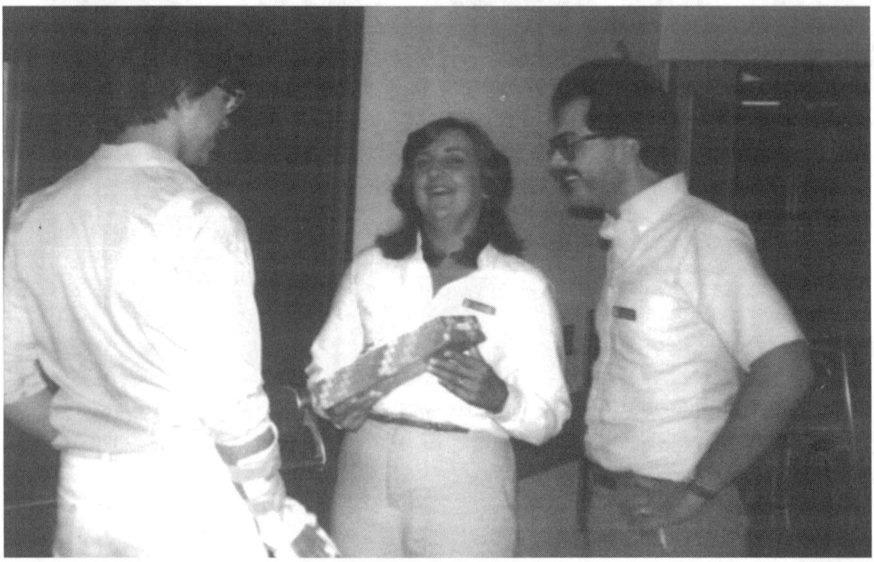

PT's Jan Alba and John Sirianni smiling, as Craig presents his physical therapist a box of candies on discharge day.

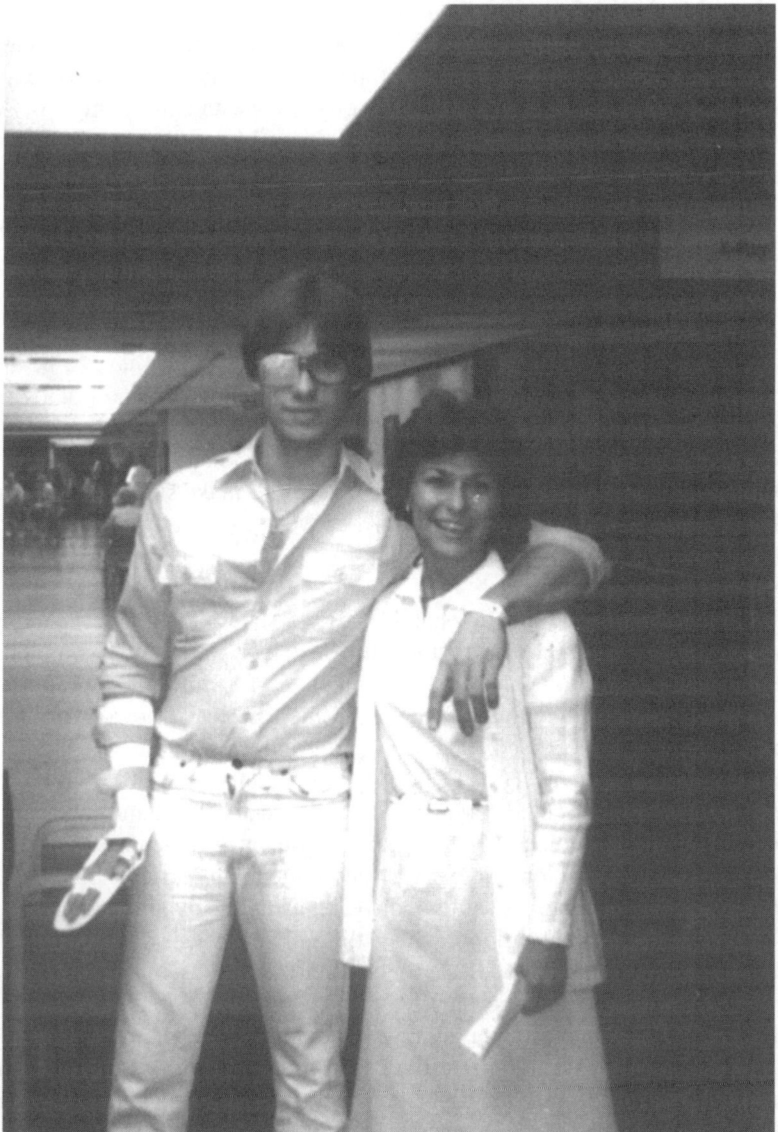

Hardly consensual, Craig wraps his arm around the Vocational Department's, Donna Sebastian.

out for me. This act alone is indicative of the character of Wendy, Ann, Stephanie, and all the rest of them, for most people would be less forgiving/understanding given the way I would gripe and blow my top at times in my hand therapy sessions.

As I sat on the mat preparing to chomp on my cake and guzzle my Kool-Aid, Wendy was standing beside me and I wouldn't have blamed her if she gave me a little kick before I left given this would be her last opportunity to get back at me for all those times I was such an irritable cuss for her. But I kind of figured that because she's such a nice professional, she'd refrain from giving me "the boot."

Like Donna a couple of minutes ago, Wendy knew that if she were going to step out of character momentarily and give me just a little punt, there's a good chance this might get caught on film, for dad was standing right there ready to take another snapshot. Despite being all bandaged up, I guess I just have to be thankful this is one of those rare days where I'm relatively photogenic, for dad's antics weren't all that I'd have to go through before I got out of here. Because I was often an aggravated cuss in her therapies—like my brother years before—maybe I should still take a close look at my Kool-Aid just to make sure that there aren't any worms floating around at the bottom that Wendy might have "accidentally" slipped in.

I should have figured they'd want a final act. I guess I ought to feel honored Harmarville thinks enough of me that I would have the spotlight flicked on me one more time, so my last moments here as an inpatient of theirs could be captured on videotape, but this is ridiculous. If they hand me a script or powder my nose, I might just wet myself because I want to go home and leave this inpatient rehab experience behind me as quickly as I can. Where's my urinal when I need it?

Directing this video, Mrs. Joy told me to go up and shake hands with some of the patients who were going to be here for a while yet and then head for the exit one last time. As I went clopping my way down the main corridor this final time, several patients and therapists said goodbye, figuring this would be the last time they'd see my hitched strut galloping down the hallway. And it was here that it was suggested to dad that he do his best Robert Redford impression and wave goodbye before he drove off into the sunset.

Not at all taking into account my urgency to hit the road, hardly being a "joy" this last day here, my psychologist strongly recommended that we run through this production two times in case the first take wasn't good enough to print. Considering all Mrs. Joy has done for me—even with my legs crossed and eyes bulging in anticipation to get going—we'd gladly retrace our steps, if this video documentary of my care at Harmarville from admission to discharge will benefit some patient here in the future. Now let's hurry up and bid "adieu" before a wardrobe consultant is brought in because they don't like the blue shirt I'm wearing and want me to try something else on.

Having been robbed of so much physically and intellectually has actually provided me with a tremendous amount of growth from a maturation standpoint. This

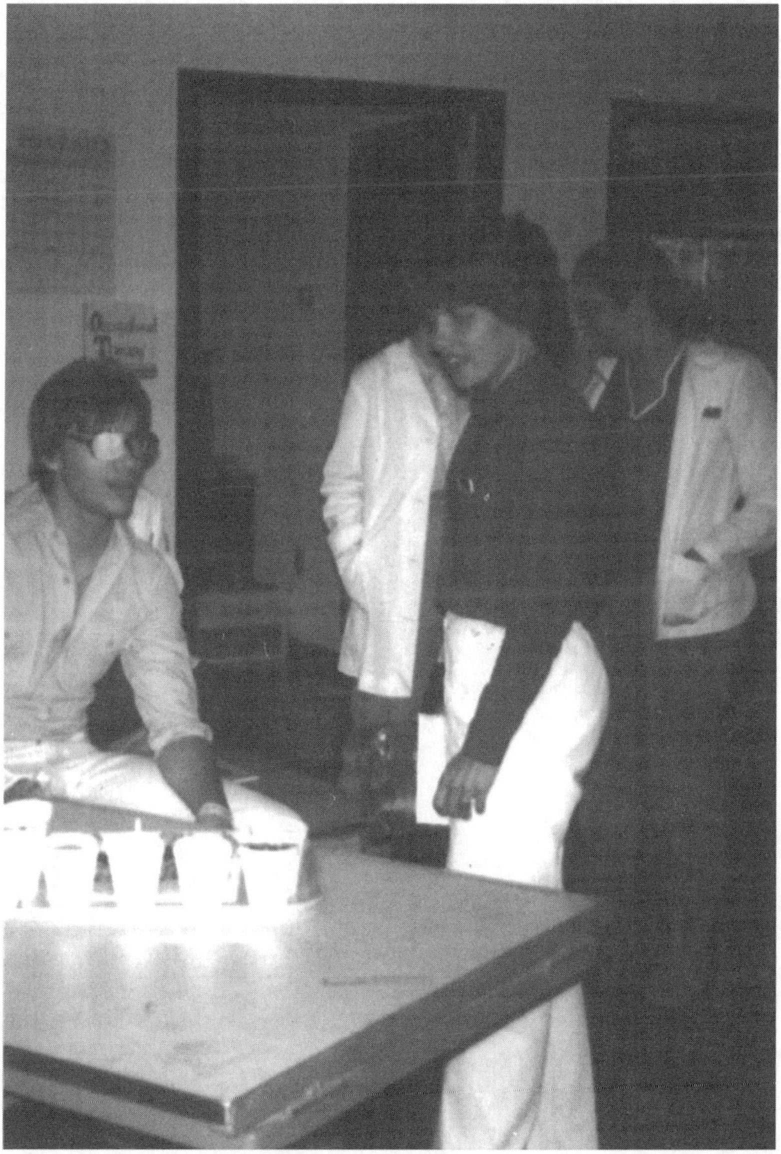

Frequently agitated in Wendy Wood's OT sessions, it spoke volumes about her professionalism that she would offer Craig a little fruit punch before this combative patient left the rehab center.

emotional "awakening" has given me the tools where I can begin constructing the frame for my future. This structure's foundation will be solidified by my enhanced perspective that the ingredients having molded me as a person are indeed special and resilient. I can now harvest a new development where the seeds of progress will sprout from this fertile understanding.

With God leading the way, my efforts and Harmarville's caring touch have transformed me from a frail boy coming in, to a rejuvenated man going out. I could never thank the staff at the rehabilitation center enough for this enlightened spirit and all they've helped me to grasp again. God bless you, Harmarville.

Chapter 6

Transition: The Long Journey Back

Slicked up modeling a suit that looks like the finest Georgio Armani has to offer, this fine-looking, distinguished gentleman with the gray sprinkled in his dark sideburns fools absolutely no one when he tries to inconspicuously look at me out the corner of his eye, as I attempt to stack these toddler blocks with my right hand for the millionth time. I've been coming to these one-hour OT sessions three times a week for many, many weeks now and at least one day during this weekly aggravation, Mr. Michaels—Paul's father—manages to step in the therapy room when I'm scheduled to work there, either to wheel in a patient or speak to the head occupational therapist. While doing this orderly duty, this spiffy gent—who looks like a million bucks—will take a peek to see how I'm doing. When I see the man face to face who is largely responsible for me being here, believe it or not, I have mixed emotions about him and all of them do not have overtones of hatred.

If there's one feeling I should reserve for myself, not one of the culprits of the crime which has left me with one workable hand, it's sympathy. Since his son bowled me into that utility pole, fearful of what the ramifications of this might be, I'm fairly confident that Mr. Michaels' life has been in a pressure cooker. No matter how much of a secondary role—if not a primary one—his parental "guidance" played in this tragedy, you have to feel at least a little sorry for someone whose reputation could be in jeopardy because of his child's actions. After spending years of study and labor honing his trade, it would be a shame if a league of professionals would come to the conclusion that, if Mr. Michaels has no authority over his own son, what business does he have working with others and having an impact on the control they exhibit in their lives?

I think Mr. Michaels watching me indicates he's at least a little concerned with my progress after his son took away the good use of my dominant hand. Because he was the one who informed my parents of some of the specifics surrounding the accident, I'd imagine his concern and interest stretches beyond how my development/progress are consequential for him. I guess he wouldn't be human if he wasn't at all interested. When I see his eyes glued to my fingers to see how they respond, I know he's concerned about something.

Being that kids are a reflection of their parents and considering the high position he holds in the human services field, I'd imagine Mr. Michaels is sweating blood right now that all this is going to be swept under the rug and forgotten about in time without causing too much damage. Putting myself in Mr. Michaels' shoes, I wouldn't be too ecstatic that the boy my offspring hurt is coming to the facility where I work, so that he can undo—as much a possible—what my son's drunkenness did to him.

Knowing that I'm not obligated to keep my mouth shut or fabricate a lie when my outpatient occupational therapists ask me about the who, what, where, and when's of the accident—more than likely—Mr. Michaels will be embarrassed and gun-shy when word gets out to the people who work with my bum hand that his boy's overindulgence devastated a family. Nor was mom indebted to keeping a tight lip.

A woman who works closely with Mrs. Michaels and goes to our church told mom that the Michaels feel horrible that their son skidded on ice and hurt me. Enraged, mom set the story straight and told Mrs. Michaels' co-worker that what really happened was that their little boy was intoxicated and couldn't keep the car he was driving from going off the road and crashing into the utility pole. Shocked to hear the true version of the story, this fellow Women's Church Organization member of mom's was speechless—at least in front of mom. She'll probably have a lot to say back at work, though.

A few weeks ago, after I finished my therapy session, I spotted Mr. Michaels walking down the other end of the floor and identified for mom who he was because they had never met and didn't know what each other looked like. A short time later, while mom was trailing me and dad to an OT session one day, she saw Mr. Michaels pointing at me and talking to someone she believed to be a doctor because of what he was wearing and the stethoscope around his neck.

Not knowing who mom was, while she was standing right there, Mr. Michaels told his medical co-worker listener that I was the one who got hurt when his son's car slid on that infamous, fictitious slab of ice that was on the road. Not wanting to create a scene with all the ailing people around, mom bit her tongue, knowing the truth would eventually come out and that the Michaels would need to be held accountable one of these days. Mom knew Mr. Michaels was not being truthful in order to preserve his son's and the family's name, but justice wasn't being served.

I can understand the difficult, no-win position my nice occupational therapists are in. They either violate their duty of maintaining patient/clinician confidentiality and compromise my treatment, or keep quiet about something I may say—but feel mutinous in the process. I can imagine how they feel and know that anything juicy I might happen to let slip would get back to Mr. Michaels, which is why I screen everything I'm asked or divulge. A rookie therapist in her early to mid-twenties, not too far along out of school who just started working in the OT department, must not have been briefed about this potentially toxic situation before she was to work with me because she gave away the department's hand.

Feeling empathy—not for the permanent deficiencies that I will always have because of this accident—but for the unbelievable pain Mr. Michaels must be experiencing, after I told this young and inexperienced worker about the circumstances surrounding the accident and Mr. Michaels' "indirect" influence, feeling a rush of power, she angrily asked me then why I got in the car with Paul. Not wanting to reveal something I may later regret, I didn't tell her anything because it wasn't any of her damned business and I couldn't be positive I wasn't being baited into saying something that later could be used against me. I think even Mrs. Joy and Diane would agree that this isn't paranoia, rather, an enhanced ability to look at a circumstance from a variety of angles and assess the meaning of each.

This setting where I have to do my therapy where the drunk driver's father is employed doesn't promote optimum comfort, but I've gotten used to this discomfort these past couple of months and it won't stop me from doing what I have to, so that I can get that right hand of mine working better. "Way to go Craig. Go get 'em!!"

While I was looking for different words hidden amongst the cluster of letters, the processes in the right hemisphere of my brain were doing their perceptual thing with increasingly more ease, as I'm starting to find these exercises overly simplistic now. To her credit—along with an assortment of her other strategies—Joni has used colored blocks, mazes, different instructional books, writing exercises, and puzzle games so masterfully that by my birthday—the middle of September—I was going through these like the child's play that they were. As a matter of fact, on around my nineteenth, Joni had seen such an improvement in my spatial/perceptual abilities, as well as my grammar/vocabulary, that she thought it might not be too soon to start thinking about taking a look around for an English college placement course somewhere. Don't know about that, but I'm happy she's pleased with my progress.

Joni's been coming to the house twice a week for the last four months, working to improve my befuddled thinking and she's really done a fabulous job moving me one step closer to going back to college. Tough, but still cool, I'm going to hate to see Joni go. She and her husband are expecting their first child in a few months, so she's taking a maternity leave from both her tutorial assignments and teaching duties in the Trinity school district.

Back in August, Harmarville stipulated that I could be discharged provided that my parents could secure the services of a tutor who was qualified to work on my cognitive deficits. If they couldn't have found a certified home-instructor to ensure that I receive cognitive retraining on a continual basis, then I would have had to stay at the rehab two more weeks than I did or—if I would be discharged—make three trips weekly to Harmarville on an outpatient basis until a private instructor could be found. Knowing that this meant I could be home full-time, mom and dad found a good one in no time and Joni was at the house doing her wonders within a week of me being discharged.

To assure my ability to better comprehend the universe in which I live does not take a prolonged sabbatical, mom and dad wasted no time looking for another tutor. Joni's last day was scheduled for Tuesday, January 4th, 1983 and the replacement tutor my parents ultimately decided on—Mrs. Rebecca Greer, B.S.—was to start Thursday, January 6th, 1983. Setting the groundwork for my return to an institution of higher education, what Joni did was provide a base which Rebecca can build from when she starts. Great job, Joni. Best of luck to you and your expanding family. "Let's go-ooooooo, Mountaineers!"

Christmas has always been special at our house, but this one will really be one to cherish because it was so close to being one that was minus one family member. Celebrating the birth of Christ will always be a special event at the Meyers', but being blessed by the touch of the Lord early this year is going to give Christmas 1982 that much more meaning for us. This religious ceremony is also a time of reflection in our household and the tragedy I have been living each moment for the past ten months—and probably will have to endure for the rest of my life—can concoct images where the misery is unforgiving.

Even with the significance this holiday plays in our lives, I wouldn't be human if I did not feel the pain and regret which comes with a loss of this magnitude. This plateau I've hit where progress is tougher to come by is particularly difficult on me now because I spend the majority of my time alone trying to restore a little of how I was before my skull had been cracked.

I know that things not only could be worse, but should be worse. Reminding myself of this has helped me during those too frequent times when I saw no end to the drought which was the absence of my happiness, but this self-encouragement only takes me so far until the multitude of defects which are who I am now bring me crashing down to the stark reality that I'm forever damned to a limited existence. Choices are no longer ample and barriers impassable to exercise the liberties that should be a given. Taking many pleasures for granted as they should, I couldn't see everything I had and that things were going pretty good during those days when choices were bountiful and barriers not so dominant. Going to therapy for my hand and receiving tutoring for my understanding, I can only hope that—in the long run—I'm able to collar some of that which I can no longer claim is mine.

Spending day after day after day by myself now fencing with the thoughts of when I was full makes this paralysis, double vision, limp, aphasias, etc., etc. increasingly harder to bear. Not that my parents' company isn't exceptional, but at least when I was at Harmarville, there was a little bit of diversity to my day. Now, it's a routine of boredom, isolation, and disappointment.

With the exception of Kevin stopping by on Fridays for a few hours, I feel I'm not in touch with anyone from the outside world because most everyone I had anything to do with is away at school somewhere. Curiosity having faded as time wore on, I rarely see anyone beyond my immediate family, those treating me, and Mr. Michaels. What a life.

I guess this is indicative of my confused and unrealistic thinking, but right before I was discharged from Harmarville, I kept contemplating to myself that I better hurry up and get better because I had the vague notion I'd be going back to W.V.U. this upcoming fall. I was really perturbed that Dr. Prostko wanted me to sit out—not just a semester—but the entire year, so I could focus on getting that damaged brain of mine to work at least at a high school level again.

I just couldn't help but think how far I was going to fall behind the rest of the Class of '81. Kevin, for example, would either be a second semester sophomore or first semester junior, if I'm able to go back to college as planned next year. Still, in essence, a first semester freshman, I'd really feel out of place and alone returning to Morgantown. Missing what will be a year-and-a-half of school because of the accident is going to force me to do a lot of catching up and won't be much fun, but I just got to remember that I should feel fortunate that my twisted thinking is becoming unravelled and I'm getting the opportunity to fight back to get where I was before academically. Many head injuries forever render a person a fraction of what they were intelligence-wise.

I hope this wasn't an omen of how things were going to turn out during my post-Harmarville era of recovery. If things weren't bad enough, eight days after being discharged, my fellow Mountaineer and Washington resident I partied with at college—Matt Wright—was also in a serious, early morning car accident where alcohol was believed to be involved.

A few weeks before Matt's accident—which he too was a passenger—Matt stopped by our house to see how I was doing. On academic probation as well, Matt had to take the next year off too from W.V.U. to get his head on straight/take his studies more seriously. After I told Matt about my condition and how some of the experiences I've had in my past have been sifted from my memory, he detailed how he, his roommate, and I got into trouble after he discharged a fire extinguisher on the PRT car we were on following an evening of partying. When Matt told me the specifics of this stupid act, it all came back to me. One weekend when I came home from Harmarville, not knowing all the details, Kevin had once vaguely mentioned this incident I'd just as soon had remained forgotten.

When I told Matt I was setting my sights on getting back to college by next year if I continue progressing, he made the suggestion that we become roommates when we both—hopefully—go back in the fall of '83. Matt sounded sincere about his intention of partying less and doing more work, but if there's one thing I don't need at this time, it's anything which will remind me of my days as a hellion because that's what got me hurt in the first place. I told Matt that, because of the trauma my brain had sustained and because of my new outlook on things, my burnout days were over. I said to Matt that my long range plans at this time are that, if he'd have me, I was going to try to get in Pierpont House with Kevin next year when I go back to West Virginia University—that is, if I'm intellectually capable of returning to school at that time.

Wishing me the best, when Matt left that mid-summer day, he told me he was happy to see I was doing so much better and that he would catch me later. But that wasn't to be, for, after he shut the door behind him, this would be the last time I'd ever see Matt because he wouldn't be as lucky as I was. Two days after his accident, August 28th, Matt passed away.

At 1:30 A.M., I lost a friend that day. A nice guy whose life was cut short at the tender age of twenty. Before he had the opportunity to mature as a man and develop through experience, Matt was gone.

Wearing my patched glasses and splint, on the 30th day of August 1982, I slapped my foot limping into the parlor of the funeral home towards Matt's closed casket with my dad by my side to help me. Having been beaten and bruised so badly, Matt was not suitable to be viewed one final time. Numb, visions of when Matt was with us flooded my conscious and a tear moistened my eye.

I thought how this tear needn't be and the agony of all the many people standing here could have been avoided had the right choices been made. Like myself, if Matt would've only been more careful in choosing who he associated with and said the word, "No," more often, our tragedies wouldn't likely have occurred. The mixture of drinking, driving, and youth can be a deadly one.

Tears pouring, Matt's brother came up to me and said that Matt would want me to keep fighting and not let my disabilities get the best of me. When he said I'm lucky to be alive and that—despite my various afflictions—I should be thankful the way things have turned out for me, I looked at Matt's coffin containing the concealed body not suitable for viewing one final time and thought how easily that could have been me.

Matt having left for the Great Beyond long before his time and me—hobbling about speaking to different members of his family—a fraction of who I was before physically, are evidence that the choices people make do have consequences. For just a little bit of fun, the stakes are far too high and far too tragic. Goodbye Matt, you're a good guy who I'm going to miss a lot.

Within two months of his dying, I went back to the setting where I really got to know Matt, so that any memory I had of West Virginia University may be sparked again. On Friday, October 15th, me and dad went south to Morgantown where Kevin was going to show me different places I had been and should remember. We go down Route 79 South from Washington to Morgantown and there are seven exits between home and the W.V.U. campus. I used to know the names of the exits, but I couldn't remember a single one until we came up to them.

The drive down the interstate to Wild, Wonderful, West Virginia this time of year is a scenic one, for all that's before you to the left of the highway and to the right is a kaleidoscope of color. I know that I've been on this route many, many times, but until I was actually here this fall afternoon amongst the amber countryside, I could not form a picture in my mind how the surroundings looked on this trip. Given its powerful beauty during the autumn season when brightly sparkled leaves blaze through the backdrop of the horizon as far as the eye can see, not remembering this spectacular view is a testament just how tattered my memory has become.

Arriving at Exit 155, I knew this was where we got off to get to the Evansdale campus where Kevin and I lived this time last year in the Towers and where my ex-roommate lives now in an apartment complex a couple hundred yards away from our freshman living arrangement. Going past the Coliseum, I knew this was where we made a left off of Monongahela Blvd. onto Patterson Dr. to get to University Avenue where Kevin was waiting.

Grumbling, not at all enthralled with having to wait to see his parents and sister, this tour director position Kevin graciously volunteered for was greatly appreciated. When we got started on this expedition that I hoped would kindle some images of when I was a pre-journalism student, it was obvious that Kevin was feeling uncomfortable with the memories the first leg of this sight-seeing excursion brought.

Passing the McDonald's I'm surprised didn't go out of business because I had been away so long, my dad, Kevin, and I then came up to Tower 4. Mom had called the Towers earlier in the week to let them know I'd like to take a look at my old dorm room this Friday. The staff at Towers, remembering when I was in critical condition, were more than happy to clear the way for my hopeful memory-jarring return. Excited to hear that I was making out so well after being hurt so badly, the Towers' staff gladly made all the arrangements, so I could go up to room 4012 and take a look around.

Smiling, the older, motherly-type clerk at the Towers' front desk said she could remember when she heard that I had been hurt and was happy to see I'm back on my feet again. After telling us the students who live there now have no objection to our stepping in and taking a look at things—armed with key in hand—Kevin, my dad, and I headed for the stairway to the room where I was hell bent for leather to be a mischievous cuss.

Although I didn't spend much time there, to my left was the T.V. lounge which, just like the Towers' lobby, looked so familiar. The heavy metal door leading to the stairwell didn't look any different than it did eight months ago when I last closed it that three-day weekend in February. I could tell the all-purpose cleaner the custodians use to wipe off the steps and walls is the same because I'd know that sickening odor anywhere.

I had hiked up these steps thousands of times, but this would be the first one where I had to cling onto the handrail to my left and concentrate strenuously to get up. Rod cutting into my leg, I slid my foot atop each step until I climbed my way up the two flights of stairs to the second metal door which separated us from that infamous floor zero where many of its inhabitants of twelve months ago are either locked up somewhere or their trials are pending. A few thuds of my right foot later, I was standing in the hallway, outside the door with the numbers 4—0—1—2 on it.

Looking to my left, I could almost see the two studly roommates who lived next door to me and Kevin putting one another in a headlock out in the hallway during one of their evening wrestling matches last year. Gazing over my left shoulder behind me in the study area which ultimately—within a day and a half—became the recreation area, I could still, unfortunately, picture this one guy who lived down the hall with his pants around his ankles taking a dump by the door. I could hear and see this one hot-looking bare-backed girl—who left her top in one of the guys' rooms—laughing/screaming as she ran around the corner of the hall. The aroma of dried puke, fecal matter, and laundry which hadn't been done since summer vacation penetrated my nasal cavity, as it had when I lived on the lowest floor of this Tower. As odd as this may seem, I couldn't be happier that some of the sights, sounds, and smells of my on-campus, higher education living experience were coming back to me. However, the best was yet to come.

Kevin then unlocked the door and flung this ingression open to our old room when, two steps later, I was standing where the foundation for this whole nightmare was set. The room was arranged a lot nicer than me and Kevin had it, but I could still visualize my unmade bed by the closets and Kevin's neatly made one by the window. Beside my bed where I threw my clothes after class, I remember the desk I never used for studying was here and this was next to my chest of drawers where my continuously running stereo was situated. Coming in—to my right—I could visualize Kevin's tidy side of the room with his chest of drawers, desk, and bed neatly arranged. Straight ahead, as if I heard, saw, and felt them yesterday, I could sense—clear as could be—Kevin's damned clock/radio which woke me up many mornings an hour before I had to get up for class, and the window sill I got hawkered on one time while I was playing my guitar there. Naturally, I was overjoyed that I could form a mental picture of the general setup of the room, but Kevin's ability to call to mind the room's arrangement made me skeptical just how good I really was progressing.

Being Mr. Perception, Kevin was able to localize where each of the thirty or so posters were on the walls and ceiling. Obviously, I didn't know if he was right or not, but after he confidently told us where each poster was plastered, I could kind of envision their placement at these spots. I don't know if it is because Kevin's been gifted with a photographic memory, I'm not as far along as I thought, or it's because he had the nightmare task of taking these posters down after I had to withdraw—helping his recollection as to where these were situated—but there's no way I could've remembered the Aerosmith poster was by the mirror, Led Zeppelin above my stereo, Scorpions beside the window, etc. I just know that if I hadn't caught my parents at a time when they were so happy to see that I was home that they'd let me get away with anything, these very posters wouldn't be up in my room in Washington as they are now. Now, about that Fender guitar they promised to get me.

After we left the room, I really felt great because my memory as to how things were once laid out had come back to me. Since I banged my head against whatever it was it hit exactly, I had no idea what our old room looked like that. Actually being in the room which the current residents gratefully allowed us to take a look at after hearing why we wanted to see it, I couldn't stop the images of the past from flooding back.

Rod digging in, stabbing into my thigh, I went up the half dozen or so steps leading from the lobby to the window of the empty cafeteria. Looking at the many long tables spread throughout and several of the circular ones in the middle, I could see the features in my mind of Kevin, Boss, Paul, and myself eating together here.

On the side, I saw the beverage machine where I was able to picture me and Kevin getting our fruit drink and the doorway where we would come out with our tray of food. If I had the "munchies," tray<u>s</u> of food.

Down the hallway, to the left, when we passed the "Blue Tick Lounge," I could form a cloudy image of the four of us sitting at a table playing quarters. Up ahead, around the corner, were the stairs leading to Paul's and Boss' cannabis quarters where I spent way too much of my time hovering with the clouds and playing guitar.

With classes ending for some at the Beechurst campus, a horde of students, who just got off the PRT, were heading our way. And it was here that I discovered one problem I was going to encounter, if and when I ever rejoin society.

Having only one good arm and hand to support me, as my right side tries not to hinder me too much, I've got to hang onto a rail to my left with my functional side when going up or down steps. It goes without saying, however, that this is the lane where people traveling the opposite direction are going to be in.

Wanting to avoid a pile-up, these multitude of Mountaineers abruptly stopped when they saw this lunatic—me—coming down the wrong side of the stairs. Darting out then back in again, if 3rd-year coach Don Nehlen had seen the fancy footwork and moves of some of these students, he may have recruited a few of them for the football team.

I wasn't only being cool getting in everybody's way, but I looked real swift staring intently at the steps to see where they were, as I went flopping down. With only a few of these students, I'd look up just long enough to catch a, "What the hell does this retard think he's doing?" look on their faces. However, the majority didn't have this annoyed expression because they realized I was having some trouble—and knew there was something wrong with me.

As I was halfway up the many, many, many, many stairs leading up to the PRT platform, one of these electricity-driven cars stopped at the station and a flock of students whose last class just finished up went flying out of these shuttles, hardly able to contain themselves from transforming into weekend warriors. Rod grinding into my leg, standing in the wrong lane again clinging onto the handrail for dear life, I just prayed I wasn't about to be barreled over. Loyal as patriots—as they did a few minutes ago while I was coming out of the Towers—dad and Kevin were standing in position to break a fall, if one of these crazed, collegiate freshman had run into me and I would have lost my balance.

With the exception of a heart palpitation, I was doing okay by the time we got to the dock where the cars pull up. While Kevin was jamming his card into the turnstile several times so dad and I could ride the shuttle for free and pressed the "Beechurst" button for the downtown campus car, I was checking the scenery out. The maze of tracks disappearing into and coming from as far as one could see looked the same as when I was last here in February. The Engineering station and the Med Center up the hill next to Mountaineer Stadium also were sites that I was no stranger to.

Returning to W.V.U. has really picked up my spirits because, before I came for this visit, I couldn't be sure that I'd be able to recognize anything. I was afraid that coming back would be like freshman orientation all over again, for I had absolutely no recollection of ever being here. When I'd look at pictures of the campus in brochures trying to revive some glimpse of my college days in my memory, I knew I had seen the halls that were photographed, but I couldn't remember actually being inside of these buildings or passing by them in my travels.

Like the first therapeutic weekend I went back to Washington from the rehabilitation center or being in our house that first time after I had my memory taken from me, I didn't know for sure if I'd know the Evansdale campus or not. But once I was here, it was as if I'd never left. Nor was the bumpy ride on the PRT something I'd forgotten completely.

Getting off at the Beechurst station and after I was slowly able to get down the steps, the three of us went into Stansbury Hall where I was taking a golf and volleyball gym class when I was hurt. I could remember the gymnasium, locker room, and even the precise locker I hung my sweaty clothes in. Like my experience visiting the greenhouse where I couldn't recollect certain things, I could remember a few details of the gymnastics course, but others were gone—likely never to be found. Strangely, for some odd reason, I couldn't develop an image in my memory some of the more major aspects of this class like who my instructor was, who any of the students were, or ever being in attendance.

After we left here, we hiked up the mountain to Woodburn Circle where I recognized Martin Hall as where I took freshman Intro Journalism and Woodburn Hall as the building I was enrolled in a history course. Across the street, I knew I was looking at the bookstore and Mountainlair. A little further to the right, Clark Hall was where I blew a Humanities I course and White Hall, where I made a "C" in my Geology class.

Despite wanting to take a closer look at these two halls and the Main Library between them, we didn't go down there because Kevin started moaning about how this week has really dragged. Before taking Kevin back to Washington for his weekend family booster shot, so he could survive the next week away from home, I took one final look at all the Mountaineer students bustling about the main campus. With the sense of my once being here returning and having just triumphantly traveled a trillion rehab miles these past eight months—which have seemed more like eight-hundred eighty—I never felt more confident that I'd be here with them again someday, however, doing well academically next time. After what I've endured during my hospitalization and rehabilitation endeavors, I now have faith in myself that I can achieve whatever I set my mind to. About the abbreviated tour that was cut short a couple of hundred yards, I didn't really care, the old Craig was never in the library anyhow.

Just finishing up college with her Bachelor's at Indiana University of Pennsylvania, like Joni, Rebecca has a good idea of the requirements necessary to get a degree. Knowing that the expression of ideas, reading comprehension, basic mathematics, handwriting, and typing are some of the elementary components needed towards successfully completing one's Bachelor's education and understanding I was having difficulty within this general realm of study, Rebecca had me working on all three of these immediately. Rebecca was due to start on Thursday, 1/6/83, but the day before my first session with her, she called the house to give me my first assignment. I've only met her briefly one time and she's already being a slave driver.

Knowing that this would help with both my brain's left hemisphere expressive language difficulty that I'm experiencing at this time and the functioning of my spastic right hand, Rebecca told me to type what my 1983 New Year's resolution would be. After my brain's right hemisphere perceptual side tried to forecast what may be in store for me within the next twelve months, it shot a signal across my corpus collusum to the left hemisphere's Department of Language Production. In turn, this office was able to eventually get the message to my left hand easy enough, but the bruise interfering with the functioning of my right hand made whacking that typewriter keyboard really tough. Spending at least fifty times longer on this homework now as opposed to when my brain worked, I still had this English lesson done by the time Rebecca came that first week of January, so I'm deserving of a little break. Not so fast.

On Rebecca's first day, she not only had me working on twenty-five arithmetic problems out of this one math book, but gave me some typing homework where I tell her what I did this week and this is to be done within two days. This might be kiddie stuff, but that's where I'm operating from at this point in time. If I can advance from the "Sesame Street" level I'm at now, to college within the next five months—which is what I'm shooting for—that will be accelerated progress at warp speed. Pile on the work Rebecca, I need to have it.

In Arithmetic—by the tail-end of the month—Rebecca not only continued to drill me with addition, subtraction, and multiplication, but had me doing division, as well as working with fractions/decimals. I was still working on my typing, but now, instead of telling my tutor what my New Year's resolution is or what I did during the week, I'm now to read a chapter from a book of my choosing and then handwrite a brief summary about that chapter before typing this review.

The moving, literary classic I decided to enmesh myself with was a biography of five innovative Australian artists whose statements are a reflection of the culture with which they've evolved and developed. Influence widespread and gripping, the canvas expressing their portrayal of life and interpretation of the world has transformed their perception of reality into gold. Their craft, a product of intrinsic examination, shall never be excused by those who understand. To some, the breadth of their message is not to question and its depth only conceivable to those which have grasped. I did not read the annals of those who merely wave a brush capturing the quintessential elements of man or delineate the foundations of the human spirit. Rather, I delved into a reading which chronicled the life and times of the hard rock band, AC/DC.

Maybe in twelve days things will be different, but right now, I couldn't feel better. With this February '83 marking the one year anniversary that my life was drastically altered, I don't think anyone could have blamed me if I would have felt depressed. But I wasn't, far from it.

Looking at things from the "here and the now," what I have today and will tomorrow is just so magnificent that loss doesn't even enter my mind. When physical pain is so much a part of one's life, the evasiveness of joy becomes trying. However, when yesterday's suffering comes to be the present day's relief, there isn't a feeling more incredible.

On February 2nd, at Allegheny General Hospital, Dr. Imbriglia removed the intramedullary rod from my femur. Free from the twitching pain delivered to my right-lower extremity by that bar that was in my leg, I felt relief the instant the anesthesia wore off and was aware of what was going on.

Eyes opening, when I could sense I was able to lie on my left side without pain—something I hadn't been able to do for almost a year—I was ecstatic. Leg feeling like a feather and free from discomfort for the first time in what seemed like forever, I rolled every which way in bed just to rediscover what it's like to lie in any position without having to brace myself for agony. Laying on my stomach for the first time since I could remember, wrapped in a ball, reclining to the left side, right side, that side, this side, I was gleaming that I didn't have to be on my back the entire night. After they've disappeared for a prolonged period of time, it's amazing the things a person can miss. To regain a little normalcy again feels fabulous.

Having a leg that clicked with misery anytime I would go up or down an incline, climbed and descended steps, or rolled over in bed was a torture I was fearful might be chronic. Taking the rod out of my femur through my right ass cheek will hopefully permit me to walk better because I won't be afraid to put weight on my right leg, fearing a titanium steel shaft will poke through it. For the first time in twelve months, I'll be able to go up some steps without preparing myself first to feel some metal ripping at my leg from the inside.

Originally, when the rod was inserted into my broken leg, it was believed that it could remain there permanently to reinforce my one-time fractured femur. But then when it started to bother me so badly, Dr. Imbriglia decided to take it out no later than April. But that was before I had a mishap at the house.

On 8/28/82, the day Matt died, I was so upset about his death and preoccupied with how easily it could have been me who was buried behind the house in the cemetery, my concentration had been broken going up the steps that evening when I turned around halfway-up this staircase to respond to a poorly-timed remark my visiting brother made that I couldn't let him get away with. As I was wheeling around ready to fire my comeback, I lost my balance on the steps and went falling back. Because of what was about to happen, I'd be making a return trip to Allegheny General to see my orthopedic surgeon in three days.

Because this failed balancing act happened just a little over a week after I had been discharged from the rehab center, my parents and I were more than a little fearful that my brain contusion was going to make spine-tingling occurrences such as this one part of the everyday routine, now that I'm away from a structured setting designed to keep obstructions to a minimum. There's a lot of obstacle courses out there in the real world.

With my left hand hanging on with all the strength it had, I clutched onto that two-inch rail which separated me from a fifteen-foot fall to the bottom flight of steps. Fearful of what might transpire here in a moment, backwards, I tumbled down uncontrollably about four of five steps. Trying to lean against the banister for support and leverage, I attempted to get out of "Reverse" and turn myself around, but I couldn't because my right arm was just dangling there, not being of any use. Trying to orient myself somehow by releasing the rail with my left hand would have been certain suicide.

Approaching the top of the seven steps leading up from the downstairs T.V. room, I was terrified because my momentum was taking me down. Not seeing where I was headed and concentrating on stopping this blind tailspin, my legs moved as fast as they could to catch my reeling upper torso before I went flying back-first into the door at the lower landing. During this violent plunge, I put tremendous force on my bad leg and it started aching with an equally fierce intensity.

Shooting off the couch, both dad and Ug ran towards me to break my fall before I stumbled down the other staircase. Taking this spill, I hurt my leg bad and thought I might have done something to shift the steel rod, or injured that bone which needs a break from all the hurting.

Because he knew wasn't that big of a deal. But still, it's a little unsettling to hear that your plans are known from someone you'd just as soon wished didn't have this information about you. However unlikely, I guess it's possible that Mr. Michaels has a few connections at Allegheny General. It's a good bet, though, that one of my occupational therapists who see me everyday did some talking.

Always careful about the way he interacts with me, a week before I was to have the pole taken out of my leg, Mr. Michaels surprised me when he came up to me one day when I was in therapy and made a comment about my upcoming leg surgery. This Rogerian/Client-Centered approach wasn't effective, for he couldn't squeeze any details about this operation out of me, but he probably knows how to get what he wants anyway.

What's a little disturbing about all this is that I'm obviously not the one who informed the father of the drunk who hurt me about the upcoming operation on my leg. More than likely, one of my hand therapists told Mr. Michaels this information about me that wasn't for publication. Putting "2 and 2" together, it doesn't take a genius to figure this out, for the details of the pin removal procedure Mr. Michaels didn't know about were the very ones that I intentionally did not divulge to my occupational therapists, such as who the doctor would be that was going to do the extraction. Not knowing if the therapists who are supposedly caring for me are double agents or my advocate is not the most soothing situation to be in.

This fraternity of health care professionals is a tightly knit web, and if anyone is in a position to disrupt this network, they're going to find out real quick where the members' loyalties are placed. For the most part, this is just how it is with any workplace circle and I suppose—*if it doesn't hurt anyone*—this is the way it should be, for professionals got to stick together, if they're to be at their best. Being a patient in this soap opera, however, I sometimes feel "on edge."

I guess I was only fooling myself believing some way, somehow, it would be different with me. I don't know if this one-sided ignorance of youth is a form of denial or just stupidity, but it's becoming more and more apparent that no matter what I do, things are never going to be the same.

Incorrectly thinking I could avoid the inevitable stagnation that occurs with other people who've had head injuries, this period of my "recovery" where nothing seems any better from the day before has been intolerable more times than I'd like to think. Isolated and feeling distanced from the world makes the deficiencies I'm experiencing with my thinking, hand, and walking all the more difficult to deal with now. You know your life stinks when all there is to look forward to anymore are outpatient evaluations at a rehabilitation center.

On 9/27/82, about five weeks after I was discharged, I had my first evaluation at Harmarville. At that time, despite spasticity and weakness still being a problem, I had shown some functional improvement of my right fingers, wrist, arm, and hand. Although my pinch was slightly less than it was when I was an inpatient, going to OT in Washington three times a week was proving to be a fruitful venture, for I was showing improvement with the operation of my hand in most other areas. However, the gains I was making with my cognitive abilities while at home were monumental.

With the bruise on my brain which controls cognitions supposedly having shrunk rapidly, coupled with the abundance of material Joni had me reading, my capability to understand and remember what I had read had improved incredibly within a little over a month's time. The readministration of the Gates-McGinitie showed that my raw and standardized scores had increased by five and the percentile score improved by sixteen. During this outpatient Speech and Language session, the pathologist found that I had a little difficulty following specific instructions, but the significant gains in my reading far overshadowed this existing difficulty.

My re-evaluation occurred 1/10/83 and it was during this second assessment that my outpatient Occupational Therapist documented that I informed her I was still having difficulty with visual scanning and tracking during this reading. While I'm doing my homework for my tutor, sometimes when I'm reading a sentence, my eyes will still dart down to the next paragraph. Or, if I'm asked to look for and focus on one particular element of a passage, my frontal lobe damage leaves me confused. However, when it came to giving a report on the functioning of my hand, the news was very good.

My grip strength increased by five kilograms to twenty-five, lateral pinch increased thirteen pounds up from two the last time this was measured during my first evaluation four months ago, chuck pinch was up to 10 pounds (an increase of eight pounds), but the best news of all was that I was showing so much more control of my right hand that I was instructed to discontinue wearing that annoying nocturnal hand splint. In September, after it was noted that my pinch had actually weakened, I strictly followed a home exercise program designed to strengthen this thumb-forefinger action.

By the first month of the year, my double vision had improved to the point that my diplopia was mainly to the extreme right side. With this lateral gaze primarily being affected, I now only wear my patch periodically and usually during the night when I'm tired. Still, it's far from soothing when everything you look at has a transparent coating surrounding it. That finger to nose exercise I wholeheartedly do appears to be helping my brain to discern between image and mirage.

Although I definitely have some deficits with my right hemibody, I'm demonstrating more involvement with my right side, as my range of motion in the lower extremities is functional and my tone has increased. Despite not having formal outpatient physical therapy, my ability to ambulate on the level and on stairs has also improved. There were also encouraging gains noted in my cognitive abilities.

To get an estimate of how well my brain's calculating function is operating, during this 1/10/83 eval, Mrs. Joy administered the WAIS-R for a third time. The results of this re-readministration yielded a Verbal IQ score of 106, Performance IQ of 85, and Full Scale IQ of 97. When I took this WAIS-R on 7/25/82, I had obtained a Verbal IQ of 108, Performance IQ of 79, and Full Scale IQ of 94. Mrs. Joy noted that, despite the Verbal IQ dropping by two, it basically remains unchanged. Extremely pleased with the improvement in my Performance score, Mrs. Joy was not real happy that I used my left hand exclusively when I manipulated objects during this portion of the WAIS-R which requires some motor dexterity. Enough of this testing already, it's now time to have a little fun.

Because she hasn't seen me since I was discharged five months ago, Diane Rosato wanted me to stop by the Communications Department before I left and spend a little time talking with her—Oh boy!!!! With my communicative abilities deemed as not being in need of extensive remediation any longer, I'm not scheduled to see my inpatient Communications' therapist during these evaluations. Diane made me late for my other outpatient programs today, but I don't mind a bit; she could've kept me all day, if she liked.

Since I haven't been verbally abused in a while, I then went down the hallway to see Jan and Mary in PT and some of the other therapists. Scarred from the emotional abuse I was just hammered with by my two physical terrorists, I then went up to Unit 3 where I was cordial (for a change) with my occupational therapists, and spoke to a lot of my old nurses whose daylight shift will almost be over. With 3:00 P.M. just a few ticks away, I could hardly wait to see my pen pal coming in with the rest of the crew that checks in for the evening.

Purse flung over her shoulder, in one of the white uniforms I was always happy to see when she'd come get me to give her a guitar lesson, I saw my short, Italian, ping-pong opponent bouncing towards me. Arms outstretched and smiling from ear to ear, Valerie gave me a hug then tapped my belly, telling my mom she must be a good cook.

When I was first discharged, I received a letter from Valerie about every 10-12 days, asking me how I'm getting along at home and telling me what she's been up to. Having written her just as much, we don't correspond with each other as frequently as we used to, but it's still really nice that a cute female keeps tabs on me once in a while and shows an interest in what I'm doing.

I haven't seen Valerie since September, when I was here for my first evaluation four months ago. Because I don't see her everyday like I used to—I must admit—it's a little awkward now when I'm around her, but that's life and life goes on. Although I don't see Valerie in person too much anymore, a little bit of her spirit will always be with me. Thank you, Valerie, I'll see you in five-and-a-half months—on May 23rd—when I'm to have my next evaluation when, in addition to my physical and cognitive abilities being monitored, I'm scheduled to have my driver's exam.

Cracking her whip, with the dual purpose of not only improving my writing ability, but my spastic hand, Rebecca continues to have me doing my writing assignments with my right hand. Seeing how slowly I write with my currently dominant left hand, my tutor knew that there was no way I'd be able to take notes fast enough to keep up with college lectures. Because some professors sound like auctioneers when they present their information in class, there's no way I could get all the important facts I'd need on paper, so I could study during test time.

I know that if someone doesn't try and practice, they'll never discover what can be achieved, but with the way my once dominant writing hand feels, it's just not possible that I can get many words on paper in a fair amount of time given the lack of dexterity in my wrist and fingers. I hate to say this word because it's a self-defeating one, but right now, with the motions my right hand are able to undertake, I simply *"can't"* realistically write right-handed at this time. With the hand Rebecca's trying to whip into shape, given it's current condition, it would be a miracle almost equal to the parting of the Red Sea if I can hold a pencil with my right hand by the time college is to start again, let alone write words with it.

Knowing that paying bills is almost as much a part of college as cracking the books, Rebecca wanted to make sure that I could do some simple mathematics and keep an account. This is one of the reasons she gives me plenty of arithmetic homework. She knew that the money required for tuition, rent, utilities, books, groceries, etc. is something parents save and bust their ass for, and she didn't want this aspiring student with a history of a head injury to blow it all because he's not prepared. Just coming off a college campus herself, Rebecca knows what it takes to survive the college grind and I'm going to "pick her mind," so that I can get back on a campus again. "Let's go-oooo, Mountaineers!!!"

Realizing that a pen and checkbook are a college student's best friend, Rebecca wanted to make sure I knew how to write a check. Having written many checks for my expenses during the two book-buying semesters I was at W.V.U. didn't make any difference because I had forgotten how to do this.

I looked at the sample check Rebecca wanted me to fill out, but I had no idea where to start. I knew I had written these many times before, but I did not have a clue what was to go on the top two lines with the number, "19" between them or what went after "PAY TO THE ORDER OF." The tiny box after this line, the space before the word "DOLLARS," the area following the word "MEMO," and the long mark at the end with no explanation were a mystery. Was the number at the top right hand corner and the digits at the very bottom just there to confuse me or do they serve a purpose?

I recognize the name and address printed on the check are mine, but I'm not sure what to do about this. The name of the bank and its address where I have the account is also on the check, but I don't think I can squeeze all this information into that little box. And when Rebecca says I need to reconcile my checkbook after making this payment, what the heck's she talking about? God help this frontal lobe of mine heal, so I can sort things out in my mind and make sense of my world again.

This is getting old. Since I was discharged, all I've been seeing are doctors, therapists, tutors, insurance people, OVR reps, and Mr. Michaels. Am I ever going to awaken from this nightmare? Deep down inside, however, I know it's more than a bad dream I'm having when this progress is harder to come by now. Working so hard, but not seeing much in the way of gains, is enough to drive one mad.

If I've done it once, I've done it a million times. The eye exercise I do to retrain my brain to see properly again where I try to focus on the distal portion of my incoming finger as I'm bringing it towards my face has helped, but my vision is still uncomfortably distorted. Everything I look at is blurred and still has a halo of two distinct objects around it.

On 10/8/82, I saw my opthalmologist, E. Ronald Salvitti, M.D., and after my eyes had been examined, he determined that my eyesight wasn't going to get any better by itself after all these months, and that my double vision is only going to improve with surgical intervention. I figured this would be inevitable given the lack of improvement in my vision, but it still sent shock waves through my system thinking of the day when a sharp scalpel will be cutting around my eye.

Hating to drive Pittsburgh, dad was quite upset to hear that this operation—where the muscle behind my eye would be snipped—was going to be done by an opthalmologist in West Penn Hospital, located in the Bloomfield section of the city. Dr. Salvitti referred us to a physician he described as the "master" of this extra-ocular resection procedure. This Pittsburgh-based eye surgeon, Dr. Albert Biglan, scheduled the surgery for June 1, 1983. I hope this miracle worker's hand is a steady one when he does that slicing on me.

While one is starting to learn any musical instrument, both the emotional and physical challenges can be overbearing at first. When you want the fingers of your left hand to do one thing, but they want to do something else and your right hand needs to undertake a totally different action at the precise same time, the frustration is so incredible most people give up pursuing this instrument-mastering endeavor in a short time. If I wasn't such an idiot and hardheaded, I probably would have done what comes natural and "hung it up" trying to relearn the guitar after my paralytic hand started giving me so much trouble. Because my infatuation with participating in sports at some level—any level—is now obviously over, letting go of another dream is just something I'm not ready to do.

The moment I could hold a wiffle ball pick and regained a sense of what was going on, I worked on getting my bad right hand to strike some strings. It might not have been music, but it was noise, and that's a start. With Kevin's help, I quickly relearned how chords were fingered and slowly became proficient enough in time that I could give Valerie some basic lessons. But, because of my bum hand, I wasn't able to demonstrate the control needed to hit single notes.

Since I've been home from Harmarville, I've been averaging close to four hours of practicing everyday, sometimes more, sometimes less depending on how many truckloads of homework Rebecca has assigned and the number of hand exercises and laps around the neighborhood I do. With the operation of my picking hand practically destroyed, the time I spend chopping at my six-string are not hours where I enjoy playing, rather, this is a period where I tirelessly practice, trying to regain a little of what I lost. It's murder when you lose something you love so much, but this guitar playing is something that—no matter how long it takes—I just can't quit. Being that playing rock 'n roll guitar is one of the few ties I have to my past which I still hope that I have a remote shot at getting back, I'm not about to lay down and die.

Knowing Rebecca has productively been working with my right writing-hand and I've been putting my right picking hand through the motions, Occupational Therapy dipped some pencils and picks into that blue "gook" that's supposed to enhance my grip. However, the responsiveness of my hand is a slow thing coming for, despite focusing most of my concentration on trying to hang onto these babies, they'll slip from my grasp more times than not.

Like I did at Harmarville, my occupational therapists in Washington were the ones who got the brunt of my agitation when my hand wasn't coming around. In therapy, despite doing everything I was asked—and then some —the progress was so minuscule that I would become almost despondent at times after I'd repeatedly lose grip of my coated pencil. A brain injury can make all the work you've put into regaining a function, effort wasted.

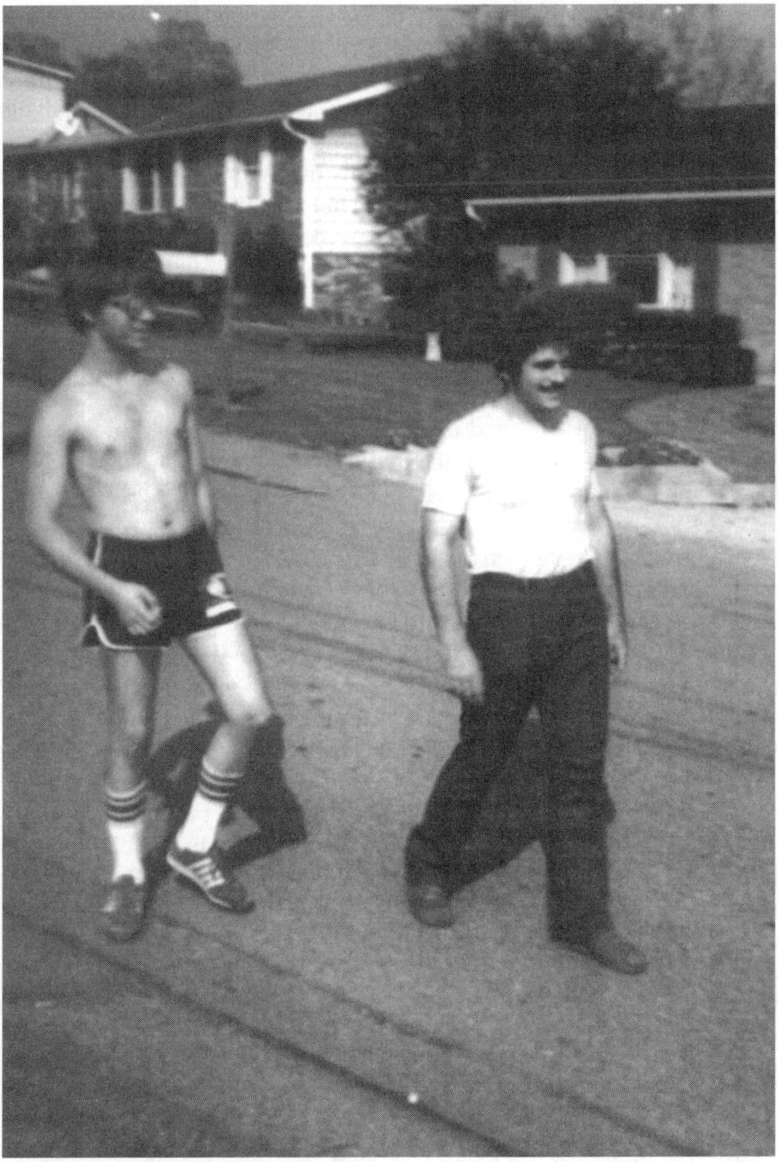

Craig and the man, the legend, Mr. Kevin Brezinski walking a therapy lap around Craig's neighborhood.

Still struggling to achieve the fine motor skills I once could do automatically, I was becoming embroiled with myself that my spastic hand wasn't progressing like I wanted. Exercising my hand with putty and with guitar playing being such an excellent therapy for the hand that wanted to be left well enough alone, I figured these workouts would make this inoperative extremity of mine better in no time. On the contrary, these drills I put my hand through were more than simple calisthenics, but that didn't seem to matter because my fingers still had the flexibility of a stone and their weakness derived from a brain which rendered no control.

On Friday, 10/22/82, my head occupational therapist had a talk with mom and expressed her concern about my increasingly deteriorating mood. Wondering if the expectations for my right hand are unrealistic, my therapist asked mom if I had any friends who distract me from my troubles. Ironically, later on this 22nd day of October 1982, eight months and eight days after my life had almost been taken from me, I got my first visit from the dude I got to know at W.V.U. and did a lot of guitar playing with.

Swaggering in on this Friday, my fellow academically-minded, freshman Mountaineer guitar playing partner, "Boss," got around to seeing me after my morning Occupational Therapy. I could understand why it took Boss so long to see me because I'm sure he had his reservations about making this visit. He didn't know how my parents or I would react to his coming in being that he was Paul's roommate/"bosom buddy" at school and was one of the players in the script which led to this whole mess. Dad, knowing of this indirect role, just kind of hung around within earshot. Also, Paul is a better friend of Boss' than I am, and maybe Boss would've felt like some kind of traitor, if he came to see me earlier.

Because Boss wasn't responsible for the accident directly in any way, we weren't really opposed to his being here. Although Boss and Paul aren't roommates anymore—anytime he wants—Boss has the means to get in touch with the person he shared a dorm room with his freshman year because Paul's back at W.V.U., attending class again. And this is part of the reason why me and my family weren't exceptionally at ease with his being in our house. After all this time, it's quite evident that Boss could have thought of other places he'd much rather be and people he'd like to be talking to instead, but knew it would look kind of funny, if he didn't at least make a courtesy stop to see me.

With the ingredients which helped foster our association—marijuana —being one of the contributors to my being hurt, there was never really a strong foundation for a friendship between me and Boss. Sure, guitar was a common interest we both shared and could have used to develop a stronger bond, but there always seemed to be a rivalry in Boss' mind when it came to playing. And when these male competitive juices start pumping, this doesn't always harvest the best of alliances. With my hand and memory being what they are now, I pose no guitar playing threat to this helpful soul whatsoever and Boss knew he had a marked advantage over me now, which was something he did not want to relinquish.

This being part of his freshman studies as well, Boss was the first one to figure out how to pay the multi-platinum, AC/DC single, "Back in Black." I can remember watching Boss play this in his dorm room before my memory "shorted out" and admiring how well it sounded. I used to be able to play some of the main riffs to this rocker, but my head being slugged against that pole knocked this out of my awareness. Wanting to learn this song myself again to help my memory and bad hand, I asked Boss during his visit, if he'd show me this tune that he used to jam to a million times. He said he didn't remember how to play it. When the use of substances is a primary component in a relationship, what you have is nothing.

Because there isn't a whole heckuva lot to do in Washington if you're under the age of twenty-one, the malls are a stomping ground for teenagers and this is where I ran into some people I went to high school with who weren't exactly expecting to see me. Always with one of my parents now when I go anywhere, these Trinity Hillers' reactions varied some, but they all had overtones of sorrow.

One day a couple of months ago, I saw our high school baseball team's right fielder—Ron "E-9" Semple—and I yelled over to him. Positioned to my left in the outfield, we had spent a lot of time together shagging flies in practice and even caught a few during the games, but he didn't know who I was because I looked so different from my high school days, sporting my patched glasses, splint, and leaning when I stand.

After Ron realized that he was approaching the only player in Trinity High School baseball's history to throw a ball over the backstop from center field during a game, he was initially shocked, before his face took on a somber look. I could very well be mistaken—because of the way he talked and carried himself—it seemed Ron wanted to be perceived as a "red-neck" hard ass. But then he left down his guard and his true colors came through that afternoon at the mall.

When I started fumbling with the bag of stuff I was trying to carry, with a look of despair that I couldn't do something as basic as holding onto a package, Ron was really concerned for me and wanted to make sure I got the help I needed, as he was more than willing to come to the rescue. Shortly after I let him know that I was okay and that everything was under control, I told Ron about my amnesia. When I said to this big boy that a lot of my memory was gone and wondered if he could help me get some of it back, Ron had an expression on his face like someone who just saw a cute little puppy dog get run over by a truck.

In a little while, after he realized I was okay with things, Ron became more relaxed and began smirking when he started to fill me in about Coach "Wild Bill," the "Pine Gang," and about some of the things that happened during the baseball season last year. Among them, my infamous throw and how one time he felt like an idiot misjudging a fly ball during a game and just laid there on his back in the middle of right field, disgusted with his misplay, so I had to run over and get the ball and relay it back into the infield.

When us two gold glovers got done talking, two things stuck with me. One, I was glad I ran into Ron, not only because he is a good guy, but because I got a little part of me back again that I had forgotten until he reminded me. Two—and this was something that kind of caught me off-guard—Ron's sad expression and response after he knew it was me he was looking at, almost made ME want to cry.

When Ron was talking about the baseball season, different visions that had been missing came back. Baseball being the only extracurricular activity I was ever involved with at school, I could picture the events Ron was talking about in my mind clear as day, therefore, I knew these images had actually occurred and weren't something my imagination had created. Being a starter in such a crucial position as center field, I know I had to be a good fielder; but why can't anybody recall some of the good plays I surely made.

Another time, I was out at Thrift Drug in the Washington Mall and I was surprised to see our high school third baseman—Steve "E-5" Oliverio—was working there as a cashier. Going up to the register, when I said, "Hey Steve," he too had a real sorry look on his face and his voice had a tone of compassion, like Ron's, that I had never heard before when he knew it was me hiding behind the patched lens of my eye glasses. It was transparent that Steve was taken back by the sight of me thin as a blade and hunched over. From the words that he spoke to the concern in his eyes, it was clear that Steve was both happy and feeling a little sad to see me. The small talk Steve tried to use to cover his emotions didn't work, for I could tell that he was choked up seeing me with my touched up designer spectacles and limping about.

Washington is a relatively small town where everyone knows each other and I've known Steve since we both played baseball on the same Pony League team at the age of thirteen. Living in close proximity to one another, sharing an interest for the outdoors and being in the same high school graduating class, I knew that Steve and Paul knew each other pretty well and were friends. Before I left the drug store this hot and humid day, I knew they had been talking about me and the accident.

Led to believe that the elements were the cause of my being hurt—not Paul's overindulgence—Steve must have been fed the Michaels' company line too, for he said something to the effect that it was tough luck that Paul's tires skidded on that glaze of ice. The stories people will resort to in order to "save face."

After I told Steve that Paul ramming into that pole wasn't because of some quirk of nature, rather, that Paul's drinking was the culprit, he wasn't sure what to say. Realizing then that it was Paul's actions which put me in critical condition, just a whisper away from death, Steve looked a little uncomfortable and seemed kind of hesitant to say anything else from there on out.

A good baseball and guitar player, Steve is one of those guys who most everyone seems to get along with because of his laid-back style and I liked Steve as well. Smiling, Steve looked as if he was really glad I was up and getting around on my own after almost "cashing in my chips." Now, I hope I can only get home this blistering summer day without dad hitting any ice patches which would cause him to lose control of his car.

It goes without saying that this dude is really on top of things which makes the actions of our valedictorian that much more puzzling. When I was out at the Franklin Mall one evening, I saw Randy for the first time since he gave his speech during commencement ceremonies. Out with his girlfriend at the time, after I called out his name and he turned around and saw me, Randy had the look of someone who had just seen a ghost. Graduating number one in our class, surely for the first time in his life, this symbol of academic brilliance was dumbfounded.

Jaws dropped and shocked that I was standing before him, at a loss for words, Randy appeared to be a little embarrassed that our reunion occurred during this chance meeting, instead of one where he made an effort to see me. In an apologetic tone, this really intelligent guy said something I will never forget: "Now that I know you're alright, I'll come see you."

Being incredibly sharp, Randy could be pretty damned witty and funny as hell sometimes which could make him an appealing person to be around. Because he takes in and absorbs information so well, I don't know, but Randy might have learned or heard some things about brain injury which would make him leery about paying me a visit. With his mind always in overdrive, possibly Randy conjured up some situation that he didn't want to deal with because he wouldn't know what to do or say. Randy being advanced in so many ways, sometimes makes it easy to forget he's still a kid.

Being that he was away at college in Cincinnati, his mom had called our house on several occasions right after I was hurt, wanting an update on my progress. First impressions are frequently lasting ones and maybe Randy formulated an image in his analytical mind early on about the state I would be in for the remainder of my days after hearing about the condition I was in at the hospital. Quite possibly, Randy could have assumed my afflictions would leave me unaware he was there anyhow, and presumed that I didn't want to be seen like that. Figuring I was still in a state where I didn't know "up from down," maybe Randy was thinking he was being kind not coming around while I was experiencing all these cognitive deficits and that's why he said what he did at the mall.

To be truthful, I have some trouble buying all that because Kevin has talked to Randy recently about how I'm faring these days and has told our classmate—who was also an exceptional offensive lineman for the football team—that I wouldn't mind a visit from him. Normally one to keep his opinion to himself, Kevin would shake his head in disbelief and express a little disappointment that Randy never stopped by.

No, Randy and I aren't spectacular friends and I know that he has a busy life with a lot of other people he'd like to spend his time with while he's home from college. But to completely ignore me when I needed as many friends in my life as possible in this time of need wasn't something I knew how to handle. For him to say he'd see me now that I'm doing better might indicate Randy was fearful for his own well-being, for the stigma which accompanies brain injury is a frightful one. Could it be anything else?

Months and months after I could have been decapitated, I finally ran into him. It was as if my friend were trying to avoid me, but I knew sooner or later our paths would cross because of how close we live to one another. However, I wouldn't have ever thought "later" would be this long.

Being the nadir of confusion, even after I saw him, I still couldn't understand how someone I thought was such a good friend could forget and discard me so easily. Spending several hours everyday during the summer playing softball and winters killing each other during our five-per-team football games—because sports was central in everything we did—Dave was practically a fixture. Since my life has taken a turn for the worse, Dave has become as inaccessible now as he was accessible when I was healthy. Misreading people is something that happens all the time, but I never thought Dave to be shallow.

There's no way I would've ever thought that I'd see this day. To be thrown in the trash by someone whom I thought I had gotten along with so well makes me wonder if the stigma associated with head injury hasn't formed a wedge between mine and Dave's friendship. I don't understand how a guy whose personality I seemed to mesh with so nicely could pretend that we weren't friends and disregard me during a time when I need to hear encouragement from the people who have been a part of my life. What Dave's doing, or rather—"not" doing—one would think we were the worst of enemies, not the best of friends. I can't even begin to imagine what's going on with Dave. Because I don't have the vaguest of notions, I'm at a loss for ideas what's going through his mind.

Dave's very sensitive and the only thing that I can think of which may explain why he didn't come to check to see how I was doing is that my currently being disabled after all those years of being a good athlete makes him aware how mortal we are as human beings. Knowing that there's no guarantees in life isn't a very comforting feeling, but I never thought an insecurity as weak as this one could render a friendship obsolete. Could it be anything else?

First, watching leaves fall, then snow melt, and finally, grass grow while I'm doing homework or my different exercises, has been the extent of my excitement these past several months. When I take a break from all this thrilling stimulation, I'll wrap myself in my music, but there's only so much guitar and stereo playing I can do in one day before looking for something else to do to keep me busy. Sitting here with my afflictions is really getting to me.

Because I don't drive, I've got to find activities to do near the house to occupy my time. My parents have been fabulous when it comes to assisting me with my various deficits, but running up in age some—even with my body broken like it is now—they can't keep up with me physically anymore since I've been progressing so rapidly. Always overprotective and fearing that I would have a seizure when no one is around, they don't let me walk around the neighborhood unless someone accompanies me. But this nonsense is going to end.

Tired of waiting and being stagnant, wanting to prove a point after my pleas to give me some independence fell on deaf ears—on 11/11/82—I snuck out of the house to do some laps around the development by myself for the first time after these appeals to stop "babying" me were ignored. When dad realized I was nowhere to be found, he shit a brick and tore off after me.

Catching up with me about halfway around, huffing and puffing, dad started hollering at me and didn't stop until he saw I was doing just fine without a guardian. Not wanting to do anything to interfere with my motivation, after realizing his older body doesn't have the second wind any longer to keep up with my younger—but defective one—dad relented and I was off on my own from now on. At the time, dad couldn't have known what he started. Nor did I know this would be my last taste of excitement for six months. If these are supposed to be the best years of my life, then I'm definitely in trouble.

Rebecca's game plan to get me back to West Virginia University has been outstanding. Making me read various books and articles, then having me write and type a report on what I went over, has helped my brain's right hemisphere prepare for the next level in the hierarchy. Highlighting the important facts in a story and reporting them in a clear and concise fashion are crucial elements with any data presenting endeavor, however, transforming expressions into a spicy account requires a little ingenuity. And it was this art form I used to have a penchant for that Rebecca had me working on next.

Effective use of the English language is essential, if one is to excel in society. It goes without saying that a journalist must have this in their tool box, if they are to productively incorporate words to convey a message. For those writers who wish to put a little flair into their reporting, these creatures of artistic creation have the ability to step outside of themselves and capture images only a mind of some depth can construct. Wanting me to operate from this sphere of creativity—so that I may regain some of this virtue—Rebecca assigned me writing projects to do now which would exercise and stretch my imagination. *I'm sure this will come in handy one of these days.*

Things weren't supposed to turn out like they have. Because of this, am I ever glad I didn't listen to everything professionals claimed I could and couldn't do, what I would and wouldn't achieve. I don't necessarily care how many degrees a person has lining the wall of their office or the number of letters that come after their name, there's no way anybody, anywhere, could know what's in a patient's heart. This determination and the make-up of the person are where any forthcoming recovery begins. A little over a year ago, I was in a decerebrate posturing position, now, I'm in position to go back to college. Who would have thought that this could be possible in such a relatively short period of time?

Without a doubt, there's a lot of people deserving of credit for how the state of affairs has turned out for me. The effort put forth by the patient can be the most important common denominator for those who go on and make something out of their lives after a tragedy. It was no different with me, for the exertion I put into getting to where I am now was of strenuous proportions. Definitely, the medical and rehabilitation personnel who have worked with me have been spectacular and deserve to take a bow, but the groundwork for the factors leading to my recovery actually occurred long before I was hurt.

My parents compliment each other nicely in their roles as motivator and support system. They both have the common goal of getting me back on my feet again—just have different philosophies of how to get there. With these diverse views of what it takes to get better feeding off each other so well, I was reaping in the benefits.

They both had this to varying degrees, but dad has been more the "rah, rah" cheerleader type when it came to me tackling something I have trouble with because he doesn't want me to get too discouraged. Whereas mom approached things from a cause and effect position. For example, I'd be in the spare room—which later became known as the "O.T. Room" because that's where I mainly work with my spastic hand—and when I'd start griping about the lack of progress I was seeing, dad would come in, rub my fingers and say, "That hand's gonna come around; you just keep working on it."

Memory back-tracking to the time when no one was certain anybody was home, dad said encouragingly, "I remember when that hand was tight under your chin, now look at how much it has improved in just a little over a year. You'll get there buddy, just try to be patient."

Doing her best Dr. Prostko, mom would tell me not to let that hand die and to use it as much as I can. Since I've been in "no man's land," I don't know how many billions of times mom's told me that the brain will develop new passageways for nerve cells to travel, as long as I do my part and practice. During those times when I'd feel I was only spinning my wheels, not accomplishing anything, both mom and dad would tell me not to throw in the towel; that my brain needs my cooperation if I'm to regain not only my physical stature, but my intelligence as well.

In a tone which sounded like a Harvard professor, mom would tell me that I needed to continue working hard because my brain needs stimulated, if I want this central nervous system to work for me again. I don't know how I could have ever survived the emotional trauma this type of injury levies on one, if it weren't for my family's involvement. For those unfortunate people who don't have this support, I don't see how they could manage. I'm just grateful from the bottom of my heart that I am getting all the rehabilitation support and emotional caring possible.

When I went back to Harmarville for my third evaluation, I was happy to find out my CNS was continuing its remarkable ascent to heightened awareness. The old adage, "Three times is a charm," does not apply to brain injury rehabilitation, for Mrs. Joy administered the WAIS-R for a fourth time on 5/23/83. Since the last time I was tested—four months ago—my Performance IQ increased by four to eighty-nine and my Verbal IQ was projected to be about 112. Because Harmarville's staff can't get enough of me, I was detained in another department and arrived a little late for Mrs. Joy's session, so she only had time to administer the digit span and arithmetic Verbal subtests of the WAIS-R. The improvement I made in these two portions of the WAIS-R were by two and three points respectively.

Aware that I would be taking a stab at re-entering college in three weeks' time, in addition to assessing how much improvement my thinking was showing since the last time I came in, Mrs. Joy wanted to see just how fast I could get those pesty little words down on paper. With the whip marks Rebecca put on my back as proof, I have been writing increasingly more with my right hand, but I'm afraid my non-dominant left hand is going to have to do the writing for me, if I want to finish the upcoming summer course *this* summer, or plan to graduate from college in the 20th Century.

Clicking on her trusty stopwatch I'd love to crush under the heel of my foot, my psychologist timed the speed which I write with both my left and right hand. Writing a short, seven-word sentence, the results showed that I just may have to abandon this ambidextrous writing venture and stick with what works best for me. Unfortunately, the only hand that can securely hold a pencil right now is the one that isn't accustomed to writing. When my left hand attempts to undertake the motions required to print or write, it feels absolutely dismal. If I'm very lucky—with the hand that at one time used to do the writing for me—I might be able to hold onto a pencil for a couple of seconds before I have to arrange it with my left hand, so that it doesn't slip out. But once I press this pencil down against paper and start to move in the direction needed for producing a letter, I always lose grip. This is misery at its tortuous worst, but you got to do, what you got to do.

Using my once dominant right hand, it took me forty-three seconds to write this simple sentence. Although, also painfully slow, I nearly cut the time in half with my functional left hand, as I got the same sentence down in twenty-four seconds. With the speed those professors give their lectures and the allotted time there is to take tests, how am I ever going to get through college putting words on paper with the hand that's not used to writing? God, please give me the strength. On your marks. . . . . . . Get set. . . . . .GO!!!!!

Eyes bulging and chin quivering, beads of sweat were forming on this assessor's forehead. Arms braced preparing for impact, a deep breath was taken—and then held, fearful of what the exhale may cause. Hair standing on end, nails dug themselves deep into the upholstery and those feet were firmly entrenched, practically burrowing a hole into the floorboard. Because I was too busy concentrating, battling the paralysis of my hand and confusion my tainted mind delivered, I couldn't be sure the fortunate one chosen to accompany me on this trip wasn't crossing herself after the tires squealed and kicked up gravel.

As I tried to steer alongside the tight bend, hugging the right side of the road near a steep embankment, the wide-eyed bundle of nerves beside me swallowed deep. Knees implanted into the dash, I could almost hear my passenger's heart pounding like thunder, scared the next Harmarville newsletter would be sending condolences to this driving instructor's surviving family members.

I wasn't responsible for a manslaughter on this Harmarville driver's exam, but I don't think that just because a potential driver being able to avoid a vehicular homicide is a prerequisite to getting a Pennsylvania Operator's License. Heart rate increasing three-fold, the driving educator who went on this joy ride where I was at the controls—Beverly Longdon—was not killed, but she possibly saw her life flashing before her several times while out on the road with me. Actually, I did okay, until the car started moving.

I scored nineteen out of twenty on the Pennsylvania Road Sign Test and my gross reaction time was rated "good," as I could complete a quick stop well. I was capable of using both upper extremities for the hand over hand steering action while I was in Harmarville's parking lot and my ability to accelerate/brake with my bad right leg were good. However, without the use of any adaptive equipment, I had trouble getting my paralytic right arm to help steer once we got into the surrounding residential/suburban areas. Possibly, with the exception of a Bomb Squad member, Beverly's job of assessing the capabilities of a "brain injured" driver may be the most dangerous and unappealing occupation around. That lady's got guts.

Nerves fried and sweating profusely, when we returned, Beverly reported that she saw I had the potential for improvement (understatement?) with some professional training, but at this time—until I learn some compensatory strategies to overcome my physical limitations—I'm not to drive. Here we go again.

With my legs being my sole source of transportation now, I was putting them to good use hiking up and down the hills around my neighborhood. Practicing a couple of hours everyday, in addition to trying to stop that damned foot slap of mine, I was attempting to smooth out my step and do something about my awkward stance. It was during these therapy laps that I was truly introduced to a world of ignorance, spawned by fear.

For the most part, my neighbors are sensational. The majority are kind, courteous, and would do most anything for you. Being of the middle-class variety, most of these folks got some real substance and backbone to them. Knowing of some of these people like I do, I can also say with a reasonable degree of confidence that there are a few who have opinions of their self-worth which could be classified as "over-inflated." Whether these select few neighbors' "uppity-up" personas are a creation of their socio-economic status, upbringing, misperception on my part, or something else, I don't know. But I found out real quick, the posture some of my neighbors have regarding those with head injuries.

Being a full-blooded, heterosexual male who is not all that tremendously unattractive now that my acne bumps have evaporated, I would occasionally do some "rapping" with some of the more appealing members of the opposite sex when these beauties would be out and about frolicking in their yards. My newfound interest in the ladies did not go unnoticed by the parents of these neighborhood girls for, when it seemed I'd just be getting to first base with these young women, their mothers would always say something to the effect of, "Missy, you've got to come inside now and help me watch television." When I'd be talking with one of these teenaged maidens, the fathers of these young females wouldn't be as crude to me as their wives were, but still, they'd just kind of putter around nearby—within screaming distance—just in case they had to leap into action to save their daughter from this "head injured" savage.

It was so obvious what was going on with them, it wasn't funny. Take it, I didn't know some of these neighbors on the other side of the development as well as those who live on our block, but living in the park for fifteen years, they surely knew I wasn't a transient serial killer. But with this brain injury I've sustained, I guess they figured they can't be sure anymore.

I didn't do anything, but I still felt like a criminal. The only crime I'm guilty of is a social stigma and a lack of knowledge. I guess I'm a victim of the, "If enough people believe something, it must be true" train of thought. I feel horrible because the attitude towards me is something I can't control right now and the cause of this stigma isn't something of my creation. It's like, because I'm not 100% healthy, I'm not even worthy of an attractive girl's attention any longer. Now that I'm believed suspect, I'm not deserving. Believed to be witches, I can sense how those who got burned at the stake in Salem must have felt.

It wasn't as if I were proposing or anything, but I guess these moms and dads don't want to take a chance and get stuck with a "brain damaged" son-in-law, if they can help it. I guess I can't blame these parents with all the fish out in the sea who don't have so many obvious defects. Such is life.

Knowing these families for years and getting along with them well didn't seem to matter now because this head injury somehow has transformed me into some crazed sadist who must enjoy inflicting pain onto others. It was like these parents were keeping an eye out on me, just waiting for me to "snap" and turn into some kind of rapist or something when I gave them absolutely no reason to have any suspicions or to be afraid of me. To tell you the truth, I feel like the one who's been raped.

Feeling as if my head were in a stock, I was immobile. Whatever it was they gave me to relax and deaden the sensation of my left eye, I was comfortably numb. I don't know if it was because I was buzzed, trying to be macho, or just being plain stupid, but I said to those preparing me for eye surgery that I wanted local anesthesia during this extra-ocular resection procedure where Dr. Biglan would be cutting the muscle behind my eye with a sharp knife. I told the pre-op staff that I didn't want to sleep through this potentially magnificent experience of a lifetime.

When I informed the doctor moments before he was to perform his surgical mastery that I wanted to be awake and aware of what was going on during the operation on this first day of June 1983, he smiled and calmly told me this would be something I would never forget. He was right.

Wearing his surgical mask, Dr. Biglan held some kind of a pointy instrument and inserted it somewhere along my eye. As I concentrated on breathing through my nose, I laid on that operating room table not at all flustered because I wasn't feeling a thing and I knew that the master of this particular procedure was the one doing the work on me. Then, things got a little strange.

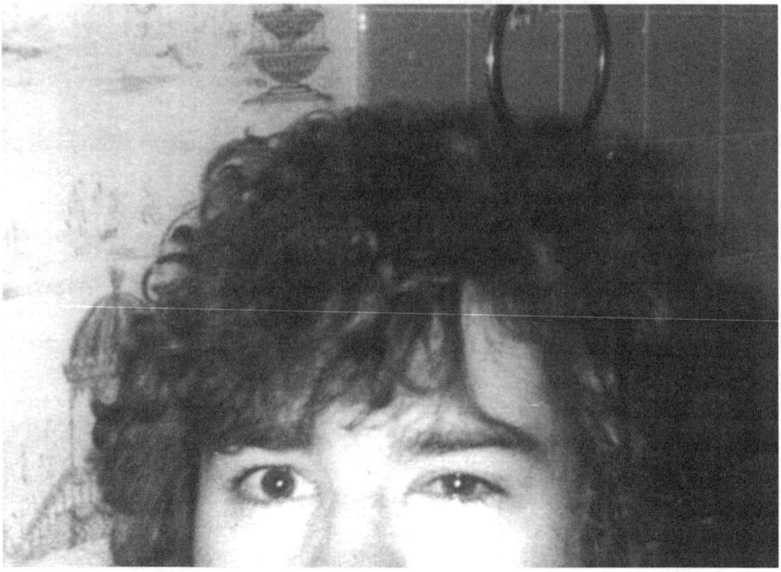

Illustrates how extra-ocular resection surgical procedure to correct Craig's paralytic strabismus/vertical diplopia rendered his left eye bloodshot several days after the operation, and disfigured permanently.

My head was braced and completely still, but when the doctor started jiggling his hand, the bright surgical light shining down on me from the ceiling started spinning. Despite staring straight ahead and my head absolutely motionless, the whole operating room and everything in it was moving. Rotating round and round, I saw the doorway and the wall to my left suddenly do an oval and end up to my right. Without so much as a flinch, the ceiling above me whisked down to the floor beneath me. Now you see it. . . . . .Now you don't.

It wasn't too extreme, but I felt a little pinch behind my eyeball as the walls and ceiling were whirling about. Twitching left then twitching right, things then stopped going around in circles and I could sense something moving around slightly inside of my head, behind my eye. In what seemed like a short time, this supposed minor operation where the eye itself is never touched, the surgery was over. But the pain would just be getting started.

Following the operation, when the drug used to render my eye numb to the snipping wore off, an incredible ache occupied my eye. This stinging throb made my head pound and stomach squeal like something one would hear coming from a torture chamber. A combination of this pain, watching my world turn while I didn't move so much as an inch, and my double vision worse now than it has ever been, my belly started to churn like a blender and I just wanted to be left alone to die in my bed. However, to pinch pennies, our medical insurance stipulated that this type of surgical treatment was one which could be done on an outpatient basis and if I wanted to go "beddy-bye," I was to do this at home.

Before we were forced to leave the hospital an hour or so after a scalpel went digging around my eye—despite my pleas of objection that I didn't want anything in my gurgling stomach, my post-op nurse—"Helga the Horrible" —insisted I drink a little soda to get something in my system before discharge. It remained in my gut until dad hit that first pothole on the way home and then I decorated the interior of his car with some bubbly pop.

Our primary payer has no idea how much time is needed to recuperate from double vision eye surgery. In and out of the hospital on a day when a patient is scheduled to have surgery to correct paralytic strabismus is ridiculous. I wouldn't know, but maybe this was the insurance company's way of compensating for being mistakenly billed for the general anesthesia procedure.

Since I have lost a good portion of the control over my life, I've put my faith in God's hands and allowed Him to guide me. Never a holy roller, in my own quiet way, I've always believed and practiced good morals. Not without sin, I try to exhibit proper behavior and ethics the great majority of the time. In this period of need, I can sense the presence of a Higher Power watching over me. Because of this, I have the confidence that, as long as I do what I can to get better, things are going to work themselves out for me. Maybe not as quickly as I would like or to the extent that I'd want to see, but with the way functions have been coming back, I have little doubt that I am going to be in charge again one day.

Regarding the eye surgery I just endured, I'm not ignorant, I knew that there were risks involved. But I had given my complete trust in the capabilities of Dr. Biglan and that God has helped him acquire the skills over the years, so that people like myself can benefit from his knowledge and expertise. For a little while—as this eye surgeon had forewarned me—immediately following the operation, my vision was atrocious. Within a short time, after the trauma of the eye muscle being disturbed had subsided, my vision has improved to the point I see things almost as they are.

With the exception of a hazed coating around objects, the extreme right or left, and when my head's tilted in certain angles, I see fine. My eyesight where I see a single object as one—not two—and a pair as it is instead of four, is a gift so tremendous, words alone do not do it justice. Appearance-wise, because of the work done to my left eye, it looks as if it is smaller than my right. But that's a small price to pay in order to rid myself of that nauseous diplopia. God bless you Dr. Biglan, you are incredible.

Initially, since my sights have always been to return to W.V.U. if I ever got my feet back on the ground, I was a little shaken when I found out that I wouldn't be heading back to Morgantown right away. However, after a little bit of thought, it wasn't too hard to understand the reasoning behind my neurosurgeon's recommendation.

Although it's questionable I was ever really there, Dr. Prostko figured that because I've been out of circulation from the university grind for some time now, it would be in my best interests if I could ease myself back into some sort of college environment and routine.

This brain surgeon feared that my going from being a one-time patient with a brain injury where my intellectual enhancement has been addressed on an individual basis these past sixteen months—to being one of a W.V.U. student body which approaches close to 20,000—would be just too big of an adjustment, making a successful return to college less likely. Dr. Prostko believed that a more intimate setting would better promote a productive readmission.

Being that I would be miles away from the family who have been so vital in my recovery up to this point, Dr. Prostko had his doubts that I could excel with my classwork while so far away from the support system who have been such a constant. Because he has had other patients who have attempted to return to their premorbid academic setting following a severe head injury, this physician understood the difficulties a student who has sustained extensive brain damage is likely to encounter.

Knowing of my family's involvement with/dedication to me and our attachment with one another, Dr. Prostko was more confident of my continued progress, if this ingredient remained intact. Despite my hesitancy at first, taking these various factors into account and the question I have of being on my own when there's so many concerns about my ability to be independent, it was agreed upon by all involved that my attempt to return to an institution of higher learning would be better served, if I would begin this first summer session at tiny Washington and Jefferson College, which is located approximately one mile from my home in Washington.

A Division III school, W and J is known for its academic standing and its capacity to provide tailored instruction. Approaching Trinity as far as the number of students who attend school there, the size of this college is similar to that of my high school. However, Washington and Jefferson College is a giant when it comes to providing its students with an education.

Everyone figured that the size and quality of the school, as well as being on my home turf, should make for an easier transition to college because my efforts can be geared towards my studies and the distractions kept to a minimum. If I should happen to stumble upon any unforeseen obstacles which may interfere with this academic pursuit, I have my incredible family, Rebecca, and OVR Counselor here in town in case I run into too much trouble.

Helping me adjust to my new academic standing as a "President"—not a returning "Mountaineer"—Rebecca walked around the small W and J grounds with me on this orientation tour as we tried to locate the building I would be registering at, the bookstore, and some of the halls I may need to know. W and J is only a fraction of the size of W.V.U. and one may think that learning how it's set up shouldn't pose too big of a problem for me then, but since my brain's right perceptual hemisphere has been bruised, any new stimulation is confusing for me now.

It's kind of funny, I've gone through W and J hundreds, if not thousands of times over the years because it's on the way to church and the Washington Mall, but I never really looked at it because it was just part of the landscape and not something I paid much attention to. Armed with my Washington and Jefferson College Campus Map, I was limping along Lincoln Street past McIlvaine Memorial Hall, approaching Lazear Hall when I saw the College Library where my first post-head injury college course would be held down in the basement. It's a little anticlimatic, but it should be a good testing ground for me.

Taught by the professor, Dr. Arnold, I will be taking W and J's four-week Economics 101 course this summer which is an equivalent to W.V.U.'s Economics 54. Enrolled in a class where I'm to learn the same coursework material in a four-week period of time that students during the fall and spring semesters have four MONTHS to absorb the information will leave very little time for anything else, but I'm positive I can do it. From June 14th to July 12th, I'll eat, sleep, and breathe such terms as "Gross National Product," "Supply and Demand," "Disposable Income," "Macro/Micro," "Full Employment," "Laissez-faire," "Equilibrium," etc., etc., etc. So much for a fun-filled summer.

Now that my main priority is this college econ course, Rebecca's role has changed from being my primary instructor who assigns aphasia-reducing/college prep homework, to being an academic support system where she'll help me with any intercollegiate hurdles I may encounter during this summer session. This may sound odd, despite the misgivings of many familiar with my situation, I have absolutely no doubt in my mind that I will succeed in my endeavor to return to college and excel. It's just a matter of discipline and this is something I've learned to incorporate during my rehabilitation. I don't care what the WAIS-R, Bender, Halstead-Reitan, Benton, or any of the other psych tests say about me and my supposed limitations because I know how clearly my thinking has become, as well as what's in my heart—and the latter can't be measured by any "mumbo jumbo" assessment.

Aware of my desire to return to the Morgantown campus in the fall and the circumstances surrounding my decision to go to W and J during the summer, my home school stipulated that I could attend college elsewhere and receive credit for my work, provided that I make at least a "C' grade. Whether I made an "A" or a "C" at W and J, my grade would not count towards my overall West Virginia University Grade Point Average, only the credits would transfer.

Also, W.V.U. requires that all core courses, which are those that deal with one's major directly, be taught by their professors and not some other school's. But this wouldn't apply to me anyhow because W and J doesn't offer a journalism program.

Washington and Jefferson definitely had their reservations about allowing me to receive instruction from their prestigious school because of my poor academic showing my first semester at W.V.U., but they still gratefully gave me a chance to prove that I could get into the "swing of things" academically. Within a little over a week after class started, I would be tested for the first time in college since my head hammered into that telephone pole and thinking had scattered. And the results of this exam would tell me something about what kind of a chance I'd have for a comeback.

After my stellar performance during the Harmarville driver's evaluation, mom and dad contracted with a professional driving instructor—Albert Reeves—to teach me how to operate a car again. Starting June 18, 1983, Mr. Reeves would be showing me little tricks, so that I would be able to manipulate a vehicle as well as somebody who didn't have paralysis of their right arm and hand. In his late fifties or early sixties, Mr. Reeves has an extensive background helping people with disabilities overcome their shortcomings.

Based on his 30+ years of experience, Mr. Reeves estimated that it would take approximately twenty-five, one-hour, driving lessons in order for me to develop into a proficient driver and learn the variety of compensatory techniques he was going to show me. It better only take this much training because that's all our secondary payer is going to reimburse us for.

Coming two to three times a week, Mr. Reeves projected that instruction would last approximately three months or until about the middle of August. Knowing that my past driving experience was practically non-existent, Mr. Reeves believed that it would take me the entire summer to understand the finer aspects of driving and be able to put them to use while finding appropriate shortcuts to alleviate the effect of my different physical limitations. Because I will be taking him out into the community repeatedly until I relearn how to drive, I was wrong about Harmarville's driving examiner having the worst job in the western hemisphere—Mr. Reeves does.

Since May 27th, my last day of Occupational Therapy, my focus now is strictly on my Economics course at W and J. When I started college right out of high school, I had no academic goals or aspirations. I was a pampered, runny-nosed kid who didn't know what was going on. If there's one thing this brain injury provided me, it was something to "shoot for."

Not all that many who've been through what I have can lay claim to being in a position where professional success is within possibility. And being afforded this chance to be a part of a mission where a milestone can be achieved is something I don't want to miss out on or forego because I did not put forth the utmost effort.

Because of this unique opportunity and my need to prove to myself—and others—that I am capable of accomplishing whatever I set my mind to, I now have the needed spark to excel. I don't know if assigning myself this responsibility is wise or something I should do, but I kind of feel that—because I was given this rare chance to make something of myself when so many others in the same situation don't—I owe something to those who have had a head injury and weren't as fortunate as myself. Specifically, to do what I can about the terrible stigma, silent or otherwise, that goes with most everyone who has had an injury to their head.

And the best way for me to start getting that message out at this time is for me to crack that Econ book. Look out "Exchange Rates," "Price System," "Public/Private Sector," because here I come.

In my short collegiate history, this is definitely a first. Because I realize there's no time to spare or slack off, once I get home from class, I open up my textbook and not my guitar case. Because of the extreme limitations my paralytic picking hand pose me now, I don't really enjoy playing too much anymore. If you look hard enough, frequently a positive can be found hidden amongst a negative and one of the pluses of this whole situation is that I have gotten a wake-up call as to what's important and what my priorities should be. Then again, I've got to take a break from reading about inflation and capitalism, now and then.

Almost immediately after I get home from class, I either start reading what's assigned on my syllabus or I play the cassette tapes which has today's three-hour lecture recorded on them. Having to write notes with my left hand now is absolute murder at its tortuous worst, not only because of the discomfort, but because I miss so many important points. Because of the painfully slow pace with which I write left-handed, I don't get all the information down in my notebook that I should. Also, focusing so strenuously on physically moving my non-dominant hand just to keep up, it's practically impossible for me to pick up all the significant facts I need to hear. Before I got into an awkward position, I addressed this problem.

Foreseeing this difficulty, Rebecca and I discussed how this situation may be resolved. We talked about how I'll need to use a tape recorder, but to first get permission from the instructor before taping him. Rebecca advised me not to get into a long, sob story where I tell my professor everything that's happened to me, but to keep it brief with a quick explanation that my dominant writing hand was affected when I was hurt in the car accident and I'll need a little help because of this physical liability. Rebecca thought it would be a good idea if I caught this college teacher during his office hours shortly before class was to begin and talk to him about my concern.

Knees shaking with the thought of actually speaking with a professor, the closest I had ever gotten to one of my college instructors at W.V.U before was when I sat in the twentieth row back one time in the auditorium at Eisland Hall during a Poli Sci class. Even then, I was sweating blood because I knew I could be seen napping.

I pictured fire shooting from Dr. Arnold's mouth scorching my eye brows and his fists clenching upon my making this request, but that didn't happen. Reading people well, because of the tone in his voice and expression on his face, I could tell my forthcoming econ professor was fairly impressed with how far I've come in my rehab and was pleased to be the initial step in my attempted return to college.

Talk about spectacular treatment. It hasn't been a year-and-a-half yet that the education therapists at Allegheny General were ecstatic that I was able to count to five and knew my name. A couple of months later, I likely would have gotten a standing ovation from Carolyn Joy and Diane Rosato had I been able to print my name and address without making a handful of mistakes. Last summer, Joni Russell probably couldn't have refrained from jumping out of her seat, if I could've consistently constructed the puzzles she put before me or found my way out of the many mazes she had me working with. When she first started working with me six months back, Rebecca would have been in all her glory and happy as a pig in mud had I been capable of picking out the important points in a passage and written a clear, descriptive sentence of what was covered.

Talk about coincidence and monumental progress. On 6/14/82, I was administered the Wide Range Achievement Test where my intelligence was equivalent to that of someone who had just started the eighth grade. On 6/14/83, I took my initial step towards returning to college, as this was my first day at Washington and Jefferson. In one year's time, my brain had healed to the extent that I could advance six grade levels.

On 6/18/82, I walked around the neighborhood for the first time without my wheelchair. And this same week a year later, I walked from a college library where I attend a summer class knowing that I had just gotten a "B" on my first college exam following a disability where no one could have ever dreamed this possible again. For all those who have worked so tenaciously with me on getting a grasp of my world once more, thank you for not giving up on me.

The investment I've put into my rehabilitation effort elevated me to a crossroad where I could either make the one-time fantasy of going back to college again reality or succumb to the fear that, because a person with a history of having severe brain damage attempting to get a degree is unheard of, this could not be possible. A patient who was once riddled with various aphasias attempting to attain their Bachelor's Degree at a major university is largely unchartered territory, but this was exactly what I was on the verge of doing. Because of the accomplishments I've made during the long, dark travels of my rehab which have helped me reach this summit, my personality has changed to the extent that I no longer feel less than others. I don't believe as if I'm deserving of entitlement in any way because of what's happened to me, but I definitely think I'm a little unique because what I'm about to embark on hasn't been done by all that many—if by anyone.

I don't know if I should interpret this as good or bad, modest or conceited, but I'm torn between two trains of thought. One, I want recognition for the special gains that I've made, but on the other, I have a part of me that has a personal desire to conform because I don't want to be different from others and stick out. However, because of what has happened to me and the visible scars it has left, I don't know if this will be possible.

Wanting a, "Hey world, see what I've done, but don't look at me!," persona during my Econ class at W and J was something that could not be possible and was a situation I struggled with initially because I didn't know how to handle the response of my collegiate peers. But from this confusion developed a valuable learning experience.

In addition to myself, there were five other students along with Dr. Arnold in the cramped library conference room where we had our "Principals of Economics" class. Within a few days' time, thinking this would get me some positive attention, I had given everyone in these cozy confines a general idea of what had happened to me. Their reactions weren't exactly what I was expecting.

Accustomed to seeing those within the rehabilitation and medical fields making a fuss over me and all that I've achieved, I was surprised my fellow summer school Presidents didn't get excited about me going from being at death's front door to a college classroom. Initially, it got their attention when I told them about how seriously I was hurt and have come in my recovery, but they didn't seem real interested beyond that and it didn't perk their curiosity much. If I had another sense and could read their minds, I know I would have been picking up something on my thought-reading scanner like, "That's nice, good for you. Now, be quiet, I got more important things to think about." Well, at least nobody screamed and none of the girls squirted my eyes with mace when I told them this.

That was an example of the, "Hey world, see what I've done" side coming out in me. The "Don't look at me" portion was what presented me with some problems and could've led to a downfall. I learned you can't have it both ways and you got to accept the good with the bad. Because the bad far outweighed the good in this particular situation, maybe I need to be a little more careful what I disclose and to whom. It might even be a good idea not to say anything—or if I do—let the person I'm divulging information to get to know, "Craig Meyers, the fellow student" first, instead of "Craig Meyers, the one-time rehab patient," because the latter may be too much of a shock to absorb "right off the bat."

Possibly, students may mistakenly think I want an unfair advantage by the professors or preferential treatment by them because of what's happened to me and I'll have to give them a little bit of time to see that this is not the case and that I just want to be one of the gang. It's quite natural to want a little bit of accolades and recognition for a job well done, but when you want to be invisible at the same time, one has to decide what's most important to them. My assertiveness and desired demeanor of being outgoing have improved incredibly since I've discovered what I'm all about, but this doesn't completely stop the remnants of my old "gun-shy" personality from coming out.

I'd have to flip tapes over a total of three times during the three-hour class. Although I don't think I was too awfully bad, I was concerned about being a bother to my fellow econ students, which was the main reason why I told them about how badly I was hurt. Hoping that they would understand the commotion I was making with my cassette player, I told my econ classmates that jiggling tapes and disturbing the silence was something I regretted, but had to do. I figured if they knew that I couldn't help being a nuisance, they wouldn't be so mad. Being different before a half-dozen probing eyes, I was about to learn a difficult, yet beneficial, lesson.

Knowing that it would be almost impossible for me NOT to get credit for my W and J econ course now that I kicked butt on that first exam, I thought this would be a good time to see if I could manage without the recorder. With my focus on alleviating the unwanted attention—and not maintaining my good grade—I paid a price that could've cost me dearly.

Admittedly, it's a hassle for me to go through the process of recording lectures and then writing in my notebook the important points I've missed once I get home. Altogether, instead of sitting through three hours of economics lecture everyday like I normally should be doing, I sit through at least six being that I'd repeatedly stop the tape, write the important details, stop the tape, write the important details, etc. Doing this everyday for six hours coupled with being away from an academic setting for so long, getting tired of being looked at, and coasting with a decent grade, I kind of burned out and let up some.

However, by the time it was all said and done, I got my "C" grade, but more importantly, I learned a lot of important things about myself. The way things have been stacking up for me and how my situation stands right now, I know I couldn't have reached this matrix unless I had a good bit of character and strength. Because of the many obstacles I have been able to stand up to and not let sidetrack me during the challenging endeavor of starting back to school after almost "flat lining" a heart monitor, I know now that my limitations can be overcome provided I not be my customary passive self and make the proper accommodations to minimize any weakness. To continue with my premorbid backward ways will not be possible anymore and in order for me to survive in this fast-paced world, I'm just going to have to speak up for myself and maintain the extra effort I've been putting forth.

Without a doubt, my tenacity and perseverance would be tested during the second summer session at W and J. My approach to this examination of will and courage brought before me will be impacted by what I have come to understand about myself. This influence will provide me with the illumination I will need to emerge from the dark chaos which I have been embroiled for almost a year-and-a-half.

Before the final leg of this W and J experience and my reorientation to W.V.U. get started, I was happy as could be with how this trial run at Washington and Jefferson was going thus far because I was seeing for myself that I can work out and execute most anything that comes my way. And it wasn't just the college studies which were coming my way for, during one hot afternoon while I was walking outside of the library, I caught a glimpse of Paul for the first time since that fateful Valentine's night.

The vast majority of the time, I'm easy-going and not all that difficult to get along with. I'm the type of person who, regardless of how well I know them, if someone acknowledges me, then I'll generally greet them back and go on my way. On this one occasion in particular, I regret being so indiscriminately friendly.

One day after econ class had just ended, I made my way out of the W and J library and was walking along Lincoln Street towards the parking lot where dad picks me up to take me home when I saw this hand wave to me from a car that was passing by. Focusing on the homework I had to do when I got back to the house and the hot girl I sit next to in class, my mind wasn't really on what was going on around me too much when I instinctively raised my hand to the person sitting in the passenger's seat of the car that drove by. Upon closer examination, I saw that I had just given my regards to the person who almost killed me and devastated my family.

Whoever was driving the car, unless it was a Michaels' family member, I could just hear Paul telling them that we're the best of friends now because I am really grateful for his heroic efforts after his car slid on that ice and crashed into the pole. Because I waved back, Paul possibly thinks that—despite disrupting my life forever—things are just fine and dandy between us. I couldn't say for sure if Paul's waving to me was an impulsive reaction as well, he wanted to get a bearing as to how I felt about him after all that has happened, was a trait of his "cocksure" personality, or something else. I just know we're not going to be getting together anytime soon to rehash the good times we've had.

If I would ever get a phone call from an ex-classmate because they wanted to revisit the good ol' days, I know it wouldn't be coming from any of my "buddies" who were involved with Ilyacoff's infamous blowout. Not that I was expecting to hear from my chums or looking forward to a reunion, when I saw Paul that afternoon close to a year-and-a-half after the accident —besides Sam—this was the first contact I had with anybody associated with the "shindig" which left me permanently disabled.

Trust is not to be foolishly gambled with and put into the hands of those who are suspect, for the penalty can be the immediate erosion of one's health and well-being. For me, the cost of pursuing a little excitement was saying goodbye to a treasure's worth of development. Sacrificing the next day's joy for a dream which may not be is a price only the desperate or a fool would pay. A bird in the hand is worth two in the bush.

Blinded by idiocy, I am guilty of drifting from that which is known. Abiding by the teachings of my past, this nightmare needn't have to be. To err is human, as people grow from the mistakes that are one's history. I am going to utilize my new understanding to propel me into a new beginning and there's no better way to start this fresh chapter of my life than to give it my all academically. Every cloud has a silver lining.

The only thing that I was ever used to reading before was my Sporting News, but since July 14th—only two days after finishing Economics 101—I've been digging into a new novel every two or three days. Equivalent to W.V.U.'s English 36, Washington and Jefferson's English 269 is a course entitled, "Tough Guys in American Literature," where I delve into several detective books a WEEK. Taught by the professor, Dr. Keen, this class is one where I not only have to read and understand several thousands pages of literary works within a month's time, but research and respond to two separate writings by a chosen author. First, in the form of a written report and then make a presentation orally to the class.

To make the probing analysis required to get a good grade on this assignment, I had to read several hours each day and concentrate on trying to "fish out" the meaningful dialogue hidden amongst an abundance of superfluous items designed to conceal. Rebecca having me practice homework like this during her tutelage is sure coming in handy now that my brain's right perceptual hemisphere needs to work for me, if I'm to continue my recovery towards this "impossible dream" of attaining a degree after sustaining a severe brain contusion.

A little over a year ago, I couldn't read a page without the paragraphs moving all over the place or scan a line because I was unable to keep my eyes from shooting "this way and that." Ironically, almost a year ago to the week that I began this detective novel class, I was administered the Gates-MacGinitie Reading Comprehension Test. Although I was showing significant improvement at the time within this realm of my cognitive rehabilitation, I still scored way below what the average aspiring college student gets on this exam.

Twelve months back, when I was having difficulty recalling what the previous sentence covered, who would've thought I would be attending a private college and taking a course where my grade was dependent on remembering themes of different passages from books that I had read? Ever having the intellectual capacity to attend a class of this nature shortly after my minds ability to concentrate had run amok, would have seemed highly unlikely when I was grappling to snare some sense of what was going on. To excel in this sphere of academic understanding and personal fortitude would not have even been worth considering a year ago at this time, however, this is exactly what I did during the final summer session 1983.

Now we're talking. English always having been my strong suit, I needed a grade such as this to start me off on the right foot prior to my returning back to West Virginia University. Only I know exactly how I'm perceiving my world and absorbing its contents, but I am hoping that what I have just done during this latter summer session will persuade the skeptics to believe that I just may pull off something that hasn't been done all that often by going back to a dominant university after having been a one-time aphasic patient.

Not expecting or receiving any favoritism, I was proud of what I had just accomplished in this intensive summer program, and this pride would be the initial block needed to build my confidence for the upcoming fall semester in Wild, Wonderful, West Virginia. Prior to classes starting on 8/22/83 at W.V.U., I needed to discover what arrangements would be necessary for my return to class and what compensatory strategies I would need to utilize in order to minimize the impact of my physical liabilities. But of equal importance, I had to find out what I was made of. To undertake this self-exploration at a small college in my hometown was an awesome idea, for I uncovered a gold mine which was my determination and fortitude to transcend "against all odds."

It is essential that one believes in their capabilities before embarking on a mission as rigorous as attempting to attain their Bachelor's Degree; particularly if the one going on this trip has sustained extensive brain damage. Because of what I have done in my rehabilitation to get this far, I now have in place this foundation necessary for academic achievement. However, because I've had something happen to my neurologic system, I'm afraid that no matter how well I do, I'm sure I will always have my doubters who will try to explain away any success I may have. But I'll deal with that when it comes. As for now, I've got to demonstrate that I *AM* capable. Always being competitive in nature, I welcome this challenge. I don't really have a choice.

Keeping my nose to the grindstone, I have proven to myself, as well as a few others I suppose, that I can excel academically now. The final paper I labored over where I compared and contrasted Dashiell Hammett's, The Thin Man and The Maltese Falcon, yielded a grade of "B+" on the written portion and an "A−" on my oral presentation. During the month of August 1982, a period of time when I had just learned how to cursively write again and still spoke in a monotone voice, not a single soul familiar with my condition would have predicted that I would receive a grade of "B" for a four-week summer lesson where I would have to read, write, and speak as much in a week's time what students during the regular academic year have five times as long to cover. I guess I fooled all the "experts."

With the summer performance I just put on—not only in the English class, but my Economics course too—despite the abundance of doomsday predictions that I'm positive are still out there, I know I'm ready to go back to W.V.U. now. I realize that there will still be some crossed fingers, but because of what I have just proven that I'm capable of doing after a forty-eight hour summer vacation, those fingers won't be mine. "Let's go-oooo, Mountaineers!"

There was never any question that once I proved I could handle college work again, I was going back to W.V.U. I have some unfinished business there and a point to prove. Specifically, I need to show myself and any detractors that I can take command of any challenge that presents itself. She had been so effective training me to be proficient and independent with my college studies that—on 7/7/83—five days before the Economics class ended, Rebecca had finished her consequential work with me. Fabulous job Rebecca, I've really benefited from you knowing your stuff so well.

Wanting me to attend W and J full-time now that I've shown I can manage college studies, mom's knees are bruised from begging me to stay home. Afraid of how I'm ever going to survive without constant monitoring, mom didn't want me to leave and to just stay put. But I would not even consider this.

In my eyes, if I were to stay in Washington and leave the school of my choice, that would mean defeat. Despite Washington and Jefferson being an outstanding institution of higher learning—since being hurt—I have always strived to get back to where I was before the accident and where I was at before being flung into the netherworld was W.V.U., not W and J. And I feel this is where I have to be in order to successfully apply any finishing touches to my rehabilitation mission.

From my vantage point, settling for anything less than going back to my old school would be "loss," for I would feel that my rehab was not complete then. The term "rehabilitation" itself means to get back what one has lost and, to me, my rehabilitation would never be fulfilled totally, if I were to be uprooted and had to revise my goal of being self-sufficient by staying home. For me to be dependent at a time when I should be autonomous and striving to break free would mean that I have lost. Because I don't take losing very well, I'm not about to let any separation anxiety keep me from finishing what I've started. "Let's go-oooo, Mountaineers!"

Blistered by the thought of me going back to school in West Virginia, I know the idea of being on my own after being dependent on others for so long just to survive is gnawing away at mom, but now is the time to find out if I'm going to "sink or swim" in this world. Mom worries a lot and I know she'll be obsessing about a variety of situations. No longer under her watchful eye or supervised by her scrutiny, I know there are going to be many situations which are going to terrify her.

Mind racing, mom could construe circumstances where, because of my bad balance and lack of coordination now, I'm going to be knocked backwards down a flight of the many stairs that are the W.V.U. campuses and suffer some kind of setback that will put me back to "Square One" again in my fight to get over what my head being banged around did to me. Because the old Craig was kind of withdrawn and didn't want to deviate from everybody else, I can understand mom being afraid that I won't ask for help when I might need it. Or that I will get despondent over the stares I'm bound to receive because I'm different now.

Mom could see me sitting at my desk in the apartment hour after hour, so frustrated with how slowly I write with my left hand that I just feel there's no use trying to keep up anymore. Because I have been slowed down so badly and can be a "klutz" at times, mom was concerned that the simple homemaking duties one is responsible for living at Pierpont House—such as cooking and cleaning—would be too taxing for me and leave me pressed for time which I didn't have. Since she's done the majority of these duties since I've been hurt, mom was scared I'd get so distraught after realizing I couldn't do the most simplistic chores with any speed that this would affect my schoolwork.

Flashing before her, not nearly close to writing down everything I know, mom could form a mental picture of a professor in a classroom telling everyone who hadn't finished to turn in their test paper while I was still frantically scribbling away. What she envisioned the days and weeks prior to this exam were not real soothing either, as a script would play in her mind where the instructor would reel off important fact after important fact, but because of my left hand's inability to write fast enough and my embarrassment over needing a tape recorder, I missed the material that was surely going to be on the final.

The W.V.U. Medical Center will be within sight of where I'll be living in Pierpont House, a fraction of a mile away, but I know mom still has pictures tucked away in her visual data banks of me shaking violently having a seizure and won't be able to get to a hospital for help. Or she'll conjure up a scene where a crowded PRT hits a bump and several students collide into me, knocking me over. Falling onto my limb that was nearly amputated, breaking the femur into pieces again, I wouldn't be nearly so lucky the second time around. However, in her revised "take" on things, severing the weakened artery this last time would result in me coming home for Christmas break wearing my new plastic leg.

The hush of night will not be a time of peace and replenishment for mom because I know images of when I was in Washington Hospital's E.R. lying unconscious on a blood-drenched gurney and Allegheny General trapped in a coma are going to twist her conscience. Because I will be attending school about forty-two miles away and living in Morgantown—instead of going to class one mile away and staying at home—it looks like mom's in for a lot of restless nights.

And daybreak won't necessarily mean the haunting visions of monitors measuring my heartbeat, an oxygen mask covering my face, or mattresses spread on the floor of my hospital room will stop from being played over and over again. Now that I won't be tied to her apron strings, when the thought of Life Flight helicopter taking me to Pittsburgh appears from the shadow of mom's subconscious, an intense fear will no doubt take her captive knowing that I won't be in the next room anymore.

As silent as mom is evident regarding my determination that a country road would take me back to where I belong, dad was more difficult to read. Never for a moment, did he stop encouraging me to plow ahead or telling me not to look back. Countless times, dad would remind me that there's a reason God gave me a chance to make something of myself and put me in this position where I could pick up where I left off. At this time, I don't see exactly how Divine Intervention played a role in my getting on my feet again or why, when so many other people—more deserving people—did not have this opportunity. I'm just happy with the way the cards have been turning up for me.

Because of the afflictions my head injury caused and how I was able to overcome them, dad would tell me time and time again that all I need to achieve anything I want is to believe in myself and not let any self-doubt get in the way. Surviving "against all odds," dad thinks God has some grand plan for me. I don't know about that, but I can say it's been a long, hard, road to get this far and dad's support, commitment, and love has meant everything. Slicked up in my cap and gown, there won't be a prouder parent at W.V.U.'s graduation ceremonies than my dad.

Despite his outward positive view on things, I can tell by the look in dad's eyes and with the way he carries himself that he's being turned inside out trying to conceal the question he has over my ability to overcome the symptoms of a brain injury and be independent. Despite telling him that my marijuana exploits are a part of my past and not something I'm going to get involved with again, dad warned me that temptation could be the end of me. When seduction beckons to embrace that which will not enhance one's prosperity, it is important not to make the same mistake I once did, for this tragic lesson of life could be the final passage of a creation which never had the opportunity to flourish.

There's a provision in the Rehabilitation Act of 1973 which would protect me from being expelled despite my academic probation status, but if I were to get horrid marks academically in the upcoming semester because I was too busy not working, I know the smoke would clear and we would all see that college just wasn't something that was ever in my playbook. However, there's no way on God's good earth I'd ever allow this to happen because of what I just went through to reach this summit.

If I would drop out of school because I couldn't or wouldn't "hack it," this would mean, in essence, that all the work I've put into my rehabilitation so this college opportunity could present itself again would be for naught. However, with the "new Craig Meyers" a refreshing and improved version from a maturity/priority standpoint, success will be within reach. I'll just have to take the stance that this enhanced attitude adjustment will more than compensate for my physical drawbacks which could pose me with some problems.

Simply put, I've just got to make "do" with what I've got in order to prevent against a future slipping from my grasp. I'm sorry, but this head injury isn't going to leave me behind. Whoever said, "One gains wisdom through suffering," sure knew what they were talking about. "Let's go-oooooooooooooo, Mountaineers!"

Chapter 7

Equal Opportunity: Fact or Fiction?

The year 1986 was supposed to be one of celebration. Come December, I would have my Bachelor of Arts from West Virginia University in its College of Arts and Sciences. Because of all I have gone through to get my Bachelor's degree, this was to be a time when the Meyers' family would be rejoicing over what I've just been able to accomplish "against all odds" and where I was headed next. However, like so many other things that have happened the past several years since I had been so gravely injured, this period which should have been one of merriment and jubilation was instead replaced by mourning only twenty-nine days into this new year.

The night sky was threatening and was the type of evening where the cold ripped to the bone. Looking out the window, the landscape was white as far as the eye could reach, for the unrelenting snow fell like a guillotine. The dark clouds above darkened the earth below, guarding against the moon's brightness from piercing the gloom and rescuing its imprisoned inhabitants from this black fall of day.

With the close of this condemned January 29th day so ugly and unforgiving, so our spirits wouldn't sink with the setting sun, my "studly" roommate—Dave "Stouff" Stouffer—and I were making fun of Kevin who now lives upstairs because of a room assignment mix-up. Interrupting our good-natured roast, my other "buck" roomie—Lieutenant David Schneeweis—came to the bedroom from the living area to tell me I was wanted on the phone and that it was my mom. Because she never calls me at school, I figured something was up, but that it was probably no big deal. I couldn't have been any more wrong. The message I was about to receive would affect me and my family for the rest of our lives.

By the tone of my voice and the laughter in the background, mom could easily sense the light-hearted mood of our fourth floor apartment at Pierpont House this evening and sounded mad I was in such a good mood because of how dreary she was feeling. Like an eclipse, the brightness of my cheer was instantly shaded by heart-felt grief when mom said, "Daddy had a heart attack while he was out shoveling snow in the driveway."

However, before this even had a chance to sink in to torment me, always doing what he could to keep distractions at a minimum for me since I've returned to college for this second tour of duty, dad got on the other phone next to he and mom's bed. Telling me not to worry, dad went on to tell me that the pain in his chest has now subsided and that he was going to see our family doctor in two days.

Despite his assurance that he's feeling fine now and thinks the whole incident was a one-time thing, I know better because it's easier for a Democratic President to get a bill through a Republican Congress—or vice versa—than to get dad to a doctor. But on 1/31/86, dad went to see Dr. Tripoli where he found out his heart was just fine. As it turns out, this normally encouraging diagnosis was just the beginning of yet another catastrophic loss.

Following the first grading period, the fact that I had made an academically successful return to West Virginia University after having sustained a severe head injury may have been pretty noteworthy. However, beyond this and my re-orientation to college life, my first semester back at W.V.U. was not extraordinary by any stretch of the imagination. But, I couldn't have hoped for anything better being that I just wanted to be part of the mix after my ingredient was almost omitted. I was just your average kind of student, average kind of guy, but being "average" considering what my mind and body have been through really took some doing.

The first half of the academic school year, rounded off, my grade point average was 2.55. Stigmatized by this status, I was needing a passing grade such as this one to get me out of "academic probation." I know that if some students came home at break with this G.P.A., they'd never see the light of day again. Because of the way my thinking had gone haywire on me there for a while after I had my bell rung, no one was going to padlock me into a box. Au contraire.

Wanting to prove I could survive outside the shadow of home and show those who believe academic achievement following a severe head injury just isn't possible that I could do well, I was proud that I was able to attain a little success when so many didn't give me a hope in hell of doing anything other than being a paper boy.

Believing this was just a fluke, I'm sure these "experts" will snicker when told I think I can do better. With a good bit of my time during my first semester back spent learning how to maneuver around my disabilities and developing confidence—now that I have incorporated these as part of the routine—I can devote more hours to my studies. All in all, I was happy with my score and how well I did. And I wasn't alone.

When I showed dad my first W.V.U. grade report since my head injury, tears bottling up in his eyes, he gave me such a big hug and yelled for joy so loud, my shoulders ached and ears rung—on top of the tinnitus—until New Year's. Dad was so elated, I thought he might give me a kiss on the cheek. But he knew that if he'd do this, I wouldn't come home again until I graduated. Always one to throw caution to the wind and not show her hand too early in the game, I know I had a good thing going when mom busted out with a huge smile.

Despite my good showing at the local college, my parents were sweating blood until I demonstrated I could do the job at W.V.U. grade-wise while concurrently tending to my independent living needs. Ecstatic, me and my parents knew I was back.

When I entered W.V.U. in '81, I hadn't any legitimate career aspirations or, as my grades would later show, a desire to even be in college. I guess because this was the only course I was really interested in or appealed to me during school, writing was the only subject within my academia that I ever excelled at. Being able to convey a message through the written word is a gift I had indulged in for quite some time, but for fear of what might be said, I used to always be silent about this experience. Because employing the English language to transmit an expression was about the only intellectual skill I ever practiced or accumulated much knowledge in, my selection of a major which utilizes this specialty—such as journalism—was a natural one. However, living rehabilitation and gaining extensive experience with the different behavioral aspects associated with rehab, I quickly realized I had a lot more to offer from my experiential tool box, if I could incorporate some of the unique and potentially invaluable events that have recently occurred in my life into a profession. My first semester back at W.V.U. was my last as a journalism student because I changed my major to Psychology. It was just a matter of time before I got the message that journalism just wasn't something I was cut out for.

I not only made this switch for the above reason, but because my physical incapacities were too much of a deterrent to continue with this occupational choice that I was never positive I wanted to pursue in the first place. To be a quality journalist, you've got to write notes quickly and type fast. My paralytic dominant right hand renders me incapable of doing either one of these with any kind of proficiency. With my experience and interests having turned a new direction, I was now preparing to delve into the Science of the Mind. Scary.

With a new major and purpose in tow, my studies now had a goal-oriented texture to them. Once again, carrying the minimum twelve credits to qualify as a full-time student, during my second post-brain damaged semester, I earned a grade point average of 2.75. I may not be a magnum caum laude, but considering I couldn't even write, "West Virginia University," a little over two years ago—let alone attend school here—I truly doubt many Rhodes Scholars have ever comprehended as much as I have within a twenty-four month period of time. I always knew I had it in me.

Missing a year-and-a-half of studies at W.V.U. rehabbing, there was little time to bask in glory over what I did my first full spring semester as a Mountaineer because—in order to make up for lost time—I would be attending Washington and Jefferson College for classes again during the summer. Being a President each summer season during the months of June, July, and August, I won't catch up to where I should be, for there has been too much time that has elapsed, but at least I know that my parents will have the opportunity to see me graduate from college which has been their primary goal after all that's happened to me. For the next couple of summers, I'll have a one-week vacation, so that doesn't give me much time to dust off my old high school French books for the upcoming first session at W and J with Mme. Scanlon. Un, deux, trois,—cinq?

To reward myself for a year well done, after the '83-'84 school year ended at W.V.U., I dug into the little savings I had accumulated over time and got a used Chevy. Five days before the W.V.U. school year started—8/17/83 to be exact—I finished my driver's training with Mr. Reeves after thirty lessons at seventeen bucks a clip, but the extent of my driving experience these past nine months has been an hour a week taking Kevin home every weekend with dad supervising.

I passed a professional driver's training course with flying colors, but until I passed my dad's, I wasn't about to get on the road by myself behind the controls of a car he bought, so I scrounged up some change and got my own. Even then, dad got volatile that I would want to drive to Pittsburgh once in a while to catch a Pirates' game at Three Rivers or a concert at the Civic Arena. Oh well, what can I say?

Academically and interpersonally, just like any other undergraduate, for me there were high points and low points during the '83-'84 school term. From a grade standpoint, during the fall semester, four classes stick out in particular which I think were representative of me in a way, for they show how I've developed as a person since I was hurt.

Light years ago, when I was a freshman Mountaineer right out of high school, I took Humanities I and promptly got an "F" because I thought this Western Civilization course was a waste of my time. Although my opinion of the class' worth hasn't changed much, my attitude about why I've got to take this subject has—which is that I have to, if I want to graduate someday. And since I don't have much of a say about it, for I want that "failing" mark deleted from my transcript, I might as well make the most of it and get this stimulating course out of the way.

With this attitude revision, I not only read, studied, and did the text work required, but I went to see a theatrical production and a musical for extra credit. Paying attention to what the instructor said the second time around and concentrating when I read material this time, I took the grade I would receive in this class seriously now since I've seen the ramifications of what can happen, if I don't. During the Holiday Season 1983, when the fall grades were mailed out, I ripped the envelope the grade report was enclosed and found out that I earned a "B" in this topic I'll probably never use again in my life. I couldn't have received a better gift. Merry Christmas!!!

I have learned that college is not only about instruction and gaining intelligence about the various course matter, but it teaches one various lessons of life. I only wish I had this maturity and understanding the first time I was here. I would have avoided a lot of hassle and heartache then.

My History 52 class was valuable, not so much in the sense that the specific names, places, dates, and occurrences reviewed were all that vitally important to me in my life, rather, its significance was that it taught me the valuable lessons of how to study and what I needed to do to overcome some of my afflictions in my development as a college student. The first test our instructor, Mr. Dawson, gave us covered 99% lecture and 1% textbook. However, for the first test, I studied many hours mainly from the book and got a low "D" on this test.

I thought I definitely put in the time required to get a solid grade, it was just my efforts that were geared in the wrong direction. From this test on, I won the brunt of the battle with my self-conscious and—concealed in my backpack so the other students couldn't see—brought my cassette recorder everyday to tape each lecture.

If my brain weren't working for me, I would have continued the study pattern of ignoring my notes in favor of the information in the texts. However, my episodic memory, which is the recollection of recent experience, allowed me to make the changes necessary to salvage this "Growth of the American Nation to 1865" course after this initial blunder. I pulled of a pretty good Sanford and Son the rest of the time, for I ended up getting a "C" for the semester. From here on out, in every class, I learned it's imperative that I take good notes and focus my energies on absorbing the information in them. I better stock up on batteries then, for it looks like my tape recorder is in for some heavy-duty work.

Since the 6th grade, I began learning how to swim. When I first started junior-high eight years ago, I could do a lot of the different strokes required to motor with the waves and have gone for dips periodically since then. However, all that was before my brain being mangled caused me to forget how to float and get moving in the water.

I always thought that once one learns how to swim, this ability is never lost. Under normal circumstances, this may be the case, but my bruised brain has forced me to relearn everything, making this far from being a normal phenomenon. Disheartened and frightened—on 12/11/82—long before any college phys ed class was being considered, I went to the YMCA in Washington with a friend to do some water therapy laps in their pool for my spastic right arm. It was here that I found out I couldn't swim anymore.

Jumping in the shallow water at the "Y," I assumed a conditioned response would occur with me where my body would sense what to do once I was in. But this brain contusion I suffered, erased any innate ability I once had to do aquatics. Because of my hesitancy, I'm sure being fearful played some role in my performance, but I also knew it was much more than my emotions which caused me to sink.

Having received some kind of certificate from the American Red Cross when I was about ten years old, I was a decent swimmer growing up. No, I may not have been the most buoyant thing skimming on the water, but I could hold my own. However, once my face went into the water at the Young Men's Christian Association that December day, I started swallowing chlorine instantly because I didn't know how to hold my breath while I was under! And I couldn't remember the motions my arms and legs needed to engage in to get me gliding through this H2O, as all I did was stand there and splash! If I would have taken it for granted I'd be able to swim and hopped in the deep end right away, I may not have been around to open my Christmas presents in two weeks. What a way to go after surviving a death-defying, violent collision with a utility pole.

Implicit memory is the mind's automatic ability to bring forth a sequence of motions in order to undertake a particular physical action. This recall is ingrained in one's perceptual field and the loss of this natural process is indicative of severe mental degeneration. For example, when I was in Harmarville, I forgot how to climb a flight of stairs because my brain didn't have any idea how to send a message to one leg to lift and then balance me on the step, as the other did the same thing and so on. The tactile sensation involved when ascending or descending stairs was now insensible to past sensory experience because the area of my brain which once controlled how to do this and stored this knowledge in its memory banks was damaged. With my cerebral automatic pilot now unaware of how to go about taking on this task, as well as many others, this adolescent toddler had to work like a fiend in order to regain this involuntary response operation.

Early on, since my brain rattled around in my skull, the instinctive and spontaneous part of me had disappeared. Because my "self-acting" switch where I engage in activities without thinking was no longer operable, I needed to reprogram my neurologic control center again, so actions I once did which were directed by will alone may return.

Like relearning how to drive, when I started swimming at W.V.U., I had to develop a "feel" again for what it was like to go through the series of motions required to propel myself through water. Because the section of my brain responsible for the faculty of knowing without the use of any cognitive process was damaged, no signal could be sent to my body what it should feel like to float, kick, and move my arms in order to swim.

However, by finals' week—December 1983—all the practice I had done in the natatorium forced something in my implicit memory to click and I was chugging around in the pool pretty good there. Before this one-credit "Beginning Swimming" physical education class ended, I had swam the length of the pool and back, from the shallow end to the deep end, back to the shallow. Doing more than a "doggie paddle" and not without its hairy moments, I got my first "A" in college. Because of the psychological obstacles I had to conquer, I only wished I could have gotten more than four grade points, for I never worked harder in my short college experience to do well, but I'll take it.

Knowing what happened to me and seeing how my bad right side affects how I move, because of the way she interacted with me, I think the instructor may have given me such a good grade, not only because of the definite improvement I had shown by the end of the semester and the effort I expended, but because she felt a little bad for me. If this was the case, things would even out in my Composition and Rhetoric class.

My English 2 writing class was an experience which benefited me, not from an academic standpoint, for the final grade I would receive was no way near to being an accurate reflection of my capabilities, rather, it enlightened me from a position of learning to keep my editorials to a minimum and being selective who receives these commentaries. Because of my freshman insensitivity and the instructor's contrasting viewpoint on the ways of the world, we didn't have the best relationship. And I'm afraid I paid the price.

I didn't intend to be controversial or rub the teacher the wrong way, but that's exactly what I did when I handed in my initial paper which did not take into account that this older grade-giver's stance on life may be different from my own. On this first writing assignment, I proceeded to write a paper about a topic which advertised some of my denominational convictions as fact. Unfortunately, my perception of things didn't exactly "jive" with this educator's, and I got one juicy "F." Because I've always been able to write and can't remember ever receiving such a horrendous mark in my life for this ability to transcribe thoughts onto paper, I was flabbergasted when I saw this grade.

Having an idea where the man responsible for my grade operates from now—in order to avoid getting a final grade which wasn't representative of my ability—I had to kiss a little ass and tailor my subsequent writings, so they wouldn't conflict in any way with his fundamental beliefs. But it was too late, for the die had been cast.

Careful not to push his buttons the remainder of the semester, I did better, but I feel I still didn't get a fair mark as things wound down. However, a "C-" sure beats a failing score. Oh, the lessons of life college can teach us.

Inching my way closer to a "B" average, the significance of the spring semester '83-'84 was that it left no doubt for me that the cognitive functions of my mind were operating just as fine as they ever have. Going to all lengths to make some sort of a statement about how my capacity to learn has returned, I needed to prove that the severe head injury that I had sustained was an unfortunate circumstance which occurred in my past that will not have any kind of bearing on my future. Among the four three-credit courses I took my second semester back, two in particular show how my brain's ability to process information and develop has remained intact.

This past summer at Washington and Jefferson when I took the equivalent of W.V.U.'s Economics 54, I made a grade equaling a "C." During the momentous second semester back at W.V.U. when my overall G.P.A. was 2.75, I took the more difficult and advanced Econ 55, but this time, earned a final grade of "B." Admittedly—unlike the case at W and J—the incentive was there to do really well this time because my final grade at West Virginia would obviously count towards my average. But still, this improved mark was indicative of my brain's current capacity to retain and retrieve data. With these two formulas being vital components to growth and enhanced intelligence, lookin' more and more like I'm getting back into the driver's seat again, I knew the makings of a successful academic return were in place.

Mr. Dawson's History 53 was not any easier than his History 52 class that I took with him in the fall, it was just a matter of understanding his style and incorporating my preparation to fit his mode of instruction. This comprehension was acquired through the process of learned experience which is a mechanism that I simply didn't have all that long ago, for the neurologic passages needed to store and obtain information were just too tattered in my brain to connect or execute any thought processes. But things were working just fine now, thank you.

Bustin' my tail all semester and taping each lecture with Mr. Dawson's permission again, I went into the final knowing the worst possible grade I could get in this "Growth of the American Nation Since 1865" class would be a "B," with a shot at getting an "A", if I aced the final. Knowing what was at stake, I pulled off one of those frenzied, finals' week studying marathons in the Medical Center library where—unless one of the many fine-looking West Virginia "snapper" nursing students walked by—I didn't take my eyes off my impeccable notes until the number of hours I had been studying had reached double digits.

As the clock was winding down, I sat in the empty Woodburn Hall classroom making my left hand write facts as quickly as it possibly could. I wasn't quite done writing down the knowledge that was in my head on this final when the instructor asked me how far along I was before I'd be finished, for everyone else in class wrapped things up awhile ago. Knowing that my injury has left me incapable of writing fast, when I told Mr. Dawson I still had some more to write, he said he'd give me "ten more minutes" which was all I'd need, anyhow.

With time running out, sensing an urgent need to use the restroom, I wrote sentence after sentence containing detail after detail in this essay portion of the final as fast as one possibly can with a hand not programmed to do this. When I eventually finished, I appreciated this older grad student giving me the added time I needed to write the answers.

I can understand the position Mr. Dawson was in. On one hand, because I was physically unable to get my "smarts" written on paper in the same amount of time healthy students can, he didn't want to intellectually penalize me by giving me a grade which didn't correspond with my knowledge or preparation. On the other, I could empathize with my history academician, if he was feeling a little uneasy giving me what he might have perceived as an unfair advantage with "bonus" time to complete this exam. The Rehabilitation Act of 1973 attempts to level out the playing field for people with disabilities by mandating that those physically compromised get every opportunity and the same chance that those who aren't have.

My diligent effort, episodic memory, and not being afraid to speak up for myself all paid off, for I almost got a perfect score on my final, as I got my first "A" in an academic course at W.V.U. for a semester. "Let's go-oooo, Mountaineers!"

Adopting this intangible was not easy, but I had to if I wanted to survive emotionally and do my job focusing on my studies these past nine months in Morgantown. Maybe not to the extreme of a lot of my peers, but like many other nineteen-year olds, I'm somewhat self-conscious of the image I portray. Having been someone who didn't really want to stick out before and grab much in the way of attention, the stares I received were not welcome nor unexpected, so I just tried to go about my own business without getting in anybody's way or let the looks bother me too much. But because I'm not exactly typical now with the way I move, I sometimes felt I was grabbing the headlines with big, black, bold-face type. By the time the fall semester concluded, however, I found out I could put these concerns aside.

Like with some classes where writing speed is an essential variable for getting a good grade, unless it was absolutely necessary for me to divulge that I was in a car accident which left me permanently compromised, I usually didn't say anything about what I've been through or how severely I had been hurt to anyone. Although this accident and the resulting symptoms have been central in my life since February 1982, I was happy to discover that other students I interacted with could see beyond my tragedy/afflictions and realize that there's more to me than being an ex-rehab patient. I was accepted as a college peer by my fellow Mountaineers—but at first—it was kind of difficult to view myself in this light, for I was always conscious of my physical unhealthiness and how different I had become because of this. Actually, I was my own worst enemy, for I was far too critical of myself again, as the large majority of students who I became friends with were positively astounded when I told them how critically I had been injured. Because of the distinctive way that I move, they figured I had done something to my leg, but had no idea that I was once cognitively "off."

With my new major and living arrangement, I met quite a few new people this year and developed an abundance of healthy relationships. Relying solely on my personality without having to explain myself for the peculiarities I have, it was evident that I had placed too much emphasis on my liabilities and didn't give myself enough credit for my strengths, as my ability to form solid interpersonal ties would indicate.

Twenty-four hours with a college student who once had a brain injury can be very much different than the norm, to say the least. Once I wake up in the morning, my schedule deviates from that of most of my other W.V.U. brethren because I start the day off by taking my anti-convulsant, Phenobarbital, so I don't have a seizure somewhere on the campus or in a classroom with a mess of horrified students.

Then I put one of these tiny little white pills in my afternoon vial and one in the evening bottle, so I can remember if I took them or not at their designated time. Because I'll more than likely be in class during the middle of the day and won't be able to get back to Pierpont House, I'll stick my afternoon sedative container in the small zippered compartment of my backpack and nonchalantly swallow my mid-day brain calmer between classes when no one is around. If there's no water fountain handy when "med time" hits, that's no big deal because I've had lots of practice taking these long-acting barbituric acid compounds the past two years without any liquid.

Taking Dilantin for a year, I lost an excessive amount of hair and it caused my face to erupt with horrible acne. In addition, this medication induced inflammation to develop around each of my toenails—so in February 1983—searching for a treatment which would have less side-effects, I switched to Phenobarbital

(30 mg, TID). However, before this change was to take place with my medication, the electrical potentials of my brain had to be recorded first.

My hair was slopped up with white cream and electrodes were glued to my scalp with tape. I was then told to close my eyes because a bright, flashing, strobe light was going to be flickering off and on a little over my head. With my scars and rigid walk, sitting there with my greased hair ready to have my brain waves amplified, I not only looked like Frankenstein's monster, but I felt like he must have waiting for the mad doctor to begin his cutting. Before I left for the hospital, I took a sedative at home that the doctor's office instructed mom to get. However, it's effectiveness got mixed reviews.

If this "soother" pill I took was to relieve any anxiety or calm my nerves about taking this Electroencephalogram (EEG), it didn't appear to be working real well because it seemed I was on red alert the whole time I was being jolted. However, this pacifier must have been able to relax the electrical impulses in my brain somewhat before they got traced, for the results of this 12/15/82 recording would work so well in my favor that by 1/9/83, I would start being weaned from Dilantin (100 mg/TID).

On 2/9/83, I stopped taking this medication which has been a major contributor towards me never having a seizure and, by this date with no interruptions, started the Phenobarbital which I can only hope will be as effective as its predecessor preventing a convulsion. I don't think I have anything to worry about though because this prophylactic dosage of Phenobarb appears to be a good calmative agent for—most everyday after class—I need to take at least one two-hour nap. Because I have to get such an inordinate amount of sleep every twenty-four hours on top of my eight hours every night, twelve-class credits is a trying workload for me.

After my alarm went off in the morning, my working memory—which allowed this tired soul to keep several things in mind at once—enabled me to zip through my routine easily. Because it took me a little longer to get moving physically, I helped myself with this sunrise rush by preparing a little of what I'd need for class the night before. Pens, pencils, highlighter, and an umbrella were always in my backpack and—depending on what day it was—my various class notebooks and tape recorder were always in the same drawer for my access to include with these other items, if I needed them. Like the acrostics mnemonics technique I often used for exams, when someone has had their head banged around, every little trick can be the difference between triumph and failure.

Living in a room on the second floor at Pierpont House with Kevin and two other guys, I fortunately only had one flight of stairs to tackle when I went to and came from class. Grateful for this convenience, I think I would have made Jan and Mary proud, if they knew I didn't take the easy way out and boarded the elevator a couple of times a day.

Going up or down these steps as well as those in the Towers, PRT stations, and the multitudes at the Beechurst campus where my classes were, I appeared kind of strange because I had to look down at where I was going, if I wanted to get there in one piece. I had to have a visual cue when I'd be climbing or going down stairs because of my brain's defective ability to sense how I was positioned. Also, because my tight right heel cord caused me to flop on each step, people would take notice of my right lower extremities, as I would be hiking my way up. Because I had to be so careful and meticulous, I moved in slow motion. Since I needed a left rail to hang onto, I was usually against the flow of traffic.

I would step aside on a landing when it was safe, so the students unfortunate enough to get behind me or ran into me head-on could get to their class without my holding them up. As luck would have it, my Psych classes were on the second and third floors of Oglebay Hall which is a building built on a very high elevation. Because I had to scale up over one-hundred steps from the PRT station alone before I'd get to my final destination, needing this head start in order to keep from lagging behind students whose bodies worked for them, I would habitually give myself about fifteen minutes more in the morning to get to class.

Flapping my foot down as I approached a car on the PRT station, I got looked at by everyone around, but it wasn't anything I could help, so I just went about doing my thing. Getting off the shuttle at the Beechurst station, I would exit the transit car after everyone else filed out because I didn't want to be an obstacle or a detour for them, as I laboriously lowered myself down steps.

After I eventually got down about four or five steps of the many that I'd need to descend, however, another car filled with students anxious to get to class would pull up to the station. Heading down as fast as my hemiparesis would allow me, I hoped that I wouldn't get flocked by any maniacs who had the potential of running into me, causing me to lose my balance and take a plunge. If I'd survive the first phase of this step-dropping expedition —finally making my descent—heavy-footed, I noisily plopped away climbing up the infinite number of cement steps to wherever I needed to go. Often, I'd clumsily bang my way towards Woodburn Circle then Oglebay Hall, before clanging away on the iron steps of this Psych building.

Able to see that I was physically having some problems, there were a few instances where students would just sort of covertly make themselves available just in case I'd need a hand with something or run into some difficulties. Like when I'd be going up or down steps, not realizing that they were putting their life in a pair of spastic hands, these Mountaineers would occasionally step aside allowing me to pass and just kind of shadow me. Because I slid my right foot on top of each step and didn't look real smooth, these students possibly figured that I was going down and their services would be needed to break a fall. I suppose a few of the more safety-conscious variety got out of the way too, but moved over because they feared I was about to do a cartwheel in reverse on the steps and didn't want me taking them for the ride.

For those who kind of hung around preparing to serve as a buffer between me and the hard steps in case I'd bite the dust, this courtesy always felt nice, but still,

I'd just as soon not be noticed. Hardheaded, the vast majority of the time, I preferred to do stuff on my own because I didn't want people to think—just because I was not the most graceful thing on this planet—that I was needy and couldn't manage. I took great pride in how hard I busted my ass to reach this level of competency after what happened to me and would do for myself everything everybody else does, even if not receiving assistance means that it would take a little longer. Stubborn as a mule, I liked to perceive myself as no different than anybody else. And, for the most part, this was how I was seen by others.

Infrequently, maybe because they felt a little bad for me, a few students would go as far as to ask me if I needed any help which is a question I always seemed to say, "No," to. More times than not, however, students would fly past me and zip up the steps without paying me any mind. After their curiosity was quenched the first time they saw me and the initial stares were out of the way, people wouldn't pay any attention to me. They were usually too busy with their own agenda than to be concerned about what I was doing or presented myself, which was just fine with me and what I wanted because this was something I'd always strived for. When this happens, I felt fabulous because this told me that I had achieved the goal I always desired which was that I wasn't all that different than most other students. The work I had to agonize over in my rehabilitation to reach this level of functioning was an effort that will benefit me throughout college and beyond.

I still limped and looked awkward writing with the hand that's not used to doing this, but if this was all that really stuck out after suffering a disability where attaining any kind of normalcy is not generally the rule, then I think I did okay. However, because of my limitations, I don't think it was all that out of the ordinary to have thoughts of myself as an "Oddball" now and again. And I couldn't have blamed my fellow Mountaineers whom I told I was hurt badly or who had seen me waddling around campus, if they had thought I were unusual and something to stay away from. But for the most part, I could sense a kind of sympathy for me, then a little admiration for what I've done and—because of this—a willingness to understand. I didn't need or look for this treatment necessarily, but I guess this just went with being different on a campus of conformity. I tried not to let these differences influence my interactions with other students or interfere with my happiness, but sometimes it was just so damned hard.

Remembering how I was once physically healthy on this campus to being disabled—early on—it was difficult assuming a positive attitude about things. Being a student with a disability, I later learned as the year wore on to "shake off" as many unpleasant circumstances as I could because many of these "goings on" were something that I simply didn't have any control over and couldn't do anything about. I just had to accept that uncomfortable events will occur when you're not the same as everybody else. Not being like most others physically, I came to realize it goes with the turf that displeasing instances are going to happen and to make the best of it. Over the course of that first school year—looking back on it—

incidents which I initially had difficulty handling were beneficial, if not essential, in accepting myself as someone who is unlike most others.

Hanging onto the pole that people who are standing clutch a hold of, so they don't get knocked over when the car hits a bump, I was on a crowded PRT going to class one day when some bearded dude who looked like a frontiersman from somewhere along the Appalachian Trail twanged at some freshman kid who was sitting in one of the eight seats to, "Get up and let that cripple sit down!"

Sensing about a dozen pairs of eyes burning into me, I concealed how upset and embarrassed I felt, as I assured the guy sitting down that I was fine and not to move. I've never been the type of person who is into semantics all that much and I know "Jed Clampett" was just trying to help, not meaning any harm by what he said, but it was still unnerving for me to know that others could see I have some difficulties when I like to think people don't make any comments about my dissimilarities because they don't notice them.

Feeling defamed at that moment, I didn't take too kindly to being labeled with such a derogatory word that has been out of circulation for quite some time because of its denigrating connotation. However, figuring "Sasquatch" just got down from the hills down yonder and this was his first glimpse of civilization in a while, I tried to let his comment slide the best I could—but it wasn't easy.

Another instance, shortly after I returned to Morgantown, I was walking from class to the PRT station when some guy who I never saw before in my life came up to me and asked if I had a stroke. Disgusted that someone I didn't even know could tell that I had something happen to my neurologic system, not saying a word, I just shook my head "no" and kept on walking. Possibly, to preserve my denial that it's not obvious I have a physical disability that is noticeable, I immediately came to the conclusion that this fellow Mountaineer was a physical therapy student and wanted to check the accuracy of his trained observation.

Maybe it was a little ignorant of a total stranger to ask me about something as personal as my health, but I don't have control of other peoples' etiquette or lack of, so I can't let it get to me, if I want to proceed in a healthy fashion emotionally. What I can do and have control over is how sensitive I allow myself to be to the spoken word. If this young man actually was in the Physical Therapy program, maybe I should have demonstrated for him the difference between how someone with a head injury walks, as opposed to someone who has sustained a CVA. I know, I've seen enough of both.

How we look at things is so important. And if I have to view myself as "special" or "unique"—instead of "strange" or "peculiar" to get over life's bumps—then I'm just going to try my best to get through things and not be so hard on myself, because what I've got is a whole lot considering how things could have—if not should have—turned out for me. It's only human nature to feel a little uneasy about being recognized for any flaws or liabilities one may have, but with practice and the "knocks" life can give us, I found out that a person can kind of get immune to things in time.

If one has a disability, it looks like the sooner a person with an affliction can develop a shell deflecting what might be said or done, the better off they'll be. Unfortunately, I didn't have the opportunity to put my shield down just because I was back at the apartment. I guess—in a way—this was a blessing in disguise, though, because this semester was a crucial time for me where I needed to concentrate on my work and not be concerned with extracurriculars, until I got clearance.

Unlike when I was an idiotic freshman the first time around and tried to be "Mr. Socialite," I almost never went out this past '83-'84 school year. I had a good many nice acquaintances here in Morgantown whom I met during the year, but not really anybody I could go out with and have a good time. My one West Virginia roommate I got along with went home every weekend to see his sweetheart and Kevin left for Washington to be with his sister once he got home from class on Friday, so that left me with the engineering major I shared the room with who I didn't "hit it off" with real well on those occasions when W.V.U. would be my weekend haven. Friday and Saturday night would come along and I'd just be sitting at my desk in my room either studying or listening to the stereo with my headphones, despite maybe wanting to check out the night life on campus a little bit, for I had forgotten what this was like.

Socially isolated almost from the very beginning, this was definitely a very depressing time for me and a situation I came to abhor, but couldn't do much about. The college environment—and at W.V.U. especially—it's almost expected that when someone is out socially, that they have a drink in hand that they're working on. However, in my case, this was taboo because I was unsure how alcohol—no matter how little—and Phenobarbital would mix. I wasn't about to chance finding out, so I just kind of stuck to myself, not doing anything. Someone could have offered me a million dollars to get toasted and I wouldn't have taken this money because I was scared to death how my brain would react to even a tiny sip of beer. Despite the grueling feelings of exclusion, I suppose—overall—this was a relatively small price to pay in order to get on track academically.

There were supposedly some really good rock 'n roll bands playing at different bars in Sunnyside that I would have liked to see, but I'd feel out of place hammering on a carbonated water club soda when everyone else was kicking back. Going to a club and possibly meeting some pretty girls would have been nice, but I don't walk too well let alone dance, so that idea was out. There were an abundance of parties somewhere every weekend at Pierpont House, but I never went to any. If I could drive and had a car during the school year, I might have wanted to take a look around at Cheat Lake or Coopers Rock for the first time, but since I don't, that's not going to happen.

Being a good friend, "Boss" transferred back home to Washington and Jefferson before the school year started and didn't bother telling his "buddy" he shared the apartment with last year—Kevin—of his plans. Fully expecting more good times partying with the "Bossman" this year, my roommate was "down in the mouth" and shell-shocked that his social schedule was going to transform from an all-out blitz to one of non-alcoholic activity with me, so Kevin didn't really bother. Being a "stickin-the-mud" and abstaining from life is a woeful situation to be in, but I wasn't going to chance having some sort of setback after all the garbage I've had to wade through just to get here. One day after I got off a PRT car, my path would cross with the guy who created this whole mess for me.

I know when I saw him this past summer, he didn't get the right message. My waving that hot day when he was in the passing car, I can only assume that—because he comes from a family with some money—he believes the rules of etiquette which apply to everybody else are different for him and he could greet the person he left comatose, as if nothing was ever wrong with this. Operating from this high-society status, Paul might have been thinking that I wouldn't have any reason to hold anything against him after all this time, which possibly is why he fashionably raised his hand high and called out, "Craig!," one day when he saw me stepping out of a car at the Towers' PRT station.

Waiting to catch a ride heading in the opposite direction—hand still high over his head—Paul yelled out my name again and I just kept on limping towards the steps, ignoring his gesture. If acknowledging me wasn't his affluent character coming out, maybe because he sensed my reaction towards him this past summer at the W and J campus was due to being caught off-guard and not an authentic response, possibly Paul wanted to see what my opinion was of him exactly. Or, it could be—as I've heard through the grapevine these past two years—Paul has now reformed after what he did to a friend and needed the opportunity to personally express his regrets to me. However, knowing him like I do now, almost killing someone isn't enough of a catalyst for Paul to alter his lifestyle.

In Hollywood, in preparation for such an encounter, the good guy always seems to somehow righteously "even the score" when this moment presents itself. Because there's a chance I would have my day in court with Paul and/or his worldly parents in the not too distant future, my day of reckoning may not be too far off, and I don't want to do or say anything which may keep me from getting my pound of flesh. Besides, I'm not Clint Eastwood.

I couldn't have known it at the time obviously, but this turned out to be an omen for me as to how I would do academically and socially the remainder of my days as a Mountaineer undergrad. The first class I took in the summer session '84 at W and J proved to be further evidence of how I've matured since my brain was spun around in my skull. The two years I took French in high school, the average grade I received was a "C" because—like my pre-head injury days at W.V.U.—I didn't take academics seriously.

Being introduced to this foreign language in senior high helped, as I would be wrestling with this subject throughout college. But I would have never guessed I would have it in me to make an "A-" in an intensive college course covering a subject that I used to joke about and couldn't have taken any more lightly. But armed with my new outlook on life and heightened discretion, that's precisely what I did during my first summer session French I course at W and J. As fate would have it, this grade would be an approximate indicator of how I would do academically the remainder of my days at W.V.U. However, this wasn't the only premonitory sign this class provided me with.

In this summer course of about ten students, as I have a habit of doing, I sat next to the prettiest girl in class and talked to this extremely nice President quite a bit everyday. With a personality and friendliness to match her looks, I became a personable acquaintance of this young lady who just finished her freshman year at Washington and Jefferson. A short time after I got to know this diamond in the rough, this madamoiselle won the Miss Teen Pennsylvania pageant.

Intelligent to boot, before I was hurt, Julie was the type of girl whom I would have avoided at all costs because I just didn't have a healthy opinion of myself. But the bold-spirited efforts I have made in my rehab and the subsequent accomplishments achieved because of this hard work have gone a long way towards opening my eyes as to who I really am and how I look at things.

Although the French II class I took the second summer session at W and J didn't have a beauty queen in it, I still had the incentive to do well because these two introductory classes to this romantic language would serve as building blocks for when I took French III and IV at W.V.U. next year. With my "awakening" as to what I stand for in place and knowing that the only thing between me and a respectable grade in any of my pursuits is the amount of effort I expend, I went all-out to get a good mark in this second phase of my college French education and promptly earned a "B+." Un, deux, trois, quatre, cinq,—sept?

Not only academically, but the experiences I had interpersonally, my second year back at W.V.U. was of premium value for me. In the Fall semester '84-'85, I finally got a 3.0 grade point average and I was off, off, and away from there. It was during the Spring semester '84-'85—with wheels at my disposal for the only time in my life—I went on my first date ever with a girl from Charleston, W.Va. who I met on campus. On this initial February 15th, 1985 courting experience at the not-so-tender age of twenty-one, I learned a valuable lesson. XOXOXOXOXOXOXOXO.

Our date started off really well. During dinner, we talked about school, our aspirations being that we were both Psych majors, our hobbies, stuff we're good at, what our hometown was like, etc. From what I understood, safe topics that people on first dates discuss. Momentarily, we hit a little turbulence when the topic of how our way of pronouncing words differ, but I was able to make the neurons in my bruised brain work for me, so that I could find a way to divert her attention away from this subject to something else pretty quickly. Letting my light-heartedness shine through, things started to pick up nicely again, however.

Experiencing a pleasurable sense of conformity, sitting at our table, talking and getting along really well, our date hit a deep pothole when my courting partner informed me—after choking down the steak dinner I bought her with no problem—that I was to pick up her female "bodyguard" friend for the rest of our rendezvous. My excitement having drastically plummeted, in a desperate attempt to change the flow this outing was headed, I thought it would be a good time to tell my new lady friend about my courageous recovery and heroic efforts in rehab after being in a coma, and figured she'd be all over me. Unfortunately for this fool who totally misjudged her reaction, the only thing that would be crawling on my date this night would be her skin.

Stunned, when I opened my big mouth and told my horrified date how messed up I had become three years ago almost to the day, her eyes got as big as a full moon and her jaws dropped to her shaking knees. Sporting a look of terror, with the date taking a nose-dive to the point of "Never again" for her, I could almost see the fun drain out of her. Rock bottom is where her mood hit and, despite her not saying anything to this effect, I could sense she wanted to go home and felt a little eerie after I told her what happened to me. When I flapped my jaws one too many times informing this Dixie Queen of my experience being a one-time critically injured patient, I could just imagine scenes of the low-budget horror film, "Night of the Living Dead," flashing in her mind with me playing one of the ghouls.

Having an escort who was probably packing a can of mace or two in her purse didn't turn out to be so bad, after all, because it seemed the southern cutie I was with appeared more at ease and able to cut loose a little better. Able to be ourselves and relax more easily, me, my date, and the security attendant were off to Pierpont House where the guys across the hall (Stouffer, Schneeweis, and Co.) were having a little powwow. Sitting in the corner of my floormates' apartment, after getting my neighbors to occupy the sentinel, my date and I had a nice time again chatting about nothing in particular.

Taking my evening companion back home, after her chaperon got out of my car, my date swallowed my face and gave me an absolutely fantastic kiss I'd never forget. Except for the disclosure blunder, because the night was an overall success, I was thinking that this pretty young woman who I had spent the past six hours or so with might like to do something during the week like lunch at the student center Mountainlair. Before she got out of my car when I asked her this, my West Virginia state capital "sweet patootie" told me to give her a call later in the week when she'd have a better idea of her schedule.

Busy signal, no answer. Busy signal, no answer. Busy signal, no answer. When I didn't get a call back and couldn't get through to this good-looking Mountaineer several days after our get-together, not having any experience with this dating game nor socially gifted with the ladies yet, I foolishly went to her apartment with the hope of getting another date set up. Not realizing she likely rinsed her mouth out with rubbing alcohol after she sucked on my face, I was in for some pain.

Not looking real thrilled when she came to the door and saw me, before I could open my mouth to ask her if another gathering would be out of the question—in an apologetic tone—my first dating experience told me she had a boyfriend back home and can't go out with me ever again. Crushed, I shouldn't have expected anything other than this, because February just isn't my month.

Assuming that members of society who are not well-versed with brain trauma will be as impressed with my accomplishments as those who are, I spoiled the potential opportunity to have a new friend. To be appropriate, I need to learn which situations will be conducive with divulging my past traumatized condition—for these instances will occur—and those that aren't. In order to be viewed as interesting, I need to continue enhancing my understanding that I have to give myself more credit for being a unique individual with my share of attributes/qualities and not someone who has to rely on telling people about my recovery from a tragedy.

Although that pretty girl I hung out with that cold, February evening was three years older than me chronologically—despite seeming to be relatively mature for her twenty-four years—her mental age probably was not prepared or equipped to handle such gore from someone she barely knew on a first date—if ever. I need to pick and choose who gets this information, what situations warrant this disclosure, where would be the most appropriate settings to reveal my background, and when would be the most beneficial time to tell my story. Maybe it's best I just keep my mouth shut because if I'm not selective, I could be in for a longer haul than it needs to be and miss chances that do not have to be foregone. But still. . . . .

The '84-'85 term was spectacular and for the first time in my life I was sorry to see a school year end. After I got the stigma of being dateless out of the way, I was literally on my way to exciting "territory" from here on out, as I took this courting experience to the next level later in the Spring semester. The friendly, lewd, outgoing guys across the hall came along just at the right time for me after last year's social withdrawal.

Before this college session began—noting how "down and out" I had become following my initial school year back where I had the social life of a monk—after asking him of the potential dangers an occasional brew would have on my neurologic system, my neurosurgeon said something to the effect that mixing Phenobarbital with any kind of alcoholic beverage wasn't advisable, but that it's probably unlikely a beer or two on the weekends would hurt me. Not out of the monastery yet, Dr. Prostko cautioned me that the more alcohol I put in my body, the greater likelihood that battered brain of mine has of suffering a seizure/convulsion or some other setback.

Accentuating the importance of moderation not excess, this brain surgeon who has helped me get so far and didn't want to see anything happen to me that could have been prevented, made sure to point out that there's a possibility if I would have a seizure on both sides of my brain simultaneously, I could have a stroke and be back where I started. I didn't have all this in mind when I decided to forego some of my more provincial and mellow friends who liked to abide by the status quo, for the more electric variety. If this is what results, I'll take "boredom" over "energy" any day.

Having devoted these past four years and four months of his life seeing that I had everything needed to reach this summit—in six more months—dad would have been the happiest and proudest person walking on earth, for this would be the time when his dream would be realized and I would get my Bachelor's Degree "against all odds." When times would get tough, and there would be more than a few, dad was there to give me the encouragement and backing necessary to pull through and come out on top. Needing affirmation of purpose and abetment during those occasions when I'd be scraping bottom over what my scarred mind no longer allowed me to do, my #1 booster put his needs second to mine and somehow had a way of making seemingly insurmountable heights a goal that I believed could be touched.

This man who asked for so little, sacrificed what he did possess, so I would have an opportunity at life. Suffering a catastrophic injury where only the lucky and fortunate have a shot at any meaningful existence, virtually no one familiar with my condition gave me much of a chance of graduating from college—except dad. Born in 1919, in one-half of a year, this consecrated advocate was about to be "throned in highest bliss" and bask in a harmony he could have never imagined in all his years. But this wasn't to happen, for on the 165th day of 1986—June 14th—dad died.

On April 3, 1986, mom and dad went to the Citizens' Library in Washington where one of the three Allegheny General Hospital cancer doctor associates who were treating dad was speaking. Not assigned to care for dad directly—therefore having no idea who he was—when dad asked this surgeon the specifics of oat cell cancer, not mincing words or realizing the impact of what he was about to say would have on the two Meyers' members in attendance, the physician lecturer happened to tell his audience that the specific type of lung cancer dad asked about—and was believed to have—has a minimal success rate with chemotherapy or any other kind of treatment and that life expectancy after the onset of this malignant growth is short. Realizing the tumor he likely had in his body was fatal, dad looked at mom and said, "Well, I guess I'm not long for this world."

For two-and-a-half more months, dad had to regularly ingest antibiotics, painkillers, and stomach medicines. From the time he experienced chest pains in January until April 18th—the day he found out he definitely had this terminal type of cancer—dad was subjected to literal misery suffering through several diagnostic tests. Having bone marrow sucked out of his hip and diseased tissue snipped out of his lungs, dad was practically tortured until doctors knew what had him.

Because I needed to take one final Psych core class before I graduated in December, I had to attend school at W.V.U. this first summer session 1986. Resting in his rocking chair which was off-limits to others when dad needed somewhere to sit, heading for the front door preparing to leave for Morgantown on the Sunday evening of June 1st, I walked over to my now frail dad and shook his hand.

Even then, when he knew his last breath was near, dad was concerned with the grip of my paralytic hand, as he insisted that I squeeze his hand tight.

Looking like a totally different person because he had lost about fifty pounds the past six weeks or so, I then put my head on dad's chest and told him that I loved him for the first time in my twenty-two years. Sensing the misery which had absorbed me—overcome with his own mixed emotions of affection and grief—forever trying to make things easier for his kids, dad tried to rid me of as much of my taunting conscience as possible for not telling him this earlier when he said in his weakened voice, "I know you do, son."

Bawling like a baby that dad was about to meet his death soon and the sun which had been his brilliance was setting, I only wished that I would have had the courage to tell dad what I thought about him when he could have really savored it. Sitting at the dining room table, tears filled mom's eyes as she witnessed this rare glimpse of emotion. No longer clinging to a hope that wasn't there, not a dry eye in the house, each of us realized that dad as we knew him was gone once his disease metastasized and reached the point where he needed to start morphine. Starting off in his lungs before invading his liver and every other organism in his body, cancer cells were rapidly overtaking dad, as his punished body was deteriorating daily.

Driving down Route 79 South, battling tears which I thought were forever dormant, I felt so selfish and shameful because if I hadn't been in that car accident, dad's time wouldn't be up. Like any father-son relationship, I did not agree with some of the things dad did or didn't do, but these pale in comparison to the infinite number of outstanding moves he did make. Things like driving a car/going out once in a while and his, "Because I said so" parenting style seem so minor and unimportant now. Dedicating his life these past couple of years since I've been hurt ensuring that a future not slip from my grasp, dad showed me what real love was.

I know that stress doesn't cause cancer cells to form, but I do realize that tension can aggravate these tiny, little bastards, leading them to spread and develop quicker than they normally would. Possibly in remission for years, I feel an incredible guilt that dad worrying and obsessing over me caused his bronchogenic carcinoma to multiply and infiltrate other areas of his body. There's not a strain more gripping for a parent than to experience the death of a child and the violent way I almost mortally exited this earth had to have awakened these death cells in dad. Living with this logic is going to be hell.

This may be a form of not wanting to accept something so catastrophic as losing a parent and feeling responsible, but when there was the slightest of chances that dad would beat this thing—to deal with the agonizing reality that the loudest rooter in my cheering section wasn't invincible and won't be around for the majority of my life—I tried to carry on as normal a routine as I could. Thinking if I don't recognize, focus on, or pay attention to dad's illness, it will somehow just go away. Hanging on to what I could, I would keep thinking that dad can't leave me because I still want him around to experience any successes I may have as a developing adult in the future and, although I could never do this fully, to pay him back at least some as he gets older for what he's done for me being my father.

Despite having quit seven years ago after retiring from his demanding job, the abuse dad's body took from years of cigarette and pipe smoking was just too much. Never feeling so alone in my life, stunned from the massive void this loss has left me with to bear, I continued the best I could at school because I knew that this was something I had to do being on the home stretch of my undergraduate days at W.V.U. and was something dad would want. Twelve years older than me, I made friends with this one fellow Psych major who was in some of my classes during the spring semester 1986 when dad was dying, and George helped me deal with some of the grief that I was experiencing being away from home, by just listening to me howl during those constant times when things got to me.

So I don't carry the burden of his demise to the grave with me, I'll try to tell myself that dad put nicotine poison in his body since he was fifteen-years-old, or twenty-eight years BEFORE I was even born. But the tears aren't likely to ever stop flowing completely until I come to my end. Goodbye buddy, words alone can't tell you how much I am going to miss you or how sorry I am. I love you.

Wanting to make a positive out of a negative so that I don't live a life of "What ifs?," lost opportunities, and regrets, I thought I'd apply for a Master's program which would allow me to integrate my rare and potentially invaluable life experience with disability into a career benefiting others in similar crisis situations. I believe people should use whatever gift they have received from God to serve others and it's important for me to use the offering of life, strength, and experience that I possess to benefit those who don't have such fortune.

According to the "experts," after one has had a severe head injury, their capability to develop intellectually will always be limited and their options—as far as what they can achieve—are also going to be restricted. Maybe if a few people like myself pop out of the woodwork who have shown that certain accomplishments can be attained by someone who has had a severe brain injury not before believed possible, this will revise some of the adverse opinions and discrimination towards this population where the facts are scarcely known. Unfortunately, it looks like these "experts" are the ones I'm going to have to rely on to get a mutually beneficial job in rehabilitation one of these days. I'm really looking forward to facing this gauntlet of prejudice.

Sick and tired of hearing that I won't be able to do this and won't be able to do that because it's unheard of that a former patient with a history of severe brain damage reaches certain heights, "against all odds," I applied for, and got accepted into W.V.U.'s accredited Rehabilitation Counseling graduate program. On an altruistic level, I want to gain some of the training, knowledge, and experience necessary in order to develop into an astute professional who not only will be able to provide clients with the textbook counselor traits required to be adequate, but also appropriately utilize the added quality of being a survivor. This potentially priceless dimension may be able to provide those who are feeling helpless and hopeless with a little extra incentive to work. Possibly, with this additional effort, the patient can gain some precious improvement that will help to ease some of their loved ones' stress.

On a personal level, being a role model and an example for those who suffered an injury where it is often unwritten and not conceded to openly that its members should not try nor won't be able to compete in a world of healthy people, I have a need to do what I can about how some segments of society falsely stereotype all people with histories of brain injuries as one vast inefficient and incompetent group. Perhaps, the best way I could alter some of this silent stigma that all people possessing such backgrounds are doomed to be forever intellectually challenged would be to get my Master's Degree and work professionally counseling patients who have sustained a neurologic impairment and provide quality therapy to their families.

If I can avoid being shoved into a closet with so many other survivors with histories of brain contusions—who are only guilty of making sensitive members of society conscious of their mortality—and work in a rewarding position which provides me with an opportunity to showcase my talents, then I would feel fulfilled and that this whole tragic ordeal would have meaning. But this isn't a storybook fairy tale where "Alice in Wonderland" goes skipping off into the sunset, rather, what's being dealt with here is the reality of society's bias and because of this unfair perception, putting this master plan to work is easier said than done.

It wasn't supposed to be this way, but I'm here. If someone would have told me when I was a fool-headed freshman back in '81 that I'd be attending grad school in pursuit of a Master's Degree, I'd have burst into tears from cracking up so hard. I might have even laughed in their face, if I were told I'd get my Bachelor's. I don't know how my life would have turned out had I not been in that accident, but I do know some good came about because of this tragedy from a personal growth standpoint and this is what I try to focus on, so that I don't become anchored in despair. Clinging onto life in a room full of mattresses has a way of influencing one's way of looking at things.

To be truthful, I believe the makings of something big could take place here for me, if all goes according to plan and I do well in my Rehabilitation Counseling schooling. Not meaning to sound egotistical, but there hasn't been a whole lot of people who've faced what I have had to endure and prevailed so well over this challenge that they could someday vie for a career that is tailor-made for them like Rehabilitation Counseling is for me. I mean, someone going from being a patient with various aphasias to a grad school student doesn't happen everyday. Unfortunately, proceeding as a former comatose patient earning their Master's and being gainfully employed in rehab, will be almost as difficult as being aphasic and getting into graduate school. As I have learned all too well, rarely do things go according to plan when it comes to head injury.

Second to none, this Rehab Counseling Master's program definitely is one of sophistication, dedication, and professionalism which has traditionally produced many top-of-the-line graduates. The cordial atmosphere created by its professors makes the Rehab Counseling endeavor one productive and enjoyable learning experience as well. The distinguished style which these instructors go about teaching their students enables the trainees to handle a wide range of situations. Depending on which track the student elects to specialize in, their coursework will either be geared towards the vocational training/evaluation aspect of rehabilitation or the counseling psychology realm. Because of my background as an undergraduate and desire to engage in psychological therapy with the rehabilitation population, incorporating my personal experience if appropriate, I chose to gain my primary training in the latter facet.

Enhanced and promoted by the Coordinator of Rehabilitation Counselor Education, Robert P. Marinelli, Ed.D., C.R.C., I was encouraged that Dr. Marinelli sounded so optimistic, even enthusiastic that people "WITH" disabilities are becoming increasingly more involved with society as a whole. Stressing that societal attitudes are improving towards those who are experiencing an incapacitating symptom or more—despite no longer seeing myself as disadvantaged because my physical ailments are so slight—I was still excited about the opportunities which lie ahead for me in the workplace because, officially, I fit into this category. However, because it's frequently impossible to discredit beliefs which are generally accepted as fact, I might not have an easy time projecting my competencies.

Being so naive as to think that I could compete on a par with those who haven't been so cognitively traumatized, however, I was given a sour taste of reality "right out of the shoot" which would leave a lasting bitterness in my mouth.

Eloquently, the fluffed tresses bounced vibrantly off her shoulders on Monday. Graced to be protruding from this sorority girl's scalp, the tight, dirty blonde ringlets flickered with a flat glow, as the light of the classroom haloed over her locks one Wednesday afternoon. The day before, trying to exemplify the beauty which she must have believed bestowed her, an alluring feathercut highlighted the swirl feature of her gifted mane. On the last day of this school week—Thursday—a wavy spiralcut flowed alongside the straight, silky bangs dangling about her forehead, charming anyone blessed enough to witness this sanctified offering. The daughter of a doctor who practices physical medicine in West Virginia, this inexperienced student's hair style changed as frequently as a chameleon's skin color.

If she were nicer looking and I still possessed an undergraduate mentality, "Penelope Rich" is the type of girl who might appeal to me. Taking personal offense to this twenty-two year old's questionable test-taking behavior because I know firsthand how important it is that rehabilitation professionals know and understand their craft, now that I'm in grad school and have experienced what quality rehabilitation connoisseurs can accomplish, my view of the significance of school has elevated to a level where I now can understand nothing is more essential to one's growth and development as academics and acquiring the needed skills to be effective. Based on what I had heard from other grad students who witnessed this female social club member's antics during mid-terms and finals, I wasn't alone in my disgust.

During my rehabilitation, if I had been exposed to professionals who took such short-cuts during their tentative years learning their trade, I would have died.

I almost became ill when I saw Penelope conferring with another student repeatedly during exams, but didn't say anything because my sole concern should be my own performance and knew it wasn't in my best interests to "point the finger" at anyone. Not my place to police anyone anyhow, on one occasion, I witnessed one of the program's professors staring at Penelope and her cohort sharing test answers during an exam.

This rehab business is serious stuff which is why I was glad to see the vast majority of the other aspiring human services workers were dedicated to grasping the skills and knowledge necessary to help others. I guess it's possible that Penelope had roving eyes only because she was curious as to how her friend's name was spelled.

However, for practically everyone else, I believe that the grad school experience influenced the other students as it did me. Unaware of what force was behind this exactly, I suppose the maturity that goes with jumping the hurdles that years of being an undergraduate present one and having the importance of responsibility/obligation stressed repeatedly were two of the ingredients which gave grad school a special aura to me. Those teaching the material in this Rehabilitation Counseling course of study had a way of making those in this class feel important and not just a number, which can frequently occur in a university of thousands upon thousands. Spearheaded by Dr. Marinelli's orientation and general overview of the various rehabilitation systems, this program coordinator's affable character went a long way towards providing the department's postgraduates with the encouragement and confidence needed to make this one fruitful discipline to study. And Bob had a quality team of masters surrounding him.

Always stressing the importance of getting to the core of one's troubles, Edward E. Jacobs, Ph.D., demonstrated different approaches and provided the practical experience/supervision which would facilitate this process. Another professional counselor, Robert L. Masson, Ed.D., taught a class covering group counseling theory and techniques. From these two professors, different methods of psychotherapy were presented which would apply to both the general population and those in rehabilitation. Relaying their years of experience working with people who have presented them with problematic situations, through role-play and lecture, these educators shared for the class a notion of what they could encounter in this field.

The Cormiers, a husband and wife doctoral counseling team, went over various theories to a variety of therapy approaches. Hats off to Michael T. Yura Ph.D., for his humorous way of presenting useful information on Psychological Testing and interventions which could work with children. A Sooner, Ranjit K. Majumder, Ph.D., shared with the class his extensive experience with research in rehabilitation. Possessing the same amount of expertise as many doctors, Barb Judy, M.A., taught a class on medical aspects of rehabilitation. And it was during this course which I learned the cherished lesson that all reactions to my personal successes with rehab will not necessarily be one of universal admiration.

As I was seated in the corner of the back row, without saying anything, Barb came up to me and placed her hand on my arm when she came in the classroom.

The day before, knowing it would be appropriate for her class and provide the Rehab Counseling program with a personalized flavor, I gave Barb the video shot of me at Harmarville to review when I was confused/agitated and still in a wheelchair. With the class as her witness just to be sure, before she started the V.C.R., Barb got my verbal permission to run this film showing me in my compromised condition. When I assured her that I was not sensitive to being shown in my "lost" state, the "Play" button was pushed and—in a matter of seconds—a few students may become shocked when they see on the television screen what I've been able to conquer in order to be a participant in this advanced course of study.

Purposefully, I was positioned in the class where I was, so I could see the reactions of my fellow grad students. Eyes glued to the screen, everyone seemed to be listening intently, as they watched me unable to make any understanding of my world. With a few looks of astonishment and maybe a trace of awe, the class viewed how I was a little over four years ago when I wasn't even of preschool mentality. While the video player showed how I was once tortured by a mind submerged with confusion, kicking the footplate of my wheelchair unable to remain still and aggrieved by the daze which controlled me, the glow from the T.V. set depicting how I was in 1982 shimmered off of Penelope's curls which had a vibrance this day that captured the meaning and essence of beauty beyond the realm of human expectation. If a picture is indeed worth a thousand words, biased or not, this moving illustration of me has to be worth at least a million.

After the twelve-minute video was over, overwhelmed, Barb and several of the students told me how amazed they were about how far I've come and what a remarkable recovery I have made. Because of the way I present myself, glistening with a slight touch of wonderment, quite a few of the students commented that they couldn't believe how critical I once was and what I've done to overcome my afflictions. However, not everyone was embraced with marvel.

My fifteen minutes of fame weren't quite up yet when—fueled by the accolades I was receiving—the anger inside this one older student who had a stroke was being turbo-charged to the point where jealousy raged into a cyclone of emotional fury. With hostility blazing from every pore and glaring at me as if I was responsible for her condition, I was surprised when this woman with a pronounced limp whom I always thought I had gotten along with well enough started to growl at me that I was "lucky" I turned out as well as I did. Seeing the chip on this lady's shoulder and my being stunned by this attack, Barb quickly intervened and pacified this single parent until she put away her battle flag.

After initially being astounded, once this emotion wore off and I saw that the class was focused on soothing my upset classmate instead of processing what was just viewed in order to prepare for clientele similar to how I once was, I became mad. I realize I was very fortunate but, in no way, did this person have the right to imply that I had gotten where I'm at only because of some chance occurrence which happened to fall in my favor. By no stretch of the imagination was my recovery a fluke, for I triumphed over this crucible by means of a conscious and unrelenting effort. I was "lucky" in the sense that I had the mental processes to figure out what I had to do to get better, but after that, it was basically all me.

Without realizing I have spent hour after hour, day after day, week after week, month after month, and year after year these past four years working my ass off trying to regain a little bit back of what I had lost—only attributing my restoration to being born under a lucky star—I was starting to boil inside. However, my selflessness allowed the empathy in me to prevail and I could then understand why the favorable attention I was receiving was so unbearable for this divorcee.

I know she must have had to endure excruciating pain, frustration, torment, depression, isolation, anger, shock, bitterness—everything that goes with acquiring a permanent disability—and I can just imagine how it must feel being worthy of some recognition and seeing another getting praised for their victories when the opportunity to champion over their loss is not likely to present itself. Witnessing a person who feels as if they are outside looking in is an experience I will always remember and yet another prized piece of equipment added to my intervention toolbox, as I plow ahead in pursuit of a career working with those experiencing the rigors of rehabilitation. So much for my fifteen minutes of fame.

Visualizing him grinning from ear to ear and a sparkle gleaming from his eye, I could hear dad cheering me on and exclaiming, "Attaboy, buddy!!," after this grad school year ended and I got G.P.A.'s during the fall and spring semesters of 3.80 and 3.81 respectively. With their tails firmly snug between their legs, I wonder what the "experts" have to say now.

With the reading, writing, and test-taking portion of the Rehab Counseling academic year out of the way, it was time to apply what I learned in the classroom to a rehabilitation setting for the next six weeks. This "Practicum" was to take place during W.V.U.'s first summer session and give me a taste of the rehabilitation workplace before deciding where to serve my "Internship" which occurs during the fall semester. After this five-month field practice has been completed, the Rehab Counseling class of '87-'88 can proudly put "M.S." after their names. And those whose history doesn't have a chapter where their awareness and understanding was once depleted, might even be able to land good jobs.

Not realizing the administrative workings of the corporation and assuming—as everyone else had—that this enterprise was what it appeared, Dr. Marinelli heaped the praises of this one particular private-for-profit head injury system which had about forty rehabilitation facilities nationwide. "For profit" organizations traditionally are those that readily have resources at their disposal to handsomely reward its employees and bountifully sustain its operation which—needless to say—make them attractive options to pursue. And nothing promotes a college department more than a high entry-level salary for its graduates, and it appeared this network of rehabilitation centers geared towards those with neurologic impairments would be any college program coordinator's dream, as well as any college student's. However, sometimes things can be too good to be true, for a wolf has been known to be in sheep's clothing.

When Dr. Marinelli described for the class some of the components of this corporate body, such as its utilizing Family Counselors who engage in rehabilitation psychology with patients and their loved ones—as well as the variety of services it has to offer—I couldn't wait to hear more about this company because this operation sounds like it would be the absolute perfect mutually beneficial fit and what I want to do in my career. I almost lost my trademark composure when told this company has a treatment program only about ten miles from my house, because then, I wouldn't have to be uprooted from home away from my recently widowed mother and pay rent somewhere while I was serving my field placement.

Locally referred to as Meadowlands Health Care Center and located to the left of and adjacent to Canonsburg Hospital on Route 519 South in Houston, Pa., I quickly realized that I had been there two or three times before with mom because this was where monthly support group meetings were held for head injury survivors and their families. However, I had absolutely no idea that it was run by such a reputable, trust-worthy, genuine, conscientious, committed, ethical, and moral establishment as—New Medico.

This was the clincher. On top of the glorified accounts I had heard of the organization in grad school, when I read several brochures on New Medico and saw the different contemporary programs it offered at a variety of appealing locations across the country, I was salivating. When I flipped through the pages seeing directors, administrators, and other executives with their gel-coated hair neatly parted to the side clad in expensive suits and beaming brightly with cheery smiles, I figured that if a rehabilitation company has management running it who look like they should be granted sainthood, then this group of seemingly empathetic professionals is something I want to be a part of. With the intent of pulling the wool over the reader's eyes, this was a situation where things were not as they appeared.

I decided that New Medico Rehabilitation and Skilled Nursing Center at Meadowlands was the place for me, not only because of the various demographic factors which would make this a productive scholastic investment, but also because much of the program's philosophy appeared to be in line with what patients need to regain as much of their premorbid functioning as possible. Having already secured a field placement site at Harmarville, I didn't feel much in the way of pressure when I was driving to the interview with the Program Director of New Medico's neurologic center at Meadowlands, Charles Goyette, Ph.D. However, being that I was warned that Goyette has a "standoffish personality" before I started my practicum site search, I knew that I had better be prepared, if I was to have any kind of shot at practicing at this facility which would enable me to benefit from the comforts of home while I still had to report back to W.V.U. periodically. With the intent of convincing The Man responsible for putting into action the New Medico Corporation's instructions on how to go about caring for patients at Meadowlands that I was worthy of volunteering my skills at the rehab center He reigned over—along with the rehearsed rhetoric I was going to impress Goyette with—I brought one of the pictures of me when I was comatose, so that I could provide a visual idea of my unique credentials and qualifications.

Pulling off of I-79 North at Exit 9, Houston/Eighty-Four, as I made the right on the way to the center for my practicum audition, I was feeling pretty good about my chances of getting approval to serve my practicum at New Medico at Meadowlands. First, because this patient population can ideally benefit from someone with my background. Secondly, after I demonstrated my effectiveness and because I live in such close proximity to the facility, I'd be viewed as a viable candidate not only to grant a temporary learning position to, but invest in a long-term commitment. Last—but as it will turn out—not least, I wasn't going to insist on being monetarily reimbursed for my work while I was acquiring the knowledge to operate within the system. Unfortunately, because of New Medico's primary agenda, this lack of insistence had as much to do with the way things turned out, as any rewards my academic or personal experience would have.

Being the Program Director, Goyette was the "head honcho" at Meadowlands who implemented the New Medico Corporation's directives, but I wasn't the least bit nervous about my interview with him. I was feeling pretty confident about my prospects of being able to attain an academic position here because I had the way I wanted to present myself fairly well outlined in my mind and would give a fine representation of what I was all about. When things didn't start out with any professional dignity, there was no way I could have known this lack of respect and honor was a sign of things to come, and the foundation for the New Medico Corporation.

When I spoke with the secretary at the front desk of the rehab center, telling her I had scheduled an appointment with the good doctor, I was told Goyette can't afford any time for me and that I'm to speak with the third in the chain of command, Administrator James O'Shea. Sitting in O'Shea's office, after pleasantly introducing myself and commenting how much I liked his tie, I started off this practicum campaign interview by telling O'Shea of my near-perfect academic score within the accredited Rehabilitation Counseling program and how this success was attributed to my desire working with those in rehabilitation, particularly patients who have sustained neurologic damage. Not mentioning a thing about my own personal experience with rehab, rather, highlighting what I have learned through role play, lecture, and books in school, I enthusiastically went on to tell O'Shea about the "*rewards*" New Medico at Meadowlands would receive by my serving an academic field practice experience here. I didn't realize it at the time, but it would appear my choice of words worked in my favor.

Asking me what sets me apart from other college graduates and why I should be considered for a placement at this facility when no student has ever trained at Meadowlands Health Care Center before, this is when I searched deep within myself to find a little bit of wisdom and articulated for this interviewer my hands-on background with head injury. When I whipped out that pic of me when I was in a coma and placed it in front of him to look at, I thought O'Shea was going to need to change his underwear when his eyes bugged out of his head like they did. In a few seconds' time, it looked like a transmutation occurred with O'Shea where he went from polite superior who graciously was going to spend a few minutes of his valued time with a hopeful intern/subordinate to someone who was thinking, "We got something here!"

After excusing himself, O'Shea rushed into Goyette's office where he spent the next five minutes or so. Proud of the way I scripted this interview production, as I was waiting in his office, O'Shea popped his head in and told me that Goyette could see me now. I thought He might see it my way.

Walking into the directorial office at Meadowlands that Goyette shared with the second in command, Associate Program Director, Donna Micklow, B.S.N., M.P.A., blood gushed through my veins at warp speed knowing that I was moments away from presenting my dialogue where the top two administrators practicing the New Medico philosophy of care here perform their magic. Not realizing at the time that it was "black magic" being performed, my excitement quickly dissolved when the expression on Goyette's face looked as if He had just gotten some bad news about alimony payments.

Crushing my paralytic hand when shaking it, I didn't know this grip was a reflection of what Goyette wanted to do to me because of the plight I was about to put Him in. I only wished that Ms. Micklow were here because her being a nurse working with the physical ailments of those having experienced trauma and the emotional disfigurement which results, this Cokeburg, Pa. native would surely have a little more compassion than someone now business-minded. However, this turning out to be a farce, I am now glad I wasn't subjected to this double-whammy.

I can only guess how busy Goyette must be. Being the Program Director running His facility the New Medico way, He barely has time to fire up His cigarettes let alone say one word to a lowly intern during his practicum. Because of my unparalled background with the disability Meadowlands claims to specialize in, I thought the extent of Goyette's interactions with me being a slight cheek flinch when our paths would cross in the big dining room or one of the hallways was a little peculiar, but I didn't think anything of this, for I had been forewarned of what He was like. For Him to take the time out to make His facial muscles move acknowledging my presence/existence, I guess I should have been eternally grateful.

Even when Goyette acted as if I were invisible, He had to have realized I was coming into His quality facility everyday providing Him with excellent freebie work well over the twenty hours a week I was scheduled during my brief practicum. Told my productive work performance was consistently being relayed upstairs, my three staff supervisors reported the fine work I was doing and how things were working out well to The Man who implemented the New Medico Corporation's orders.

Also, my academic practicum site supervisor, Dr. Marinelli, said the work I was doing with clients was exceptional and surely he mentioned my prime counseling performance to his fellow doctoral cohort who has the final say on who gets hired at Meadowlands. Although New Medico at Meadowlands understood—before I started my field practice—that I was to experience the same routine as regular staff, not everyone was obliging. Out of my control because of my subordinate ranking, this would one day be used as a trump card against me.

Goyette would meet with the Family Counselors approximately once a week in His office to go over what I thought was the progress of the particular patients assigned to be reviewed that week. Because Goyette possesses a Ph.D. and had been involved in a field which emphasizes the psychology of human behavior/interactions, I assumed He wanted briefed about how the various patients being staffed were emotionally adjusting to their disability, before proceeding to develop measures/strateegies to enhance these individuals' livelihoods. This very well could be part of what went on, but the aura of secrecy which seemed to surround these closed-door conferences make one wonder if this was all that was taking place.

Almost right off the bat, I've noticed the New Medico staff I am exposed to have a way of saying what's politically correct and turning things around, making black seem white. Knowing that I just better keep my trap shut about things I don't understand or occurrences I perceive as a little questionable, I know I'll only be accused of having brain injury-induced paranoia by those who ultimately report to Goyette. If there's any suspicion that I have not fully recovered cognitively from my head injury, I won't have a hope in Hell of landing a position here. Helping patients who could benefit from my skills, knowledge, and rare experience, I'm going to do my utmost to make this dream a reality. Anyway, if I choose to be trained here for my internship, once I settle in after a few weeks, I'm sure I will feel foolish that I let my imagination run wild on me after I learn the workings of New Medico better.

Despite my numerous face to face interactions and productive counseling sessions with the various patients who were scheduled to be reviewed, I was never invited to offer the information I had on these different people in these Program Director/Family Counselor meetings. Instead, I had to inform any events of substance to the Family Counselor assigned to be my primary supervisor ("Berkowitz"). Never given a formal explanation of why I was excluded from these discussions, despite my incomparable experience with rehabilitation and figuring Goyette did have the personality He was reputed to possess, I just assumed that because I haven't earned my academic stripes yet, I wasn't thought of as being worthy to confer about the welfare of patients with a purist such as Goyette.

Other than being shunned from these weekly conferences, everything else seemed to be working really well at Meadowlands, making me extremely happy about my choice to serve my practicum here. Feeling a little intimidated that I was working with established New Medico professionals and conscious of my relative youth/minimal workplace experience, during the first week of my practicum—so that I'd be viewed as equally qualified—I'd almost immediately tell the respective patients and families of my personal crusade beating this disability. Eager to maximize my personal experience and utilize this quality to its fullest, the staff Neuropsychologist and my Family Counselor supervisors thought it best if I would first present myself in a professional fashion with those seeking services before divulging my special experience with head injury, so that sharing my background would have the greatest positive impact possible on my clientele.

Also, despite the abundance of ways I may have proven my proficiencies, it was pointed out that prejudicial attitudes towards those with brain injuries may take away from my ability to project myself as a quality professional, for there will be a few who have reservations accepting what a "brain damaged" counselor has to say. However, as things would develop, before this first leg of my New Medico experience at Meadowlands wound down, I would discover that my concerns about any oppositional reactions towards me by patients and their families were not warranted. Unfortunately, this is not to say that unfavorable notions of the "brain injured" population did not exist or that misleading stereotypes of those once having head injuries were nowhere to be found within these Meadowlands' walls. Disgracefully, divisive attitudes could be found screened behind the villainous veil of deception which was the administrative office of Goyette and Micklow. The stratagem schemed by these two New Medico four-star generals was an artifice which led me to believe that I was part of a design which would enable me to seize a dream.

Not only was I feeling comfortable counseling patients and their kin—but as I was hoping—their response to me was, for the most part, one where they were feeling more optimistic about what rehabilitation could do for them. Subsequently, their prospects for the future weren't so counter-productive which resulted in their addressing hurdles in a more beneficial manner. With this enhanced outlook, I was feeling pretty good that I could provide a number of people with some incentive to utilize the needed approach to make the most of a seemingly impossible situation. Actually, this description of me feeling, "pretty good," would not be entirely true because I was on top of the world that I could make a little bit of difference. And those staff members whom I reported to directly were aware of the effective way I was providing services to my limited practicum caseload.

Recognizing the attributes of having someone like myself on board, coupled with the excellent relationship I have developed with them, my supervising Neuropsychologist and three Family Counselor supervisors were hoping that I'd be so moved by the care Meadowlands provides its patients that I would choose their facility to serve my internship over Harmarville. Expecting me to spend this five-month internship training period with them, Harmarville already had prepared a training schedule for me, anticipating my arrival as an intern. Because the Rehabilitation Counseling Department in my "home" rehab center of Harmarville is geared 99.5% towards the vocational realm of rehab, despite the program arranged for me supposedly being personalized to make the most of my once being a patient here and desire to counsel, this blueprint of duties I was to engage in was top-heavy in vocational evaluation tasks with hardly any time set aside for psychological therapy with patients/families. Realizing the potential rewards working in the center which once cared for me as a patient, I was greatly disappointed that my rehabilitation experience with Harmarville was hardly going to be utilized. Home sweet home.

Outside of the directorial office, as far as I could see, staff at Meadowlands were very professional and approachable. Getting a taste of the New Medico system during my month-and-a-half practicum, I was very impressed with the treatment the therapists at Meadowlands provide their patients. Though difficult to be impartial because of my natural fondness for Harmarville, the quality of therapeutic services offered by New Medico at Meadowlands appear comparable to those of the facility which did so much for me. Early on, during my practicum—because of my disastrous personal experience with this program—when I saw the emphasis and importance New Medico placed on Recreational Therapy, I was initially doubtful of the merits of Meadowlands.

However, I soon realized the degree of excellence at New Medico was equal to that of Harmarville in most respects and, in the case of RT for example, even surpassed it. With the quality of care being on a par with Harmarville, their extensive utilization of adjustment counselors, previous exposure to many of the operations of the Family Counselor position, and Meadowlands practically being in my backyard, there was never any real question that New Medico would serve as an excellent training ground for me in my pursuit to attain the skills needed to be an effective counselor. So, I made the easy decision that I'd serve my internship at New Medico rather than Harmarville. Oh, if the cat were only out of the bag when I made this choice, things just might have worked to my advantage.

What the hell's going on around here? Despite my eagerness to assume the same caseload/responsibilities as the Family Counselors during my internship and desire to ease some of the volume of work they have on their hands, I was only given about 65%-70% of the workload as the other counselors. Because my practicum was only a basic means to introduce me to a rehab field workplace, I could kind of understand why every little nuance of the Meadowlands' facility wasn't thrown my way, but now that I've been here everyday, at least forty hours a week and will continue to do so for the next five months as a full-time member of the staff, I don't quite understand what the problem is.

Still as warm and friendly as a rabid pit bull, although I've shown that I am capable of doing a good job these past few months, Goyette was still excessively distant, as He still didn't want me to attend those weekly meetings with the Family Counselors. Because of the short-term nature of my practicum, I could sort of empathize with Him not wanting to risk patients' long-term confidentiality with a student trainee who very well could be here today and gone tomorrow, but now that I'll be more of a fixture around this place, I don't know what to make of this. With the exception of the most superficial things, it seems I'm still purposefully being kept in the dark about this operation for some reason.

I guess because I'm not a paid employee who has earned their work site badge of honor yet, I'm not viewed as qualified to sit in on these huddles where I'm told an interchange of views are bandied about. I have been praised many, many times for my interviewing ability with my various people, as the staff most familiar with my work were quite pleased when I decided to serve my internship at Meadowlands. However, despite my excellent work performance and attendance, no one has ever said a peep about me someday working here after I graduate, which is something I've let staff know I desire.

At Meadowlands, every patient is assigned to a group of caregivers known as a "team." With one staff member usually representing the respective departments, each team is comprised of professionals from all of the various disciplines. During my practicum, there were three teams, meaning only that many counselors were employed. I'm not a math whiz, but I know that when one puts together three Family Counselors already on the payroll and myself, you come up with "four," or one too many. Being on the bottom rung of the Meadowlands' seniority list, it's not too hard to figure out who gets the short end of the stick, if the number of teams remain the same. But, during my internship, Meadowlands added a new team and intended to hire one representative for each of the different programs. "Happy days are here again."

Mistakenly thinking my short tenure here and triumphs within head injury rehabilitation would make me a front-runner for this Family Counselor position, I concealed how badly I was hurt when Meadowlands hired someone unfamiliar with the New Medico system I have learned so well. Although nowhere near as qualified to work with those having sustained a head injury as myself, knowing the man they did hire ("Patton") was an effective professional and a veteran of the armed forces, took some of the sting out of the bite. But it left some deep scars. Down on my luck, this baptism of fire would not be the last.

Because I've been exposed to the personable staffs at Harmarville and the Counseling graduate program at W.V.U., I'm accustomed to rehabilitation professionals being open and genuine which makes the tight-lipped nature of those working for New Medico at Meadowlands seem very puzzling and out of the ordinary. At Harmarville, when speaking with one of their staff, one can expect to get an immediate response leaving no doubt the honesty and sincerity of what's said. But here at the New Medico Rehabilitation and Skilled Nursing Center at Meadowlands, with the speaker frequently looking down at the floor unable to make eye contact when replying, after a lengthy pause and a couple of, "Well, uhhhhhs," you seem to get a dialogue that sounds like a politician's who is being investigated for a scandal. I may not be in the annals of rehabilitation lore, but I think I'm at least worthy of a little more respect than I've gotten so far from the executive branch here at New Medico at Meadowlands. A severe head injury too often leaves its survivors forever whirling in a torrent of lost comprehension—if it hasn't rung out a death knell to toll the passing of another victim—and I think I'm deserving of some credit from the upper tier at Meadowlands for what I've been able to accomplish in the face of this tragedy. But I guess New Medico has its own way of doing things.

It's amazing what they can do. Meadowlands is only a small fraction the size of Harmarville and I can easily understand that—because New Medico specializes in only one type of disability and has to compete with more comprehensive centers for patients—the Corporation must employ some highly virtuous strategies at their headquarters in Massachusetts in order to stay afloat. Because of my primary focus/concern being on what I've got to do to fulfill the requirements necessary to get my Master's and the hush burning from the administrative office, I have absolutely no idea how Meadowlands goes about keeping its head above water. Because of this need to generate revenue, I could appreciate a strategy that creates as much inpatient space as possible.

During my practicum, there was a room designated as the "Family Room" where the counselors would talk with the patients and their families discussing issues of concern, answering questions, providing different information, etc. This liaison role was a much-needed and essential component in one's rehab, but by the time my internship rolled around, this vital area was converted into another patient room. This move created a lot of "space stress," but I just viewed it as something Meadowlands had to do to survive.

The person assigned this room furthest away from the nurses' station and closest to the frequently noisy dining area was a really nice Afro-American lady from all the way down in—South Carolina—who had suffered an aneurysm and was in need of some extensive care. Unable to speak nor capable of engaging in many purposeful motor activities, this admission needed to interact with compassionate people as much as she required Physical or Speech Therapy. Mentally aware of what was going on around her and that she was trapped in a body which no longer rendered any control, tears never seemed to stop running down this woman's face. Placed in a somewhat secluded rehab center on foreign soil and assigned such an out-of-the-way room does not appear conducive with optimum care, however.

Assured that this patient whose suffering was her only companion was getting the best of care, Berkowitz told me that administration was searching for a nursing home down South for "Katy" that was better equipped to care for her because these execs realized she would only deteriorate while at Meadowlands. I hope a facility is found soon because her strength to endure has been heading south for awhile now and nothing is more saddening than to witness such a friendly person wanting to "check out" because they feel so alone in their battle with their ravaging disability. May God bless you, Charlie Goyette and Donna Micklow for your careful planning and swift effort.

Feeling the magnificent pain of these patients, Berkowitz appeared overtaken by a deep sorrow when he told me one day that he just can't understand why there are so many patients at Meadowlands from so far away. Knowing that these inpatients need the healing only a family can provide, he remarked how some admissions were just taking up space and were being ignored because they've been at New Medico at Meadowlands for so long. This was said in reference to a patient better suited for a geriatric home who needed to be consoled on a daily basis because the stroke which leveled him caused him to stagnate to the point of no return a long time ago. Like Katy, with most functions having shut down and not at all ignorant of the catastrophic condition which has forever taken refuge in his body, the loneliness and agitation which simmered within this patient was of seething proportions.

Withdrawn from all that he knows and cherishes, this man's sad eyes tell the story of one held captive in a lonely vigil. Voice having all but abandoned him did not stop "Ben" from communicating how angry he was about the grief tangled within him nary taking a reprieve. Taunted with isolation, his fist pounding on the wheelchair tray rung out loud and clear that he was not too pleased with the way things have fallen "out of place" for him. Always by himself, being supplanted from his home of—New York, depression's grip was inhumane.

If it weren't for my family's spectacular involvement with me, there's a chance I probably would have never come out of my coma. The disturbing lack of family interactions with patients here at New Medico at Meadowlands made me start wondering why many of the people filling these vacancies live so far away. Mind you, not fifty or sixty miles, but several hundred. However, my primary supervisor quelled any queries I might have had about this distance issue by saying that there just weren't any suitable facilities in these new admissions' hometowns to properly accommodate them and that the administration at New Medico Rehabilitation and Skilled Nursing Center at Meadowlands were gracious enough to let these needy folks come to their program for treatment, no matter what inconvenience this may pose for the facility. May God bless you, Charlie Goyette and Donna Micklow for having such kind hearts.

Not thinking anything of this at the time because it was an administrative issue only the talents of Goyette and Micklow could set into motion, but there weren't that many Pittsburgh area patients at Meadowlands compared to the out-of-staters. And after these Pennsylvanians were admitted, they didn't seem to stay that long. Meadowlands was starting to resemble an embassy of sorts with the abundance of out-of-state inpatients receiving the New Medico treatment. Thinking back on it, the discharge criteria of these patients living outside of the Keystone State (Pa.) varied as much as the symptoms they were experiencing.

Some who were progressing nicely appeared as if they could have been released from Meadowlands' bondage a long time ago to a hospital near their own stomping grounds for outpatient care, but never were. Because I've never been invited to attend the weekly meetings held with the Family Counselors in the privacy of the Goyette/Micklow administrative office, with a background in nursing, I can only guess the second in command—Ms. Micklow—determined it would be in these patients' best interests, if Meadowlands would hold onto them for medical observation. Whatever purpose the Goyette/Micklow tag team have for keeping these vulnerable admissions hostage in an environment so far away from their home better be good because it's creating an incredible amount of tension in the lives of these inpatients and their families.

Extremely intelligent people, I wouldn't be surprised, however, if Goyette and Micklow have a stellar plan up their sleeves for the many patients who have put their trust and care in these two New Medico administrators' hands. May God bless you, Charlie Goyette and Donna Micklow for keeping the well-being of patients as your top priority.

One of these patients who was doing rather well was from—West Virginia. If suffering a disabling head injury which left his future in doubt wasn't enough of a stressor, the many miles between his apartment he shared with his wife and the New Medico center created some difficult moments in an otherwise good marriage. Because of the healthy nature of their relationship, this inpatient's wife would have loved to spend each visiting day with her husband at the center, facilitating his rehabilitation and helping him to progress during this crucial, early stage of a brain injury which has definite consequences for the long-term.

But this wasn't feasible because of the five-and-one-half hour drive New Medico at Meadowlands was from their home. The financial concerns of their situation at the time made paying for one of the rooms that New Medico rents out to visiting families a less-than-appealing idea as well.

Not employed during his admission and not having any children, the opportunity was available for this caring spousal partner to be by her husband's side as often as possible, helping him cope with the emotional rigors that being away from family and home usually present a patient. However, now that she's scheduled to be working again shortly, the frequency of her visits are going to be curtailed significantly because of the amount of time involved to get to the center where her husband will be working to regain his life.

Exactly what kind of impact this absence will have on this kindly gentleman who has benefited greatly from the skills of Meadowlands' direct care workers is unclear. Hopefully, the increased mileage and subsequent times spent in isolation won't have too excessive of a detrimental effect or cause too much regression. But keep those fingers crossed.

With the success of any rehabilitation venture boiling down to what the patient does or does not do, it wouldn't be too hard to imagine that being so removed from familiar surroundings could present a patient with emotional difficulties that could ultimately influence the degree of restoration experienced. But I guess administration has figured this factor into a formula which provides their patients with the best care possible. May God bless you, Charlie Goyette and Donna Micklow for having such foresight.

Nice kid. Only a little younger than myself when I was hurt, there was this one adolescent who had suffered a severe head injury when the car he was a passenger in wrecked after the driver had lost control of the vehicle. Circumstances very similar to my own mishap, this inpatient was comatose for about a week-and-a-half when in the hospital and—as a result of his losing consciousness for such an extended period of time—contractures formed.

Pointing downward in such a fashion that it hurt just looking at this deformity, this teen's feet were so severely contracted when he was admitted to Meadowlands

Health Care Center that he was restricted to a bed all day unless pushed by someone in his wheelchair. Once a participant in team sports, this state of inactivity was a situation that was extremely trying on the nerves of this outgoing youth, not to mention his caring/helpful family who couldn't come as often as they wanted. Requiring a lot of time and attention, addressing this friendly boy's feelings of detachment from the world were not easy.

Struggling to form words, his erratic breathing and brain contusion made it very difficult for "Bobby" to be understood. Missing his parents and sisters, one concern that came out crystal clear, however, was how much he dreaded dealing with his immobility and shocked senses so far from his loved family who lived in—Kentucky.

That's quite some hike from Pennsylvania, but I guess the administration at New Medico at Meadowlands are willing to endure any hardships which may pose itself rehabbing a patient from such a far-off state. May God bless you, Charlie Goyette and Donna Micklow for enduring such personal sacrifice, just so suffering patients can benefit from the most accommodating services available.

Not done scavenging prey from the western horizon, New Medico found another patient to transfer out of their home state and stick in Meadowlands. Having already locked up the patient from West Virginia with a commitment to be treated and previously snatching a young female from the state of Ohio, New Medico's philosophy of, "Go West, Young Man," was put into effect again as they seized one more person from the Buckeye state.

This new admission netted from our westerly neighbors and hauled into Meadowlands was not real happy being taken away from his spouse and home. An absolutely fantastic lady, I felt bad for this patient's wife because she had some legitimate concerns and difficulties being separated so far from the husband she loved so very much.

Shelling out dollars either to New Medico or various hotels a couple of days a week for a room while she was visiting, not one to complain, "Mrs. Smith" would express how uneasy she felt about being so far displaced from her husband while he is in his severely agitated state and can be a threat to others because of his husky stature. Temperamental because of the severe head injury sustained, Mrs. Smith's husband improved dramatically when he saw her in the dining area, as his affect would brighten like no other time when he saw his wife after she made the long trek from Ohio. Unfortunately, because of the many landscapes and countrysides which separate this loving couple, Mrs. Smith's husband isn't going to get as many respites from his irritability as he should. May God bless you, Charlie Goyette and Donna Micklow for a game plan which must be outstanding.

The command Meadowlands' therapists exhibit with their respective specialties has helped more-than-a-few patients make up lost ground because of what their neurologic impairment had done to them. Proud to be part of this corps of restoration engineers, although nowhere near to being accomplished yet nor receiving as much as a whisper of encouragement from Goyette that someone with a background such as mine could prove invaluable—if not ideal to His facility—I was still feeling pretty good about my prospects of landing a Family Counselor position at Meadowlands; figuring Goyette's lack of regard was just His style and that He'd eventually come to his senses.

The patients and families that I was assigned to counsel were a conglomeration of admissions from three of the four Meadowlands' teams. Electing not to serve in a supervisory role, a compassionate, female Family Counselor on staff whom I got along with well when we did talk ("Thelma"), for some strange reason did not hand over any of her caseload for me to work with and kept her interactions with me to a minimum. Being a W.V.U. Rehab Counseling graduate whom Dr. Marinelli spoke of as being extremely intelligent and having a heart to match, this well-paid New Medico employee's minimal involvement with me was kind of puzzling because I knew she had a lot to offer, as far as helping me to understand the New Medico way of providing services. Just a little on the reserved side, the only thing I could figure out which may have explained her limited participation with me was that she didn't feel comfortable telling a head injury survivor about a disability they already know all too well. Could it be anything else?

I guess because of my inexperience with head injury, administration must have decided not to give me my own team where I not only would engage in top-of-the-line psychological therapy with my population, but undertake the various other corresponding duties that are required with those receiving the New Medico treatment. My receiving only select fragments of the other counselors' people really bothered me because I didn't want my training to be compromised, if all works as I am hoping and I were to work at Meadowlands one day. I couldn't imagine why there would be any reason for the New Medico administration not wanting me to know and understand the "ins and outs" of the different patients' care.

This restricted allotment of patients and corresponding tasks signed over to me was something that troubled me greatly because—despite my being their first trainee—when Meadowlands agreed to provide a Rehabilitation Counseling internship, they realized they were to give the student the same experience as their regular staff. Voicing concern about this limited assignment, all Berkowitz said was that Meadowlands was appreciative of my patience with them while these student placement supervisory kinks get worked out. A rat's ass there were kinks.

I was afraid that my once having a head injury influenced Goyette and Micklow to think I couldn't handle the full Family Counselor responsibilities of counseling, paperwork, addressing family issues, conferring with Case Managers about discharge planning/insurance concerns, etc. I was just told that I needed to do the best I could with my counseling interventions and the paperwork that goes along with it. As far as understanding the inner workings of insurance coverage and discharge planning with the patients on my "caseload," Berkowitz would only say, "I'll take care of that." Yeah, I just bet he will.

I'm not sure what to make of this. One minute, I get another feather put in my cap for helping a patient take a step towards the important goal of acceptance who, otherwise, wanted to lay down and die. The next, New Medico at Meadowlands is pulling some stunts with me that I can't make any sense of because they defy logical explanation.

A month after I started my internship, my experience with head injury rehab was featured in the first installment of Meadowlands' newsletter, "Access," which was due to come out every other month. Entitled, "A Student Intern's Courageous Recovery, An Interview with Craig Meyers," this printed periodical report was made available to patients and families at the center, making the attempt to conceal my history with this disability very difficult. Three-quarters of this newsletter was dedicated to some of my experiences with head injury, as a snapshot of me counseling a patient donned the front page. Not doing a whole lot for their egos, on the back page tucked away in the upper right hand corner was a pic of Goyette and O'Shea's replacement, Mr. Jeff Grimm, briefly describing Grimm's accomplishments.

Because of my notable background with head injury, I'm able to do some things that your average Family Counselor could not. Now that the "jig is up" and my involvement with rehab has been exposed for anyone interested to take a look at, my supervisors thought it would be advantageous—in select cases—to utilize my personal experience with disability, so that it can be beneficial to those who have a reasonable prognosis. This disclosure was something I wanted all along, so I could make use of my extensive rehabilitation adventures to benefit others when appropriate. With the triumphs I've made in the face of this rehabilitation challenge being "hung out to dry," it was decided by my placement supervisors that it might not be such a bad idea if I were to be present while some patients are working in therapies where they frequently are not real responsive. Now we're talkin'.

During one of Berkowitz's team meetings, my head was starting to swell some because I was receiving quite a bit of praise from the different professionals that my presence during their therapies served as the added "push" some of their patients needed to be less combative and work a little harder. Embarrassed to be "dogging it," this patient reaction to my being in the same room with them while they were struggling to overcome many of the same obstacles I once faced was something I was hoping would happen. Not really taken by surprise when the increased effort did occur, I thought I had found my niche in life.

Orchestrated by the respective team's Case Manager, these meetings occurred once a week on different patients assigned to be staffed. Because Berkowitz's Team Leader/Case Manager was none other than the Program Director's newest wife, I was ecstatic that these compliments came during Her review. Surely, Goyette could find out in the course of "pillow talk" how effective my unrivaled interventions have been with patients and that it would be essential not to let me go elsewhere upon completion of my training. Logic not serving as the base for Meadowlands' governing body, who's to say what New Medico is going to do next. But, I'd find out soon enough.

Now this was very strange. If a written article describing some of my achievements during my Harmarville rehab was beneficial to more-than-a-few Meadowlands' patients/families, I could just imagine how these folks are going to react when the day comes that I show the video of how I once was in a similar predicament. A visual depiction showing that it's possible to overcome many of the symptoms of head injury could be a fundamental component in a person's making progress during his or her rehab. But in a move which shocked me and left me overwhelmed with disbelief, my primary supervisor told me that Goyette does not want me to present this moving illustration of me to any survivors or their loved ones. At a loss for words, I had absolutely no idea what was going on and felt destroyed.

Reflecting on His decision, I could almost understand Goyette not wanting to have inpatients or their kin seeing a video which promotes a rival rehab center and running the risk of losing the almighty New Medico dollar. Furthermore, I could appreciate not showing a video showcasing a comeback to a patient who has little chance of making much of a recovery, for this would only make things worse for them emotionally. Running the risk of falling out of favor with the patients who don't have a very bright prognosis wouldn't make much sense, however, most of the patients and families could benefit from seeing this tape.

I thought those that could gain some inspiration from seeing this documentation of what I was like when I was fighting my head injury should have had arrangements made for them, so they could view it, if they wanted. Being in absolutely no position to question New Medico management's tactics, I could only surmise that all moves are made with the patients' welfare at the forefront. Whatever, Meadowlands' administration wasn't done yet digging into their bag of tricks.

After receiving instruction from Goyette, giving no explanation, my primary supervisor also told me not to show this video to any of the staff besides the Family Counselors. Although very much aware of how important their work is, this decision seemed very peculiar because even the best therapy professionals could use a little encouragement and a "picker-upper" once in a while that the work they do can have long-term fruitful consequences because—all too frequently with the rehab population—things can run into a dead end.

Because each head injury is different, even the most experienced professional can gain a little added knowledge seeing a success story unfolding before their eyes in a telecast. But the opportunity to utilize this tape as an educational tool wasn't going to happen. So much for thinking my experience with rehabilitation could benefit others here at Meadowlands.

However, my Harmarville Neuropsychologist—Dr. Ratcliff—had at least found good academic use of my video tape, for he showed my film to the graduate students he teaches at the University of Pittsburgh. Dr. Ratcliff had nothing to lose and everything to gain, though, because Harmarville was where he did his consultation work. Patients at Meadowlands could "profit" from such a presentation as well, but this doesn't look like the type of return New Medico had on its mind. $$$$$.

Although this is in no way a reflection of my attitude towards myself or those working around me, maybe New Medico administration thought that my peerless achievements with head injury rehab would compromise the experience of the other Family Counselors. Like my field practices, I thought that maybe New Medico at Meadowlands wanted to limit who gets to know about my one-time Ranchos 4-5 state which this video depicts because—when they did hire me—I could make the most of my personal experience with head injury after I proved myself professionally first.

Having the exceptional trait of being a survivor on the verge of attaining professional status within the rehabilitation field, I thought that possibly Meadowlands was strangely hiding me in the closet with the intent of springing a surprise of what they had on the Corporation, and would arrange somewhere down the line for me to speak at a headquarters' conference in Massachusetts. I don't know why else they'd be so intent on making light of my experience which has proven so effective with the people I have interacted because—otherwise—Meadowlands would be like the government's high-security Area 51 in Roswell, New Mexico where it is believed top-secret activity occurs. But I couldn't possibly fathom that New Medico would have anything to hide.

What exactly is the story around this place? If reading about my victories in rehab made any kind of impression, I know this video of me battling my way across rugged rehabilitation terrain was going to have a tremendous impact on the Commander in Chief of the New Medico facility at Meadowlands. When I walked past our noontime gathering place, joining myself, the four Family Counselors, and the Neuropsychologist in the latter's office for our daily review of patients during lunch break, Goyette was seated, preparing to witness the video documentary of my recovery while I was at Harmarville.

In a few moments' time—after I retrieve the magnetic strip storing images of what I was like when I was hurt—Goyette would see for Himself just how qualified I would be for a Meadowlands' Family Counselor position, if and when one becomes available in the future. My cerebral cortex, which is the portion of the brain that controls emotion, was sure busy firing off electrically-charged excitement impulses as I headed back to the office where this New Medico facility's program director would see the premiere Meadowlands' showing of my video.

When I walked into the office, everyone was there—except Goyette. Not worthy of such grace, Goyette couldn't wait two minutes until I got the tape which would show Him just how extraordinary a reclamation project I had become. Noncommittal, the other staff members just went about setting up the equipment as if nothing strange had just happened. It was at this point that my amygdala—that system of the brain which controls fear—was beginning to tell me that this whole New Medico Rehabilitation and Skilled Nursing Center experience was looking more and more like a sham.

Seeing me in a condition where I was so close to being "toe-tagged," the warmhearted Meadowlands' Neuropsychologist began crying after the video finished and demanded that I pursue my doctorate upon realizing just how severely deranged I once was and how far I've progressed with my recovery. Viewing how reality eluded me after I got caught in the crossfire of another person's drinking and driving, with the exception of the counselor possessing the longest tenure at New Medico ("Butch"), all of the Family Counselor staff members remarked something to the effect that I am a medical miracle and would be an asset to any facility I worked for. Hinting that this possible place of employment could be Meadowlands, Berkowitz was sporting his cotton candy smile. Maybe there is hope.

Grinding his teeth that someone has light years more experience than he does with head injury despite his lengthy association abiding by the New Medico Corporation's directive, referring to the Van Halen and AC/DC shirts I was wearing when the video was shot, all the veteran of all New Medico veteran counselors could comment on was my attire. Wanting a report of what the tape showed, I guess it will be Butch's misguided account that Goyette will selectively remember. The chemical in my brain which signals risk or danger—serotonin—was pumping wildly with this thought.

I didn't want to see it, but the writing's been on the wall the whole time. Having the metal of a Volkswagen twisted around my body hasn't made me stupid or blind, I just couldn't understand why anyone would want to shuffle me aside and sweep me under the rug considering how effective my work has been at Meadowlands and what I can offer the people who could use a little hope. I suppose I have overrated and miscalculated the value of my personal experience with head injury and rehabilitation because different signs have been popping up at New Medico ever since I've been here. In addition to being excluded from the Family Counselor meetings with the top brass and having my experiences censored, more trash was starting to build up.

Goyette knew I couldn't hold a pen/cil with my dominant right hand any longer, forcing me to write left-handed these past seven years and that the paralysis of my right hand made typing very difficult, but that didn't stop Him from picking. Through my primary supervisor/messenger, I was told Goyette was pretty pissed that I had done something so sacrilegious as not presenting Him with a typescript layout of my field training requests. Insulted that I'd present His Lordship with such an ugly hand-written document, Goyette demanded that the list of duties I would like to undertake be typed. This "crime" occurred at the beginning of my internship placement and, considering the unattractiveness of my handwriting, I could understand His objections and it was no real big deal that I peck on a typewriter. Please forgive me, "Oh Great One," for I have sinned.

Not done grasping for straws, once again through Berkowitz, I was informed Goyette wasn't too happy either with the way I signed off my progress notes on my caseload—as if I had full-fledged experience with head injury—and He wanted me to put "FC Intern" after my name indicating my student status. That's understandable for I'm not qualified enough to be a regular New Medico staff member yet because of my lack of knowledge about the symptoms which result from a bruise on the brain. Nor have I been taught to this point by New

Medico staff how a patient will react to the emotional fury which accompanies a brain injury.

Before we started practicing at our respective training sites, Dr. Marinelli warned the Rehab Counseling class about how some self-serving facilities' top guns may try to take advantage of its interns by not offering them any kind of respectable monetary wage for their work and/or making the student do inappropriate tasks not related to counseling whatsoever. Giving an example of how one intern was seen mowing the lawn of the center where he was training, Dr. Marinelli emphasized to class that we are not to engage in manual labor at our placement sites or any duties not affiliated with enhancing our professional growth, for agreeing to this sort of activity only makes the trainee vulnerable to future abuses.

Claiming that I was getting paid in the form of the knowledge I would gain from Meadowlands' staff and turning things around by saying that I won't be charged for taking up these experts' time—a day or so after I started my internship—Goyette denied me any cash reimbursement out of New Medico's private-for-profit pot of gold, figuring that a subservient student can't possibly offer His facility anything other than getting in the way, no matter what their experience. The Man in charge of seeing that the New Medico method of service provision at Meadowlands was followed through did not appear to be miffed that I would even think of doing such a thing as try to dig my hands into His alligator shoe reserve, but I do know by the tone of displeasure in His voice that Goyette wasn't real thrilled by my refusal of a "request" He made of me.

I suppose Goyette was fully expecting me to bow my head with gratitude that He went to all that trouble to give me a telephone call at my house. Even after the manner in which this New Medico commander has operated with me since I've been at Meadowlands—personifying distance and disrespect—I think He was stunned when I said that I wouldn't pass out name tags or pour lemonade at the Meadowlands' picnic. Caught between a rock and a hard place, I remembered what I had been told about the Program Director's personality, and with this, I assumed that His narcissistic disposition could very easily translate a refused request as insubordination. Simultaneously, I was thinking about how Dr. Marinelli told the Rehab Counseling class not to subject ourselves to mistreatment of any kind. Not wanting to clean the bird shit off of Meadowlands' roof or empty His ashtrays nightly, I wasn't about to "brownnose" Goyette because that's His most recent wife's job.

Responsible for the smile on Goyette's face, Shirley Goyette knew she could sit "cushy-comfy" in Her Case Manager's chair after she was able to entice Her Husband to accept the head managerial position at New Medico at Meadowlands. Upon the completion of each work day, a grinning Goyette would come in to rub His bleached-blonde newlywed's back and shoulders. Legs quivering, although one never forgets their first love, Goyette acted as if he couldn't wait until they got home.

Accountable for The Program Director's nocturnal cheer, Shirley G. knew there would be no way She'd ever be called on the carpet—at least to be reprimanded. Sittin' high and mighty in the facility Her Hubby ran by the New Medico guideline, staff knew to keep their lid shut about any comments which didn't stroke The Man the right away because—seated at a desk near the center of the program office—there was a bug which had a direct line to Goyette's tender ear which liked nibbled. Knowing the hormonal power She had over the Program Director, Shirley G. must have felt immune to the etiquette which applied to everyone else.

Because of my hemiparesis and tight heel cord, even seven years after my accident, my right foot still slapped down hard on the ground when limping my way along. At the beginning of my internship, not knowing that I have trouble controlling or balancing objects with my hands when I walk because my entire body recoils and shakes after my right foot thuds following a step, my primary supervisor asked me to get two cups of coffee out of the percolator in the break room for a family. With all the queer things that seem to be characteristic of Meadowlands Health Care Center, I was afraid to speak up for myself and divulge my problem, so I just told myself that I'd just be careful and make the best of it because I didn't want to be seen as incompetent, which is something that very well could take place here given the way events have occurred thus far.

I was sweating blood when there weren't any plastic lids to be found to put on top of the Styrofoam cups. Everyone was extremely busy in the kitchen, so forcing myself to solicit any help there wasn't an option. Even with my Meadowlands' work "above and beyond the call of duty" the majority of the time, I still didn't know exactly what the opinion of me was coming out of the Goyette bedroom—but I was about to get a helluva clue.

Demonstrating the compassion only a Program Director's wife of an anarchistic facility could possess, when Shirley G. saw me coming out of the tiny break room looking like a tightrope walker splashing coffee all over myself—having a good ol' time seeing me struggle—She made sure that I saw Her smirk at me and heard the subsequent laughter. Always making sure I'd pick up on Her snicker when a reference about my gallant recovery were made—for some reason I did not understand—from the very beginning, Goyette and His follow-up wife seemed to be trying to make this New Medico experience an absolute nightmare for me. It was like they made things as miserable for me as they possibly could, so they wouldn't have to worry about me applying for a job at Meadowlands someday and having to contend with the idea of interviewing a person who once had a head injury. Having already shown my qualifications for a Family Counselor position, after they would reject me, the center might have a tough time formulating a believable excuse as to how they could do such a thing. Instead of an impeccable reference, New Medico would have to cover their tracks and explain away why someone with my background and experience wasn't hired. Smelling like a ruse, this New Medico charade shall unfold one day.

It's kind of hard to understand why there's such a massive turnover of personnel at New Medico when they pay so well. Despite everyone most familiar with my work realizing how effective my interventions have been, rarely was a word ever said to me about my being hired here one of these days as a professional. I have made it known my desire to work as a Family Counselor at New Medico Rehabilitation and Skilled Nursing Center at Meadowlands and I believe this resulted in the occurrence of some rather odd circumstances.

Approximating me in age, there was this one female cognitive therapist whom I would usually talk to a little each day. Being engaged and knowing she was not too hard on the eyes, as may be expected, generally it was me who approached her for a chat. By the time my New Medico internship was drawing to a close and it was universally known throughout the center that I wanted to work at Meadowlands, this goddess only came up to me one time to talk. But it was a conversation I wasn't about to forget.

During my practicum, this therapist told me that Meadowlands pays "great," but at the tail-end of my internship training when I'd be looking to jump in somewhere for full-time paid employment, this same staff member said that New Medico *DOESN'T* provide its employees with a very rewarding wage. Obviously having forgotten that we had talked about this money issue earlier, she didn't realize she had just deepened the New Medico mystery that much more.

With no openings presenting itself in New Medico at Meadowlands, I had to resign myself to the fact that I would more than likely have to move elsewhere. If I could find a rewarding position close to home so I wouldn't have to leave mom by herself, that would be preferable, but relocating would be an option I wouldn't oppose, as long as I knew I'd have a career secured working in head injury rehabilitation. Knowing of my desire to move South away from snow and to an environment where the temperature during the winter isn't so hard on my once fractured right leg, Goyette helped arrange an interview for me with His buddy and fellow New Medico program director cohort, Phillip Barry, Ph.D., in—Cortland, New York.

Paying for my own plane ticket to go up there several hundred miles NORTH of Pittsburgh to this tundra was a waste of money, for I doubt I was given serious consideration for the opening, as I found out shortly thereafter that New Medico found someone who knew more about head injury rehab than myself. Figuring this would keep my mouth shut for awhile, after a snide remark from Butch that my experience with head injury hadn't been helpful landing me a job in the direction I wanted to go, I was given the National Head Injury Foundation's 1988 Edition of the National Directory of Head Injury Rehabilitation Services as a resource to find a job in the rehabilitation field. Gee, why am I getting a feeling that I'm not in New Medico at Meadowlands' future plans?

Why in God's name am I being led to believe I've done something gravely wrong? After I gathered my personal belongings off the stall where I did my documentation and other paperwork in the Meadowlands' program office, with no job leads in sight, I said my good-byes to everyone and was offered the best of luck in my search for employment. Walking out towards the front desk on my way out one final time during my internship, I just so happened to cross paths with the New Medico at Meadowlands' Grand Dragon one final time. And Goyette made sure He didn't waste this last chance to express His regards for me and—underneath it all—send a message about my prospects for working at Meadowlands as long as He were King.

Swallowing my pride and expecting to be pained by another crushing grip, when I extended my hand for a handshake and thanked Him for the opportunity to train at His facility, Goyette didn't flinch or say a word. Not willing to make the effort to take His right claw out of His pocket, as if my work performance were not productive and I wasn't dedicated to helping those who have suffered as I once did, Goyette just stood there looking down at my outstretched paralytic hand. Heading towards the program office, He could have been getting ready to see His case manager wife and was playing a little pocket-pool, but this wasn't it, for I knew that His attitude towards me was being telegraphed loud and clear.

Over the course of my rehabilitation, more than a few people have made a comment, saying in essence, that I'm a thaumaturgical marvel. Flattered, even with this miracle quality attributed to me, given the way the New Medico Rehabilitation and Skilled Nursing Center at Meadowlands' administration have functioned with me throughout my training, I guess I shouldn't have been caught too off-guard by the silence and still before me. I obviously couldn't have realized it at the time, but this was only being done to serve as a smoke screen.

Forcing myself not to see that which had been occurring around me all this time and wanting to believe that my frequently superb work performance would be enough to keep me in the running for a Family Counselor position at Meadowlands when one became available—still holding out hope that things could be worked out—I reiterated my desire to be employed at Meadowlands because I believed in the work the counselors did here and what little I knew of the New Medico system. Giving myself a little blue ribbon, so that this may stick in His mind for the long-term, the last thing I told Goyette was how I have productively influenced and impacted the lives of people I had the opportunity to work with while at Meadowlands. Despite earning high marks in most every facet of my field training, Goyette never stopped trying to employ His minor-league manipulation tactics, so that I'd be influenced to think that my conduct throughout this New Medico experience was improper somehow.

Taking this signal to mean that I wasn't worthy of His time or effort, Goyette limply "shook" my hand for a second or two before saying, "Thank you," in such an icy/exaggerated way that I knew He wasn't sincere. Maybe I'm just reading too much into things because New Medico wouldn't do anything to hurt someone who has already had more than their fair share of devastation in their life.

Not familiar with the trauma a patient and/or their family will experience after the onset of a head injury, I was not qualified for a Family Counselor position at Meadowlands Health Care Center, but I did not allow that to dissuade me from my attempts to get in a New Medico facility somewhere else in the country.

Hard-headed, figuring that possibly it was only the administration's own personal attitudes toward those having sustained head injuries which prevented me from getting a shot at the Meadowlands' job, I went about scanning the directory I had, searching for facilities around the country where my knowledge and experience may be better appreciated and utilized to benefit their patients and families of those hurt. All the while, I was foolishly hoping that my internship site would be calling about a newly-developed Family Counselor opening.

Visualizing myself helping people in a first-rate rehabilitation center closer to the equator where the temperature rarely drops below the 70's, if I did have to pack up and leave, I wasn't totally depressed about my inability to acquire a position right away working with those who have had head injuries because I believed that once I got "discovered," centers would be beating down the door to get to me. To find the ideal workplace site, utilizing the directory I was surprised New Medico didn't charge me for, I first acquired information on what services the various facilities offered and then I'd delve to see if the geographical location and climate of these different centers was appealing. Thinking that already having had a bit of exposure to the Corporation might help me land a job with them, despite the sour taste I got in my mouth from Meadowlands' administration, New Medico centers near an ocean or The Gulf were my first choice to work. But I didn't limit myself to only this one system of care, for I also applied at independent treatment programs, hospitals, and other head injury companies such as Rebound Inc., NeuroCare, Mediplex, HEALTHSOUTH, and REACH.

Thinking it would be beneficial if I concisely documented my achievements following my hideous accident to let these industries know I wasn't just your average, everyday, college grad looking for a job—in the envelope I sent—I enclosed my cover letter, resume, grad school grade report, the Meadowlands article featuring me, a picture of when I was in a coma, and one as I currently look. I was absolutely positive that different centers would line up and compete for the opportunity to bring me on board after they saw what a valuable commodity I would be. But I would be extremely lucky, if I'd even get a smidgeon of interest.

I told my W.V.U. academic internship site supervisor—Roy H. Tunick, Ed.D.—about the contents I sent to these prospective places of employment and he didn't get real excited about the manner in which I relayed my experience. Not seeing me in person and how well-off I am now—only having a picture to go by—this Vocational Evaluation instructor said that I just may scare off some employers about my ongoing condition. Bullheaded, not wanting to believe programs treating those with head injuries would do a thing such as deny "one of their own" the opportunity at a chance to better themselves, I kept on doing the same thing and basically got the same results.

I found out awhile ago that if an employer doesn't want to hire you, they've got a handful of ambiguous "trick questions" or approaches that'll be asked/used with you which will leave the applicant with absolutely no chance of getting hired. After I got my Bachelor's, I applied at and interviewed with this one drug and alcohol facility in town only a couple of miles from the house I call "home."

Conscious that my Psychology degree wasn't worth a hell of a lot and thinking that my experience being hurt because of a substance being abused would give me an "edge," during the questioning—like a dumb ass—I yapped about how I had sustained a severe head injury after a drunk driver went off the road and totaled the car I was in, leaving me comatose. Shocked by my disclosure, with a horrified expression on her face which resembled how my first date at W.V.U. looked when I told her, I doubt if this interviewer heard me say that I wanted to serve as a role model for teens who may subject themselves to risk by drinking, just so they feel that they belong to a peer group.

Not previously advertising this as a prerequisite for the post I was interviewing for, she then told me that the organization was really looking for someone with their Master's, but that if I wanted to volunteer, arrangements could be made. No thanks, I didn't bust my tail for four years in college and in my Harmarville rehab, so I could wipe some addict's toxic asshole free of charge. Even after I did kick butt in grad school, only a less conservative state was willing to give me a chance at proving what I could do. Well, at least at first.

I had a telephone interview three time zones west with a New Medico facility in Apple Valley, California. Articulating myself well and having what I thought were all the right answers, this background hunt was going real smooth. But then things took a dramatic turn.

Apparently, the snapshot of me comatose at Allegheny General Hospital was before the interviewer and the C.V. documenting my history with head injury was being reviewed a little closer by this community-reentry facility's "head" when the questions started getting real picky and insignificant. In the midst of explaining what I would do if confronted with a particular situation, I used the term, "crisis intervention," and this administrator had a field day harping on what I meant by this exactly. When I didn't give him the answer he was seeking precisely, overlooking the multitude of attributes I possessed which we had previously discussed, disappointment overflowed the phone lines and I knew then that I didn't have a chance at getting my foot in the door of this facility. With the way New Medico's administrations have interacted with me, one could almost get the idea that the industry really isn't all that concerned about helping one-time patients get back into the community as quickly as possible with the highest degree of independence. With this thought, I could just hear various New Medico professionals who I've had the pleasure of meeting claiming, "Well uhhhhh, that's only a delusional symptom of Craig's head injury coming out."

Why take what could be perceived as a chance, when you don't have to? I've never been naive and I've always known it's tough out there. Thinking that I actually could be a little notable with all that I've been able to master again after being "off my rocker" for what seemed an eternity, I assumed some rehabilitation doors might be opened for me that, otherwise, would have been closed. But, because my brain being jarred within my "brain box" had left me blundering like an invalid at one time, these doorways to a life of promise weren't only shut, they were locked and bolted.

Don't call us, we'll call you! The welcome I had received from the real world was indeed a chilling one because—for the past two-and-one-half months—if I hadn't gotten a, "The position which you have applied has been filled by someone who knows more about brain injury than you" letter from the dozens of head injury rehabilitation programs which I had applied in the surrounding area and across the country, I wouldn't have gotten any news at all. Apparently, it looks like I had either overestimated the value of my rehabilitation experience or underestimated the prejudice which exists in the offices of rehabilitation administrators who are responsible for the development of staffs. Maybe someone going from being comatose to attaining professional status isn't that unusual, after all.

Focused primarily on what I have accomplished in rehab and my subsequent effort thereafter, when I attempted to become a member of the rehabilitation work force, I incorrectly assumed that rehab execs would think, "Since this guy has overcome so much to get where he's at now and has acquired so much knowledge that can't be appreciated from reading a textbook, he must have exceptional strength, character, and expertise. And we would feel honored having a person of this nature on our staff."

Reflecting back on this phantom belief of how I expected to be perceived, I have felt like a fool on more than one occasion because I had received countless response letters with an underlying message, stating in essence, "Your qualifications and credentials are very impressive and you're one of a kind, but we're still never going to call you in for an interview, or for God's sake, consider hiring you because of all the unanswered questions which exist with people who have bumped their heads."

Instead of the previously mentioned healthy qualities being attributed to me—more than likely—a rehab employer is going to think, "We can't take a risk hiring someone that could jack up our insurance rates or has the potential of going 'bonkers' on us."

If one has had a head injury and has applied for a position of responsibility within the field of rehabilitation, it's far too easy for a treatment facility to put your record on file and forget about you, hoping that you'll forget about wanting to work for them or change your mind. Or, to lose track of the cover letter/resume you've sent in and ask you to send in these again, for yet another six-month run-around.

With the golden experience I have with head injury rehab and not a single soul taking a serious look at the bait that I've cast, it's looking increasingly more like unfounded fear is guiding those who head rehabilitation services. It appears as if one has sustained a severe head injury, the vast majority of rehabilitation employers are not going to abide by their equal opportunity obligations, even if they surmise that a high percentage of patients and families could benefit. Conveniently misplacing one's C.V. and resume must be a practice utilized by quite a few head injury rehabilitation center's Human Resources Departments, if the applicant interested in a professional position was once a patient whose thinking had decayed at one time. Like an idiot, I always thought E.O.E. stood for "Equal Opportunity Employer," not "Evil Office Executives."

Getting the feeling one senses when they're being brushed aside, it seemed that in the eyes of rehabilitation higher echelon, if one has earned their Master's Degree but once had sustained a severe head injury, the traumatized person will then be viewed as someone who has the intellectual capacity of a person not quite smart enough to get a G.E.D. Never to be conceded to, it looked as if it was much too easy for an employer to overlook a person's qualifications, credentials, and abilities if they're seen as damaged goods. Earning a Master's from an accredited program with fabulous grades and serving a very solid—if not sometimes spectacular—field practice is usually enough to get a well-paying position with a reputable company, but this academic standing and work performance seems to get rescinded, if the person attaining these has had a head injury.

In the short time I have looked for a job, I soon discovered that Mental Health/rehabilitation employers who know of my history with brain injury would offer this Master's-trained graduate a Bachelor's level wage. I knew that within this counseling field that Robin Leach would never interview me for a forthcoming episode of, "Lifestyles of the Rich and Famous," nor did I try to take anyone to the bank, but I would have liked a salary commensurate with my abilities and academic experience. It just seemed that having a Master's coupled with a head injury, I could command a Bachelor's level salary and if I only had this undergraduate degree coupled with my past aphasic history, I could have commanded minimum wage. Regretfully, it's looking as if any degree I may have or experience I've accrued gets canceled out after it's learned I had sustained a head injury.

I didn't think I should have had to fear rejection from a potential employer because of my past history with head injury—especially a rehab center dealing with this group of patients—but with the way things had materialized, it looked as if I'd have to hide my experience with rehab, if I wanted a job. Coming so close to being charred in a Volkswagen, I thought I should have been proud of what I had been able to accomplish in my therapies and use it to benefit others when appropriate. Apparently, however, this wasn't the way things were seen by those seeking personnel to fill job vacancies because, although counseling those with head injuries was my primary objective, I hadn't restricted myself to this specialty altogether.

Those places of employment which *DIDN'T* deal with the head injury population had actually been more receptive to my overtures for employment than rehab centers because, I believe, I didn't mention my "brain damaged" history, only my academic and field practice training experiences. Defeating the purpose of getting into Rehab Counseling in the first place, I was shocked and felt betrayed by the insidious way I was being discriminated against by rehab centers across the land. I guess a mindset was being assumed where executives were thinking, "Because a person attaining a professional level job after the onset of a severe head injury just doesn't occur, it can never happen." Not with that attitude, it can't.

With the "Craig Meyers Head Injury Package" where I have included information on my rehab background not exactly selling to the Dixie rehab centers I have applied or putting much of a dent of curiosity in these programs, I then sent correspondence of interest to facilities not so deep in the South and also closer to home in the regions surrounding Pittsburgh, which wouldn't be at all bad because then I wouldn't have to leave my beloved Pirates and Steelers. But this expanded arena which I was applying to utilize my services didn't change much, for rehab centers were still avoiding me like I had the plague. Sadly, to the various Human Resource Directors who have read my drama, it seemed that having once sustained a severe head injury and contracting the plague are one and the same.

If there's that many people out there more qualified to work with the head injury population than myself, I'd like to shake their hands because I know then that they must possess some remarkable abilities. Knowing that head injury systems like New Medico exist out there, initially, I felt confident about my chances of starting a fruitful career where I'd professionally be involved with "my population." But I would soon find out that empathy doesn't go too far in rehab managerial offices because this head injury I sustained many years ago had actually prevented me from landing a REWARDING job working with this disability.

Sustaining a brain injury, it seems I've been "blackballed" from getting a good job with head injury rehabilitation because former patients who had been hurt so bad that their mental processes had once decomposed are usually viewed as always trying to snare a sense of balance and must be approached with caution/reserve. The saddest thing about this whole tragedy had nothing to do with me permanently losing my good physical health or even any of the number of things that happened to me during my hospitalization or rehab, rather, it turned out to be that the real catastrophe lies with rehabilitation professionals who claim they want the best for people who once suffered through a head injury, but do just the opposite to one of its members, prolonging their agony. There seems to be an unwritten code and long-standing belief that hiring a "brain injured" person for a professional position is unheard of, so this doctrine is closely adhered to by rehabilitation managements.

Because of the way things had been going, the writing on the wall appeared to be that one will be judged by their head injury, making it easy to overlook their advanced academic standing. Forever looked at as a one-time patient permanently affected by unforeseen symptoms of a brain injury, rather than a person with a history of a head injury, prosperity wouldn't be coming my way. Because I was in control of the effort I put into my recovery, good things happened. But once I had to be dependent on the objectivity of head injury rehabilitation employers for continued progress, my world stagnated.

And here I thought, because they didn't have in their experiential tool box the personal struggles and background with rehab I possess, that various staff which I've been exposed to in my young "career" were only threatened by my experience and that's why I was told to be quiet about my history. With the alarmed way I was reacted to by the different rehabilitation programs which I had applied, one could easily think I was institutionalized and sent my notifications of interest from an insane asylum.

Detecting what I believed to be high-octane discrimination and/or nepotism, despite feeling I would constantly be under the microscope working for them, I decided to fall back on my trusty "home" rehab center of Harmarville, egotistically thinking that they might do something so outrageous as create some kind of unique, not-yet-developed position where a former patient's encouraging personal experience with them and counseling abilities could be utilized. After my brain had hammered against my skull and I needed a life preserver thrown to me so I could stay afloat amidst the tidal wave which is stigma, I soon learned how alone I was.

Plain and simple, I wouldn't be at all surprised and would not blame them one bit, if Harmarville were a little "ticked" at me for deciding to serve my field practices with a competing rehab center after all the "trouble" they put into developing a personalized training schedule for me. Personally witnessing my perseveration and hemiparesis, I could understand 100% if my "home" rehab center wasn't real thrilled with the prospect of distributing some of their non-profit funds to an employee whom they have images of as being incoherent and not capable of doing much of anything physically. 100%.

It's important that a patient strives to attain everything they can and maintaining a workable attitude is essential in order for them to be achieved. Employed in a full-time professional capacity, Harmarville may not want to have me limping around their facility, for fear that their current patients could get depressed seeing what a brain injury can do to a person's long-term physical stature. And that is completely understandable. Completely.

Hypothetically, in the course of my employment with them, if Harmarville would "talk me up"—highlighting some of my virtues which wouldn't have been possible had it not been for the efficiencies of their therapies—and then I'd have that first seizure somewhere along their busy hallway or in the crowded dining room, I wouldn't exactly be an ideal role-model. Having a lot of explaining to do, then, Harmarville surely would just as soon avoid this potentially humiliating circumstance. If a quivering man so many years after they've been hurt is the best that Harmarville can do for someone who has had a head injury, what does that say about the facility and the prognosis for that particular condition? To avoid this concern is totally understandable. Totally.

With all the beauties running around Harmarville, one could think Hugh Hefner were the Personnel Director. Given the universally accepted belief that health and beauty are interpreted as competence—and disability as incompetence—the avulsion of my right ear, bum right side, and subsequent sorry gait wouldn't exactly help me with my job search here. Knowing I didn't fit in because of this prerequisite, I could never blame Harmarville in any way were this approach followed, for I know if I was the one responsible for hiring at my "home" rehab center, I'd much rather look at an attractive female with some brains over someone who limps that may be qualified. But I thought I'd give it my best anyhow. Not employing staff who remind patients of their own vulnerability and mortality is entirely understandable. Entirely.

Adding it to my collection, because they knew me best when I was almost a "goner," I wasn't too surprised when I got the, "Thanks, but not thanks" reply from

Harmarville. Being passed over and passed along by programs that I could easily assume hadn't found people more experienced for the different head injury rehab jobs which I've applied had me starting to question whether I would actually be as good as I thought working within the rehabilitation realm and, if indeed, I was at all marketable. As dangerous as it is to doubt one's own ability, these past refusals of my pursuits for employment would be nothing, for I was about to get a neutron bomb dropped right on me.

Sunday, April 9, 1989 would develop into my day of infamy. In the Pittsburgh Press Classifieds on this morning was an ad from the New Medico Rehabilitation and Skilled Nursing Center at Meadowlands publicizing a job opening for the Family Counselor position. Approximating five months, it looked as if my battle with the many rehab centers—feverishly trying to establish my stability and effectiveness as a given—was going to end because these New Medico guys already knew how valuable of an employee I would be, having already shown my abilities at this treatment facility. With my previous orientation to Meadowlands Health Care Center, the multitude of rare skills I've proven to possess, and the stellar rehabilitation background in my history, I believed I was a "lock" to get this job after the administration at New Medico went through the formality of interviewing those who had only learned about head injury recovery by reading the pages of a Rehab 101 text. Overflowing with excitement, that very night I typed up a cover letter addressing it to the person "The Press" instructed applicants to mail their correspondence to—Associate Program Director, Donna Micklow. Highlighting my many unique attributes which could go a long way towards helping a patient/family and expressing my long-term desire for employment at Meadowlands didn't really matter, for the administration had other ideas.

One week went by and when I didn't see the classified from Meadowlands in the following Sunday edition of the Pittsburgh Press, self-centered, I figured that this New Medico facility didn't need to put anymore "Help Wanted" ads in this paper because they already knew that I would be the absolute perfect candidate for the job when they saw that I had applied. With one of Goyette's arms thrown over my shoulders, picturing a caption which read, "Program Director welcomes accomplished survivor as newest member of New Medico at Meadowlands' staff," I could almost see a photograph of us smiling together like father and son on the cover of a National Head Injury Foundation newsletter. Spirit about to be shred, was I ever in for a shocker of a New Medico surprise.

Weeks dragged by and I didn't hear a word about anything pertaining to this vacancy. Feeling a little slighted, not receiving any message from the facility where I already had proven my dedication to the well-being of their patients and families as a student not demanding so much as a nickel of monetary reimbursement, I was still waiting for that infamous phone call from Meadowlands. Not taking into account the way New Medico at Meadowlands' administration gave me the "cold shoulder" throughout my training, nor willing to totally accept that there may be a reason management behaved in this fashion, I still expected to be contacted any minute by them telling me to come into the center, so they could formally offer me the Family Counselor opening. Created when the employee New Medico hired during my internship was let go, following this dream of working as a Meadowlands' Family Counselor would take me to the reality where the forces of prejudice and partisanism hail.

It had been a good month since it was advertised that the Family Counselor job at Meadowlands which I already had experience working was made available to the public, and I still hadn't heard anything from the center whether or not this position had been filled. As a general rule, if one has applied for a job with a company which had advertised the need for someone and the applicant doesn't hear from that place of employment within a week or two, the employer probably has found other candidates who they like better and feel are more qualified. Given the special circumstances of this New Medico field training experience and the crazy notion that I just may be unique—knowing Goyette's New Medico at Meadowlands' phone number—I gave them a call hoping to speak with a staff member I knew who might be able to fill me in as to what was going on. What I was about to hear from New Medico would send me back to the hospital.

It just so happened that I was able to get through to Butch. Surely recognizing my voice, I probably didn't have to pleasantly identify that it was me who was calling—but I did anyhow—and even inquired how his new, New Medico baby was doing to be polite. After the small talk was said and done, it was time to get down to business and find out where I stood—or didn't stand—with the New Medico employment situation. Having a hunch that this dreaded moment might one day be before him where this azygous survivor would inquire about whether or not the job which I had been trained for all these months had been filled, this long-time New Medico practitioner had a reply ready, dangling from the tip of his forked tongue after I finished dialing the number and made the connection. Because of the devastating impact that this would have on my life, the dialogue which transpired will forever be etched in my memory.

When I asked the "$64,000 Question" if anyone was hired for the New Medico Family Counselor slot which had been opened, he said in a tone of apparent rehearsed excitement, "Yeah, we hired a real experienced therapist."

At that moment, I could feel my heart crashing down deep inside of me because of the despair and disappointment which had ahold of me. Stopping his answer there, not volunteering any more information, I then asked what this person's name was, thinking that if someone had more experience with head injury than myself, they should be dead and must be a mummy.

This New Medico vet claimed he didn't know her last name, but said her first name was "Penelope." When I heard this name, it then felt like my heart had been set ablaze.

Praying to God that this Family Counselor who lives and breathes New Medico would say "no" to my next bit of detective work, I immediately said in an inquisitive tone, "Penelope Rich?"

"Yeah, do you know her?," he told me in such a fashion that I couldn't tell if he already knew that she was a fellow W.V.U. graduate or not because I was in utter shock when I heard the affirmation.

The very instant I realized who was deemed more capable of fulfilling the Family Counselor job requirements and seen as possessing superior knowledge/skills to my own, I was done hiding the sharpened misery which stung into me and became outraged when I answered Mr. New Medico's question if I knew Penelope with, "She's not an experienced therapist, she was in my grad school class at W.V.U.!"

Getting Penelope Rich to work as a New Medico Rehabilitation and Skilled Nursing Center at Meadowlands' Family Counselor—what a feigned.

To think that a person—whose only real experience with rehab was more than likely limited to twisting her ankle once when crawling out of her daddy's whirlpool—got the Family Counselor job working with those affected by head injury over someone who had plowed ahead "against all odds" to attain two college degrees following a severe brain injury, left me feeling numb, hopeless, and discriminated against. Receiving the news that a girl not fit to handle the Family Counselor responsibilities long-term or deserving of such an opportunity was given my "dream job" I had earned, I almost wished that my life had been taken that February night over seven years ago. I was that much of a "wreck" because I couldn't believe New Medico would do anything to harm someone so badly who once had a head injury. What I didn't know then.

Wanting some consoling, I called Dr. Marinelli at school and this professor who consistently stressed throughout the school year that people "WITH" disabilities are receiving the same equality as those more fortunate, didn't have much to say. In a no-win situation, for this New Medico fallacy dealt with two students taking his rehab course, all this rehabilitation instructor could say when he heard who would be gainfully employed at Meadowlands and who wouldn't be was that he was "surprised" that I didn't get the job after all the productive hours I put into learning the Family Counselor position and that Goyette's opinion of Penelope's physical appearance might have done the hiring. My academic practicum site supervisor tried to tell me that maybe because I identify so well with Harmarville, that this may be why I didn't get the job. Whatever, I guess if Meadowlands' patients and families got questions about head injury, they are asking the most qualified person possible when they go to Penelope.

You gotta be hungry if you want to get better. Just so that some semblance of a normal step could be taken again—clinging onto a parallel bar for dear life—I first had to diligently concentrate and focus in order to reteach that brain of mine how to bend the front part of my foot up, so I could place the heel down first. But Penelope understands the emotional strain Physical Therapy has on those whose brain injury has rendered them unable to move.

Having forgotten how to walk, after recapturing the elementary function of lifting my foot off the ground, I strained and strained so I could relearn how to do something so basic as throw my leg out to the side with the hope that it might end up in front of me. Regaining this lost ability to take one lousy step, I knew that a magic wand wasn't going to be waved over my head making me better, but that I'd have to endlessly practice until tears of frustration ran down my face. But Penelope can tell a patient what it's like to work so hard for something and not reap any rewards from the effort.

Not capable of standing by myself or knowing if this would ever be possible again, I fought like a dog to rid myself of this disablement by going for the jugular of this problem which entailed overcoming the emotional barriers that stand in the way of a patient with a brain injury trying to reach a goal. But Penelope knows all about that and can tell a patient/family member all about her experience with this; that should take about a second-and-a-half.

Relearning the basic skill of getting my feet situated properly, it was then time to balance myself and get a "position sense" of where I was in relation to the world. Withstanding the emotional pain which accompanies forgetting how to do something so fundamental is grueling. A doctor having made her, Penelope would no doubt have more knowledge about the psychological warfare a patient endures with their disability than anyone else could—including a person who may have personally experienced this trauma at one time.

To think that New Medico hired somebody who didn't even bother reading the chapter about head injury recovery in the Rehab 101 text, rather, skimmed through the cliff notes, is unconscionable. However, as things would evolve, unscrupulous behavior would be the framework of the New Medico Corporation's covert operation.

In many ways, this head injury had allowed me to find peace within myself. Owning a new confidence and assertiveness because of my fresh outlook, I was getting set to assemble a life for myself that most thought wouldn't ever be possible after what had happened to me. New Medico crumbling the foundation which I had been piecing for myself from the first moment Paul's getting sauced resulted in me being bounced off that telephone pole, was nothing short of sadistic and criminal. Apparently, Butch told the Associate Program Director that I had called the center wanting officially notified about the position which I had applied for almost a month-and-a-half ago because, a few days after I made the call—May 19, 1989 to be exact—I received that formal letter stating they had found someone who would better suit the needs of the facility.

Quickly glancing at the letter, I saw that the salutation started of with a warm and fuzzy, "Dear Craig." After noticing the informal opening, I was relieved it didn't identify me as "head injured dreamer," "shunned," or "gullible idiot." Reflecting our tight-knit bond, this note's introduction also bubbled.

Reading on, this letter signed by Donna Micklow starts off with a sweet, how much it was a pleasure receiving my resume regarding possible employment at Meadowlands. Given the frigid tactics utilized by administration to dissuade me from seeking a Family Counselor position with the New Medico Rehabilitation and Skilled Nursing Center at Meadowlands, I just bet Micklow was dancing in the street after she scanned the envelopes in her mailbox during application time and saw that one had my name/return address on it.

Getting to the meat of this lovely document, in the second paragraph, it tells a fairy tale that after all the applicants' credentials, experience, and professional interests had been reviewed, Meadowlands determined that Penelope would be the best person to fill the counselor opening. According to the Third Printing of The American Heritage Dictionary of the English Language, "credential" means: That which entitles one to confidence, credit, or authority. I think Penelope's antics in graduate school and what her slithering into this New Medico job has the potential of doing to the spirits of patients and their families who need to see someone who has triumphed over this disability are enough to question if these three attributes apply.

Seeing the PR video of me recovering at Harmarville in Barb's "Med Aspects" grad school class, Penelope knew she would be stealing from the Meadowlands' clientele fortunate enough to be on her caseload any faith or confidence that would have been gained viewing my tape and being exposed to an experienced counselor who has a pretty good idea of what a person goes through with a head injury. But the needs of those suffering through the rigors of disability didn't appear to be the top priority for this novice student of rehab whom New Medico deemed most capable of delivering the best services possible.

Comparing Penelope's "experience" with head injury rehab to my own is a joke and not even worth a moment's thought, nor a breath to comment on. And if her "professional interest" exceeded mine, she wouldn't have geared her studies so much towards the vocational realm of rehab and could have asked daddy to secure a spot at Meadowlands for her to train. But it looks like this wasn't the type of securing the Rich family had on their mind.

Because of what occurred at Goyette's New Medico neurologic center at Meadowlands, for three months, I couldn't stop obsessing about how I got the "shaft" at His facility, as I was too sick and upset to make much of a dent in the job search front. Calls made to Meadowlands wanting to speak with this Program Director so I could ascertain what I needed to do in the future to secure a position at the center one day should one become available, were never returned. Although not yet sending applications of employment to such tropical paradises as Fairbanks, Alaska, I expanded the number of states significantly where I would consider living and working, but this didn't make a whole lot of difference because my background/personal experience with head injury was apparently continuing to "turn off" all the places where I had applied.

Straight one day, teased the next, I couldn't get the thought out of my mind that Penelope's locks were adorning the center where I had more than proven myself. In addition to knowing that patients/families were being unfairly cheated getting a counselor who couldn't render a fraction of the impact that I could, the notion that possibly Penelope got the position because of "who" she knows not

New Medico Rehabilitation and Skilled Nursing Center at Meadowlands

May 19, 1989

Mr. Craig Meyers

Washington, PA 15301

Dear Craig:

It was a pleasure receiving your resume recently regarding possible employment as a Family Counselor with the New Medico Rehabilitation and Skilled Nursing Center at Meadowlands.

Following a careful review of all the applicants' credentials, experience, and professional interests, we selected another candidate to fill the position. We will keep your resume on file for one year.

Thank you again for the interest you expressed in seeking employment with us.

Sincerely,

Donna Micklow

Donna Micklow, B.S.N., M.P.A.
Associate Program Director

DM/jld

R.D. 1, Box 146, Route 519 South
Canonsburg, Pennsylvania
15317

Telephone
(412) 745-8000
(800) 346-8391

"what" she knows, weighed constantly on my mind and this never-ceasing torment of not getting the job I deserved had an effect on my physical health.

In the years since my head rapped against that utility pole, I'd never had a seizure. Because of this fortune, since 1/13/87, I had stopped taking Phenobarbital, for Dr. Prostko believed that continuing with anti-convulsant medication of any kind—given the prolonged relative calm of my brain—was no longer necessary. On 1/7/88 and 7/7/88 prophylactic appointments were set up so that I could be checked to see how my forever bruised brain was responding to being medication-free for the first time in five years. As it turned out, everything was working as fine as could be expected. New Medico doing what they did to me only a short time after my dad died from metastatic undifferentiated lung cancer played so heavily on my neurologic system—which had been through enough already—that my brain started to rebel to the stress those fuckin' bastards created for me.

Every waking hour, I focused on my bogus training practice at Meadowlands Health Care Center and would become despondent thinking about how the sorority girl who ultimately acquired this New Medico position could get the job over someone with my training and experience. Penelope's exposure to the rehab population was "zilch" compared to mine and more than likely was limited to when the hunk on her favorite soap opera would wreck his motorcycle and needed treatment. A recurring, taunting nightmare where the Family Counselor position would have been Penelope's all along from the very beginning—no matter how effective this noteworthy survivor would have been in his training—twisted my conscious.

If a case of nepotism was the reason why I was ordered not to make the most of my personal experience with head injury—such as refraining from showing my video to patients/families/staff, and told to narrow what I was to divulge—New Medico not only robbed me of the opportunity to build a prosperous career which I would be dynamically qualified, but took a little piece of heart from those whose eyes would have lit up and worked a little harder upon seeing a survivor come so far in their recovery. Treated with such disregard by New Medico at Meadowlands' administration, I also couldn't help but think that Goyette and Micklow believed that they had every right to act as they did because no former "head injured" patient is worthy of the same professional respect and opportunity as one who has never personally experienced disability.

Dismembering the stability which I had captured through seven years of hard work, I just couldn't stop thinking and thinking about how this New Medico organization underhandedly mistreated this one-time patient who was representative of the disability population they claim to advocate so well for. Unable to make sense of the clandestine way which I was approached by Meadowlands Health Care Center staff, in an unsuccessful attempt to avoid being psychologically overthrown by them and maintain my physical orientation the best I could, I just wanted to keep believing that New Medico wouldn't lie.

Nighttime was Hell. After a day troubled by thoughts of New Medico round-the-clock, when I'd put my head down on the pillow at bedtime and close my eyes to escape this punishing memory, violent white flashes exploding before me would not allow me to sleep. Attacking the darkness, I was terrified because I didn't know if this bright flare of light meant I was about to have a seizure, so an appointment was scheduled with my neurosurgeon for the first time in over a year to find out what was going on. Prior to these fireworks blazing inside of my head, I was never to see a neurosurgeon again, as the July 7th check-up was to forever be my last.

My brain doctor is an absolutely fantastic person, but I wouldn't have minded one bit if I'd have never caught a glimpse of Dr. Prostko again because this would have meant everything was working fine for me upstairs. On 8/24/89, I had an appointment with my neurosurgeon and told him about the night flashes I had been experiencing because of what the farce at New Medico had done to me. Always cautious and thorough, this highly-skilled physician—who sure knows how to settle a brain down—made an appointment for me to have an EEG done at Washington Hospital to ascertain what, if anything, was happening with my brain. An experience I thought I would be over with, I wasn't looking forward to being subjected to a strobe light and having more brilliant lights blowing up before me, but I definitely wanted an answer as to why my mind was detonating nightly.

On 9/6/89, I went to Washington Hospital for this EEG adventure which I thought may possibly result in me going back on anti-convulsants. However, a few days after they slopped my hair up with cream and stuck electrodes on my scalp, I was relieved when informed that there was no sign of any seizure activity. This New Medico-induced trauma would be but one reaction to what was once my promise being incinerated to ash.

Rather than entering the job hunt frontier with the outstanding reference I was deserving—without scruples—New Medico just dumped me in a scrap heap, hoping to never hear from me again. Leaving me to fight the wolves of discrimination without the weapon of support I'd need to disprove long-standing stigmas and prejudice, I was in for a battle that I couldn't possibly win.

After running into walls for so long, trying to locate a rehabilitation employer who would help me and trust my abilities as an aspiring professional, I just got tired of being beaten and bruised. The enthusiasm about my significant background just about dwindling to something bordering embarrassment over what had happened to me, I had just about "burnt out." The more I tried to "get in" with different rehabilitation programs, the more I sensed that companies' horrific presumed inferences about what people with histories of head injury are like kept me from landing a professional position.

Sustaining a belief that there are no exceptions because *all* people with head injuries are the same, it would be a pretty safe bet to assume that employers were unjustly scared when someone surfaces who doesn't meet the standard criteria of what "everybody knows" a person with a T.B.I. history is like. Because I am a member of this unfortunate group, my individual strengths and character were apparently not being considered by employers who probably thought that attaining my Master's was somehow just a fluke. If this generalization and lack of recognition wasn't what guided personnel execs, then a pretty good chance could have existed that employers just didn't want to bother hiring someone so unique because they didn't need the hassle entailed with developing a personalized program to utilize a survivor's potentially invaluable skills and experience. Give an employer a graduate from an ordinary social work program that they can be reasonably certain about or someone who could be incredible, but the literature doesn't support, and there's a good chance the former is going to be chosen every time. I could be positive, given the way I had been dealt with by various rehabilitation managements, that fear had swayed attitudes not to work in my favor.

With misunderstanding and generally accepted beliefs the major influences leading employers astray, I had been unable to utilize the gift of life and strength that God allowed me to earn since my accident, to benefit others. Wanting to do some good for those whose mind had been disturbed did not matter because every rehabilitation door had been closed that I had pursued and the one at New Medico had even slammed in my face. Craving to aid those whose confusion hadn't ceased to linger, head injury and comprehensive rehabilitation program's resistance to me was never-dying.

I felt like David taking on Goliath. In my case, instead of Goliath being a Philistine, the giant was prejudice and discrimination. Because a patient traumatized by a brain injury and recovering to the level which I have been able to triumph to is virtually an unknown, I sensed that rehabilitation directorial bodies would just as soon "give my flesh to the fowls of the air and to the beasts of the field" than to give me the opportunity to work with those who have hurt as I once did. Believing I was presented with the opportunity to make something of myself, so that I could do some good for patients/loved ones in their time of need and not being able to because of the bias that is so widespread amongst rehabilitation professionals, made me want to cry and rip those son of a bitches' eyes out.

Goliath came to David with a shield, spear, and sword, and when I confronted my behemoth, this less-than-tactful foe was armed with the same weaponry. However, being less conspicuous, these tools of destruction were more damaging than any blade could be because I could not see the armor I was up against nor could I even prove its existence because of the hidden, unseen nature this enemy needs to survive. For employers, this concealed property must be preserved at all costs.

The shield used by rehabilitation administrators is the denial that any unsubstantiated, preconceived ideas of any condition exists or unfair action based on this belief is undertaken. Racism is the impression that other ethnic stocks are inferior to one's own, and because of brain injury's characteristic mental deficiency trait, a person with a history of this disorder will be looked upon as always delegated to assume a subordinate position in life. With this global attitude about brain injury no doubt existing within the majority of rehabilitation settings, this "disabilityism" has been my lethal adversary. What really cuts deep is when the governing uppertiers of rehab facilities try to give the impression that they don't discriminate. But given the squiggly lines of the letters in their signatures after "Sincerely yours," and the perspiration droplets soaked in these "There's no way we're going to hire someone like you, so get out of our hair" letters, it wouldn't be too hard to picture these execs—who claim not to grant preferential treatment—sporting "Captain Crunch" social worker smiles when scribbling their name. All the while, they're shaking in their boots and sweating profusely, visualizing a former "head injured" patient decked out in a shirt and tie working for them in a professional capacity.

The spear used by rehabilitation Human Resources Departments is the continued rejections, claiming that so many other applicants are far and away more qualified. Or, they offer the person with a disability an insulting, newly-revised pay scale to fit the job seeker's incapacity. With the hopes that those searching for equality will turn back and retreat, this sharpened shaft will be thrown in order to slow down the pursuer seeking fair consideration. The intention is to bloody the one making the assault on equal opportunity, so they won't persist in their quest to assume a position a healthy person could man. Sometimes this spear will catch its target square, stopping the advance completely. When it doesn't, the cold steel is drawn.

The sword used by rehabilitation Personnel Departments is the refusal to change adverse judgments about—and irrational behaviors towards—a disability group, even after examination of the facts show that there is no basis for holding such an illogical opinion and behaving so unreasonably. It's definitely looking like—regardless of what I've been able to overcome or what potentially tremendous work I could do in the future for those having sustained a disability—it won't matter what impact I may be able to levy for those needing help because those two words, "brain injury," take away every attribute I've ever earned and replaces them with suspicion.

David ultimately triumphed over Goliath with a stone and sling before taking off this favored force's head. My stone is the competence I know that I possess and my sling is the communicative abilities I have to get the message across that fears without a foundation shall collapse and this instability does far too much damage. I can only hope that the sword raised against me shall one day be used to behead my evil opponent as well.

It had been one month shy of a year since I had completed my New Medico internship, earning my Master's, and still rehab centers nationwide were keeping their distance from me. Not willing to consider the possibility that a former patient might just be out there who could offer to those reeling from the effects of a head injury something more than, "You must be feeling upset" counseling, I'd continuously run into walls to no avail, trying to prove that my *former* condition wouldn't be a hindrance. I must have had two strikes against me—if not three—when rehabilitation places where I had applied wanting work reviewed the material on my "brain injured" background. Hypocritically, I'm sure these same rehabilitation execs had a glorious smile on their faces when they spoke with their own admissions about all the opportunities out there for them because of the revised attitude about those who had suffered disabilities involving the mind.

I know that if I were in various rehabilitation administrator's shoes and saw my cover letter highlighting all that I've done following a head injury, I'd be thinking, "If there weren't anything wrong with this guy and he actually had the competence and ability to make the impact he claims, a system like New Medico which could optimally benefit from someone like this would have never let him get away in the first place." But if any sneaking suspicions about questionable tactics were ever voiced by me about New Medico, I could be positive fellow rehabilitation programs would jump to the defense of their rehab cohort and use this as another example of why they shouldn't give me a break. The saddest thing about this whole ordeal is that patients who would have improved seeing someone similarly traumatized will likely never experience such an enhanced outlook and what could have resulted from this optimism. Because of what the Corporation has the potential of doing to these folks and myself, the ghastly governing bodies seeing that the New Medico way is followed through can rot in Hell.

New Medico staff would probably have the view that I ought to be grateful Meadowlands allowed me to serve my practice with them and that I should just stop whining and being a sniveling ingrate. As hard as this may be to believe coming from a former patient who once suffered a brain injury, I didn't pursue a Master's Degree and begin diligently learning some of the methods incoporated within a head injury system just so I could do freebie work, providing my skills during two field practices without expecting a little reciprocation in the form of advancement into the paying work world. For Meadowlands Health Care Center to proceed with me as if I could be laying a foundation for a career—only to destroy this base of support by hiring a kid grossly inferior to myself—was immoral given the way New Medico administration knew what all I've had to endure in my young life already to get this far. Hurt bad enough, the Goyettes and Micklow had absolutely no right to inflict me with further devastation.

Feminists could claim that because three of the four counselors were male, it was imperative that Meadowlands hire a female. The male who got fired by New Medico to create the Family Counselor position—if not "for" Penelope then conveniently timed where this could appear to be the case —might have had a case of sexual discrimination on his hands because Penelope couldn't hold Patton's jock strap when it came to skills and abilities, let alone mine. Hiring Penelope looks like it had nothing to do with a gender issue or quotas, rather, a case where New Medico could either hire a miraculous survivor once afflicted with the disability they treat to speak with those the effects of head injury has knifed, or a healthy "bush league" counselor whose daddy might be able to fill some beds generating some revenue for the facility. But New Medico wouldn't do something so heinous as to put dollars before the quality of care for their patients. Would they?

With the phobia about employing a former "head injured" patient polluting the executive offices of rehabilitation centers and the subsequent unwillingness to overcome faulty judgments about this population, reason would dictate not to reveal the history about oneself, if it doesn't work to their advantage. Headstrong and perseverant as they come, if I think something is worth standing up for—despite maybe more-than-a-few rehab centers perceiving me as a former patient foremost and then a highly-skilled graduate a distant second—I didn't think I should be hiding my extraordinary accomplishments overcoming the symptoms of a brain injury disability, even if head injury rehab Human Resource Managers find it inconceivable that one could do something so unimaginable. Fearful of what this may do to generally accepted guidelines of what a victim of a head injury can ultimately accomplish, rehabilitation facilities from ocean to ocean may not have wanted to deal with me because they didn't understand what was going on exactly and why I wasn't fitting the mold of what was universally recognized as fact about a person's capabilities after one sustains a head injury.

People who know me first as a person as I present myself to them interpersonally, and then discover I was once a former patient suffering from the symptoms of a severe brain injury, are amazed by the recovery I have made, as they have a hard time believing my claims. Unfortunately, like the many rehabs I had been in contact with, people who know me first as a patient either don't care who I am as a person, or will be so judgmental of me that my attributes get clouded. With every little nuance of my behavior under such remarkable scrutiny, it would be impossible to be regarded in an objective or favorable fashion.

If it's God's will for those with histories of a brain contusion to stop living an existence of secrecy because some segments of society want to keep them in the background, mere mortals like Goyette, Micklow, and other New Medico execs are not going to be able to interfere. As unflattering as it may be to look at myself in this manner, if this fear of the unknown premise does exist, New Medico at Meadowlands may have actually been Area 51 where a few extraterrestrials are believed to be stored and I'm one of the aliens being kept from sight because standard beliefs of the way things have evolved over time may need some serious restructuring. If you got questions about head injury, go ask Penelope.

I had two formats of cover letters: one went with the "Craig Meyers Head Injury Package" containing all the goodies about my personal experience with this disability, designed for both comprehensive rehab programs/centers, as well as those specializing in neurologic impairments. And the other to counseling services offered to the general public. One day, in one of my grad school classes, the topic of careers within rehab was looked at and discussed. With the intent of introducing students to an array of specialties within the field, this review covered those arenas desirable to get involved with and those that were not so attractive.

Because of the financial rewards and the skills required to work the job, private-for-profit companies such as New Medico, vocational corporations like Crawford, and a variety of others were deemed as being highly coveted. We were told that on the other end of the spectrum were such outfits as Supported Employment Services (SES) agencies which teach people with an assortment of disabilities how to undertake the various duties required in a low-level job. Being a job coach doesn't require an advanced degree, but I figured since I don't know enough about head injury or disability, working professionally in a rehab center wasn't going to happen, so I took this SES job concluding that my attaining a career position wasn't going to occur, as long as employers maintain their baseless opinions about *all* people with histories of a head injury.

It's quite apparent that when an applicant has sustained a brain injury, this dilutes every accomplishment they've ever made in their life; not only those that occurred *before* the trauma, but *since*. In the view of rehabilitation employers, brain injury and professional standing are two ingredients which "everybody knows" just don't mix.

November 1989, I got my first post-head injury job working full-time in the shadow of my high school in Washington as a "temporary" for a Supported Employment Services agency. Receiving no benefits because of this interim standing, I'd be out of a job again in a couple of months once the regular employee got over his illness. Paying $7 an hour, or a small fraction of what Penelope has been making at New Medico these past seven months being more qualified than myself to work with those whose head injury has put them in a tailspin, I was just glad somebody who actually knew about my head injury had no objection to hiring me. Because of my history with head injury, regardless of my academic background, I guess I should have just been happy someone was willing to give me a few bucks more than minimum wage.

The role of SES is to train and get people with handicaps gainful employment, so they can be contributing tax-paying members of society. Hiring me not only exemplified the purpose of the agency, but got them a Master's-trained student for practically nothing. Wanting to rid myself of this "handicapped" label and be viewed as a graduate school professional whose rare abilities/accomplishments can make a difference for those lives experiencing the rehabilitation world, I was earmarked for depression, as my gloom hit mercurial proportions. Having once had a severe brain injury, I guess I shouldn't have set my sights so high as to think that I should be treated with the same courtesy as those who don't have disabilities. If it weren't for the absolutely fantastic people working for the SES agency and my trying to stay focused on the fact that I was helping a person acquire some skills which could enhance their life, this job training experience would have been unbearable. Wondering how things might have turned out had the circumstances been different with New Medico, I couldn't stop boiling, however.

Shortly after Cyl gave me a tour of different restaurants and grocers approximately twenty-five miles east of Washington in the Mon Valley where I might do some job training, I got my first case teaching a guy who had a mental illness. Breaking in this rookie Vocational Specialist by giving me an assignment only about three miles from home, I was to show my consumer how to go about properly packing and stacking cardboard boxes in the stock room of a department store. Having been "head injured," I just had to learn to be content that I had a job because the type of injury I sustained looks like one where I am going to be approached with leeriness—or at best—indifference. Having a personal history where I had sustained a brain contusion, I suppose I shouldn't have anticipated anything other than working the bottom rung of rehab employment and being overlooked for a promotion into the paying work world. In order to work professionally as a counselor in a rehabilitation program which includes those who have survived a neurological impairment, how much more suffering do I have to endure before my dues get paid?

In a couple of weeks—with my guidance helping him along somewhat—my hard-working, energetic client had learned this warehouse job sufficiently enough where he could more or less do it on his own without me intervening any longer. Physically and intellectually, this big dude could handle the job—but emotionally—he had some trouble relating to his co-workers. And learning how to deal with this difficulty was an issue we had discussed. He denied any symptoms of his disorder were taking place which may have prevented him from being as affable with the others as he was to me, and I had no reason not to believe him.

However, one thing that did occur was that nobody made any overtures to be this trainee's friend and those in the back room with him seemed to have a tough time even being cordial towards this guy who was seeking a permanent position. "Tony" was very keen and he knew he wasn't being approved of by the storage room clique, which was an unfair initiation that would make anybody mad and take away his desire to develop any kind of rapport with anyone. Adding to my client's worries was the fact that the time was approaching where I wouldn't be needed too much longer, leaving this consumer with no one to associate with.

Training sites are not permitted to inquire what an SES client's particular affliction is, so the fellow employees don't know what the person's difficulty may be, only that they're different because they need someone to "show them the ropes." To not be accepted because of something outside of one's control is a hard pill to swallow.

I felt bad about my trainee's interpersonal situation, for he wanted to be received by those in the storage room with him, but I sensed they withdrew and kept their distance because they couldn't be "sure" about him. Being unlike everyone else can be threatening to those who would just as soon live in a conforming planet where no one deviates from the norm. Also harvesting intimidation, like Butch was at Meadowlands with me, insecure co-workers could have their self-concept bruised and egos deflated seeing someone who has had a prior history of being mentally stunted doing a job at a level of efficiency equal to their own, if not surpassing it in some respects.

In many ways, mirroring my own experience, I could assume a similar plight could have existed with the places of employment where I had applied a little under a year ago who knew of my history being seriously hurt and felt it would be too big of a risk to take "someone like me" on board. Tenacious about my pursuit to get into a head injury rehabilitation program as a counselor/advocate where I know I would be stupendous and establish some prominence, I set on another merry-go-round endeavor attempting to "hook on" with a rehabilitation establishment that would prove to be mutually satisfying for both administration and myself. With misgiving running rampant and prejudicial skepticism the fuel driving this apprehension, no rehab center was willing to take a look at me, as an unbroken string of written rejection replies continued to pour in from every head injury treatment facility where I had applied.

Very much aware of my deficits, I could have very easily been accused of being overly self-conscious of those physical functions that I no longer have and of my one-time history being intellectually incapacitated, but rehabilitation employers sure didn't do anything to change my thinking. Their continued paranoia and subsequent resistance hiring me was very difficult to battle after a year of their prejudice, but I had to, if I were to continue believing in myself.

Fighting off the self-doubt that could have stirred within me that rehabilitation center's managements could be right thinking that I wouldn't be an effective professional—because there's a very good chance my record never made it to their file in the first place—I re-sent my cover letter, resume, and all the other information on my personal experience I still wanted to believe would "set me apart" from every other applicant to many of the same rehab centers across the country to let them know I was still available and interested. By the, "We're never going to have an opening for a former patient like you," responses I continued to get from these same quality facilities twelve months later, I can almost be sure that when they saw my correspondence, the fear of God bolted into the hearts of those saints running the show at the different rehab centers where I had re-applied. Surely hoping that they could "pass me on," so I could be someone else's problem, those righteous personnel execs responsible for hiring applicants who I've had the pleasure of corresponding with, likely wished that I had died from some complication of my brain injury this past year.

I realized that if all counseling/advocacy positions within a rehab center are capably manned and there's no need for anymore employees, a company isn't going to terminate a competent professional just so "someone like me" has a place to put their suitcase. Almost every, "Someone with your brain injury history doesn't have to bother applying here again," rebuff response I received from the numerous rehab centers where I had applied made the claim that, if a position does become available which I'd be qualified, I would be contacted. Right, tell me another one.

Within the dozens of rehab programs where I sent my letters of interest and notified them of my credentials, common sense would dictate that over the course of the past year, openings had developed that were filled by people who didn't have a fraction of the knowledge I possessed about disability or the intensive background I own with rehab. Despite my correspondence documenting my qualifications for a position helping those affected by head injury probably being trashed within twenty-four hours of their receiving it, the fire within me to work full-time in a facility treating head injury had yet to be extinguished.

Persistent as ever to be a representative of and an advocate for those whose head injury will change how they are looked upon by society, my unwavering attempts to work with persons suffering through a brain injury condition led me in another direction. Unable to crack into individual rehabilitation centers, I devised another cover letter style and promptly sent it to an organization which could possibly get me some mass exposure. Subsequently, alleviating fears which obviously exist about this former "brain injured" person, I could then attempt to perform my magic with patients and their relatives or friends.

Like when I sent the information on my encouraging recovery and subsequent achievements to the separate rehab centers across the frontier, I was excited because I anticipated that this group would marvel over what I've been able to do and wouldn't want to waste any time "signing me up," for I would be so invaluable. Writing the President of this body which supposedly represents and supports those who have sustained the same disability I once had to endure, I figured it was only a matter of time until I got that phone call instructing me to gather my gear because I was moving to the nation's capital. But instead of this "Welcome aboard!" call, I got hammered with yet another "Don't bug us again"/unwilling to hire me letter.

Sitting on their hands, not willing to assist this survivor who found that his one-time condition was actually preventing him from gaining admission into the rehabilitation marketplace, the National Head Injury Foundation sent me a declination epistle which—paraphrasing and interpreting once again—had an underlying message stating in essence: "Your background/experience are very impressive and inspirational, but don't count on us to help you develop a career working with those who we claim to advocate for, because we're just going to look the other way."

At wit's end, if I had read anymore "Get lost, idealist" notices from head injury programs not willing to help me—but wishing me the best of luck in my continued job search—I would have screamed, "Foul!" I have a real solid understanding of R.E.T., but it's getting increasingly more difficult not to get furious over the apprehensive attitudes centers and organizations have towards this one-time patient who once was a member of the disability population they declare to stand by and promote. But this advocacy claim, I have found, is nothing but a crock of shit.

Turning their back on me, when these institutions decided to give me "the boot" out their rehabilitation doors, they paradoxically symbolized everything they claim to stand up against. Just waiting for me to "snap," figuring something's gotta give, treatment facilities and N.H.I.F. were the last places I thought would react to me in a fashion of guarded bigotry. Unfavorable responses to those who have had head injuries is something that I've personally come to call "The Goyette Syndrome" and this condition has taught me all too well about the widespread inclination of treatment facilities towards those with histories of severe brain damage. This preposterous behavior had left me with no other option than to try to keep quiet about my head injury. But this would make me boil.

One time while I was typing a cover letter to a head injury rehabilitation center and got to thinking about New Medico's claim that Penelope was more qualified than myself to work with those having head injuries, I became so outraged about the universal discrimination which I had been getting slaughtered by that I pounded the card table the electric typewriter rested on so angrily that I knocked it off, damaging it significantly. Not taking into account that there may be justification for such a reaction, the rehabilitation administrations whose centers I have sought employment would probably blame my neurologic impairment for this spurt of agitation or any action they could not understand or wouldn't accept, and point to this as another reason for not giving me a chance to prove that someone so unprecedented could exist and be productive.

One evening, following a day where I spent a good part of the time filling boxes with cartons of feminine hygiene products, I ran into one administrator heading the macabre operation at New Medico at Meadowlands whom I was never able to get in contact with. But being practically hand-delivered to me, I wanted to make the most of this rare opportunity to be heard. Largely responsible for the misery which had suffocated me these past twelve months since December 1988, I needed to wish this New Medico exec a very Merry Christmas '89 and express my fondness for the Corporation.

Almost immediately after walking into Hess's department store in the Franklin Mall, I looked to my left and spotted a reptilian-like figure dodging from the aisle displaying the outlandishly-priced imported perfume to the glass enclosures where the pearl necklaces and diamond pendants were ostentatiously exhibited. No question I was seen, this snake's head was tilted back just far enough back so I'd still be within the bounds of her peripheral vision, yet not so obvious as to not make it look like she was actually looking at the expensive jewelry only an extortionist or a New Medico exec could afford.

With a charm that bubbled with the same glee as the letter she sent me stating that Meadowlands had found someone more qualified than myself to work with their patients, I cheerily said, "Hi, Donna! How are you doing?," to the woman who was more than likely in the administrative office at the time when New Medico at Meadowlands' Family Counselors were coached to do the unbelievable by instructing me to keep my disclosures about my personal experience with the disability they treat to a bare minimum.

With a poorly-acted performance that I caught her off-guard and surprised her with my appearance, understandably not real thrilled she wasn't able to duck out of sight, Ms. Micklow really dug deep to put on a production. Trying to wear her fake New Medico smile and iron out her quivering voice, this New Medico jewel asked me how I was doing as well.

Before she could tell me how the New Medico family was continuing its, "Patients are our number one priority" operation, I asked this Associate Program Director, "How the hell do you figure 'Penelope Rich' is more qualified to work with patients and families at Meadowlands than myself?"

Eyes floating in her head, shocked that I would do something so unimaginable as question the New Medico theater of operation, Micklow got stiff as a board and couldn't keep her voice from shaking when she started off this answer search with a patented New Medico, "Well uhhhhh,. . . . . . . "

Not able to find a believable response, Micklow shirked the responsibility of being knowledgeable about the people administration find to fill vacancies at Meadowlands and passed it off to the New Medico Program Director above her, telling me that she'd let Goyette know that I was upset and that He would give me a call explaining the basis behind His decision. Yeah, right.

Knowing that Goyette doesn't have the swingin' beef to stand up to me, I knew I was never going to hear from Him, so I pushed onward now that I had this sneaking administrator cornered. Saying that Meadowlands discriminated against me and only hired the far-less competent Penelope because her daddy could possibly refer patients her employer's way, this stunned New Medico check-collector would brush this off as an absurd idea coming from someone who has had a brain injury.

Stinking sweat poolin' on her forehead, Micklow tried to drop a bomb on me, only to show Meadowlands' hand and definitively reveal one of the New Medico tactics that I could only previously assume was used against me. When she told me that I wasn't qualified enough for a paid Family Counselor position with Meadowlands because I didn't fully experience the requirements of the job when I served my field practice there, some things started becoming crystal clear.

Micklow told me that, because of my restricted caseload during my seven-month training, New Medico at Meadowlands could not be sure I'd be able to handle all the tasks asked of a Family Counselor. Although she served her placement at another site which had nothing to do with inpatient head injury rehab, determined Penelope could deal with these duties based on a forty-five minute interview.

At least Penelope had the opportunity to express her desire for the Family Counselor position; I was told not to bother coming for this face-to-face meeting because New Medico administration already knew what I could do. Not given the number of people I desired to work with, told to refrain from disclosing anything about my potentially invaluable history, and it being demanded of me that I was not to show my video, Goyette and Micklow had no idea what I could do or the impact I would have because my training was compromised. Feeling as though my hands were tied behind my back and blindfolded the entire time I was at Meadowlands, there would be no way I could fully utilize my value and prove myself. But this apparently was the way New Medico wanted it.

Surely anticipating that I was about to accuse her of purposely limiting my training experience at New Medico when I was there and slighting me because administration knew damn well who would be prancing in the next Family Counselor shoes when a pair hit market—running out of lies—Micklow commented that it was inappropriate discussing New Medico administrative issues in a department store and went worming off into the night, quickly excusing herself. As fate would have it, this month I would read that someone else I know all too well had once again inflicted destruction on a life; possibly as a result of nepotism's favor as well.

If he could have only held out three more days, the 80's could have passed without him killing someone. If he would have only stuck with his first love, to be a forest ranger when he grew up, a woman in her late 60's would likely still be with us. Knowing what strings to pull, mommy Michaels knew how to get her sonny-boy set up in the profession.

Although probably not due to his tendency to abuse alcohol, rather, the culprit could have been his only being on the job approximately six months as a part-time employee. At it again, Paul made another critical mistake, one which would prove fatal to a senior citizen. The Pennsylvania State Health Department and Washington County Coroner's Office investigated the death and a jury ruled the killing accidental, but that Paul was negligent in his treatment. These findings were partially based on the results of a toxicology test done on the elderly victim. If this exam were conducted on the caregiver instead to see what may have been ingested in his system, possibly the verdict could have been different. Tarnished be the soul of those not willing to repent.

After I finished up with my first SES consumer, showing him the right way to fill cardboard boxes and then how to place them on shelves, I was then "promoted" to work with my next client as a bagger in a grocery store. Located in a dying, closed steel mill, rust town, the environment surrounding this food market was symbolic of my outlook, for my enthusiasm about my prospects of one day working in rehab were just about "shot." Like when I duct-taped boxes shut and hauled these heavy, pasteboard containers up on rafts, my spirit quickly hit rock-bottom when the extent of my decision-making was limited to determining if I should use paper or plastic bags for certain items. Earning an advanced degree that gets canceled out by a prior history of a head injury, I was inclined to believe that I shouldn't have expected anything more challenging.

Wearing a smile the best I could, for I didn't want to let my fellow bagger/trainee know how I was truly feeling, too often, some old battle-axe would snap her fingers at this pouchfiller, letting me know I wasn't moving fast enough before telling me she wanted the other type of bag. If I put all her food in a plastic bag and she wanted "paper in plastic," I'd have to take everything out and start all over again, much to the annoyance of the eighteen customers angry at me behind her in the checkout.

Ripping me up inside that securing a position for Penelope in a head injury treatment facility and loading a cart full of groceries wasn't why I got my Master's, role-modeling appropriate behavior for my SES trainee was particularly difficult this one day when three prissy girl students from the college down the road—California University of Pennsylvania—came up to the cashier. Sticking what they perceived as their more advanced, bachelor's-educated noses in the air, they laughed at me seeing what they believed to be a twenty-six year old who was only intellectually capable of demonstrating to a novice food packer the proper technique of how not to put a can of corn on top of a bag of potato chips. The rage I felt being swindled out of working for Goyette's New Medico facility was at a fever pitch.

In addition to filling up bags and putting them in wheeled food carriers, another duty required of the bagger was to collect stray carts out in the plaza's parking lot and put them in a station where shoppers could get them when they came in. Away from the others, while I was alone scavenging the lot for any bastard four-wheeled food carriages one rainy afternoon, my mind regressed and revisited the New Medico fabrication once again.

Herding these buggies together, I hadn't only been getting drenched with droplets of rainwater, but with agony thinking of what New Medico and other rehab organizations had been doing to me since I had needed them for continued progress and assistance in the development of my happiness. Being repeatedly snubbed, I headed into the work force feeling cheated, bitter, and angry.

I felt cheated by the reprehensible means which New Medico at Meadowlands used to underhand me, after all the unselfish, productive work I had done for them as a student. I felt bitter because it was looking like—if I wanted to get anywhere in the vocational world—I had to keep quiet about my fascinating personal experience with head injury that I should be proud of and bellow about because of the gains a good many people could get being counseled by someone coming so far after sustaining a disability of this magnitude. I felt angry because my history of once having a head injury was actually preventing me from attaining a quality job working with those whose brain contusion left them barren of hope. Judgments based on hearsay and actions undertaken without individual examination of the person were evidently continuing to take place in rehabs across the land.

I tried not to rewind the grossly wicked tape of the vile New Medico Corporation and my abominable experience with them, but because I was bitten bad in the "dog eat dog" world of rehab employer's twisted predetermination, this ongoing curse would give me little peace. Coming to a "head" this one dark and dreary mid-day, tormenting thoughts of how this position I was trained for had been swiped from me recurred with a staggering blow.

A few months ago when I was talking to Micklow at Hess's, that angel tried to turn things around and tell me that if I couldn't get over Penelope getting hired instead of me, I had no business thinking that I could counsel patients with head injuries the principle of "acceptance" as a Meadowlands' Family Counselor. Whereas it is essential that conditions following a severe brain injury are recognized if one is to progress, if social injustices such as prejudice, discrimination, and cruel nepotism are approved of without recourse, these unhealthy actions/attitudes shall become sanctioned. Symbolic of the images which formed in my mind, the precipitation outside the grocery continued, as no clearing was in sight.

Divulging my incredible experience with head injury and showing my video would have revealed just how inferior Penelope would be to me for the available Family Counselor position and Meadowlands' administration knew this which evidently was one reason—if not the main one—I was told to limit my abilities and restrict my expertise. In the planning stages, with no deadline date in sight, my primary supervisor unsuccessfully tried to do some consoling over the phone when I called by telling me that, "Well uhhhhh. . . . ," one day Meadowlands MAY start a vocational program and would want someone with a vocational background already in place for the long-term. C'mon, I think most people with any kind of sensitivity would agree that there's no way a head injury neurologic center with any kind of fiber is going to view a student fresh out of school possessing a scant, "anyone with the desire can learn" vocational background as desirable over a survivor who has "been there" and "come out on top." What was New Medico thinking?

Winding back the script to when Butch told me that Meadowlands hired, "a real experienced therapist" when they got Penelope Rich and how—void of any emotion—he flatly said, "Oh," after I informed him that she was only a recent W.V.U. grad/a novice in the field of rehab, questions began filling my mind. First, did this veteran New Medico Family Counselor actually believe Penelope was "experienced" or did he only say this hoping that I wouldn't press the issue and ask him who was seen as more qualified than myself by New Medico administration for the Family Counselor job working with those traumatized by a brain injury? Over the phone, Butch claimed he didn't know Penelope's last name and was this true, or was he being dishonest, knowing that if I knew a fellow student who couldn't hold my jock strap when it came to knowledge about head injury was hired over me, I could cause some flak?

If he did actually believe Penelope was "experienced," did Meadowlands' administration or New Medico top brass in Massachusetts tell this lie? And, if they did, where did they claim Penelope was a paid employee at and for how many years because she was so young, both chronologically and emotionally? Is there a possibility that—in her pursuits to attain a position with a private-for-profit company where the standard of living she was accustomed to could be maintained—Penelope falsified her resume, so that it appeared she wasn't a rookie in the world of rehab?

I'd talk on the phone with this one really friendly, pretty, Meadowlands' employee quite a bit after work while I was training there, just to shoot the breeze and see how things were going with her. Not working in a professional capacity—therefore having no exposure to any administrative coaching on "what" or "what not" to say pertaining to this issue—she claimed one time when we spoke on the phone after I got the big, "New Medico Ripoff," that Penelope wasn't too well-liked and was talked about quite frequently amongst many of the people at Meadowlands. Never one to take much credence in rumor, I wasn't sure what to make of this. Knowing the subjectivity of this situation from my phone pal's perspective and how it doesn't correspond with the partiality of what those in program purport, this anti-Penelope sentiment would be one image my scarred right hemisphere could easily bring into focus, however.

In my opinion, Penelope could almost pass as a younger Shirley Goyette and maybe Program Director Chuck liked this stimulation. Wheels creaking as I was bouncing those empty grocery carts through puddles of water, I thought maybe Shirley G. laughing at me spilling coffee all over my hands and on the floor was a demonstration purposely done to show no compassion or regard existed for me at Meadowlands. As a means to dissuade me from applying at this New Medico three-ring circus, the disrespect exhibited by the Meadowlands ringmaster's wife would be telling.

Not about to kiss Goyette's ivory ass after the way I was dealt with by Him all through my training, may have been a situation that this New Medico Program Director's "standoffish personality" wasn't used to and He wasn't about to hire someone not willing to put Him on a pedestal. Not having the equipment in His narcissistic toolbox to handle someone so enlightened who wasn't going to bow at His New Medico feet, could have been a situation Goyette didn't know how to master. Not worshipping Him surely being sacriligious from His view of things, Goyette could have wanted to hurt me and knew hiring a fellow grad student from the same program I worked so hard in would be an effective way to get even with me. Foremost in New Medico at Meadowlands' mind, it appeared that I first was—and always would be—a former patient whose thinking at one time had gone abroad and an aspiring professional with some uncanny abilities a distant second.

Picking up some wet, loose papers fluttering about with the wind off the asphalt in the lot closest to the Mon Valley Health Center, I couldn't help but think that money talked and daddy Rich's position of wealth and influence had a bearing on New Medico's personnel decision at Meadowlands. Having young families and starting new ones, some of the professionals I was exposed to at New Medico at Meadowlands would naturally want to have an income where they could afford presents at Toys "R" Us as opposed to some discount store. Possibly, from these New Medico professionals' vantage point, sacrificing the demeanors of a few "bruised brain" patients like I once was who don't know what the hell was going on anyhow was a small price to pay, if these name-brand gifts were going to bring smiles on their kiddies' faces.

Surely realizing that a shady deal was going down which would rob patients of the opportunity experiencing a role model who had beaten a head injury and me of the chance to fulfill this capacity, New Medico staff who I worked with shouldn't have been able to look me in the eye. Given what would be done to admissions as I once appeared and how I was about to be personally and professionally disemboweled, the money must have been spectacular, if these Meadowlands' accessories were able to come across as being part of a reputable organization. Because of the inevitability of this discovery, could the conscience of the one female, New Medico Family Counselor been bothering her and this was why Thelma elected not to serve in a supervisory capacity with me during my field placement? Refraining from this guidance, did Thelma think this would absolve her from acting in a hypocritical fashion? Or could there be more trash coming out of the New Medico closet?

Nothing short of crooked—potentially—Goyette and Micklow may yet devastate a multitude of their patients for personal gain, if they hadn't already. If this personnel determination was financially driven, I believed it was an isolated incident only the somewhat remote/rural Meadowlands facility could engage in. Not suspecting that other New Medico operations would design their respective programs to maximize stockholder value, I had no doubt that the overall workings of the Corporation did what was best for its patients. Oh, it's painful to fathom what people do to other people.

Nowhere near to utilizing the counseling skills that I had developed during my grad school training in this SES position, I continued to apply at various rehab centers across the country/in the surrounding region and research the Pittsburgh Press Classifieds for job openings. Tickling their fancy with my "Craig Meyers Head Injury Package," yet obviously not convincing them that I wasn't "goony" anymore, many rehabilitation programs where I had applied would give me a bogus phone call telling me that they didn't have a need for anyone at the time, but would leave suggestions hanging where I would have to use my mental processes and communicative abilities to complete the thought. I deducted that this was done because they couldn't believe my recovery claims and just wanted to hear what I sounded like/ascertain my reasoning abilities.

Or, I'd be asked open-ended questions not pertinent to the job which I applied, as the telephone "interviewer" would just prod me on to use my brain's left hemisphere and express myself. If interrogating me wasn't the method used to establish my sanity, those undertaking this covert investigation also would say something like, "We don't have room for anymore staff right now, but things can change within a couple of months' time."

Stopping there, waiting for my brain's right perceptual hemisphere to pick up that nothing else was going to be said and that this was my cue to fill in the "dead air" blanks by articulating my desire/qualifications for the job and attitude about relocation, these skeptics had to be very anxious to hear what I had to say. Looking for some way—any way—to let me know not to get my hopes up that I actually had a chance to "hook on" with their respective treatment programs, some managements of different head injury rehab centers would say something to the effect that my verbal dialogue resembled my cover letter too closely. Given hell for mentally rehearsing facts that I wanted to make sure I covered. What's next?

Ethnic cleansing is the attempted elimination of social, religious, economic, and cultural factions by a predominant group in society which is threatened/intimidated by the differing standards practiced by this minority class. Hitler tried to do this in Nazi Germany by mass extermination of its Jewish people and rehabilitation employers' preconceived fears that all "head injured" people are incompetent and actions to keep this order of citizens "in their place" were no doubt keeping this somewhat amazing survivor who doesn't come along everyday "under wraps" and out of the rehabilitation workplace.

A head injury disability is an unknown condition which strikes intense fear into the hearts of employers and the terror experienced because of this ailment creates a vocational annihilation of this population bordering genocidal proportions. To exclude hiring someone "you can't be certain about" is a common practice and—because of the universality of this policy—will be generally accepted at all points on the compass. With symptoms of my head injury that have never occurred—and likely never will—being customarily attributed to me by those rehabilitation personnel departments where I had applied nationwide, these Human Resource managements have definitely been my Hitler. "Heil, New Medico."

Thinking that my personal experience with disability would help me secure a job in rehabilitation was a belief that I could not have been any more wrong about. It definitely looked like comprehensive and head injury treatment programs would just as soon prefer that a counseling applicant possess a run-of-the-mill human services background and not anything special because these "open-minded" places weren't exactly sure what to make of my history, or else didn't know how to go about managing someone so optimally qualified.

Left with no other option than to come across as your everyday, popsicle job hunter since possessing "extraordinary" qualification is seen as "extraterrestrial" by rehabilitation employers, I was able to get an interview with a family services' counseling agency in downtown Pittsburgh apparently because the generic resume/cover letter I sent in highlighting my minimal experience was exactly what this non-profit, service provider was looking for in an applicant. Advertising in the Pittsburgh Press the need for a Family Therapist, although it had absolutely nothing to do with rehab, this job sounded like one where I could truly utilize the counseling abilities I had been developing and satisfy my desire to engage in psychological therapy with a challenging population.

Knowing that I was able to land this audition partially because I didn't mention anything about my "brain damaged" history, I was very self-conscious of my hemiparesis and limp. Waiting for the two older, Catholic ladies to call me in for this interrogation, I wasn't so much worried about how I would present myself because I was prepared, rather, I was afraid my obvious physical limitations would prove to be a handicap which couldn't be overlooked. But knowing that I had the skills for this therapy position and the confidence to express my credentials, I was ready to "wing it" and let the chips fall as they may.

Seated in the waiting area of this impressive, metropolitan office, I was sweating blood filling out the application before the interview. I was tense, not because this form had a section requiring verification whether any type of affliction would present me with difficulty performing the duties of the job or if compensatory devices would be needed—for there wouldn't be any—rather, I was scared someone would actually see me filling out this questionnaire. Although I had been doing it for eight years—because my brain's programmed in such a way that I am to be a right-hander—I still physically struggle when moving my left hand along to write, and the letters that eventually get down on paper look like they've been written by someone who has a developmental disability. Fire burning in my stomach thinking about how I obviously have had employment doors slammed in my face by those who were aware of my brain injury disability history and that there aren't too many therapists out there who have been writing their particular way the same length of time as a third grader, I knew my verbal presentation had to be better than my written one, if I was to attain this therapy position. In the back of my mind, I was aware that I had to hide my physical incapacities the best I could, if I was to capture this job, but I tried not to allow this to distract me from what I had to do.

One of the women who would be interviewing me at this Pittsburgh agency headquarters was an administrator and the other, a member of mid-management who was to be my supervisor, if I'd be the one chosen to fill this family counselor slot. After the phone at the front desk rang, the clerical worker stationed there told me that I could be seen now and that she'd show me the way to the office where I was to be questioned. Always conscious of the abnormal way I walk—especially if I want to be inconspicuous—I purposely allowed the secretary to lead the way and walk in front of me, so she wouldn't get an up-close, posterior view of my paralytic gait. Because of my past experience with employers, I feared that these two trained observers of human postures/reactions would take note of my chopped-up right ear, my waddling in, and censored presentation, and come to the conclusion that I was damaged goods who was not deserving of fair consideration.

However, during the course of the interview, judging by the correct responses I had ready for them and the frequent smiles on their faces indicating that I had given them the answer they were looking for, I felt pretty confident about my chances of acquiring this counseling post after this drilling ended and even a little stunned that I was treated so fairly. I guess my hair was at such a length it covered my 120-stitch scarred right ear and limped into the room at a time when the ceiling light was dim, not reflecting much of my funny walk.

Although never inappropriate or the least bit intimidating during this question and answer prerequisite for this family therapy job, when inquiries were delivered my way by these two sharp ladies, I had to battle back thoughts that weren't going to do me any good which made me my own worst enemy again. When asked about my experience working with adolescents, for example, my mind wavered from my training at New Medico where I shared with the teen from Kentucky some of my personal experience with head injury which I confronted as a traumatized youth, to me, as an eighteen-year-old, lying comatose on mattresses. If these ladies only knew that it had only been a little over a handful of years that I wasn't even able to talk, write, move, or make sense of my surroundings, there would be no way I would be given this opportunity for a position of such responsibility.

Gut churning, sensing that these two social worker, mind readers' piercing eyes could read me like an open book, my frayed nerves tried to seize control over me, but I fought hard to keep my composure. I dueled the thought that I wouldn't even be here trying to convince these two senior therapists of my capabilities for this important therapy job, if I hadn't concealed the brain injury chapter of my life, with images of all that I've had to accomplish "against all odds" just to be in this envied position and how any agency should be honored to staff an employee so determined.

With select snatches of my New Medico rehab experience edited for survival's sake, with my mind reviewing what would be safe to divulge, I highlighted the favorable points of the interaction with this blue-grass teen which brought expressions of approval to the faces of those putting me under the microscope. All in the eye of the beholder, what one may perceive as true character and strength under magnification, another may see as bacteria. Having the foresight not to self-disclose helped me acquire this position located in the young professional's haven of Monroeville where, coincidentally, was the exit my oldest brother got off at the turnpike to see me when I was comatose at Allegheny General Hospital. Talk about an omen.

This long-standing counseling agency was going through a period of reorganization where tenured therapists who had been at their respective locations for eons were being transplanted. And a few of these counselors—who were reluctant to retire and had adhered to some outdated modes of therapy which didn't work so well in today's complicated society—were subtly being asked to reconsider their longevity plans and if they really wanted to go through a transition period, putting off their pensions. Opposed to change, some of these therapists—liking to classify themselves as Neo-Freudians practicing psychoanalysis—certainly had to have viewed the arrival of fresh, young blood in their prime being hailed into jobs once habitually reserved for the "over 55" club as a sign that the time had arrived to start a new chapter, for the "status quo" was no longer going to be accepted. It was a given that an alteration in the philosophy of the way things were done had to occur, if the agency were to be marketable. Balking at the notion that therapists actually do more than sit on their "duff" and reflect how the client was feeling, several Rogerian/client-centered practitioners weren't all that pleased with the agency's desire to adopt a brief treatment, more action-oriented approach utilizing modern methods. Among other things, abandoning prehistoric counseling styles was undertaken in order to appease insurance carriers and managed care organizations providing financial support for client policy holders.

It wouldn't have shocked me too much, if I'd have heard one of the war-horse therapists—comfortable with the way sessions had been conducted for the past twenty-five years and reluctant to change their "Did your mother breast feed you?" approach—say something like, "You can keep your new-fangled, contemporary, psychedelic principles which supposedly have proven to be effective. Give me the traditional, old-fashioned way of going about business any day that I'm used to and things'll be fine." It looked like the day had dawned where oldies were no longer necessarily being viewed as goodies, and it appeared I had been designated as a symbol of this trend to do away with the old and bring in the new by the "mid-20th century" staffers.

I wouldn't think of "making light" of or take away from the trying difficulties of yesteryear which has allowed today's generation to enjoy many fruits of previous era's labor, however, with all the demands of today's more technologically advanced world and the subsequent increased abundance of choices/obligations, the everyday stress on a family now is that much more incredible. This is evident by the escalating divorce rate, number of single parent households, incidence of mixed families, behavioral difficulties with children at school, and problems in the workplace. Because of the diverse nature of difficulties nowadays, the agency was going through a revision process where therapists were delegated to focus on and work within particular specialty dilemmas. Those established, well-read, vets of the agency being shuffled about the organization and no longer free to counsel those experiencing a vast array of problems was seen as regression/a harnessing of their abilities by these seasoned troops who didn't like the writing they were seeing on the wall. Such was the environment this twenty-six year old therapy professional, approximately ten to thirty years younger than most of his family services' cohorts, was welcomed into.

What a person feels about another—more times than can be seen—has nothing at all to do with any actions or background of the one being judged, rather, what the one "on trial" reminds their peer(s) of will determine how they will be received. In someone's perception, if a total stranger is somehow symbolic of a good quality, it's human nature to accept this individual as one who represents healthy attributes without really investigating the facts. Based on one's impression, either favorable or adverse, opinions/assumptions will be "transferred" onto the unwitting recipient being revered/ostracized. Bearing a psychological resemblance to an image which exists in one's mind of another person, event, or idea—many times—will lead to unfair criticisms and unwarranted judgments.

One's character being approved of or not has a lot to do with what's going on internally and externally at the time with the person assigning those positive or negative traits. "Transference" is the unconscious identification of characteristics to a person/principle and this unsubstantiiated association could influence one's overall attitude about someone/something. For example, the feeling towards a person may have absolutely nothing to do with the one being examined's predisposition or how they generally present themselves, rather, the mood created within the arbitrator can often be dependent on what has happened in their history and/or is presently occurring in their life. My arrival at this agency coincided with the emotional tone of upheaval which can frequently occur when an establishment is being organized differently.

Being affiliated with the turbulence which can occur with change didn't help matters much when it came to me being recognized as a professional possessing a multitude of abilities. A little on the peculiar side to begin with, as many of their own questionable personal life histories may indicate, some of these therapy professionals seemed to have had a tough time of it exhibiting the necessity they must demonstrate with their clients—unconditional positive regard—when a newcomer, who unintentionally represented overhaul, arrived on the scene.

If being symbolic of agency-wide renovation wasn't why I was being approved of by several of the older therapists right from the start, I could only hope that it didn't have anything to do with an accurate, highly-educated guess as to what my disability could be, for a few of my physical symptoms resulting from my brain injury screamed for attention. It didn't take long for me to find out how I was being looked at by a certain faction of therapists who had to be better with the people who came to them for counseling services.

There was this group of seasoned, male, professional employees who would congregate in an arbitrarily chosen office at the Monroeville agency and have private discussions which apparently spawned a lot of humor given the cackling that could be heard clear on the South Side of town. Calling themselves, "The Boys'

Club," this social clique comprised of a handful of professionals who would get together when they could, laughing about a variety of topics which I would soon find out didn't exclude me and told me something about how I was thought of. Knowing of my background as a greenhouse employee before I headed off to college and surely to make light of my limited experience as a counselor, a few derogatory comments were made over the course of a short time which didn't do a lot to make me feel welcomed.

I selected the counseling profession as a career to pursue because it matched many traits of my individual personality and not so much for any monetary rewards, thank God. Just out of school and not exactly floating in cash with all the debts/expenses that life will accrue for someone, with this therapy position paying a Social Worker wage, I just made "do" with what I already had until the cash flow picked up a little bit.

With spring knocking on the front door, the weather outside went from being miserably cold to chilly, so I had to wear the black, leather jacket my dad got me for Christmas several years ago when I was a W.V.U. student. This attire and knowing of my guitar playing history earned me a nickname by these same therapists who suggest to their clients that they not ridicule others' individual differences. Asking him not to refer to me in this manner, this one Boys' Club member therapist repeatedly called me another name which—to my face—would appear to be one friendly in nature, but behind the underage Boys' Club's closed doors, could very easily have been sexually construed into something else like a cartoon in the back of a "Mad" magazine. Mind you, these weren't uneducated people, rather, world-wise counseling professionals making these snide remarks. Maybe because they hadn't thought of it, I never overheard if I had been referred to as "Cripple Craig."

Realizing that I didn't have too many therapy allies on my side, being the first therapist in their twenties hired to work in the Monroeville office during the reorganization, I wasn't going to complain to anyone about something which could be seen as trivial. I could have been viewed as a "scab" by some of the old-timers in the agency who perceived me as representative of the new wave of counselors gaining admittance into the program which previously had been stationed by those who had completed their apprenticeship decades before, so I wasn't going to gripe. Possibly, a few of these therapists mistakenly assumed that I was hired only because administration assigned to fill available positions felt sorry for me being so young and hobbling around. If these therapists wise in the ways of the world thought that their long-time family counseling peers weren't being recycled in order to create space for a "sympathy case," I knew the road ahead would be a hard one.

I started working this family counseling post in February 1990 and by the time April rolled around, only two months into my new job, I would be confronted with two obstacles which I would have to overcome in order to preserve my professional well-being. Not being seen in the most favorable of terms as it was, talk about horrendous timing.

The agency employed a Bachelor's-educated intake counselor whose responsibility it was to answer incoming calls from people in the community requesting counseling services and to document some information on these potential clients-to-be. Depending on the area they were calling from and the nature of the problem, these persons seeking help were assigned to a therapist within the agency, if their difficulty didn't have anything to do with severe substance abuse or a profound mental illness (psychosis, personality disorder, or chronic depression). In these cases, future counselees would be referred to organizations better equipped to provide these specialty services.

One week, this phone counselor was off which meant that the therapists on staff had to take turns answering calls from these prospective therapy customers. As luck would have it, one day in-between the clients I had scheduled that afternoon, I was available to answer one of these calls and what I'd be told by this upset woman put me in a difficult predicament.

Distraught about the veteran therapist this lady found out she would be counseled by, voice trembling, this woman told me that there would be no way she'd go see this service provider because she knew of a former client who had accused this worker of engaging in unthinkable behavior with her while she was in the therapy office. Being the new employee in town and given that I wasn't exactly being embraced by senior members of staff, I couldn't believe this was happening. Feeling like my first consumer at SES who worked in the stockroom of that department store and wasn't being revered by his co-employees because his having a handicap seemed to have hurt the pride of those he worked with, the last thing I needed was to be put in a position where I could cause some static for someone who was very popular amongst the other workers in the agency.

After this troubling conversation ended and I hung up the phone, on the daily time sheet therapists are required to fill out indicating what their duties entailed within the last twenty-four hours and with whom—in addition to marking the length of time in minutes of this interaction—I jotted down this shaken woman's name and the code numbers stipulating that the service provided was an intake call, as well as what office she would have been seen had there not been any trouble. Now for the tough part.

Immediately, one wants to believe that a fellow counselor wouldn't take advantage of a client and that the only reason an accuser would make such a charge would be because of something that was discussed in a session that they—or a member of their party—didn't care for. On the other hand, because of the regard that is essential and must take place within a counselor-client interaction, as difficult as this may be, a therapist can't completely discount a consumer allegation. Pulling at me, I battled with this quandary.

The first thing that came to mind was that, if I did tell someone of this incriminating exchange and it more than likely proved false, I'd be seen as the new kid on the block, troublemaker who must have thought that this well-liked, tenured suspect might have been guilty or else I wouldn't have reported it in the first place. My second thought was that if I didn't tell anyone of this complaint and word filtered back to administrative management about these misgivings and that I was the one who took the call, I'd be setting myself up to be the "fall guy" because nobody would lose any sleep, if anything happened to this limping, new worker. Either way, I knew I was in a no-win situation.

A source of merriment, humor, and relief for many, I could just picture this therapist's friends making life at the agency that much more difficult for me, figuring that I was deserving of being on the "hot seat," for a young therapist isn't to report any allegations involving a senior staff member. Struggling to do what was best, because this woman felt she needed help and trusted me to do the right thing, I had to "make good" by her. After this difficult internal deliberation, I reported this unsettling incident to my mid-management supervisor because this was an issue to be addressed by the executive branch of the agency, not a beginning therapist.

"Fluffing it off" as if it were nothing to be concerned about and never happened—at least as far as this long-time job-holder was concerned—my supervisor told me that clients will get mad at their therapists on occasion and try to get back at them for something. Faster than one could say, "No big deal," the whole incident was viewed as an unjust personal vendetta and quickly forgotten about.

The two things which sold me on this job when I elected to work here were—first and foremost—the abundance of adjustment counseling that I would be engaged in, and secondly, the appealing bonus of working in the attractive, bustling suburb of Monroeville where I was told I would be counseling single parents and/or their children four-and-a-half days out of five. There's this one run-down district within the Pittsburgh city limits where, if you're a male who wants to make something out of themselves, your life expectancy is ten days—two weeks tops—if you can run fast. With my name inked on a contract, considerable thought was directed towards permanently placing me in this area for the indigent full-time after I had only worked at the agency approximately a month. Talk about a bait and switch.

I didn't know if I should've perceived this assignment to work in the slums and the callous way I was approached by counseling professionals early on as an intentional means to hasten this lame person's exit out of the agency, but I did. I thought that possibly some influential members of staff sensed/"got wind" that something happened to my neurological system, as my "one hemisphere's not working" walk and handwriting could have spilled my secret that this young counselor once had severe brain damage. If being sickened by suspicion that I had a neurological dysfunction affecting various abilities at one time wasn't why things weren't clicking at first, for my own peace of mind, I just had to convince myself that the transfer consideration and lukewarm reception were simply due to disorganization/a needed period of adjustment until things settled.

Whether it was these couple of things or possibly transference, I knew I could be perceived as prejudiced myself and not a team player refusing to work in the ghetto, for this area could be a gold mine of income for the agency. With the crime rate against innocent victims in this poverty-infested neighborhood so incredibly high and with only half of my body working to defend myself, I didn't want to be a sitting duck. Talk about making a good first impression.

Human Services Development Fund (HSDF). So that people who normally couldn't afford counseling would have the opportunity to receive therapy, our agency was granted HSDF money as reimbursement for providing freebie services to clients. At a rate of $90 an hour, the agency could have really cashed in with the HSDF dollar had I not been so concerned with self- preservation and went jovially skipping along into skid row. Already having one near-death experience during my young life, I felt deserving of taking a break from risk for a little while.

Because of the agency's reorganization, my role hadn't been clearly defined yet. Once a week, I tagged along with a senior therapist to some HSDF-haven projects where she'd discuss with residents issues such as how these subsidized housing "lifers" were going to catch the world on fire and be successful in their pursuits to attain independence and how—with their welfare check incomes—they could get their little ones through med school. With most of the sparse crowd wanting to be left well enough alone, my task during this educational enterprise was to get two dozen cinnamon sweet rolls for about five bucks at the restaurant down the road, so somebody would bother to show up. At ninety government dollars a head, the agency sure got a good return on this expenditure. And usually, there were a mess of goodies left over.

After a few more weeks of relative stagnation, the brain trust at the downtown office developed a better idea of how to delegate/utilize its manpower and became a little more focused on how to situate the schedule/assignments. After this tall order had been chipped away some, amongst an abundance of other reorganizational matters, the top brass figured out better ways of how to go about using me. With things picking up on the administrative end, coupled with students being home for summer vacation to get in their parents' hair instead of the teachers', my caseload boosted and kept me pretty busy. With more people coming for therapy, it was finally time to get down to business and incorporate the techniques I had learned all through my training.

One primary aspect of our job as therapists was to get an understanding of how clients' actions relate to what's going on in their environment or how the client PERCEIVES what's taking place, for these can be two very different things. A productive outcome of therapy would be one where the therapist allows the client to see what they can do to improve their situation. Depending on the circumstance, I'd use a variety of approaches.

For difficulties requiring immediate attention, I'd utilize a brief treatment modality. For example, examining a situation in search of solutions to a dilemma, sometimes it's valuable to go over the elements of an ordeal so that, hopefully, a client will ultimately begin incorporating appropriate problem-solving skills. Looking at the various dynamics of an event and weighing the aftermath of particular decisions is an invaluable aspect of Reality Therapy.

If a person encounters a problem with a decision that they don't know what to do, in order for clients to see the potential consequences of their actions, having them make a pros and cons checklist could prove beneficial because they wouldn't only be thinking about their troublesome situation and how to go about taking the steps necessary to address the issue while sitting in the therapy room, but give them a tangible object which to refer later at home when they're not in the counselor's office. When clients can discover for themselves the nature or basis of a particular circumstance which is giving them some concern, sometimes with the therapist helping these folks along to dig underneath what may appear to be occurring on the surface, the impact of this search can be long-lasting and serve as a model for future encounters. One thing an effective therapist does is help their clients develop skills to handle tomorrow's undertakings.

If a client is having troubles with certain people they can't avoid, sometimes recreating a drama and effectively handling the turbulence in a reenactment has the best chance of sticking in the minds of those seeking assistance when they come face-to-face with a problematic situation again. Whether it be parents, peers, teachers, bosses, or a host of other members of society, an approach which incorporates this role-play can work wonders for those experiencing interactional difficulties. Because they have practiced how to go about dealing with certain troubles, there's an increased likelihood clients will have a better understanding of how to handle an intense encounter, if it presents itself again. Instead of only speaking of a situation, the Gestalt characteristic of actually trying to put the client in the dysfunctional environment is how this counseling technique gets its trademark effectiveness.

To get a client to relive an emotionally trying event isn't always easy because of the pain involved and, especially for some who are overly self-absorbed, people can feel silly thinking that they're in a theater production without realizing the benefits of actually placing themselves in the eye of the hurricane again and practicing ways to address what's bugging them. I could just see some of the self-proclaimed Neo-Freudian, senior therapists laughing at me about my use of this "hallucinogenic" approach during the staffings with the consulting psychiatrist and dismiss its effectiveness. Gimme a break.

The psychodynamic method of counseling—cognitive therapy—operates under the basic premise that one has control of their life and emotional reactions, not some extraneous variable like another person or thing, because "*You feel how you think.*" Since the person doing the thinking is the only one who can ultimately produce what occurs with their thought processes, the person with the power to create dialogue in the mind has control of their emotions and subsequent actions, not any perceived manipulative force. This approach stresses that thoughts create feeling which ultimately influence behavior. Therefore, thoughts are the generator of one's affect, with this emotional tone leading one to operate in a particular fashion.

It's important to stress to clients that they do have a say over what goes on in their life because, too often, they don't take responsibility for what happens because they can have a tendency of always assuming the victim role and assigning control of what occurs to everyone and everything, but themselves. Also, it's noteworthy to point out that this "thoughts create feelings which produce behaviors" train of thought can be an inverse process influencing mood because, if one changes their behavior, this can alter how they perceive or think about a variety of situations. This revised way of taking note of the world can enhance one's outlook as well. Ask any dieter who has lost a good bit of weight.

Along with employing this foundation for Rational Emotive Therapy's Action, Beliefs, and Consequences substitution of dysfunctional thoughts platform, Transactional Analysis would be another therapeutic mode I would customarily take out of my intervention toolbox to try and make some sense out of why my clients may react/respond as they do. Every person, according to Eric Berne, is comprised of three parts which he alludes to as ego states. Dividing the personality into Parent, Adult, and Child segments, a person operates from each one of these states given a particular situation. Each individual has these three modes of operation and, depending on the nature of the event, which function gets activated can very likely determine the outcome. If the results aren't what is desired, a client may want to develop a conscious understanding of what state they were operating from at the time and attempt to make the appropriate adjustment.

If a person is in a situation where it would be most beneficial to think, feel, and act like a parent might (such as when the traits of discipline, nurturing, and authority are needed), they are best served, if they are in their "Parent" style of interacting. Situations which require the use of facts and information such as those characteristic of incorporating compromise, negotiation, and logic, the person needs to be in their "Adult" ego state. When having fun, possessing no cares, being impulsive, and self-centered are what's necessary to make a circumstance right—like a vacation or picnic—the "Child" function is what needs to come to the forefront. From birth to adulthood, the transactional analyst believes that there are four lifestyle positions based on a person's experience and degree of acceptance of self and others, with the "I'm O.K., you're O.K." position being the optimal, "adult" phase.

Frequently, parents would call in for counseling because they wanted the therapist to "fix" their kid and, in some cases, initially I'd give them just enough of what they'd want, so they could be enticed with a carrot to come in for more counseling to work on the real core of most child problems—the parents themselves. Operating under the premise that, "We are the way we are because that's how our parents made us," it's essential then that—after the behavioral techniques are employed which may provide some temporary relief remedying the immediate problem—the real "nitty gritty" of the issue gets focused on.

This is where the sometimes painful "scripts" and "messages" of early childhood need to be taken out of the trunk, dusted off, and looked at, so the client can understand themselves better and move on with an enhanced acceptance of how they "came to be" in their luggage. Often, a parent would request therapy services saying that they want counseling for their child/teen because their offspring is exhibiting behavioral problems when, in fact, these fathers and mothers may actually have a strong hunch that the core of their problem(s) is a much deeper developmental history issue which is causing much of the unhappiness being experienced within the family. In order that they can proceed in a more stable and productive fashion, many of these admirable people seeking help for their difficulties really want their influential past explored, so they can make better sense out of things.

For instance, a little kid might be referred because s/he is fighting, having trouble in school, disobedient/not listening, and/or smoking when this is only the tip of the iceberg. An adolescent may be at risk for drug use, dropping out of school, running away, pregnancy, or continued truancy and this is why mom or dad say that they want some guidance. More times than not though, this is only part of the story.

Often, because of their inability to communicate effectively, kids will let an adult know that something's bothering them by their actions. And here is where therapists need to be sensitive and tie in the child's responses to what's actually going on in their surroundings, so they can help the family see the dynamics of a situation. With an enhanced realization of what's really occurring, caring families will usually find the ability to keep their head above water and weather the storm together.

For example, usually when little kids start smoking, that's more than likely a sign for a therapist that something negative is going on with them. A therapist who works with families knows that, from a child's perspective, negative attention is better than no attention. To find out why a kid may feel that this vital, nurturing ingredient is missing in their life, a therapist must examine the home environment to find out what is and isn't happening there first before any remedial action/treatment can take place.

Many of my single parent clients had strong parenting skills, however, more than a few lacked these essentials because they didn't have solid parental role models themselves to form a base of how to go about resolving problems. With an abundance who had fallen into the repeating patterns cycle of single parenthood, some elementary strategies which would have been learned and incorporated in their own approach had they witnessed them in use during their own formative years, needed to be taught to those caregivers hungry for information. Fundamental rules and approaches that a parent needs to know to be effective aren't genetically inherited, rather, these learned behaviors are attained from observing prior generations at work with their children. If this nurturing relationship was missing from a parent's own homelife, they'd have little or nothing to fall back on from their own childhood experience.

So many parents came into therapy because they needed help disciplining their children. Quite a few allowed their "rug rats" to take over the house, figuring if they let their little tikes run wild and do what they pleased, this would be an expression of their parental love. When kids sense that there are no controls, that's when all hell breaks loose, making life absolutely miserable for mom—and if there's one around—sometimes dad, too. Many parents came into counseling claiming that they wanted a little bit of insight into what could be done to alleviate some of their kids' hellion antics, but many realized they needed to work on themselves as well, and were a little "gun-shy" at times to concede this.

Tossing these parents a smidgen of the bait they wanted, so that they could see a few immediate results and be enticed to come in again, I'd implement a behavioral chart or a behavioral checklist which would often bring expressions of satisfaction to their faces. Discussing this token system of rewards and punishments, I'd be able to get a little flavor of how some of the mechanics of this parent-child association operates and look into what the parents' primary role was with this impaired union. A good bit of the time, these parents just simply needed to establish some basic guidelines with their children about what is to be expected of them and here was where I'd try to help some.

In order for kids to develop in a healthy manner, they must experience "security." To be able to predict what's going to happen in their life gives children a sense of safety and stability in this world overflowing with intimidating grown-ups. When a child is at ease/comfortable with their surroundings and what occurs within it because set guidelines have been established, this can greatly assist in the promotion of a well-rounded upbringing. Because these are the first people a child is exposed to and identifies with, parents are the ones who develop their little ones' perception of themselves and what impression they have of the world. Consistency is essential in the fostering of this initial identification.

In the parent/child interaction—without a doubt—children want disciplined because this is a parental sign that these tiny people are loved and cared about, and hence, important in this planet which can have its threatening moments. With approximately 98% of the single parents I'd work with being female, often, they'd feel guilty about not providing their child with a paternal figure, believing that this omission would somehow inevitably interfere with their baby's development. And, as a sort of consolation prize for not giving their child a daddy, these moms believed they could "make it up" to their son(s) or daughter(s) by giving their fatherless offspring the "run of the house."

It would then be important for me to stress that the "quantity" of sources this love came from wasn't what was necessarily important, rather, the "quality" of the love received was the significant factor in the eyes of a child. With the discipline equaling security equation in mind, it was imperative to stress that kids need to see what the consequences are going to be for their actions for—if this pillar is weak—the frame which is growth and development could come crashing down.

Any healthy kid is going to test limits because they want to know who the *boss* is. And if these limit-testers get the notion that they're the ones in charge—"look out"—because the walls are going to start tumbling down. It's vital that a parent not only lay down the law, but just as importantly if not more, enforce the rules of the house *each and every time* they are broken. If a child can get away with something one time, but the next, there are punitive repercussions for the misbehavior, they don't know what to make of things and this uncertainty about what "gives" makes life miserable for everyone involved.

Like when demonstrating how to use the behavioral chart and checklist, I'd go about explaining to a parent how to go about using a very simple, but effective, strategy which could help them discipline their rambunctious little darlings called the "What's the Rule?" technique. This method entails that a parent tells their child what behavior is expected of them, and that if they intentionally do something bad/opposite of what they've been told instead, certain negative consequences are going to follow *every time* the parent's orders are not followed through. After the parent explains to the child how they are to behave—so they know that they've been heard correctly—the law-making parent will ask their child to verbalize back what rule has been set.

Focused on the specifics of this behavioral exercise—without realizing it—a parent would frequently divulge some information about the dynamics of the relationship with their child that they normally may not in a question and answer counseling framework. Trying to get a sense of how the parent and their child connect, knowing that children are reactive because of their minimal life experience, the real cause of any dysfunction would, 99.9% of the time, point back to those raising the easily-manipulated child. And here is where it would be important to tie in what has formed the parent as they are.

Digging beneath the surface of this parent-child interaction dysfunction, sometimes painful themes which have occurred during these authority figures' lives become exhumed such as guilt, shame, feelings of omission, abuse, etc. And this is where some exploration of the chronic baggage which may have been so skillfully hidden in a parent's closet needs to be looked at and sometimes dissected. Frequently, in this hunt for answers to long-standing problems which usually have been "gaining steam" by tapes of past turbulence, this search could uncover some skeletons the client didn't even know about.

It's important to find out how clients currently perceive things, what "messages" they got from their own parents about themself/life in general when they were impressionable children, and—with the client's input always a given—try to revise any faulty perceptions/private logic if possible, which could contribute to any dysfunction that interferes with the attainment of happiness. Finding the factors which may interrupt feelings of joy can sometimes be facilitated, if the client is permitted to take the ball and run with it.

There will be a fair share of occasions when an action-oriented method of intervention isn't going to be as effective as one which utilizes a Rogerian/client-centered approach where the client is guided to discuss pertinent issues through reflection, empathy, and unconditional positive regard. Especially with clients who appear easily intimidated with a standard inquiry/respond format, it would be best to establish a style of interaction where the client is free to talk without being questioned. With people who are the survivors of incest, for example, this delicate delivery can particularly be effective in helping a client to master some of the psychological hardships that will hit them head-on.

Employing a more direct methodology to ascertain how past experiences influence current functioning could be viewed as therapist insensitivity on the part of the client and these counseling service patrons who came to the agency in the first place to better cope with their particular dysfunction may just "clam up" again, keeping everyone at a safe distance. If a client is going to open up the floodgates and let uncomfortable feelings which have been harbored—sometimes for a lifetime—gush forward, they must feel comfortable with the person they are discussing issues with and not feel pressured. Troubles left to simmer can flame into an inferno later on.

Once in a great while, because the vast majority of these single parent women have had more than their fair share of troubles with their male counterparts, a client may tell me that she'd feel better talking over certain sensitive topics with a female therapist. Realizing their opinion of this therapist's gender had been blackened, I would assure my tentative client that this could be arranged, if she found it absolutely essential that this would be the only way progress could be made. However, I'd also ask these ladies, before they made their final decision, to give me a chance to work with them because if they talk with a member of the opposite sex who possesses a few traits that they didn't think any male had, this role-modeling therapeutic benefit could be more advantageous than any technique that may be set into motion.

Seeing it from this vantage point, these open-minded female clientele would always reconsider this transfer request and stick it out with me. This acceptance would be a major step in the direction of healing because many of these women had impenetrable walls, keeping out anyone who had anything to do with the male gender.

A few female clients could have held an anti-male position and tried to cover this viewpoint up by saying that they could not see a therapist who didn't have any kids themself being able to relate to them. Or if they did actually believe this faulty assumption, I'd be quick to point out that, although I had no children in my personal life, my experience counseling a multitude of others' throughout Allegheny County made me more than capable. Using the analogy that a doctor never had to have a particular disease to treat it, clients would look at it from this perspective and realize that if a professional wasn't qualified, they wouldn't be engaging in these type of services.

Not being in the client's shoes, I could also understand completely that there would be no way I could fully appreciate all the relationship turbulence—from the identification with father to the disruption with their children to the obstacles that can occur within intimate relationships—which can be so characteristic of single parenthood. However, working with so many people who have to raise their children by themselves, I could get an accurate approximation of the emotional overtone of the situation—but by no means—not an out-and-out comprehension of their ordeal. Whether the origin of their difficulty stems from a paternal figure background history issue or a romantic relationship circumstance, innocent children twisted in this entanglement often suffered dearly.

Not possessing the know-how, experience, maturity, or language concepts of an adult, trying to get an impression of what may be happening in the mind of a child or teen can pose an abundance of obstacles. A counselor needs to interact with their younger client in a manner which these youths can relate to, and not say something like, "We are going to look at the interchange between the superego and the id; while simultaneously attempting to acquire a comprehension of how this association is being manifested within the psychological constructs of the reality principle's ego." With a look on their face void of any expression, a little kid isn't going to know what the hell you're talking about and an adolescent is going to turn you off faster than you can say, "Get away from me, asshole."

By the same token, if a therapist is too anxious to get on the same wavelength and tune in on their young client's frequency, the kid is going to read these motives too and slam their hatches down tight. There's a fine line between being an insincere fake and so sophisticated that talking over someone's head had been such a trademark ritual that viewing the world from a young client's vantage point could not be possible. Being able to respond to both children and teenagers on their level, I could make an identification with them that they could sense. And because of this, develop a rapport which could harvest some productive results.

Concurrent Play would be something I would have absolutely no objection to and wouldn't feel the least bit awkward engaging in because I could very easily transform into a big kid, if I needed to. In order to help take these small guys' awareness away from being in a therapist's office, if I had to drop to the floor and play paper football on the low-set coffee table in my office in order to help a tot relax and take their mind off of the fact that they were talking to an adult stranger about what's happening with them, down I'd go trying to get the corners of these celluose pulp pigskins to hang over the edge of the table. I didn't know if I was supposed to react in this way because I was to be professionally focused on creating therapeutic movement within the session, but I would have fun too sometimes with these games. Being viewed as a young "whipper-snapper" with an assortment of radical approaches to therapy wasn't pleasant, but I'd try not to focus on this.

While trying to get these distracted youngsters to feed me a little information at a time, while I'd be touching my two index fingers together and putting my thumbs straight up to make a field goal post, I would reflect how lonely it must be not having a daddy to do this with anymore. A few would give me a prolonged hesitation, looking at me with a blank stare as if I were nuts, before talking about this sensitive topic. And some of these little fellows would be happy to be presented with the opportunity to dump their feelings of absence onto someone who wanted to know how badly they really were being cut up inside. Having an adult flop down to their eye level and be goofy playing a game (which is what these little dudes new life is all about), can help reduce the intimidation of talking with a man about touchy issues. And the kick is up and—Good!

Because they want to be seen as adults and in control, teens would try not to show their vincibility about being in a professional's office, which made their shell a particularly tough one to crack sometimes. But like the younger versions, away they would talk if they felt comfortable with you. If you're a phony with a teenager, they'll know it and cut you off faster than one can say, "Oedipus Complex." Whereas if a therapist is "real" and authentic with them, they can pick this up too and trust what you're all about a little more.

If there are words or terms not characteristic of one's dialogue that a professional forces into their verbal exchange with a juvenile, this is going to be so obvious to these wizards that they'll be skeptical about everything you're trying to represent before shutting you down altogether. With those hormones zipping around like they do, a lot of teens are going to close their doors and turn away from therapists merely because it's these adult counselors' jobs to help if they can, and no other reason.

Like a minefield, if these minors give someone a path where they can be safely reached and this explorer goes off course and "blows it," another chance isn't likely to present itself again anytime soon, so it's important to tread softly and be in touch with how you're being perceived by these adult hopefuls who are just waiting for you to "foul up." Chronologically, with only a decade or so separating me from some of my pubescent clients —although growing up in the 90's is unlike any other time in the history of mankind—I could get a pretty good sense of where these young people were coming from and how things were being looked at. Because I had been improving steadily, I was feeling reasonably content with this family therapy position, as my comfort zone about what I was doing had settled in some.

Social work counseling with parents, children, and teens was something I was trained and qualified to do because of the extensive practice geared towards this population I had undergone to attain my Masters Degree in Rehabilitation Counseling. But I never would have expected that I'd have to engage in this type of psychological therapy in a work environment because I was deemed not qualified enough to work in the arena of rehabilitation.

However, in a relatively short time, I came to like family counseling almost as much as rehab counseling because—in many ways—working with family systems and the dynamics involved with this was just as challenging—if not more so—than engaging in mental health therapy with patients having head injuries and their loved ones. Unlike family therapy, the quality of utilizing all my abilities was not always present when working with patients having had sustained brain injuries because, often, their neurological impairment resulted in my having to significantly curtail my dialogue and approach, so they'd understand.

Although it was frequently a challenge to break down what I wanted to present in an elementary fashion, to make light of the situation the best I could that I wasn't using and could not use my potentially invaluable personal experience with head trauma in this family counseling endeavor, I successfully told myself that the enhanced cognizance/intellect of the clientele I had been working with would offset any feelings of non-fullfillment I may have experienced not being able to serve as a role model for those similarly traumatized. But, sometimes it was hard to keep this focus.

It seemed to me that if I wanted to continue receiving the respect from my family service's clients that I had already earned—and not create further distance from my therapy cohorts who weren't all that happy with the "transition" theme I must have been identified with where older therapists were being put on waivers—I had to keep quiet about my sensational head injury experience/recovery. I felt bitter that my therapeutic expertise might be questioned because of an unfounded attitude about this disability which can permanently affect the mental processes of many.

To help ease me through this wave of biting emotion, I'd just have to try to pat myself on the back a little and say in my mind that I've made such a fascinating, unheard of comeback after sustaining a brain contusion that nobody knew how badly I had been hurt. And if someone would find out that I was less than mentally and physically retarded only a handful of years ago, they'd be utterly shocked. All in all, with the exception of this fear factor of being "discovered" weighing constantly on my conscious, things were going pretty good at this therapy office, as I was able to conceal my deep, dark secret—or so I thought.

Being in the counseling field so long, my supervisor, "Emily Sue," and many of the other therapists had quite a bit to offer professionally that I could learn from and this was outstanding. Things started to develop ever so slightly on the interpersonal front too, as I even had someone to talk to on occasion. The agency hired a therapist in his early to mid-40's, "Luke," shortly before I was brought on board whom I discovered was also an avid baseball and football Pittsburgh sports fan like myself and who did not adhere to the "Boys' Club's" ideals of the world either.

Needing to get an idea if the book on my disability history had remained sealed and wanting to witness firsthand how someone not involved with rehabilitation may react to my "shocking" revelation I once was severely brain damaged—assured first that what I had to say wouldn't leak to any of the staff members—I felt comfortable telling Luke about my history with head injury because of his confidentiality promise. I was either not as smart as I thought or pretty gullible thinking my associates wouldn't be able to tell that I had been seriously messed up.

It had been pointed out to me that I might have been able to fool my clients because of the professional manner which I present myself to them and the wisdom I can exhibit at times, but that—seeing me move around like I do everyday instead of once a week for an hour like my clients—staff could sense something much more serious than a broken leg had happened to me, which is what I tried to let on was the only injury I had sustained in my car accident because it was obvious that I had a "bum" leg. Luke told me that the other therapists weren't stupid and picked up right away my avoidance of the issue when the topic of my car accident came up, sensing that I had some grave secret I didn't want to let out, as they could tell something about me "just wasn't right." Uh oh, I knew I was behind the 8-ball then.

This therapy job had two spectrums for me. One was the professional counseling I undertook with clients which I thoroughly enjoyed because I could see that my efficiency as a therapist was growing by leaps and bounds, in part because of the substantial experience of those around me who usually offered to share their wealth of wisdom with me. Right or wrong, the other range of values had a great impact on the way I looked at things overall and ultimately influenced my feelings about my position with the agency. And this was how I—with my personal characteristics—could respond to the individual personalities of those professionals surrounding me, given their very unique traits, and if we could mutually relate one day to one another.

My direct, mid-management boss—"Emily Sue"—wouldn't let one of our supervisory meetings go by without reminding me how young I was and the lack of hands-on work experience I possessed compared to the Social Worker therapists in the agency. Feeling pretty powerful because of her senior status within the agency, essentially telling me that I would be prone to jumping to conclusions and making faulty determinations during my therapies because of my minimal life exposure to misfortune, I'd have to snicker to myself when my supervisor would make this hypocritical statement.

Unaware of the experience I had to keep hidden in my hip pocket, when Emily Sue would stress that it doesn't do anybody any good making hasty judgments and that I'd need to gather as much relevant information about my clients as possible in order to keep from developing erroneous deductions which hinder progress, I would have to fight hard to keep from blurting out my extensive contact with the ways of the world. Not having a clue as to who this therapist really was sitting before her, I'd just play my role and be in awe of the treasure chest of rare knowledge she possessed. Not realizing the feelings of intense guilt which hammered at me believing I was more than indirectly responsible for my mom being a widow and alone in the homestead —without fully understanding even a fraction of the whole story—my supervisor was quick to pass judgment on me, cutting on me and questioning why I'd commute 115 miles round trip from Washington to Monroeville everyday.

Also, hearing the crack of that voice and seeing those eyebrows going up, it didn't take a rocket scientist or nuclear engineer to tell that my supervisor was disappointed because of the small amount of money I'd donate out of my paycheck every two weeks to the non-profit agency's corporate headquarters. But given that I was on the bottom rung of the therapist pay scale because of my novice status, I just wasn't comfortable giving what might have been expected. Until I found somewhere to live closer to work—in my mind—the wear and tear on my seven-year-old used car, cost of gasoline, and the two-hour, fifteen minutes travel time everyday just to get to and come back from work were enough of an expense. Staff could not see why I wouldn't want to escape out of "little Washington" as soon as I could, given that these non-biased therapists believed my hometown didn't have much to offer.

Because it's largely agricultural, Washington County may not have the abundance of technological and material amenities that Allegheny County does, but it's still a nice place to live and grow up. The majority of therapists in Monroeville, however, didn't see it this way, as these urban dwellers were more than happy to insult my home and refer to me as a rural country bumpkin. With this suburbanite's exposure to corn stalks being limited to the County fair, I normally wouldn't even bother to contest these perfect human beings' preconceived impressions about what it was like where I lived, not only because I was outnumbered, but because I knew that they were only trying to make me mad.

Surely warning their own clients about the dangers of baseless prejudice and being judgmental, these understanding professionals who frequently had the duty of enhancing client self-esteem should have known better than to degrade someone, just so they could experience some personal feelings of superiority. If I'd have made equally critical comments about the cultural backgrounds of some members of staff who didn't have anglo-saxon family histories—given the way this paralytic counselor was customarily approached—you better believe a double standard would have occurred where I'd have been reprimanded. Not only would I have been "called on the carpet" if any similarly ridiculing comments had been made by me, but this employee who could have embarrassed a lot of associates with his poor gait would have been given "the boot" faster than one could be accused of being two-faced, if I'd have made disparaging remarks on the same footing about the personal lives of various workers.

All hell would have come down on me, if I'd have commented that the multitudes of divorcees in the agency had no business counseling couples on how to go about maintaining a loving marriage, old maid therapists better stick to watching T.V. on Saturday nights instead of working with their clients on how to form relationships, or well-to-do employees in the agency who live in some of the more affluent areas of Pittsburgh don't have the sensitivity to talk with the less fortunate experiencing the hardships of life that being in financial straits can cause.

In reference to me only being in my mid-twenties, in the short time I had been with the agency, I had heard endless comments from more "advanced" therapists that once I experienced more of the bumps life can deliver someone and how to go about properly handling tragedy, I'd be deserving of being classified as something more than a "Beginning Therapist." Knowing that I had likely come face-to-face with more character-building catastrophe in the first eighteen years of my life alone than all these worldly therapists combined will ever likely encounter, and being stepped on repeatedly by these almighty human services providers, made this person with a physical disability want to throw up his arms on more than one occasion and ask, "What's the use?" Cut me a break.

I know that I had better keep my mouth shut about what exactly happened to me in the car accident because I knew these counselors' overly-analytical minds would start pumping and they'd mistakenly calculate that—as badly as I was hurt—some cognitive mechanisms must have been rendered permanently inoperable and that something's got to be seriously wrong with this guy. Being looked at as a "special needs" therapist and one-time secure employees sensing that they were going to be given their "unconditional release" in the not-so-distant future, it felt to this recently-hired laborer like I had to "scrap and fight" for every ounce of consideration I could snare. I had to just keep my fingers crossed that things would eventually become less rocky because it had started to wear on me being the whipping boy of those therapists who were upset about what the reorganization would mean to them. Flinging shots at me much too often, even something out of my control like picking my days off this summer was met with displaced contempt.

The pay in this counseling operation may not have been the very best, but some aspects of the benefits package were attractive. For this rookie therapist, every month I had worked at the agency, I received two-days vacation time. After my six-month probationary period ended and before the new fiscal year officially started for me, I had to take the accrued time I had earned or else lose these paid days off. Not being on a vacation since I was twelve-years-old, I looked forward to this break. But wouldn't you know, one of the tenured therapists purposely tried to do what she could to replace this excitement with a feeling of shame. Since I started this counseling job in February, I had almost two weeks respite time coming to me which just so happened I had to take during the best weather month of the summer. Even a situation as benign as choosing some solstice days of ease wouldn't immunize me from wrath.

With the message obviously intended for my ears to hear—while I was standing right there—this one experienced therapist who was a vocal opponent to the reorganization told our supervisor, "Why does the new employee get to take his vacation in the prime month of July when everyone else in the agency—who've been here for years—have to take theirs in June when the weather's not real good yet?"

This is the kind of stuff one would expect to hear from a junior high kid, not someone who's supposed to be geared to help people lessen the strain of life and teach others to deal with members of society directly. But I guess this was this lovely human being's way of welcoming me to the agency. Before those enchanting counselors who were legitimate candidates themselves to be labeled with a DSM-III diagnosis drove me crazy, I needed to get out of that agency.

I think southwestern Pennsylvania is an exceptional place to be the majority of the time, but I'd have to admit, I've never been a big fan of snow, cold weather, or an aching leg. Had it not been for therapists who supposedly adhere to a higher standard ripping on my home in an attempt to upset me and rarely giving me credit for knowing much about anything, I'd have been more than willing to put up with the meteorological inconveniences. Having already consistently tore into my home and various individual traits, I was not about to wait for further character assassination so—after my summer vacation days off had been determined—I went ahead and made arrangements which, hopefully, would lay the groundwork for a warm-weather career in rehabilitation and get me the hell out of Dodge.

Not exactly rubbing up against the equator, the furthest south I had ever been was Virginia Beach, Virginia and I wanted to see if Florida was what it was all cracked up to be. Influencing my imagination to one day take up residency there, I understood that the weather in this "snow bird" state is absolutely spectacular during the winter months when it seems I can routinely have eight layers of clothing on, but an unbearable frypan during the summer. However, being a hot-weather kind of guy, this sounded very appealing to me, so I planned a megawatt vacation in this paradise during the scorching month of July to experience exactly what it was like down there this time of year. Seeing if I could stand it, I thought I'd take a look at a couple of head injury treatment facilities I had gathered some information about that were down there. Having never been in Florida either and knowing she would never ask to go with me, as a birthday present, this sweet son invited his 67-year-old mom to "tag along." Paying for over half of everything, this didn't turn out to be such a bad drawback, after all. I love you, mom.

Because of rehabilitation Human Resource Department's ignorance and closed-mindedness regarding what can be achieved by a person after they've sustained a head injury, I was almost prepared to accept that I'd never be able to professionally work with those who have experienced similar symptoms of a brain trauma as myself, so I thought I might as well become content working in family therapy where I'd just have to forget about using my potentially inspiring recovery background. If it hadn't been for the disturbed nature of so many of the staff members at the counseling agency and the odd fashion which many of the family therapists viewed the world, my dream to attain an awesome position in a rehab center would have—more than likely—only been another fantasy I'd have to forego.

Believing the abundance of rejections by head injury trauma programs were designed to pass me on and keep me out of sight—never given any serious consideration for a prominent position in rehab—I wasn't about to let the biases of program directors in centers keep me down, if I could do something about it. Settling for a job any aspiring book-trained professional could handle may not have been the most fulfilling, but I would have been willing to take it because it was apparent rehab managements either were negatively influenced by what they previously understood about head injury or else didn't have the entrepreneurial ability to utilize someone who had attained much more than a degree.

Despite rehabilitation companies' antics which would normally dissuade most from their pursuit to begin a career professionally counseling those having disabilities, my heart was still very much striving to excel in this field. The incentive to continue attempting to get in the rehab industry would come about not only because I'm not like everyone else, but because I have a point to prove to rehab execs who wouldn't give me the opportunity to be accomplished and to the many who doubted my ability to succeed after my head injury. Unfortunately, desire alone cannot overcome prejudice and discrimination, if a chance never presents itself. So what I was forced to do was try to pound down some rehab doors that serving my field training at New Medico should have opened up wide for me. The key word here is "try."

With the hope that I could appear in the flesh at some of the Florida rehabs where I had applied for work corresponding through the mail—after reviewing my arrival date and time—I scheduled to speak and show my video at two hospital, head injury rehab programs in Orlando for free while I was down there. Figuring I couldn't possibly receive any money for my time or effort because of my "head injured" history, I didn't ask for any monetary reimbursement basically because my primary purposes for giving these presentations were—not intending to sound vain—to reach some Floridians who wouldn't normally have had the opportunity to see a unique survivor like myself and to allow these employer-hopefuls get an up-close and personal look at me to alleviate any fears they probably have about my competency. I guess Mickey and Donald were appealing enough, but the main reason I went to this heaven was, not to experience my initial airplane flight or see palm trees for the first time, but to check out the head injury treatment regimens at Sand Lake Hospital and Rebound Inc. of Florida Hospital firsthand.

If there is such a thing, it appeared that the demeanors of these "sunshine state" patients, families and department staff (no administrators) who came to hear and see me could be classified as polite skepticism. I really couldn't tell if the smiles sported or the enthusiasm displayed were authentic towards this guy slicked up in his formal attire who supposedly knows a thing or two about what a head injury can do to a person, but if these presentation patrons did have some doubts of my expertise, I couldn't have asked for anything better. Possibly assuming that I had sustained *only* a minor head injury, slicked up in my formal duds, not being able to definitively tell that I was once in critical condition/potentially irreversibly aphasic was indeed very complimentary to me given all that I've been through to get this far "against all odds." If these Disney residents—starving for any kind of reassurance that something could be done in the face of this disabling tragedy—would be able to take some small steps towards improvement because they had seen something favorable in my video, this would also be a gift of encouraging proportions.

With the way I approached patients and families while at New Medico in the back of my mind where people got to know me first as an effective counselor prior to understanding some aspects of my history as a former patient—after I thanked these Florida health care facilities for giving me the opportunity to speak—I wanted to first allow my audience to witness firsthand my dignified, post-traumatized mannerisms before I rolled the video, depicting just how personal my escapades with brain trauma were. I believed it was important to initially leave an impression of professionalism before this congregation could only identify their speaker as some sort of rehabilitation prodigy. Trying to give a viewpoint from a patient's perspective, I advocated for the overall effectiveness of rehabilitation and the importance that patients work hard at their therapies in order to see some improvement.

Accentuating what the skills, knowledge, and experience of various rehabilitation professionals *can* result in—prior to introducing my video documentary covering some of the struggles I encountered during my own rehab—to disprove the widely held administrative belief that all people with head injuries can be rolled up in one tight ball and deemed communicatively inept, I articulated for my "class" a generic explanation of what happens to someone who's had their brain injured, some background information of the events leading up to my accident, and a few details of the video itself.

Like when I showed the video in grad school, following this portrayal of my rehab experience which had captured some stunning moments, the reaction of those who had seen me dangling from the brink of disaster was largely one of astonishment about what I've had to overcome to be in a position where I could attain a few goals. Unfortunately, for those staff members who saw the tape of how I struggled to cognitively capture my world and could have relayed my employment wishes to the "higher-ups" of these two hospitals, they likely thought that all the claims about my current intellectual capabilities were too good to be true.

Amazement and respect over what I've been able to accomplish were the general reactions of the viewers who had seen my clip. The main focus of this talk was not a self-serving one where I would "toot my own horn" and take a few bows, rather, I quickly diverted the focus off of me onto these southern folks seeking some answers to their questions that possibly only a survivor of this injury could respond to best. Using my personal experience with this disability to further solidify my stance as someone who knows a little something about brain injury, appeared to be an approach which had a profound effect on quite a few of the people in attendance. With the images of how I once looked and responded to various stimuli fresh in their minds, having mentioned earlier some biological reasons as to why some people may experience more restoration than others—such as spontaneous recovery—I went on then to emphasize the importance of some environmental factors which contribute greatly to a patient's rejuvenation.

One of the most appealing aspects of this video is when it captures my late father following me out of Harmarville on discharge day and—while pointing to my mom who was sitting in the room amongst the others—I'd talk about "support" being a vital ingredient in a patient's psychological healing. Giving my parents and brother an abundance of credit for helping me come as far as I have, I emphasized that this backing can also come from a variety of sources outside of one's immediate family such as friends, the professionals who work with a patient, and from God—who is available anytime, anywhere, twenty-four hours a day, seven days a week, weekends and holidays.

Saving the best of all possible Advocates for last, following my look at how the power of this all-encompassing, everloving, deistic backer cannot be exceeded, I talked about how so much can be taken away from a survivor —but that hopefully—one still has control over the amount of effort they put in their rehabilitation. I stressed that it's important to grieve, but that it is essential that one not mope for a prolonged period of time when diligent work is such an urgent necessity. Most head injury professionals agree that a large majority of a patient's recovery is going to occur within the first two years after the injury, so time is of the essence to get down to business and bust some tail.

Using myself as an example—because I continued to keep "hacking away" after that generally assigned two-year healing period deadline—I pointed out that I think, walk, talk, move better than I once did, and that many of these gains occurred many years later. Highlighting how many improvements have appeared following this cut-off date, encouragement was given not to give up, if there's still a glimmer of hope. Stressing the importance of compensatory strategies to address limitations and how perseverance is the only way many skills are going to return, I then discussed my favorite topic in the world—my guitar playing—and the many improvements I've made these past eight years with my musical instrument since my accident left me with paralysis of my picking hand.

Capable of fingering just fine, making my right hand keep up with my healthy left one was very difficult physically, but ten times as hard emotionally for me given my love of rock music and my desire to be a proficient musician. To get over these psychological hurdles, I just had to keep after it and repeatedly tell myself that I can do anything, provided I set my mind to it. If I wanted to triumphantly overcome the barriers my bruised brain left me to battle, I had to remind myself that tough times don't last, but tough people do.

Not being able to get my right hand to localize on one string to pick one note because the dexterity just wasn't there at one time to do this basic fine motor skill, was agony for me. Using my playing as a longitudinal study example of how functions can return in time, I proudly boasted that I kept at it and went from not being capable of playing single notes early on to jamming out some pretty vicious Judas Priest and AC/DC chops. Shifting gears some, I spoke of how it is essential that one tries to set their dejection aside and focus on what needs done to climb the next mountain, but that it is also important to "accept" that some abilities aren't likely to appear or reappear.

With my six-string, for example, I told my listeners that I realized the stiffness of my paralytic right wrist prevented me from doing basic things required of a rock guitarist, with the most prominent being unable to play while standing up. Even while sitting, I was pretty much incapable of holding a standard, flat pick for any length of time with any comfort as the pick would still slip out of my grasp, so I had to use an enlarged triangle pick just to hold on. But even this didn't work too well if I had to continuously play a song for over three minutes, so I would be back to feeling the blues again. Back to the drawing board, I was not accustomed to the "feel" of a thumb pick nor able to finger pick because those rigid right fingers of mine just wouldn't listen to me, so I had to come to grips with the fact that I wasn't going to be the player I wanted to be and would just have to settle for the fact that what I could do was still pretty good and much, much, much, more than anybody would have thought considering how badly I was hurt.

In addition to having trouble clutching onto a pick for any extended period of time and my right wrist not being flexible enough to strike strings while I was on my feet, more advanced right-handed picking techniques like artificial harmonics, palm muting, whammy bar dives, and Van Halen's tapping/ tapped harmonics were methods I could not do, as they were simply out of reach. Keeping my nose to the grindstone, however, notice the word "never" was never used.

Wrapping up this exhibition of instruction and self-disclosure before opening it up to questions, I talked about how all people—younger people especially—want to be accepted socially; but that society's reaction towards those having sustained head injuries may not be one of an accepting nature because of fear, suspicion, and misunderstanding. Using various events of my life as an illustration, I went on to say that when I was in rehab, I was praised for my strong therapeutic work ethic and subsequent gains and figured that society would give me the same praise/admiration/accolades as those familiar with trauma. However, I was also quick to highlight that the response to me outside of the rehab setting was generally one where I was approached with caution, anxiety, and mistrust.

Re-entering society, I reviewed how it was more than likely that the average, everyday, person isn't going to know too much about brain injury and—because of this—could imagine an assortment of different things that aren't true. Largely, because of misleading portrayals and what's commonly accepted as fact about those of us who have suffered through a neurological impairment, it would not be too hard to understand why those not acquainted with brain disorders—as well as those who are—might be leery of us and maybe more than a little scared. With these two parties in mind, I spoke of my experience with my first W.V.U. date who almost shit herself when I told her about me being in a coma and how New Medico, of all places, soiled themselves.

Subsequently, I stressed the importance of not divulging right away one's experience with brain injury in certain situations and to let others know—by their example—that just because an individual has had a head injury doesn't mean that they can't possess a multitude of special attributes. I told my crowd that if they insist on being primarily received as a former patient and a "regular Joe" second with the individual strengths they possess outside of their rehabilitation comeback, they very possibly could run the risk of subjecting every move they make to being examined under close scrutiny, as if under a microscope. I professed that every mistake, indiscretion, or any nuance of behavior which deviates ever so slightly from what is prescribed as "normal" practice, will be blamed on their head injury and the knowledge of their brain injury disability history could very likely cause them problems they don't need.

Another environmental variable I went over which should promote optimal mental health after the onset of a disability is to "socialize" with people, both friends and strangers who appear trustworthy. To be isolated with and constantly focused on limitations which very well could be a part of one's being for the rest of their life would cause any person to feel trapped with misery. Having the slightest control, a survivor of any disability needs to avoid the unneeded setback of merciless emotional torture by being amongst people whom they feel comfortable with. To be agoraphobic at a time when sharing is essential for balance, could do some significant harm that need not occur.

The onset of permanent afflictions caused by head trauma renders enough damage, so creating further disabling symptoms by giving up cognitive control is ill-advised because of the psychological danger this will levy. To contend with the rehab necessary after a brain injury is enough of a struggle which is why it's important not to make the therapeutic excursion the patient has to travel any more damaging. Just ask New Medico's Penelope Rich, she's had extensive experience with this.

Despite my bitter experience practicing at Charles Goyette's New Medico facility at Meadowlands, the second tier of my vacation took us a couple hours south where I would not only be sucking up some sun, but give my third and final Florida presentation at the New Medico rehab in Palm Beach. So incredibly desperate to get out of that family counseling agency and still very much hungry to work in rehabilitation, I was willing to give New Medico another "go" despite the horrendous experience I had at the center in Pennsylvania. Hoping so much to impress the directorial faculty at this New Medico utopia located on the ocean-side land of milk and honey with my post-TBI talents, that I'd no doubt be offered a satisfying position here, I still believed that this head injury corporation overall was a fundamentally sound one and that the tragedy which occurred at Meadowlands Health Care Center was only an isolated incident created because of a groundless administrative prejudice that my head injury somehow left me mentally "out of kilter."

Given short notice of what days off I would have coming to me this summer, I was unaware of my exact summer vacation plans until shortly before I left, so not much in the way of advanced warning was given to the Palm Beach center as to when I'd be available to provide New Medico with additional volunteer services. Possibly, no New Medico administrative policy planners/personnel management types bothered to show up for my "no reimbursement required" talk because they either weren't aware of my proposal until it was too late, or else just assumed someone once in an aphasic condition didn't have much to offer that they hadn't already seen or heard about before. No matter what gains I've been able to make following my head injury, it appeared New Medico rehabilitation employers merely viewed me as some quirk of nature. Discrediting my standing and experience as if I didn't know enough about neurological impairments or disability to be able to work for them, I wouldn't be afforded the opportunity I deserved to benefit their patients.

Ironically, the month that I had planned to continue hammering away on those New Medico doors with a freebie/Atlantic Coast presentation, the humanitarian program director—who determined that someone I believe resembles a younger version of his wife would be more qualified to work in head injury rehab than this former patient—was getting some print in our Nation's Capital.

Under the headline, "Beltway Victim Transferred to Pa.; Improved Patient Taken for Rehabilitation," in the Washington Post Final Edition dated June 27, 1990, on page G7 of the Metro section, staff writer Debbie M. Price penned an article where New Medico's Goyette described the types of (time effective?) treatment this soon-to-be Meadowlands patient would be receiving and the prognosis for (a speedy?) recovery. Attempting to do some New Medico damage control, I then jabbered on to my Florida gathering about the benefits that can be received from various therapeutic delivery systems.

The encouraging reception/response I received from the sparse New Medico Rehabilitation and Skilled Nursing Center at Palm Beach crowd of a dozen or so who had heard me speak and saw my video, foolishly led me to believe that these corporate guys would finally come to their senses and give me a call once I got back up north to offer me a permanent, full-time position with them. Unfortunately, my desire to engage in work such as giving presentations to people affected by brain contusion and believing that I was cut out for this type of counseling job would not be enough to spark any interest at these Florida programs.

As it turned out, not only was this lack of consideration by New Medico once again devastating to me, but our healthy schnauzer—Fritz—was neglected by the kennel where we left him to be cared for when we departed for Florida and he died the day we came back home. Describing an account of affection for a little dog might sound strange to someone who isn't an animal lover, but Fritz dying from starvation was an emotional wrecking ball for mom and I. Because of our infatuation with dogs and his being more my dad's dog than anyone else's, Fritz was such an integral part of our small, immediate family. Representing a lot of history and because of the joy he filled in all of our lives, the way Fritz suffered was unforgiving.

Skin and bones when me and mom picked Fritz up before rushing him off to a different vet, we couldn't understand why this animal clinic didn't call my brother because we left his phone number with these "caregivers" in case of an emergency. Only living about three miles away from where Fritz was to receive medical care should anything happen to our canine while we were away, Ug didn't bother to check on our family pet because he was preoccupied with his second wife and mom told him not to worry about it. Not accepted in the field of rehab in Florida possibly because these shoreline professionals mistakenly believed my head injury would cause serious, ongoing physical problems and losing my buddy—life isn't fair.

"Who told her to do that?" Holding an anti-choice position, when these exact words were spoken to me in a stern fashion by my supervisor at the counseling agency when she had heard a teen-aged client of mine had an abortion, I knew I was in trouble.

Feeling like I was on trial, knowing her view on things, I thought I had better quickly defend and explain myself by saying that everybody is an advocate for life, as anything artificially done to prevent the arrival of a new resident in this world is catastrophic—but that unfortunately—sometimes people elect to have this done. Emily Sue obviously not being in this accredited class, I could remember the stance that was professed to us in grad school that those providing counseling services are not to tell a client what to do, not only because the counselors aren't the ones who have to live with the ultimate determination, but for the reason that the patrons of counseling services have their own denominational standards, insights, and convictions about what's right and wrong. Stuck in an agency where subjective ideals frequently prevailed, the position where professionals are never to impose their personal values onto the lives of their clients would be something that apparently was not always to be adhered to.

Free-falling back into the reality that I was no closer to working in a head injury treatment facility than before I left for Florida, and that I was back to umpiring inter-family grumblings, I was definitely fed some mixed messages by my fellow therapy professionals. Told that our job is not to advise a client on what to do, rather, to help them look at *all* possible options and then weigh the consequences of their various decisions before acting them out, so the one searching for answers can decide for themselves the most beneficial action to take.

But the way things had developed, it appeared that I was being prosecuted for not telling this girl and her mother that the option they were considering of their own free will—and ultimately chose—would not be acceptable. Sweating blood by the end of this supervisory meeting, I guess even the rule that a counselor not encroach upon a client's fixed opinion had conditions, depending on the deep-rooted belief held by mid-management. Oxymorons anyone?

Without a doubt, Emily Sue's multitude of skills and knowledge did help me form an approach which enhanced my understanding of various family dynamics essential for counseling this population. In addition to the assortment of counseling methods and the different elementary components of therapy I learned in my graduate studies, theoretical principles such as the comfort of familiarity, rewriting scripts, mixed messages, we are the way we are because that's how our parents made us, past behavior is the best indicator for future behavior, shifting the blame, rewriting history, repeating patterns, etc. that I incorporated with this family services' position would be further elements I was grateful that I could apply in my work.

Also, I developed a growing understanding about such items as children's responses to separation, misogynistic relationship "hooks," characteristics of birth orders, and psychological effects of marital discord because of my first therapeutic instructor's efforts. However, with the reorganization's shifting of philosophy where rearrangements and demotions were occurring, my initial supervisor would no longer be serving in this capacity or even operating in the same locale as myself. In this organization's quest to revise and reload, a replacement would have to be named to work with me and others.

Along with another recently-hired employee, Luke was assigned to be one of my supervisors. From my point of view, when Luke was slated to be my primary supervisor, this altered the chemistry of our relationship from his being the only person within the agency I found fairly comfortable talking about things not necessarily related to therapy, to someone with boundary parameters because he had become my boss. Because he was definitely a trustworthy man, I had no real concerns that a member of mid-management knew that maybe I was some sort of a head injury disability phenomenon. But I'd have to concede that the thought did cross my mind that maybc I just should have never said anything about my altercations with the symptoms of a brain injury disability.

In Counseling 101, a student will learn within the first week or two of class that one person can't change another person. With acceptance being the optimal remedy, if Person A doesn't like a nuance of behavior Person B is exhibiting because this action doesn't fit the mold of what Person A idealizes how the world should be, that's too bad until Person B sees the need to modify their way of doing things. Not acknowledging the need for change, a person isn't going to alter their mode of operation just so somebody else—who wants to feel more "bubbly" in their environment—demands they do so. Like the abortion issue where I was to incorporate my supervisor's moral doctrines in my counseling session with the pregnant teen and her mother, I quickly learned that commonly accepted standards of practice seem to have a condition here where senior staff members attempt to sway their influence when they can.

Luke had a female therapist buddy in the downtown Pittsburgh office who must have believed that it was her right—because of her tenured standing—to voice objections about how this novice therapist stuck so much to himself and didn't try hard enough for her to be cordial with senior employees when the entire therapy team would gather at the agency headquarters smack in the middle of town. Not exactly experienced with the metropolitan way of life yet or all that comfortable partaking in a reunion with veteran therapists who were mad at the world because they saw themselves as spinning in a downward spiral because of "young bucks" such as myself having been brought on board, this rookie therapist would make it a point to schedule my share of clients and other duties in my home base of Monroeville on these in-service days, so I would have a reason to leave right away.

Unaware that too many members of this "elite" veteran group irreversibly rubbed me the wrong way by continuously ridiculing the people where I was from as being "hicks" and not having a clue as to the fire which burned inside of me being discriminated against by New Medico, this middle-aged worker whom I barely knew and wasn't aware had any kind of "beef" with me had to have realized she could utilize her friendship with the therapist who had become my supervisor to assure that this opinion of me got heard in her attempt to revamp my way of going about my business.

Talking about this harmony issue later with my one-time friend turned supervisor, because this message which got back to me was relayed by a practical stranger who could sense that I was bothered, I could appreciate the viewpoint that I needed to "loosen up." Deciding to make a commitment of doing what I could, not being so distant with my co-workers whom I assumed would have just as soon kept this "invalid" at arm's length, would backfire, however.

Admittedly, because of my efforts to make myself more available and to be anything but aloof, I did feel a lot better for a short time. However, as it would turn out, my attempts to approach people in a more hearty fashion who only were in a festive mood with select members of their clique would turn out to be a big mistake.

When I first started working at the counseling agency and prior to being cast off, because she was the only one around who approximated me in chronological age, on occasion I'd talk with this clerical worker four years my junior who supposedly was being groomed to one day assume the immaculate office manager position. In the short time before I was looked at as some kind of threat by some of the older therapists—in no way inappropriate or flirtatious—I would be able to kid around with this secretary who gratefully helped me to learn how to fill out different forms and go about completing some of the paperwork required for filing at the beginning, when I first started.

"Rose" never once complained about our matches of good-natured barbs, as she would poke more than her fair share of cracks at me as well. Not at all dense, in time, I know that this Associate Degree-educated typing specialist could see that the therapists who had been with the agency since the beginning of the 20th Century millennium had little consideration for this physically-challenged therapist. In her early twenties and apparently still bogged in the "need to be accepted" stage of development, I think Rose felt that her attitude toward this disapproved of "disabled" employee had to correspond with the others' generally pompous style of interacting with me, if she was to remain popular. And here was where I wore a kind of scarlet letter for twenty-four hours and a black mark on my name indefinitely.

Compensating for the paralytic right side of my body these past nine years, my overworked left shoulder started to rebel and began subluxating. This incomplete or partial dislocation worried me because the clicking in my shoulder went from being annoying to aching pretty bad. Despite the pain continuing to shoot down my arm, I remember being told by Luke that I had better start becoming "Mr. Cheer," if I didn't want to suffer any unpleasant repercussions. Putting aside the pronounced discomfort my cracking shoulder caused me, I tried to wear a bubbling personality which would make a lot of Miss America contestants proud. But here at the Addams' family counseling agency, it was obvious I couldn't win for losing.

One day in particular, my shoulder was bugging me pretty bad, so I went up to the front desk just outside my office door where Rose was sitting and—tongue firmly planted in my cheek as every indication was given by my tone of voice and delivery that I wasn't serious—jokingly asked the young employee I used to be able to kid around with to rub my shoulder. Not noticing the scowl on Rose's face at the time, I figured she knew I was just goofing around with her again, so when she told me to stop, I didn't bother to listen because I had no idea that I had caught her at a wrong moment.

The next day, Luke called me into his office to tell me that Rose filed a sexual harassment claim against me. Like a tsunami hitting me square in the face, I couldn't believe this bogus charge and went on to tell my supervisor how silly and unfounded this accusation was. I told Luke there was nothing to this indictment and that making me an easy target occurred in the first place because this youthful office worker just wanted to be seen on some kind of a par as those therapists around her. Knowing that the feminist movement was armament which not only would be loaded and ready to fire so those legitimately violated could be rightfully protected, but also unjustly used as an assault weapon, I realized my new cordial approach was seen as excessive.

Despite understanding full-well that the inalienable right of safe-guarding against mistreatment could be twisted to make it look like an offense, without taking into account that maybe Rose just wanted to use the feminist armor granted her to feel less secondary in the overall scope of the counseling operation and that I wasn't guilty of this abuse—as so many people in society are quick to do—Luke concluded that my once having a head injury was why I didn't know when to stop tormenting. It was at this point that I definitely started to worry that a member of mid-management knew of my once having a severe head injury and that counterfeit marks such as the assault Rose lauched could one day be used against this one-time seriously "brain damaged" counselor.

The following morning, I would be told that this word processor whiz—who would be appealing enough from a football field's view away—had cooled off and saw this benign situation for what it definitely was. A short time after this whole circumstance got started, Rose contacted the upper-brass, conceding that there were no foul intentions on my part/that I truly didn't mean anything and dropped the charge. By this time—with regards to trying to "fit in" here and becoming established at this agency—I began asking myself, "Why even bother?"

I have a photograph which illustrates, from the very beginning, how I was widely approached and regarded by a not-so-small segment of this counseling operation's senior therapy faculty. For the most part, when I'd go over different issues with, or occasionally just chat with the staff's older therapists on a one-on-one basis—not only was I generally received with regard, but as a peer—as many of them didn't appear to be so strange, after all. However, once another elder member of the "advanced" therapy team was added to the mix who possessed similar characteristics such as age, racial background, "Boy's Club" status, and/or duration working for the agency as the senior staffer I would be talking to, the respect took a 180` nosedive where I was back to being seen as a hobbling subordinate and not really someone to be considered.

This snapshot highlights how I must have been perceived as a "scab" by tenured employees who apparently weren't comfortable with what I had to have come to symbolize because they weren't prepared for the forthcoming organizational restructuring. No question, this pic nabs a perfect photobiographical representation of how this youngster was generally looked upon by those members of a bygone era of therapeutic interventions. No doubt, I know that if this rookie counselor had been seen doing something so professional as give another therapist "the bird", or if an intake call had been made by a potential client claiming that unimaginable behavior had taken place in my office, I'd have been gone in a flash.

When I first began working for the agency, I had a pretty small office in the middle of the counseling department's floor with no view besides the four walls within this tight enclosure. After about a year, one of the long-time employees left the agency for greener pastures, so I got her appealing area to do my therapy work. In addition to being assigned to work within another program because I had proven I was capable of handling the caseload delegated to me during my probationary period, I was proud to have a spacious office with a nice view of Monroeville to do my counseling because this was a tangible representation of the progress that I had been making since I started working at this operation.

Wanting to capture an image of the room where I would be utilizing my professional training, I brought a camera along to work with me one day, excited that I had been able to achieve such a distinguished professional position "against all odds" after having been in the silent emptiness of a coma. While I was taking some pictures of my work area and the view I had from this upper floor of the office building, I spotted one of those seasoned therapists just outside of my office whom I'd be able to talk to individually, as long as no one else from the veteran therapy clique were around.

With only Rose around sitting in the background at her desk, I said this "Boys' Club" therapist's name, so he'd give me a friendly pose. I wanted to snare an image of someone whom I thought I had gotten along with. But instead, I unfortunately snapped a portrayal of my relationship with veteran staff.

Glaring me down as if I were responsible for the reorginization, the very instant I flicked down the camera button, I was shocked and hurt when this professional therapist flicked me "the bird" with his middle finger. This hand gesture, indicating "Fuck you," was done in response to my request of this counselor to be civil to this "scab" for an instant, so I could get a mug shot freezing some history. However, once again, my overtures to be personable with senior staff were met with callous disdain. Directly analogical to my overall attitude which had slowly burned working at this place and the repugnant manner which I was frequently dealt with by tenured staff, the excitement which I should have experienced because of my new standing and accomplishment was quickly replaced by question. But the astonishment as to the reason for this disrespect would only last for a fraction of an instant.

Out of my sight when I decided to take this photo, popping out of nowhere from around the corner was the "Boys' Club's" senior dignitary. Positioned in such a way that this professional giving me "the finger" could see his "Boy's Club" fraternity brother coming and I couldn't, this therapist's longest digit pointed skyward and stared at me in such a way so as to leave the impression for this shirt and tie superior that he and the new "scab" never had any moments where we got along.

Headed back to his office while I was given this disturbing memento, possessing corresponding ethnic lines and cultural attitudes as the gentleman presenting me with the salutation, this snapshot captures half the profile of this white-bearded heavyweight in full-stride and the rest obstructed by the wall. Exemplified by this frozen frame of time, the professional manner which these counselors wanted to portray where empathy would occur for those who ran into some misfortune and how way too many of them really were, a picture's worth a thousand words.

Another fall, winter, and spring of this reject the "scab" nonsense, I was more than ready to embark on another tropical paradise summer vacation in June 1991. Whether it was desperation to get out of that counseling agency where it appeared many of the veteran therapists weren't real comfortable that a young "cripple" was trying to be successful within their organization, stupidity thinking that I actually might know a little something about rehab, or just plain fortitude and reserve, I thought I'd give it another shot and try to kick in those New Medico doors with another "no dollars necessary" presentation at their Palm Beach facility again.

Since the overall response to me was such a welcomed one last summer and because I knew I could do so much good working for a corporation which specializes in head injury, possibly a form of denial, I thought I'd give it another "go" to get in with New Medico. Having had a brain injury, I also realized that I had to fight and give one extreme effort over and above the call of duty, if I wanted to be treated equitably and make working in a good-paying job with rehabilitation a reality.

Knowing my sunny days of relaxation well in advance during this summer's intermission from my parental/child counseling work, I gave the New Medico at Palm Beach center a call several weeks ahead of my arrival down there, so they'd have ample opportunity to prepare for my talk this time around. Hopefully able to do something to alleviate the corporation's faulty generalizations which apparently had a hold on me, I thought I'd professionally demonstrate my qualifications one more time. Wanting so dearly to work for this windfall operation, I only hoped this would be the case given that I had basically done all that I could.

The interference with my potential having the capacity to harm others, it got to be pretty upsetting when the biases of rehabilitation employers prevented me from fulfilling this promise. Five years ago, at the age of twenty-two and six months from attaining my Bachelor's degree "against all odds"—when I closed my dad's eyes that last time when he died—this signified the end of an era which I assumed was only just beginning. Likewise, I wasn't about to let New Medico pass away my career before my vocational era was set to begin, if I could do something about it.

Unlike last year when I mixed business with pleasure during both tiers of my vacation, this summer's first respite stop was one where I only swam in the ocean everyday having fun in the sun for a week and mom just kind of checked out the various sites in Myrtle Beach, South Carolina. On 6/22/91, however, the day had arrived where I would set into motion the purpose for taking this time off, as I found myself once again standing at the podium in the main dining room of the New Medico Rehabilitation and Skilled Nursing Center at Palm Beach.

About 10:30 A.M. on this Saturday morning, as I looked out into the crowded eating area packed with tanned faces eager to hear what this survivor had to say, I admittedly felt relieved and happy because I couldn't be sure of the interest that my background/experience would generate given the small number in attendance of my 7/21/90 talk last year. Brainwashed by my employer that I was some second-rate counselor whose competency was in question and New Medico's past antics with me, I didn't know what the story would be, but I was keeping my fingers crossed that things would work in my favor because I really liked the Florida heat last summer the short time I was in this wonderland. However, this occasion would be much different.

With flyers having been spread throughout the treatment facility for this year's appearance, New Medico had advertised my arrival for about a month and the response was overwhelming to me, as about four times as many people came to find out what I was all about because they were made aware of my speaking at this family seminar. Unfortunately, like last year, it cut real bad when no management members from this center's Human Resource Department bothered to show up this weekend amongst all those listeners and viewers of my video who came to learn about me. With no word of mouth to be passed along as to my potential value to corporate "royalty" who could make a difference with regard to my employment status, I would be back to "Square One" in my aspirations to fill a promising position with this rehabilitation firm, as I wondered just how many people would flock here at this Florida center to hear Penelope speak. In God's name, what have I done to be treated like this by New Medico?

If one can't find an answer, they might be asking the wrong question.

Following my second oceanview leave in two years, I went about my family counseling business anxiously expecting to finally receive that rehabilitation job-offer call from someone representing New Medico, and hopefully from those boys down along the seaboard I had just spent a few days with. For about two weeks, the area of the brain responsible for happiness—left portion of the frontal lobe—was sure busy firing off joyous electrical impulses for me because I was fully anticipating to be thrown a New Medico life preserver, so I could be rescued from that family counseling job that I was fearful its members saw me as some sort of "vegetable." However, after seven days short of a month, the "logic" process located in my brain's right hemisphere took over when I didn't hear a peep from anyone where I had given my second critically-acclaimed waterfront presentation, and I figured that New Medico was back to their standard operating procedure of banishing this head injury survivor who was seeking a little bit of reciprocation for his efforts.

My ghastly exposure to New Medico had led me to believe that, because a rehabilitation employer can't visually see right away traits which could prove impeccable to their facility—but would notice a limp and paralysis immediately—the latter physical symptoms would be attributed to the "handicapped" job applicant as a character and/or intellectual flaw. After voicing my despondency not being able to enter the rehabilitation work force as a professional counselor where I knew I'd be perfectly suited, my family would try to console me by saying that no matter how many times I'd get "the shaft" by rehabilitation employers, they can't take away my Master's degree or the stellar recovery I've made after sustaining a head injury. But unless I'd be able to overcome faulty employer actions where they do not give a former patient a chance due to feeling uneasy about a professional position being manned by a head injury survivor, instead hiring a far-less qualified applicant merely because they have had no history with trauma, this pair of achievements wouldn't be optimally fulfilling until I'd be able to utilize these two accomplishments to benefit those with disabilities.

When I'd think back to how my New Medico at Meadowlands staff supervisors basically told me not to use my personal experience with head trauma so that I'd develop the skills required of a rehabilitation adjustment counselor, I'd be cooking inside knowing that the ulterior motive behind this instruction was one where my amazing experience with head injury rehab could be kept in the dark. Therefore, no questions would arise as to why the far-less experienced Penelope got hired for the job this survivor had already been trained for. Such is life, but I wasn't about to quit because God wouldn't want me to give up my pursuits and ambitions to be a rehabilitation professional with the ability to help a multitude of people, just so prejudicial New Medico execs and advanced family therapists symbolically flicking me "the finger" could feel powerful.

Feeling down but not out, combating any sense which could have developed that I was underemployed or treading stagnated waters at the counseling agency, was a more focused idea of how to better address certain aspects of my job and an enhanced manner of how to go about using me. Although a good number were very solid people, the individual personalities of the caseload population I was assigned to see was the primary contributing factor as to why I'd encounter the cancellations and "no shows" that I did. In time, though it is important the therapist is aware of the impression they're leaving, I learned not to take it so personally and be so self-focused as to why a particular individual might not have come in for a scheduled meeting without notifying me first or to scratch out an appointment altogether, because I came to accept that I am only a minute fraction of the counseling patrons' overall lives.

Over the course of a couple of weeks, I learned not to obsess with the notion that possibly something about this therapist didn't meet a potential client's fancy, developing an understanding that a lot more is happening with these people than a one-hour-a-week counseling session. With this enhanced appreciation that I wasn't necessarily a central figure in peoples' everyday life, I could also see that maybe someone didn't bother to attend a session because I was "getting too close" to a sensitive issue that they didn't feel comfortable talking about or simply would rather not disclose any knowledge about those crimes I would be obligated to report to the appropriate authorities (homicide, suicide, or child abuse).

Learning a good bit about the dynamics of therapy was definitely a plus, but feeling that I had to hide my traumatized history in order to remain employed and not being on the same frequency as most of the influential therapists, had me starting to take inventory once more whether the pros of working at this outfit outweighed the cons. Bouncing from one locale to another didn't exactly do much for my sense of security or cultivate my satisfaction working here either, but things would at least pick up on this front some. Juggled about, not knowing what exactly to do with me early on, administration finally cooked up a better idea of how I'd fit into the mix.

Because of the uncertainty of how to best utilize my abilities, during my probationary year, I was introduced and assigned to quite a few areas in and around Allegheny County until management found a way to fit my pieces into the puzzle my second twelve months. Following early stints in McKeesport and two projects in the Allegheny Valley, after a temporary assignment to work with grade school students at an elementary school in Homestead to get a taste of the tasks a school-based counselor engaged in, I had been permanently scheduled to work in Tarentum one day a week. And it was while I was there that I started to do some investigative work.

In a very short time, after I had become reasonably familiar with some of the surrounding communities in the Allegheny Valley, I thought I'd make some connections with a few old acquaintances. The increased amount of duties for which I was responsible and the corresponding confidence shown in me, no doubt made me feel like I had become more of a contributing member of the family service's staff and helped somewhat to ease a few doubts which may have emerged about my standing with the agency. However, even with the new assignment on the shores of the Allegheny River and things picking up as far as keeping busy with counseling work—from my point of view—this would be too little too late.

Like when I'd do those countless laps in my wheelchair up and down that long Harmarville hallway, my heart and determination were always set on rehabilitation. I just had to duel the thought that I was unjustly treated with apprehension by rehabilitation personnel departments because my head injury made me suspect, with the fact that things were slowly starting to settle in a little at this family aid agency.

The additional duties/caseload and the enhanced feeling that I was starting to "belong" slightly more helped some to lessen the stress that I experienced about being employed in this outfit. Also, getting an apartment a mile from work in Monroeville after seven months of commuting one hundred fifteen miles round trip everyday understandably did a lot towards alleviating a lot of the tension. On Thursdays from Monroeville, I would travel on the Pennsylvania Turnpike—Route 76 West—to Exit 5/Allegheny Valley, which is where my "home" rehab of Harmarville just so happens to be located.

A few brief weeks following my second sunshiny/whirlwind furlough a month shy of a year, one day after I finished up with my family service's work in Tarentum—on my way back to Monroeville—I got off of Route 28 South and headed towards the Harmarville turnpike to make a sort of unexpected reunion visit. With this decision to get my courage up to say "hello" being a spontaneous judgment call, I didn't know who would be around to welcome me.

All in all, as things would materialize—not that this would do much good—I at least got my "application hat" thrown into the ring and continued professional rehabilitation interest known. I joyfully discovered that some of my '82 therapists I hadn't seen in approximately eight years had continued to climb the status ladder and became administrative "big-wigs." Saying that they were happy to see me, these professionals whom I hadn't run into since the last time I was evaluated here, assumed I was doing well because of my "slicked up" duds and polished delivery. In no time, however, I was sure they deducted that all was not as it seemed when this Harmarville rehabilitation matador inquired if the rehab—which had been using the video of my recovery all these years as a public relations promo for their head injury treatment program—were looking for somebody to fill a job position with some experience which couldn't be thoroughly grasped by answering the multiple-choice questions in a Disability 101 workbook.

After I was told that they weren't aware of any openings for which this brain injury survivor would be qualified, I asked these professionals if they knew of any "leads" anywhere which might finally get my foot into that rehabilitation door which only appeared to be reserved for females wiggling 36"-24"-36" figures around. Told they would keep their eyes open for any rehab posts which might become available around the areas east of Pittsburgh out there for me, I knew that this was their way of bidding me adieu and not to call them, but that they'd call me if something would come up. Empathizing with these good- hearted souls, seeing me aphasic big-time and during a period when I had to "get with the program," I could totally appreciate this reputable center's hesitancy to deal with me when the topic of job placement within a rehabilitation organization was discussed. Totally.

Not even vaguely comparable to the calamity occurring 2/14/82 which had me coming to blows with the symptoms of a brain injury at this rehabilitation center, nonetheless, the July 17, 1991 car accident I would be in a short time after this Harmarville visit would cause some very dark moments for me as well.

After an all-important in-service meeting at the newer Lawrenceville office on this Wednesday morning, I drove a therapist back to the Monroeville agency and then headed to the mall to have lunch before I was to see my scheduled clients later in the day. What would transpire after this mid-day break would force the cancellation of my appointments and have me revisiting the four-wheeled catastrophe of nine years ago.

My belly full and ready to see clients for the next few hours, I crawled into my eight-year old Chevy for what would be the last time this mid-July afternoon. Chugging along on Mall Boulevard, I flicked up my right turn signal indicating I wanted to go up the Oxford Drive hill which was where I caught Monroeville Boulevard on my way back to work. Located between Mall and Monroeville Boulevards, connecting the two, Oxford Drive is situated shortly after the right of the entrance to a K-Mart/Shop 'n Save plaza. Well, this sixteen-year old girl who had been driving only a couple of months took it upon herself to assume that my right signal flicking meant that I was going to pull into this shopping plaza she was coming out of, and gunned her car to beat the forthcoming traffic a little bit behind me. BOOM!!!

Seeing this car fly out at me and nobody coming opposite of me, I immediately slammed down my brake and veered my car in the other lane, so that this kamikaze could have a fraction of a second longer to stop her missiled jalopy. But she was accelerating too fast.

Crashing into my right front fender, my head violently bounced off the steering wheel with a snapping force, as my glasses gashed into my forehead. Speedometer, brake light, oil/gas level indicator—everything on my dashboard panel—brightly flashed on for an instant before turning dark. The humming characteristic of a running automobile died an eerily, still silence. With this wreck happening so lightning-fast, I was too numb to what just happened and everything around me to be scared.

Barking a tad more than a few expletives to myself as a means to rid the terror which had started to surface, I got out of my disabled car and saw that my right front end was thoroughly smashed, as the indentation reached far into the bent-up hood.

With pieces of what used to be my car's body strewn all over the boulevard, sitting in the driver's seat of her banged up car sobbing, I battled the intense consternation and anger which raged within me as I walked up to the driver's side of this girl's car.

My glasses irreparably bent and my guts turned upside down/inside out from the fear which started to build, the therapist in me somehow emerged from the terrified emotions which clung onto me, as I calmly asked this young female if she was okay. Telling me that she wasn't hurt physically, I knew that this apologizing teen would be in for an emotionally-thrilling surprise after she "snapped out" of her frozen psychological state and examined what she did.

Getting out of her car and seeing the damage to my Chevy she caused, this inexperienced motor vehicle operator who didn't bother to wait to definitively ascertain where I was going, then started bawling. Seeing the mess she made out of my transportation and the hell that would probably be waiting for her at home after she told her parents, her reaction was such that it could have easily been assumed she was the one almost left dead in the water that February 1982 night, not me.

Knowing the disaster which could have transpired from her mistake and seeing how she was utterly devastated about "totaling" my car, I fought hard to come to grips with my own turmoil, as I put my hand on her shoulder and said that the important thing was that nobody was hurt. Looking at me through watery eyes, she said, "Really?," but I didn't want to lie, so I let this question pass.

Too preoccupied with their own lives and concerned about avoiding the glass scattered about this busy street, cars whizzed about, as nobody stopped to offer any assistance. Apparently however, just when I started thinking that these suburbanites would rather not get involved and see if everyone was alright, one of the many businesses in the surrounding area must have called for assistance, as a tow truck and police cruiser arrived.

Without any "wheels" at my disposal, after I exchanged the necessary license/insurance information with this adolescent driver and those who could've given me a ride back to either my apartment or work having left, I walked back to the mall shaken and called Luke back at the office from a pay phone to tell him what had happened to me. The only staff member fully aware of the extent of the trauma I had experienced back in '82—possibly thinking that I was accident prone or cursed—my supervisor not only arranged to cancel my appointments for this seventeenth day of the month, but the following day as well, despite my fabricated macho protest that I would be alright to come in the next afternoon.

Hands shaking from the thought of being involved in another collision, I didn't want to cause Luke any more friction being that he dealt with a bogus sexual harassment claim against me. Nor did I want him to know that this formerly "brain injured" employee could still be emotionally traumatized by an accident which occurred many years ago, so I didn't make any waves and this mind-reader saw to it that I had some much-needed time to recuperate.

Too mentally bent out of shape to work, I felt that I could not talk to my fellow therapy "brethern" about how shook up I was because of the way I interpreted being regarded by so many of my cohorts. Although it was these counseling professionals' jobs to help people who were being eaten alive by occurrences from the past, possessing the firm belief that I needed to continue keeping my one-time brain injury condition hidden, dealing with this adversity myself wouldn't be possible. Because utility pole splinters were pricking my short-term memory banks during the instant of time when my '82 automobile mishap should have been registering in my long-term recollection data recorder, absolutely no images of ever being pounded into that wooden monster exist.

More than likely, it was merely due to my knowing what happened to me previously and the subsequent pictures I conjured in my mind because of this awareness and not some kind of flashback, but some process within my darkened neurological subconscious appeared to sense that I had experienced a moment of time where this occurred before. With the lack of close ties with counseling staff and my perception that I had to keep my once being twisted a secret, I thought I'd explode not being able to exorcise these fragmented images of my past which resurfaced. Unfortunately, it would be these two deductions of mine which would cause me another problem.

I wish I would have heeded my own warnings that I had given a few of my clients not to act when emotions are running high, because this can cloud all rationality and create volatile circumstances. But I didn't, and paid the price.

Veteran therapists being ousted at a time when the agency was gaining a little prominence because of their efforts, definitely made quite a few of the long-time staff members I was around disenchanted with the reorganization. I could almost understand their displaced disaffection toward this "new employee" because it appeared I would be benefiting from—and "cashing in" on—senior therapists' prior efforts/sweat at the expense of these ripened workers.

Being held somewhat accountable for older staff being given their walking papers at a time when they should have been harvesting the fruits of their labor wasn't this "scab's" fault, but it looked like I had somehow been viewed as a little responsible for the agency's planned extensive philosphical/personnel turnover, which created an environment for me where success at this outfit would be remote. Not exactly seen in the most favorable of terms during this period of inevitable dismissals, with so many things I'd do or say being ridiculed to the point where I knew that the only way to avoid censored commentary about me would to pull away and be alone, I felt this situation was hopeless.

Knowing that lightning can strike the same place twice and given my previous history with the trauma a mishap in a car can render, I was really in shock about the Monroeville accident although—with the exception of a temporarily throbbing face—I wouldn't be hurt physically. Imprinted into a telephone pole and gravely injured less than ten years ago, feeling as though counseling staff were largely unavailable to me and I couldn't solicit their help, desperate to talk with someone and not wanting to worry my family any more than I had to, I made a big mistake resorting to a client whom I had seen twice and developed a positive speaking rapport with to help me with the stress I was experiencing.

Idiotically thinking that I could gain some peace of mind contacting someone who came to see me for the same reason was highly unprofessional and something I'd regret deeply once I was able to think more clearly. With an all-too-frequent tendency to read too much into things, overly analytical therapists could possibly claim that my thoughtless blunder was caused by head injury-induced impulsivity, rather than the basic human need to release corralled feelings which could otherwise burst unproductively. Walk a mile in my shoes before judging me.

After being dropped off at my apartment by the taxi I had arranged to take me home and having informed mom that I wasn't hurt in another car accident which left my vehicle nothing but twisted metal, being a practical stranger in this town and not really knowing anyone besides those I try to assist, I sat alone in my apartment needing someone to talk to because I had become really scared thinking that I might have only been inches away from another helicopter ride to Allegheny General or a mile per hour faster from a return trip to another hospital room full of mattresses.

Being that she had only recently come in for services and I had made the initial contact with her only about a week or two before, this lady's number was still fairly fresh in my mind and I foolishly proceeded to hit those digits which I knew would reach someone that I shouldn't have had to rely on to talk about a personal issue. I knew it wasn't proper for it to have affected me this way, but the empathetic things this woman said over the phone when I told her about the accident I was just in and how I felt like climbing the walls, relieved some of the tension that had bottled up inside of me trying to pretend I was not bothered all that much.

Realizing that I had crossed a boundary when I called this person at the spur of the moment to talk about a personal matter which was disturbing me instead of the other way around, wrongfully, I didn't feel much in the way of discomfort when this good listener came over to help me through my ordeal because those trained to help people encountering tough times—my maverick therapy cohorts who could have soothed this shaken co-worker—were emotionally inaccessible to me. I was fully aware of the risk I took calling this person to help me overcome the nerves which pulled at me, but with the discourteous way things were going at work, it got to the point where I just stopped being so concerned.

Between the time when I asked if she wouldn't mind talking with me about how bent out of shape I had become over the Monroeville crash which had me rehashing some of the events surrounding the '82 tragedy and when she arrived, I thankfully had second thoughts about divulging how I was once critically injured. Because I was uncertain as to what her response may be to this disclosure, I thought better of it to tell her about my one-time demented history, so I didn't say a word about my former condition.

My request of this light-haired mother of an adolescent to dump my sorrows on was an imprudent and rash action on my part. Not guided or influenced by discretion, feeling as though I had been put into exile by so many of my therapy buddies and barely knowing anyone outside of work, I selfishly felt I had to get the pent-up heightened emotions off my chest before it weighed me down and the source of this purge didn't really matter. I'd soon find out that one can never have enough friends at the agency for—unlike the situation where alleged abuses occurred within the office of a senior therapist beloved by those who had been with the agency since The Dark Ages—I knew that my injudicious move of contacting someone I shouldn't have to help me get over a troubling relapse wouldn't get swept under the rug and forgotten. Far from it.

Having a meal with this older, still good-looking, bubbly, blonde was a real treat. Because of the unusual circumstances surrounding this rendezvous, there seemed to be a little bit of odd tension in the air when I saw her in the parking lot of the fast food restaurant, standing by her car waiting for me. But things eventually picked up once the initial jitters subsided. In no time, as if a moment hadn't passed where our lives pointed us in different directions—like old buddies—we laughed and picked up on where some of the travels our lives have taken us the last time we saw each other.

On Thursday, 8/22/91, I had a little time coming to me, so I arranged to take an extended mid-day break to meet with someone whom I knew lived in neighboring Lower Burrell. In the nearby Tarentum office during this particular afternoon, about 12:30 P.M., I planned to be traveling on the bridge crossing the Allegheny River to have lunch with an attractive female I hadn't seen for what seemed an eternity. Out from under the watchful eye of management, I knew I would not get caught.

Knowing me when the insult to my brain caused wholesale damage and rescuing me from having a fork scratch the surface lining of my brain (dura) when that cognitively-impaired lady wanted to whip her silverware at "Christ's son" in the Harmarville nurses' station during dinner, my rehab center nurse/buddy who was part of my very first long-term memory following my head injury—the former Miss Janice Goga—was about to see me for the first time since I rose from those ashes that brain injury smothered me in.

Coincidentally, if we'd have had this reunion get-together only ninety-six hours ago, it would have been nine years to the day that I was discharged from Harmarville. That's a long time not to have contact with someone who left a lasting impression with you and had a major impact on your life at one time. Accompanied by her restless, grade school and preschool children, we caught up the best we could on what had been going on with our lives a year shy of a decade. Grateful that Jan's husband didn't object that this once "bruised brain" patient wanted to see her again after all this time, I also wanted to see if one of my leading advocates while I was a mangled patient could point me to any rehab places that were looking for a "one-in-a-million" professional like myself.

Proceeding my claims that work was alright and having been informed that Jan wasn't aware of any rehabs needing any help, I got on my high horse again and griped about how rehabilitation personnel execs still approach me as if I were "not all there," assuming that former "head injured" patients aren't supposed to be capable of doing all that I had claimed to have achieved. Referring to my internship and practicum at Charles Goyette's New Medico at Meadowlands' facility, after an argument broke out between her little ones whether "Scooby-Dooby-Doo" or "The Adventures of Yogi Bear" would be the cartoon of choice this upcoming Saturday morning, I talked about how my life experience with head injury appeared to have canceled out my advanced degree/textbook experience I earned in grad school. As if they had already known what was to transpire, I dejectedly went over how none of the New Medico Family Counselors, nor the Neuropsychologist, seemed to be all that surprised someone with my personal experience with disability didn't get the Meadowlands Health Care Center job over a girl with inferior credentials.

Ducking a flying box of french fries, I spoke of how rehabilitation personnel staff members have shown that they don't want a person who walks and moves like they've sustained a neurological impairment on their payroll collecting a good paycheck, no matter what treasure trove of information the survivor's experience could provide their treatment program. Pepper shaker bouncing off my forehead, I told Jan how upsetting it was not being considered for paid employment at all these rehab facilities and corporations, but being in high-demand by these same outfits to give "freebie" volunteer services because of my "one-of-a-kind" experience.

Ketchup squirted on my dress shirt and a piece of dried nasal mucous flicked on my tie, in addition to mastering the curriculum in my Master's program, I screamed over the ruckus that despite almost paying the ultimate price trusting someone who had been drinking to drive and sustaining a debilitating brain injury, I was still being viewed by both comprehensive and head injury rehabilitation facilities' Human Resource Departments as someone who had not yet "earned my stripes" to be able to work for them in a professional capacity. Salt tossed in my eyes, it burned even more talking about how rehab centers' various administrations must have just taken it for granted that my work must be inefficient because of my one-time neurologically impaired history. I spoke of how it was quite evident that I didn't have much hope of attaining a bountiful counseling position with any center, as long as program directors had misgivings about this survivor's intellect.

Beef patty twirling towards me, I told Jan that I was wrapped in a massive web of fury having rehab employment doors slammed in my face because—of all things—my experience with disability where I had been so close to "kicking the bucket" had led employers to believe that I was "compromised." Discouraged and exhausted—but not down for the count—dodging a pickle whipped my way, I assured Jan that rehab personnel exec's biases weren't going to suffocate me because of the "know-how" I possessed and that it would take a lot more than their prejudice/discrimination to completely take the wind out of my sails.

I relayed to Jan that—point blank—it had been my experience that if I was given a puppy dog smile by an employer who said that it wouldn't be held against me that I once had a brain injury affliction, I knew not to believe this for an instant because they're lying. Likewise, if I received a flowery response letter from a facility aware of my once deranged condition stating that no position which I would be qualified currently exists—but that once an opening would arise, I'd be contacted for an interview—I knew to take this with a grain of salt as well, for I realized my resume would find its way into the trash. Knowing that I wouldn't have a chance at these rehabilitation jobs—even if I'd accept a reduced salary—was disheartening, but I wasn't about to stop believing in myself or stoop to a level where I knew that not being reimbursed fairly would make me miserable in time.

Telling Jan that it appeared rehabilitation employers already had their minds made up that all people with histories of a head injury disability were incompetent "across the board," with the expletive whispered so only the two of us could hear, I then said to her that I didn't have a "hope in Hell" of ever attaining a fruitful position in rehab, as long as this opinion was held and actions taken because of this globally accepted belief. After trying to dry off the pop which ended up in my hair, I finished up my delivery by telling my nurse well-wisher that legislators who drew up and regulators enforcing "The Americans with Disabilities Act" were being scoffed at as foolish idiots by rehabilitation personnel executives and most other employers since its inception. The "voice" of those with disabilities barely being audible and with this population being in the minority, plain and simple, this law always will be regarded as a joke. There's a lot of Charles Goyettes out there.

Asking me if I had tried applying for a professional position at the rehab center where I got to know her, with a stream of mustard headed in my direction, I said to Jan that Harmarville's extensive vocational program was designed with the intention of helping their inpatients attain gainful employment with other organizations—not their operation—so that really wouldn't be a realistic option. One last sesame seed bun flung at me, I told my one-time LPN pal—"retired" into the sanctimony which is motherhood—that I could whole-heartedly understand my "home" rehab center feeling as if they had done enough for me already and that it was more in line with their needs/deemed more preferable hiring a Rehabilitation Counselor possessing classroom lecture experience with vocational training/ evaluation over someone who had life experience with disability at their facility. Whole-heartedly.

If the government intended HSDF money allocated to different service providers be primarily used to maximize profits for the respective organizations, rather than to assure that clients who required some financial assistance received help when they needed it, then our counseling agency utilized this grant pretty well. Being in the single-parent program, because more than a few one-parent households experience some cash flow problems and find it a necessity to pinch pennies, about half of the clients I saw were eligible for this government-subsidized counseling. Some barely hovering over the poverty line and a few trying to climb out of the welfare hole, these therapy patrons' incomes weren't usually a reflection of their dedication to work on their problems. For those concerned with their quality of life, these folks were loyal to keeping their scheduled counseling appointments. Obligated to adhere to administrative directives, I wasn't always to be so committed.

Seeing it as a HSDF dollar bonanza, an executive order came down from headquarters that I was not to set aside any time for my devoted, regularly-scheduled, government-assisted clientele—who quite possibly could have benefited from speaking with me this one particular day—so that I could make arrangements to give a talk about an assortment of issues on a speeding bus with a group of women who did not request this service. With the destination being a prison north of the city, I not only felt like I was a trespasser infringing on these ladies' private time when they'd just as soon be gathering their thoughts about a range of personal issues that they'd only feel comfortable their imprisoned loved ones would hear, but almost like a thief when I passed out the HSDF applications to these trapped females for this forced-upon presentation. Unless they wanted to flee out of the back emergency door of a bus going up a highway at 60 m.p.h., they had no choice but to sit in attendance for the HSDF role call and listen to my words of wisdom.

Already having had my skull cracked once, I stood at the front of this HSDF-mobile clinging onto the back of a seat, fearing that my head's infrastructure was once again going to be whipped around, as that bus went flying up I-79 to Mercer County. Sweating blood that I was about to make a return trip to A.G.H. because my brain's bruised "position sense" function would send me on my backside, I was still able to manage to get about half the group of travelers to discuss how they go about best mentally preparing for this inmate encounter, while the other half just wanted to be absorbed with quiet and couldn't care less what the hell this intruding stranger had to say. Regardless if these inmates' loved ones were concerned or not, the agency sure made some solid dollars.

As I kept looking up at the sky praying that this lecture vehicle wouldn't hit one of those infamous Pennsylvania potholes—landing me on my seat beltless buttocks—I expected to hear some choppers and see some clerical workers armed with more HSDF applications parachute from these whirly birds, if it was somehow noted that I didn't have enough of these income forms. Like when I didn't take the "bait and switch" transfer consideration that was cast my way when I first started at the agency, voicing my objections later on about this "regular clients-be-damned" HSDF tactic didn't exactly earn me any "brownie points." Hell hath no fury like a "disabled" person scorned.

It's hard to say if my invitation of a single parent to help me address a problem that I felt staff wouldn't empathize with was any less appropriate than the way the agency pocketed the government's HSDF grant. Regardless, I would find myself on the "hot seat" six months after my ill-advised call of someone I shouldn't have to assist me regain my composure after the Monroeville brush with fate.

In a relationship where the turbulence too frequently exceeded the pleasure, not all that pleased his woman was coming in to work on their troubled union in the first place, this lady's partner saw to it that I'd be reprimanded for my witless phone offer when learning about this visit after all this time had passed. Not aware of what this confidante I inappropriately resorted to told administration or her boyfriend, I knew that I would be on "thin ice," if the agency found out about my call of this friendly mom.

Coming down hard on me for setting myself up like I did for any kind of accusation, despite my plea that I was not guilty of any wrong-doing, Luke told me that a client's presence in my quarters would more than likely be enough to "send me packing." Insisting that I did not take advantage of this client while she was there and what we did do was talk about how lucky it was that I was not hurt in the Monroeville accident as well as her relationship, I would be told that it didn't look good that this lady stopped her therapy after those initial two sessions and that the previous strikes against me weren't going to work in my favor.

Explaining that her continued attendance was on shaky ground from the beginning as it was because not everybody in her party was exactly thrilled with the idea of her talking to a counselor, I'd only be able to guess that she could have been feeling some pressure to drop out of therapy, or felt tense talking to a male about sensitive topics which were characteristic of her relationship. Assigned to read Dr. Susan Forward's classic book about women in painful relationships entitled, Men Who Hate Women and the Women Who Love Them, in classic misogynyst fashion, I was told that this client's male companion would tell her—upon finding out of this homework—that I was going to teach her how to hate him.

Given that I had been regarded with general disfavor because of the timing of my admittance into the organization, the belief that what I would "bring to the table" of this counseling operation as far as life experience was minimal, could have put a well-liked senior therapist in some "hot water" reporting that I had received an intake call laden with allegations about this employee, was reluctant to work in an area where the non-profit agency could have prospered with the HSDF dollar, probably agitated some authoritative figure griping about how the revenue-generating bus trip shouldn't have been seen as priority at the expense of my faithful clients, didn't make much of a donation out of my paycheck to the corporation every two weeks, didn't address that abortion issue like my supervisor would have liked, had been associated with an artificial sexual harassment charge, and was suspected by more than a few staff of once being put "out of commission" by a neurological ailment that I wanted to portray as not being serious, this phone message where I reversed the roles of helper and helpee would be the straw which broke the camel's back.

Knowing that administration was informed of my stupid action, before any determination would be made regarding my continued employment—so that I could speak for myself—I scheduled to meet with the two personnel who would ultimately decide my destiny with the operation. With a dark cloud of question hanging over me as to whether or not there was once a time when I wasn't "playing with a full deck" and fears possibly having existed that a thinking disorder could still be an element of my future, I realized my chance of "sticking" were slim.

I believed that if I were to continue working at this organization, keeping my one-time "brain injured" condition secret had to be preserved. Not feeling as if I could disclose that the reason for my need to talk with someone about the "minor" smash-up in Monroeville was because it brought back memories of the events surrounding my brain injury, I knew that I didn't have much ammunition to defend myself with and lost my job. Always darkest before the dawn?

A little more than two months had passed when I interviewed for this new, residential/treatment program position only about twenty miles from home in

Washington. Located in southern Allegheny County, the partial hospitalization component of the treatment center where I would be working was—overall—generally more in line with the philosophy of care I was accustomed to in my personal life and the fundamentals of my Rehabilitation Counseling education.

While a patient in Harmarville, the open and personable demeanors of the staff working with me was a major ingredient in my rehabilitation recovery. Medical staff and therapists having such affable, down-to-earth personalities not only promoted their own healthy, formidable personal lives, but motivated those whom their character touched to give an utmost effort, so that improvement could occur. Being treated with such warmth and respect by rehabilitation professionals at a time when this once mentally-mutilated patient couldn't understand what was going on around him, limitlessly fostered my restoration and meant so much to me.

Although the importance of operating within professional limits had always been emphasized, the rehabilitation field allows for a more open/not-so-aloof association with its patients than straight-laced, traditional psychotherapy does with its clients. And the way the philosophical rudiments of the latter were presented to me was something that this new member of the therapy work force just found too unnatural to feel comfortable with. Being required to let go of an approach which I had repeatedly witnessed to be so beneficial for the masses in the disability population and personally experienced myself in my rehabilitation, was hardly soothing.

Naturally, my primary focus had always been to work in rehabilitation, but there would be some definite regrets being "shown the door" of this counseling operation. Living there for sixteen months and becoming acclimated to the area's many amenities, I developed a fondness for Monroeville that would be sorely missed. Having become accustomed to the faster pace of this Pittsburgh suburb's lifestyle, I wasted little time not only attempting to remain in this "happening" community, but tried to acquire a job where I could utilize my quality of being a rehabilitation titan of sorts, just up the road from the counseling program I had an axe to grind with.

Like my speaking displays in Florida, I gave a "no charge necessary" head injury rehabilitation talk and showed the video of me when I had intellectually "missed the boat" on many counts to a sizable crowd of people associated with the Greater Pittsburgh Rehabilitation Hospital in Monroeville. So that patients, families, and staff who weren't able to attend this evening January 1992 presentation could witness how cognitively intact and physically presentable a person could be after having been stampeded by the symptoms of a severe brain injury, my "lecture" would be saved on videotape for future use at the facility while I would—more than likely—be back home trying to pound my way into that rehabilitation work force where I should have already been prospering at these past four years.

Amongst the group of interested listeners who were hanging on to my every word, I spotted a recreational therapist formerly employed in the same capacity at Goyette's New Medico at Meadowlands madhouse whom I wanted to inform of the shabby manner in which this survivor was treated by her employer. The caliber of my recovery being kept from the vast majority of New Medico staff, I saw this presentation as an opportunity to finally give the center's administration and Penelope Rich's potentially influential affluent background some free advertising to someone in "program" who worked there when I was training.

Viewing my rehabilitation history on that tape New Medico administration didn't want their employees to see, this worker appeared to be more-than-mildly surprised and even slightly amazed of the extent with which I had been incapacitated/the recovery I had made because the degree which I had been hurt and the positive impact my background could have had on those I would have been around were hidden so well. This one-time New Medico employee had quite a bit to ask when I opened up my talk to questions because, with the exception of a scant article written about me and my struggles, there would have been no way she could have realized just how potentially valuable my miraculous comeback could have been for those who needed some light at the end of their tunnel. In early 1992, coinciding with this Monroeville rehabilitation exhibition, light would also be blazing upon the New Medico Corporation by those who shared in my abomination for this heinous company.

Chapter 8

New Medico

Long before the New Medico operations' dark strategy of burning patients' candles at both ends was anywhere close yet to setting off an alarm and becoming common knowledge, a week after I was made out to be a bad guy and dumped by the agency that could have very easily been intimidated that a bachelor male therapist was counseling female single parents, my tenacity to get with the corporation which I already had proven I'd be perfectly tailored for, would be resurrected. Always sensing that he had felt bad for me not deservedly getting the Meadowlands' job I had worked so hard for and wanted in the worst way, my primary supervisor when I served my unpaid student internship with Meadowlands—Berkowitz—had a promising tone to his voice when telling me the good news. My supposed New Medico advocate told me that, not only did Penelope quit the Family Counselor job which I believed I'd have been the long-term solution to after only about a year, but Program Director Charles Goyette got fired!!!!!!!!!!!!

It would be tough containing myself when told that the one-time Meadowlands' cognitive department's supervisor, who had always seemed to be impressed with my work as an intern, had become responsible for the clinical program. Thinking that this professional who was aware of my incomparable background and subsequent capabilities would be overseeing the personnel staffed at the facility, I mailed this staff member a cover letter and an updated resume, feeling as though I had finally gotten a break from the Corporation. However, on 1/29/92, a mere thirteen days after I got my hopes up sending this "sales pitch" letter to the doctor whom I had been told became clinical director and assumed would be doing the hiring at Meadowlands, New Medico ripped out my heart and shoved it up my ass again.

Like the New Medico 5/19/89, "We treat those with head injuries, not hire them," rejection letter I received informing me that Penelope's credentials, experience, and professional interests were deemed as superior to mine, the Meadowlands' notice I received the first month of 1992 began with a cuddly, "Dear Craig, it was a pleasure receiving your resume recently regarding employment with New Medico Rehabilitation and Skilled Nursing Center at Meadowlands. Thank you for your continued interest with our organization."

The warmth which glowed inside of me reading this eloquent opening quickly turned to frigid ice when I looked at the bottom of the page and saw that Donna Micklow hadn't yet been canned along with Goyette, as She continued to obediently adhere to New Medico's tactics of generating revenue/patient care. With Her reward being advancement upwards on the Corporation's hierarchical progression, my hopes of being a working cog within the New Medico system would be thoroughly dashed. Unlike the first notification I received from Meadowlands in May 1989 that a sorority sister would be more suitable working with those having sustained the disability which would always be a part of me and was more prepared to counsel the New Medico head injury population despite my already having been trained there, Micklow's latest spurn response had Program Director under Her name and a new set of initials (CRRN: Certified Rehabilitation Registered Nurse) after it, to indicate just how far Her concern for patients' well-being had taken Her.

After being informed once again that Meadowlands found yet another person more qualified than myself to work with the "brain contused" disability population and thanking me for my continued interest, the passion of the New Medico "refusal to hire one of their own" document reached exciting proportions when Micklow signed off only using Her first name. I took this informal signature, validating the contents of this New Medico message to be the whole truth and nothing but the truth so help me God, to mean that this righteous administrator had no hard feeling towards me because of my relentless pursuit of Her Corporation not to discriminate against me.

Calling Berkowitz a short time later for an "insider's scoop" of what was taking place within the ethical walls of Meadowlands, this Corporate employee who still seemed to weigh his words so heavily before speaking, sounded stunned when hearing my voice after my most recent bout with New Medico. Surely hoping that I would exhibit some behavior that they could fabricate as being attributable to my brain injury, when bringing me on board in the first place to serve my academic training, New Medico probably assumed it was only a matter of time before some sequelae of my head injury would surface that they could use as a reason not to hire me, if the day would arrive when I'd seek reciprocation in the form of paid, equal opportunity for employment at their company.

However, being a productive intern who doesn't have—therefore couldn't exhibit—any abnormal behavioral symptoms of once having his senses sabotaged by a bruise on the brain, a feeling of administrative worry/panic likely evolved once I proved myself and showed no ill-effects from my contusion existed and that the only consequence of almost being brain dead would be one which would benefit their similarly traumatized patients. Unable to find or secure any legitimate grounds for not hiring this survivor, turning things around to make it look like my confrontational outburst in Hess's at the Franklin Mall was a result of my head injury and not a reaction to being victimized by discrimination or possibly even nepotism, I was told by my primary supervisor that Micklow used this incident as a lame excuse not to give this "head injured" applicant with inestimable value, proper consideration.

New Medico Rehabilitation and Skilled Nursing Center at Meadowlands

January 29, 1992

Mr. Craig Meyers

Washington, PA 15301

Dear Craig,

It was a pleasure receiving your resume recently regarding employment with New Medico Rehabilitation and Skilled Nursing Center at Meadowlands. Thank you for your continued interest wih our organization.

At this time, the Family Counselor position has been filled. We will keep your resume on file for one year, and in the event that another comparable position becomes available, we will contact you to discuss future opportunities with New Medico.

Thank you again for your interest in seeking employment with Meadowlands.

Sincerely,

Donna

Donna Micklow, BSN, MPA, CRRN
Program Director

DM/jld

R.D. 1, Box 146, Route 519 South
Canonsburg, Pennsylvania
15317

Telephone
(412) 745-8000

Micklow knowing that I had commendably undertook all the duties for which I was assigned and responsible during my New Medico field training —like when She had the gall to blame me for the size of my Meadowlands' caseload in the department store—this administrator with the fantasy moral guidelines scraped the bottom of the barrel and grasped for straws with this latest conniving alibi. With all the double talk and the evasive approach so characteristic of the Meadowlands' personnel I had the fortune of being around, I didn't know what was going on, but one could almost assume New Medico wasn't on the "up and up."

It had been ten years ago to the month that my perception of the world had disintegrated and the jaws of death nearly claimed me as another one of its victims. Forever leaving an impact with me, before I left the area of Monroeville, I wanted to offer my oratorical skills on this anniversary date of sorts to the "home" rehabilitation facility that helped me dig myself out of the rubble that accident buried me in a decade ago. Giving this freebie demonstration, I wanted to pay back Harmarville at least a little bit for their stupendous therapy work with me when I was "three bricks shy of a load."

In addition to wanting to give the center which had done so much for me a little something in return for their talents, admittedly, I also gave this complimentary talk, so that my name would be fresh in the minds of those drawing from my "home" rehab's personnel application pool and because of my burning desire to remain in this part of Pittsburgh. Despite the many gallant cognitive victories I had made since my awareness could only be inferred, I suppose the continued hunch in my gait would be an embarrassing sight for anyone from Harmarville's staff who may have promoted my restoration as being a direct result of their therapist's skills and knowledge. I could thoroughly comprehend if Harmarville had reservations about employing a former "head injured" patient of theirs who still had a gimp in his walk after all these years, for this could be discouraging for some of their recent admissions who may see me. Thoroughly.

Although the dozens of applications for employment I sent out again to various comprehensive and head injury treatment facilities across the nation all resulted in my receiving a "Not him again" shunned response, I was still able to manage to keep a stiff upper lip and continued to slug away at those rehabilitation employment doors. However, with those entranceways to a prosperous career professionally working with those who had suffered disabilities reinforced by steel bars of discrimination, I could assume applicants were getting the very jobs which I would be more qualified merely because—along with 36"-24"36" sugar plum fairies—fantasy symptoms were dancing in the heads of personnel administrators who worried that my once having been "knocked out" created some maddened lunatic. But try to prove prejudice exists.

My giving voluntary presentations at all those treatment programs, hoping that some rehab employment position might fling open for me, hadn't done any good. And if anything, could have validated different administrators' prejudices towards people with neurological impairments. These center's managements possibly figured my contusion created someone who had fallen from grace so badly that I wouldn't be bright enough to ask for any reimbursement for my time, skills, or effort.

Training at New Medico, I discovered that if a head injury survivor does freebie work, it will be believed of these unfortunate souls that they are "out of their mind" and so intellectually stunted that they'd be too dumb to ask for any money for their labor. Not wanting to live a life behind the bars of suspicion and rejected opportunity, I thought I'd approach things from a different angle.

I wouldn't have a clue as to how many people out there have sustained head trauma to the extent that I have and could get their experience jotted down in written form, so I thought I just might start trying to work on a fairly unique book project, detailing many of the traumatic events which are part of my history that could help out others in similar circumstances. I have always been your average kind of guy whom no one in their right mind would ever label a "holy roller" or be mistaken for ever attending a theology seminar, but I firmly believe that I survived that accident "against all odds" for a reason. Maybe a perspective being offered from someone down-to-earth could reach a few "commoners" like myself who otherwise might not be real receptive to anything but meat and potatoes rehab effort. So, here goes.

When so many people simply took the time out from their schedules to use the most potent force available to them—the power of prayer—and said a few silent hopes/wishes for me when I was teetering between life and death, without a moment's doubt, I will always acknowledge that God responded by tipping the scales in my favor. Giving this lucky recipient the strength that I logically should have never expected, I think I should share this gift to those who were just as deserving and more so, but may not have fullly grasped this fortune. If the biases of people like those navigating the pirate ship which is New Medico are going to prevent me from doing my work, another means will need to be utilized.

With my previous pursuits to be significant having been misguided and meaningless in the general scope of things, I know that I now have a purpose in tow and it wasn't to tell parents that the reason their kids don't like them is because some of these caregivers had threatened to lock their little ones in the kitchen cupboard all week. Although there's a definite need to help people whose life has had some heavy emotional baggage in it dragging them down, I wouldn't suppose I was given an opportunity to achieve, just so I could umpire inter-family grumblings.

My recovery pointing me in the direction that it has, I wouldn't imagine it would be too hard to understand that I'd be inclined to think my "calling" was one where I was to share my incredible experience in whatever way I could, so that my story could be reached for those who need to grasp to some kind of message. If I must hide my recuperation from administrators like those at the counseling agency who frowned on me referring to myself as a "family therapist" until I gained as much life experience as those "advanced" counselors around me, then my struggles to return to a state of normalcy would not have the meaning that it could and its impact non-existent, or seriously compromised. If it is not possible for me to be "heard" in the traditional fashion made available to "healthy" people in the form of attaining and maintaining influential employment, then I'd just have to slip in a back door somehow.

For this survivor who was almost mortally wounded and later tortured within a brain injury's chamber of horrors, being in a tragedy helped me to gain an enhanced appreciation for, and an elevated understanding of what is important in life. This conceptualization had facilitated an understanding that my "calling" was one where I could be meaningful to a number of people because of my exclusive trials with a horrifying disability.

A pen as my brush, I thought I would paint a portrait of words capturing a time in my history which could be savored by a few and might just serve as the key I'd need to escape my concealed existence. With this excursion highlighting my insider's perspective of a treacherous condition stewing on the back burner, not sure if this assignment of self-disclosure would be beneficial, I continued to search for a position where I wouldn't have to isolate my trials with trauma.

In addition to continuing to apply for different jobs advertised in the Pittsburgh classifieds and attempting to convince many of the rehab facilities listed in the N.H.I.F. directory that my head injury hadn't permanently wilted away my intellect—while I waited for management to get approval from the government to begin operations at the new, MH/MR treatment facility where I would ultimately attain the first full-time therapist position—I thought I'd also start digging in the closet and gather some of the files needed to start working on a writing project highlighting my unique, symptomatic adventures through the dark continent known as brain injury. Knowing the experience of being hurt so bad that it had left me comatose and the subsequent comeback I made doesn't happen everyday with everyone—realizing this trauma affects hundreds of thousands of people every year—I thought there might be an audience out there interested in what I had to say and have been through. Since my unlikely return from a neurologically disconnected state where I was unbalanced and not sound, I had wanted to express my phenomenon through the perils of brain injury in a tangible form.

God bless my parents for being "pack rats" and never throwing anything away, because I would need all the documentation that I could get my hands on which had been collecting dust these past ten years. Writing this autobiographical self-portrayal—because I learned so much about the dynamics of family systems in the Monroeville therapy job/my graduate studies which assisted me in my understanding of who I am as a person—I thought I'd start near the beginning and review some of the influences and factors that developed my personality which could leave a useful impression on readers, if anyone outside of my family or friends ever decide to read my writing endeavor. I kicked around different titles for the book and thought that because I was given another shot at life to make something out of myself, I'd naturally call my project, "Second Chance." However, this sounding like something any divorcee who remarried might pen, calling my enterprise by this name wouldn't be etched in stone.

Having a vague idea of how I wanted to arrange my worded venture into the unexplored territory of chronicling a passage marking the events of a life after severe head injury, I had to first mentally outline how to go about setting things up before any kind of a formal layout could be developed. I knew that this project would consume not only a massive amount of time, but peace of mind, for I'd have to unleash some painful emotions which I'd chained out of awareness and wrapped into the safety net of my unconscious.

Freeing repressed shadows would not be the only psychological blade tearing at me, but physically getting my ideas down on paper with my non-dominant left hand, before struggling at the typewriter constructing the final form to be submitted, would literally be hell. Having basically started this book in February 1992—with the excruciatingly slow and trying manner in which I wrote—if things hadn't materialized as they had, I may not have gotten this undertaking done until the year 2020. I thought I had better start getting this book written because, by the time I'd finish, if I had waited too long, there may be a cure for those with head injuries. A capsule could be developed where coming out of a coma to being a professional wouldn't be all that out of the ordinary, making this achievement more the rule than the exception and my book anything but interesting. One never knows.

Appreciating why personnel departments may hold the wary position that they do towards me given what's understood about brain injury, receiving the gift of having a life with the potential of promise, I felt I had to reciprocate and do what I could to lessen the onus associated with head injury. Feeling as though I had some insight and experience about what the predetermined judgments linked to people with brain injuries can do, I thought I'd crawl out of the disability scrap heap where the "brain injured" are left to rot and possibly revise some thinking.

The time and energy entailed in working on a project of this magnitude would be excessive. Soliciting the skills of a professional writer to help me co-author this manifesto of exertion, who knows the "ins" and "outs" of the publishing business, would likely be seen as advantageous by a neutral source unaware that the intention of my plan is to heighten awareness. To have someone coming up with different ideas and concepts for my written expose, who didn't have a brain injury, would defeat one of the major purposes of the book. If this project wouldn't be approved of and falls flat on its face, I could accept the failures for which I was responsible. However—even to the slightest degree—if my work would be received somewhat favorably, I'd want the majority of credit for this marginal acceptance and not someone serving in a role as a contributor.

I thought it would add the flavor of authenticity and validation, if the book's sole writer had experienced the anguish of brain trauma and were the only one to pen a record of this frequently misunderstood disability. Because of the horrific stigma associated with head injury, I could just hear cynics—like many of the rehab execs I've had the fortune of encountering—making the remark, "That passage required some thought and creativity, the guy with the head injury must not have written that part."

I realized that tackling a work of this nature would come at the cost of an employment gap in my resume, but the strong impulse God gave me to catalogue my experience would seem to make this sacrifice worthwhile. The size of this work void would be the result of a double-edged sword because I wouldn't want the period between jobs to be miles apart, yet, neither would I want to rush through this documentation, for a "chop job" may not only leave a poor impression as to the capabilities of the head injury disability population in general, but me as an individual once having this affliction and seeking status of some sort.

Without question, it's important to be cautious, but to generalize can also render extreme harm to those being given a label, as well as those their life affects. Merits difficult to come by for a disability not usually substantiated by known fact, regardless of content, I anticipate this depiction would no doubt be subjected to being maligned. Those calumniators out there who may review my effort surely could crow, "That book wasn't bad considering it was put together by somebody who was once goony."

No doubt, the toughest obstacle I've had to contend with since my brain trauma hadn't been coming out of a coma, relearning how to think, move, and write, or the terrifying psychological strain of acquiring a disability and accepting this affliction as a permanent part of myself, because "I" had control of how much effort was put into addressing those deficits. Rather, the hardest hurdle I've had to encounter is one largely outside of my control because it is dependent on the attitudes of others and that universalized obstruction has been taking prejudice/discrimination on the chin, not only from prospective employers, but from various members of society in general. But I suppose my brain being bruised has caused me to miscalculate the motives of employers because nobody discriminates—just ask those filling job vacancies.

Along with the altruistic striving to record my accounts of the struggles I faced following my seriously brain damaged past that could benefit patients/families scuffling with many of the same dilemmas, knowing that my cognitive capabilities are more than firmly in place and not wanting my life to be a sediment of past errors, I had the desire to circulate my expressive/comprehensive abilities to a few employers who might have been previously directed by false stereotypes when learning of this job applicant's one-time, "brain contused," mentally-paralytic history.

Never having an ailment characterized by assumption and fear, most job applicants can attain a rewarding position, if they have had the educational requirements and experience background necessary for fulfilling a professional post. However, with the way things had been developing on the job battle front for me, it looked more and more like I'd have to go that extra mile because of my head injury, if I wanted treated equally/fairly. My way of going about putting in that extra effort is by writing this review, so that maybe someday I'd be given the same chance by rehabilitation administrators at acquiring a rewarding job, as someone who hadn't had a head injury.

In addition to my taboo criticism of New Medico execs, if my book would get published and someone outside of my relatives reads it, prospective employers likely would use the excuse that too many people are aware of my history to be a respected and effective counselor; using my printed attempts to reach out and help some people as a reason why this "head injured victim" could never be hired to occupy a professional capacity. Viewing this equal opportunity as taking a risk, there's a slew of imaginary justifications disability-conscious human resource department's can use to segregate the physically vibrant from those not so fortunate. With the way my entrance into the work world stalled for me, I could be reasonably sure personnel department darlings were shaking in their booties when thinking about the prospects of a former "brain damaged" patient wanting a fruitful position with their respective establishments.

Like when I enrolled for the W.V.U. Rehab Counseling program in the first place to assist me in my pursuits to attain a higher-level head injury rehabilitation job—helping people similarly afflicted and provide me with the opportunity to sustain a respectable livelihood—I thought I'd try to make a positive out of a negative and write about my personal confrontations with brain injury, so that the whole experience wouldn't feel so meaningless and be utterly counter-productive to me then. Hopefully, the latter will reap some opportunities that the former hadn't.

If the attitudes of rehabilitation execs prevent me from attaining a prominent position helping patients having sustained disabilities, I thought maybe writing a book—and hopefully getting it out to a few people other than personal acquaintances—might be able to reduce some of the damage that preconceived notions which exist about people with histories of a brain impairment have caused. With rehabilitation administrator's biases keeping me from assisting patients having sustained head injuries and their loved ones—while concurrently trying to gain admission into some acute head injury treatment care program—I thought I'd get serious and focus a good bit on getting this introspective project started, with the hopes of reaching some folks who aren't ever going to see me in a professional realm.

Locking horns with rehab bosses who quietly held the position that professionally employing this scarred job applicant was a risky proposition because of my history of once being tangled within the mesh of neurological damage, I just had to dig deep within myself and find the constitution to prevail. Possibly feeling threatened that I was putting a gun to their head, forcing them to abide by their equal opportunity obligation, I sensed the rehab vocational world closing in on me. With the Equal Employment Opportunity Commission not returning my phone calls or making any kind of effort to be helpful, if a rehabilitation facility is going to pass judgment on someone they designate as a "disabled vegetable" and not consider the "cripple" because of this perception, nobody is going to be able to stop them, for seemingly sound warrants for their actions will be concocted.

As if it were my fault and a sign of a character flaw, I don't know how many job tryouts I'd gone on where I had been questioned as to why it took me so long to land a job after I served my internship and got my Master's. Liable to be taking note of my paralytic right side, not wanting to divulge to the interviewer that I had been discriminated against by my training site because my claims of prejudice would obviously indicate that something definitely had happened to me, I would be at a loss for words. Needing to keep my one-time aphasic condition secret at all costs, if I wanted an opportunity for the particular position, this limping applicant could only say that the job market is tough out there. "Duh."

Like New Medico's Micklow before them, if I'd have said to those questioning me about my background that it took a great deal of time to get over seeing a far-less qualified/fellow student get the rehab job for which I had been trained, the prospective employer would have surely turned things around on me to make "up" seem "down," so that this physically damaged job hopeful wouldn't have any chance of gaining employment. Those responsible for finding personnel would likely say something to the effect that I must be emotionally weak because it's quite evident that I have trouble accepting unpleasant circumstances. Subsequently, staff seeking available human resource candidates would devise the conclusion that I had no business thinking I could help people instill a little strength in their lives because I obviously had no experience handling discomforting incidents that life can tax one with.

In some respects, rehabilitation health care facilities' response to this brain injury survivor's search of gaining professional employment with them corresponded with a situation where a particular establishment wasn't to begin operations because residents owned a "not in our neighborhood" attitude. Nervously shuffled off with the hopes that I'd forget I wanted employment with them or had found somewhere else to settle in, head injury trauma operations had been passing me on from one to another because recent college graduate applicants had been found who were deemed more knowledgeable about brain injury rehabilitation than myself.

If one day my head injury disability struggles would somehow get a trace of exposure, I could just hear a former interviewer, unaware of my bruised brain history at the time of my work audition, breathing a deep sigh of relief before exclaiming, "Whew, that was a close one. We could've hired that guy." Stockpiling a roster of employees who could be suspect would not be wise, however, assigning an unfounded and incorrect "questionable" designation to one whose travels through life could enlighten so many, is tragic.

More than likely, I wasn't given a shot of acquiring any available rehabilitation stations in life because "fear of the unknown" potentially guided directors to set their sights elsewhere when seeking capable bodies to fill their payroll. Accepting that a "head injured" applicant possessing the mandated credentials for a job slot couldn't be medically possible, it would hardly be a long shot to assume that rehab execs running facilities and in charge of personnel went for the "candy store twinkie" possessing the stated prerequisites—whom they could feel safe and cozy with—despite knowing in the back of their minds that someone with the experiential elixirs in his cabinet that this survivor supposedly had at his disposal could be optimally prosperous for patients.

Publications such as the various annals of medicine not supporting such claims, managements must have figured that there had to be some sort of a hitch or condition smearing this "Eighth Wonder's" fairy tale recovery because "everyone knows" that after one has hit their head as severely as I had, only so much can be accomplished then. This "suspect's" attempts to gain passage into the rehabilitation work place serving as an example, it looked to be a given that administrators wouldn't deviate from what is regarded as acknowledged fact. Because some of these principles accepted as fundamental understanding rest on shaky foundations, my war has been with those rehabilitation commanding tiers who will do what they can to preserve dubious beliefs/ practices which had always been adhered to. Suspicion about this former patient's competency aside, factors personal in nature may have incited human resource "heads" to operate as they did.

Conceding that one is wrong doesn't come easy for a lot of people, especially those driven by professional vanity, rather than logic. Feeling as if they aren't obliged to answer to anyone, the rehab facilities' upper echelon which I have been exposed to customarily seem to take this stance. It almost appeared that those disability professionals who previously had professed I wouldn't be able to get my Bachelor's Degree, let alone my Master's, would do what they could to prevent me from attaining any more goals which they heretofore declared couldn't—anyway under the sun—be possible. Attributing this statement to paranoia manifested by my head injury and not objectivity supported by the record, I could almost hear those New Medico "buttercups" I had the enchanting experience of meeting, snicker at my inability to crack into the rehabilitation work force.

Given the type of injury I had sustained and the extent of its severity, for me to make these "shirt and tie" executives eat their words/swallow their pride again by being much more than efficient at a rehabilitation job site, would definitely be a humbling experience for them. This brain injury survivor's performance corresponding with my competency claims, proving stately administrators were incorrect once more, would be a situation managements simply were not going to allow to happen. While waiting for the dust to settle on the rehabilitation employment front where treatment centers' personnel execs were my "Achilles heel," I had been making solid—if not speedy—progress in my pursuits to leave some sort of a signature in the book-writing world.

After having cognitively pieced together a general outline of how I thought various events of my experience could be sequenced, I wrestled with the reasons as to why I might want to write a book and came to the conclusion that the pros would outweigh any cons. After determining the potential for servicing others would compensate for the misgivings, I had to formulate the project's content and how I wanted it presented.

Having just worked in the same agency as many social workers who liked to classify themselves as psychoanalysts, I know people of this nature in society possibly could be offended by the segments I plan to incorporate in my written work which I feel need to be graphic in order to give the reader a real sense of experience. Knowing that you can't please everyone and somebody's bound to be disgusted, I thought it would be more important to make a connection with people who weren't odd, so that those who would want and need an accurate depiction of some of the struggles one is up against when crossing swords with the symptoms of a brain injury can get this representation. Being in such sad shape I ended up in a head trauma rehabilitation unit was often an utterly embarrassing and humiliating nightmare, with the only way to get a real taste of what one goes through is to detail various events vividly and not sugarcoat things because someone with a delicate tummy may be insulted. I wasn't about to compromise the experience.

As far as those components of my book where I thought I'd wind my jack-in-the-box and utilize my interpretation of humor, I believed that a format which conveyed a light-hearted mood/overtone could be advantageous. It's quite natural for both the patient and those who care for the one stricken with the head injury to obsess about how the brain being jolted or pierced within the skull will affect personality. For those overflowing with concern whether or not laughter will ever be heard again coming from the one with a glitch in their thinking, role-modeling my rendition of what I thought might be on the funny side, I calculated it might be helpful to try and write some quasi-comical parts on occasion to show that—just because someone has had their brain rattled or shaken—doesn't necessarily mean they'll never perceive things in a joking manner ever again.

I figured that reading word after word, sentence after sentence, paragraph after paragraph, and page after page about an accident, hospitalization, and rehabilitation can kind of put a gloom over one's hunger to cuddle up next to a book near the fireplace, so I thought I'd better intermittently sprinkle just a little of what I classify as "humor" here and there. I knew I needed to be careful with this because there would be some incidents which I would want to intentionally create an atmosphere of dark somberness. Knowing that Ug likes to repeatedly practice a dialogue consisting of his version of humor, if I would be tired and somehow couldn't come up with anything better, maybe I'd use a disparaging remark or two branded into my brain's right perceptual hemisphere that he's flung at me in the past—or would no doubt say—to lighten up an otherwise sour moment. Before the reader would think about taking the anti-depressant, Prozac, upon reading a dismal account of my experience, I reasoned that I had better let the one reviewing my book know that things will ultimately turn out okay by using a little dash of cheer.

One's ability to laugh at themself being a healthy sign of growth, I came to the conclusion that if I directed some barbs at myself, this could be beneficial. Kicking around the idea that if I could get the point across that the day can come when one might be able to look back when things were tragic and take a different perspective of the one-time calamity, this could provide some much-needed relief for those who could use a little promise with which to grasp.

The message to my brain's deportment function as to what was and wasn't appropriate behavior being scrambled, when I wasn't exactly keen about what in the world was going on around me, I did some very outrageous/uncharacteristic things not within the framework of normal conduct which wouldn't be comforting for anyone to find out about. Discovering that I routinely started yanking out my wang for anyone to gawk/marvel at and knowing that I had been defecating daily in front of an audience wasn't exactly consoling. To ignore aspects of my embarrassing rehabilitation history not being an option because such editing would undermine the experience in my mind, I needed to present an accurate portrayal of a disability which has a wide range of symptoms. And since I would want to display an all-encompassing depiction of brain injury disability with the least possible amount of personal abasement, I'd just have to joke about this part of my past the best I could.

I played with the idea of not including the act of brain damaged immodesty where I'd reach underneath my hospital gown and whip out my plank, no matter how many spectators were around or their gender, but to do so would rob readers of an index symbolizing just how inclusive the effects of a brain injury can be. With the concept that someone is bound to be offended no matter what I would write in the back of my mind, I was sure that there would be some "bookworms" out there who wouldn't mind this type of theft, but I thought it would be more important to accurately portray the confusion of a mind hampered by lost perspective. Or maybe I would just be making some excuses for my being so crude!!!!

I didn't feel right that I had to hide my tremendous recovery coming back from a disability which forever ransacks its victims of their competency in the eyes of employers. It's torture having a wondrous experience nobody knows about and needing to preserve this as "classified information" in order to have a chance at life. Being a fortunate person who had lived through a blockbuster excursion of will, managing to ignite an electrifying comeback, is just too valuable of an experience to be forced to keep tight-lipped about.

Deleting my purpose of pursuing an advanced degree, it would wear on me no more that I had to refrain from disclosing amazing events associated with my trauma merely because exposing my former disabling condition secret had rendered me as a risk from the perspective of personnel managements. With rehab administrators previous experience up to this point supporting the claim that a one-time severely "head injured" patient aspiring to be a rehabilitation professional couldn't possibly be productive, these execs weren't about to "chance it" and hire someone from this population. Rehabilitation employers must think that a past "head injured victim," whose central nervous system once served as a buffer between a car and a telephone pole, couldn't in any way be skilled at a professional position because they've never heard of such an event occurring, as they would surely howl that "brain contused" patients "just can't do that."

Point blank, it was much more than apparent that my sustaining a neurological impairment "burned the bridges" for me in the eyes of those rehabilitation directors heading centers where I wanted to be professionally employed. The words "brain" and "injury," when used in conjunction with one another to describe a condition sustained by a former patient, subjects the survivor to a "leaves a lot to be desired" label. It not being real complimentary that rehab supervisory personnel assume that a head injury survivor must be a moron, I've had a lot of emotional hardship accepting the fact that rehabilitation employers had deemed my attempts to work professionally in a rehab facility as a goal that is not realistic.

My interactions with prejudicial administrative life forms being a "Close Encounter of the 7th Kind," I got tired of waiting for rehab employers to abide by their E.O.E. obligations/make things happen for me in order to enhance my life, so I thought I'd just use a written method of operation to try to pound down those "good 'ol boy" rehab employment doors. Learning that I couldn't count on rehab managements to "cut me a break" and that I'd have to find some way to make luck for myself, if I was ever going to turn potential into production—if I wouldn't attempt to use a different ticket to achieve admittance into the rehab work place—the status quo of shunning "the disabled" would continue to be upheld and I could expect to be introduced to little prosperity.

Concealing my restoration history, which should put me in a position of being "looked up to" and not "down upon," would not eviscerate me any longer. Without a doubt, moments of pain and regret are going to resurface which I'd just as soon leave submerged assembling this saga, but I had to do something to fill the massive void of injustice being forbidden from working with those encountering the same hazards I once battled. I believe too many people have the potential to prosper from what I could share.

I would stand to gain from this project in the sense that I need an attitude adjustment. Because I was treated like dirt by New Medico, I've been miserable for a long time. Brought down so hard before my career could ever get started, made me a "grouch" entering the work force and manifested the pessimistic outlook I developed about my place in the employment world. Having such a profoundly dysfunctional influence on my well-being, I had to exorcise the sadness built up inside of me before it did any more damage.

In order to progress, we often have to let go of our past, so that tomorrow can be welcomed in an anticipatory fashion. I thought I'd follow the approach which had worked so well with many of my counseling clients and purge the history that interfered with happiness. My pursuits to work in rehabilitation/be happy dealt a major blow by New Medico, I've turned anger inward for a long time and the moment had arrived where I needed to extract the depression which had been cooking inside of me. Exclusion from life does not promote happiness and "being on the sidelines" as the rehab occupational world goes around, would not erode my spirit or resolve, if I could leave a mark somehow. I did not want to believe that I couldn't be successful after my head injury so, having an appetite to succeed to my utmost abilities, I would just have to gear my efforts elsewhere. Now, if my brain healing could only come close to my resolution.

Given the "short end of the stick" by rehabilitation employers, it wouldn't be tough to put myself in the shoes of readers who may grow weary of my going over numerous accounts where I harp about executive maneuvers generated from fear, ignorance, and a general directorial viewpoint that people with disabilities are needy "basket cases." No problem, I could empathize with those sick and tired of absorbing my complaints about how I felt beaten, kicked, and dumped on by managements. On the other hand, I would hope those fatigued by my griping about administrative policy could try to understand the merciless predicament that I encountered on every corner of my rehab job hunt where I wasn't given any chance at attaining a gainful therapy employment vacancy. After fighting like a damned dog for my life at Allegheny General Hospital in a bedroom full of mattresses and pushing the limits during my rehabilitation just so I could be a functional human being, it's so unfair the caution which I had been approached with resulted in my being on the outside looking in. Saturating their virtues, hypocrisy universally adorned executive masters of deceit.

There could be no way those hearing me grumble and feeling as if I had gone to the "bickering well" one too many times could ever feel as "fed up" as I had become repeatedly being informed that I wasn't qualified, nor had enough knowledge, to be able to work with the head injury disability population and that someone had been found for an employment position who would be more suitable and better serve the needs of patients. Feeling as though I had to get graphic during some instances of my confrontation with the symptoms of a brain injury in order to give the reader a real sense of experience, likewise, I believed making a non-stop review of my inability to "hook on" with a quality rehabilitation establishment could bring to life the most frustrating obstacle I've had to overcome since my brain injury. With this being the effect I'd desire, if those digesting my frustrations get ill over my redundancy, this nausea would parallel how I've felt since getting my Master's and being told that I don't have the substance or backbone to be able to work with those suffering disabilities.

Not deserving to be held in such a light of ill-favor, upon reading my candid experience with them, rehabilitation human resource directors would likely use my exposing their practices/tactics as another weapon against me without taking into account that I had justification for my bitterness. Having no idea the lumps that I've taken since getting my Master's, those rehab personnel execs would probably think that I should maliciously title my book, "<u>Settle the Score</u>," "<u>Pay Back Time</u>," or "'<u>Tis my Day of Reckoning</u>." Without taking into consideration the reasons for my acrimonious language pointed their way, those doing the hiring at rehab facilities would likely "black ball" me so that they wouldn't have to bother worrying about employing someone who once had "bats in their belfry." I'm no fool, I know it's "tough out there," but it had become more and more obvious that when prospective employers observed the way I moved and made an educated hunch as to what might have happened to me, I knew that any respect the interview or my resume earned me would be out the window faster than one could say, "Good luck in your job search."

How one approaches a tragedy is so vital in their pursuits to "bounce back." Developing mental toughness and a "refusal to give in" attitude is imperative, if one is to make any kind of recovery. My primary consideration when I depict how hard I worked to get back some of what I had lost will not be one of self-promotion, rather, if any patients ever decide to read my book, I would want to stress the importance of practice, if one is to see any improvement. It is essential that a survivor knows their limitations and formulates the strength to work around them, so that the extent with which the deficits impede one could be minimized.

Since I've been hurt, I had been told more times than I'd like to remember that the "old Craig" is forever gone, as if I could never be as good as I once was. My physical limitations being permanent, it may be true that many of the athletic abilities I was once skilled will never return, but I need to view the situation from the angle that—because of my injury—I will be able to excel in arenas not before possible, like writing my book. When those times would surface when I'd feel "down and out," I would just have to remind myself that accomplishments such as getting my Master's would not likely have occurred had I not met with my twist of fate.

I couldn't say for sure if being told that I wouldn't ever be able to do certain things again by those who supposedly know best motivated me to prove people wrong, but I can certainly claim that my need to be a semblance of my premorbid self definitely pushed me. In my writing, I don't think it can be stressed enough the importance of approaching dilemmas with a positive mental framework in order to have a fighting chance. Desire only being a foundation, I would need to punctuate how vital it is to act on aspirations.

The crushed wreckage of that VW almost sending me to my tomb, corresponding with the plight of anyone in rehabilitation, I just had to summon the strength within me in order to make a life for myself, because I wasn't prepared to forego all that which had been a part of me. One of the first therapeutic weekends I was home from Harmarville was extremely agonizing for me because I listened to an 8-track tape of me playing some original tunes on my guitar that I had recorded before I was hurt and had become discombobulated. Not appreciating the solid ability I possessed at the time that I laid these rhythms down, misery grabbed ahold of me because these songs I completely had forgotten I taped sounded pretty damned good, if I may say so myself.

At the time I listened to these ghosts of how I once flew across the fretboard, I was barely capable of moving the wrist of my right hand, not able to pick single notes, and unable to even hold a flat pick. Hearing how I once had the ability to attack strings without giving it a second thought and just taking it for granted that I automatically could do this, I hit "rock bottom" and really got depressed because of my infatuation/obsession with hard rock guitar. But this anguish served as a turning point for me.

Like anyone who has had a head injury, if any strides toward regaining a function are going to be made, I was just going to have to "tighten my chin strap" and make the most of the cards that I had been dealt. Anyone suffering through a disability, who wants to reach a pinnacle where promise can be seen, must be tenacious in their restoration efforts and try to make inner voices work in their favor. If these self-dialogue, message tapes "trip up" a survivor too badly during a "do or die" situation when one needs to tap into all of the positive thinking reserve possible, one's prospects become dimmed.

A benchmark of my earnest duty, I had to construct my thinking in such a way that I could amass as much psychological willpower as possible, so I'd be freed to exert a zealous effort. Submission of my desire to be a top-quality counselor wouldn't be something I was prepared to do, for surrendering my hope of becoming an accomplished rehab professional and recognizing this endeavor as one which "just wasn't in the cards" would—in my mind—force me to sit out life. Holding out hope that I could play my occupational hand to the best of my ability and come out on top before what happened to me at New Medico made me any more rabid, in order to proceed in a healthy fashion, I'd just have to tell myself that some good did come of my not getting the available Meadowlands' Family Counselor vacancy.

Regarding the numerous fortunes which presented itself to me throughout my perils, I couldn't know exactly what God had in mind for me by the way so many things had turned out in my favor, but I knew for a fact that the period devoted to effort during my rehab was "put up or shut up" time. Maybe He knew that my personality was one where my perseverance would lead me towards undertaking a written project after all my other role-modeling attempts to do some good for the head injury population had failed at the judgmental hands of rehabilitation human resource departments. With my blood at their feet, possibly God realized that my drive would shift into a gear where my focus would lead me into a direction other than trying to enter rehab personnel execs' individual rehabilitation facilities; exposed to a select fragment of this disability population, towards something more global in nature.

Following a chartered path which possibly could ease the burden of more than a restricted few, it's highly unlikely that I would have considered writing a book had I gotten the New Medico or Florida/Pittsburgh presentation jobs. For example, when I gave my talks at these different rehab sites and opened it up to questions—wanting an insider's view—each speaking engagement, I was asked most often questions which started with, "How long did it take you to. . . . . . . ?"

After prefacing my answer that no two head injuries are alike and that recovery—if it occurs at all—varies in duration and extent of rejuvenation, I would then tell my "crowd" of no more than a few dozen at the most, approximately how long it took me to regain those functions which I had been able to grasp again.

However, with this worded expose I had begun, the dates will be precise because I would have my dad's daily memoirs/diary which chronologically outlines what happened to me each day I was in a coma at the hospital, as well as everyday I had done something noteworthy at home after I was allowed to visit Washington on weekends from Harmarville and after being discharged. Also, at my disposal for detailed review of my history when I was unhinged were copies of the Harmarville progress notes which—like my dad's documentation—largely chronicle a time my personal recollection was "cease and desist."

Because my parents lived through the Great Depression when it was a sin if anything got wasted or made its way into the garbage without first going through an extensive inspection, very little got thrown into the trash at the Meyers' house which had the slightest chance of one day being put to good use. Double digits in years had gone by, but always filed away in a drawer throughout the better part of the 80's—and beyond—were 1982 hospital/doctor records, prescription tags, therapy reports, psych statements, receipts, appointment notices, bills, canceled checks, letters to insurance companies, travel mile records, personal notifications from medical and rehabilitation staff, etc. Wanting to give a well-defined time line, along with mom available for verification and interpretation, I had the means to break down events to an absolute science. My thoughts with those ensnared in the midst of desperation and having an insatiable craving for answers, providing unerring testimony to a broader circulation could reap rewards which may not have otherwise blossomed.

I was happy to personally answer inquiries and share my experience during those presentations, however, for me to isolate my potentially invaluable reclamation experience to only a limited gathering who had an opportunity to see yours truly, would leave this survivor with a deep sense of under- achievement. I thought starting on a book to reach patients and families who could benefit from witnessing the work and capabilities of a head injury survivor would be something crisp and fresh. However, no sooner had I got my narrative project rolling, I had to close down shop.

Driving to work a mile up the secluded, windy, country off-road, when I had reached the plain closer to the top of the hill and all I could see were a condemned farm house, groundhogs, and a youth detention center a couple of hundred yards to my left, it really hit home just how far off-track I was from a career position where I could best utilize my experience. Instead of hearing the exciting commotion associated with a bustling suburban area and seeing speeding cars of commuters scurrying off to work, I listened to pheasants squawk and watched them flutter just above the black tree line into dense, empty woods. With my hometown somewhere in-between, culturally, Monroeville and this section of South Fayette Township were on opposite ends of the universe spectrum.

Five months ago, I was a therapist in a progressive business community just outside one of the larger metropolitan areas in the United States, but now I'd just have to be content spending about forty hours a week in rural surroundings that time forgot between home and Pittsburgh. At first, it wasn't easy to view my new, work environment situation from a perspective other than one where I had taken a hard fall, but events over time would alter this hard-line stance.

Not being a part of the scenery I desired and a void in my sense of independence, I was absolutely miserable starting off. However, in a relatively short time, I could better appreciate that I was reaping quite a few long-term benefits not only professionally, but physically, which wouldn't have occurred had I remained east of the city.

As the first full-time therapist hired for this new treatment facility, I primarily utilized a group therapy approach for a dozen or so residents with mental illness where support, education, and discussion modalities were used. Providing counseling to the MH/MR population would be a new experience for me because any referrals with a diagnosis of a mental disorder made to my previous employer would be assigned elsewhere to a program such as this one, specializing in the treatment of this type of illness.

The philosophical makeup of the program was unique and original because it provided both therapeutic and residential services within the same setting. Designed with the intent of reducing chronic patients dependency on the hospitalization system for care and to facilitate independence, my serving as this particular center's initial therapist, I played an important role in the development of this transitional operations' partial program.

Broadening the scope of people with which I was to help to include the seriously mentally ill and—to a lesser extent—mild MR, was prosperous not only from an academic standpoint, for this approximated some of the population studied in my Rehabilitation Counseling grad work, but from the vantage point that I would be gaining experience with an illness which requires a specialized approach. With the exception of watching moneymaking, group services being provided at those projects, my therapy involvement at the Monoeville agency was always done on an individual basis with clients. But here in this open-field, residential/treatment operation, I'd finally be able to hone my skills on an average of two to six hours a day as a group leader, which was an aspect of my graduate training I was happy I could develop further.

One of the major challenges of this therapy position was presenting serviceable material and discussing topics that could be understood by an intellectually diverse population of previously institutionalized patients with varying attention spans, comprehensive abilities, and interest levels. Not in any immediate danger to hurt themselves or harm others because many of the symptomatic behaviors of their complications were largely in remission, structuring interventions in order to enhance the lives of those having a diagnosis of a psychosis, personality disorder, depression, and/or a dual diagnosis of MI/substance abuse was another fruitful piece of equipment I could add to my counseling basket. I soon discovered that, in many ways, engaging in therapy with those having a mental illness required a different breed of methodologies.

For example, those residents with the common diagnoses of Paranoid Schizophrenia (295.30 DSM-III) and Schizoaffective Disorder (295.70 DSM-III)—in addition to strictly following their medication regimen of treatment—would need to be shown rational strategies in group on how to minimize the occurrence of their malady, as well as how to behaviorally address the different effects of their affliction when they may appear in an attempt to lessen the dysfunctional impact this condition may have on one's life. Genetics play a key role as to whether or not one will be predisposed to the arrival of a mental illness, and taking prescribed drugs in their proper dosage/time of day for this element of the sickness with its chemically imbalanced/neurologically-impaired roots is the action one must engage in order to treat the "nature" component of the psychosis.

Because of the surroundings one may be in, taking a pill to remedy the potentially unproductive "nurture" influence of an illness wouldn't be possible, so it would be important to teach the residents how to efficiently deal with difficult situations which could not be avoided. And this would be where the cognitive therapy technique stressing that one's thinking influences feelings/behavior needed to be elementary broken down and presented in a utilitarian context where it could be accessed. With so much of residents' thoughts/perceptions outside of the control of their mind, it would be comforting for many of them to know that they may be able to manage certain attitude aspects of their life which could help them to deal with various symptoms of their perceptual organization defect.

Residents experiencing auditory hallucinations, for example, would need to be educated and re-educated over again how these frequently destructive "voices" that are truly being heard has nothing to do with what is actually going on with them or their environment, rather, it would need to be repeatedly accentuated that this deviation from reality was purely a trademark effect of their ailment. Tormented by unwanted dialogue, this lack of solicitation could cause the one hearing spoken words void of a source to feel as if they are possessed. Often identified as a signal from Hell, haunting passages with no core of meaning or sense of purpose mystifies the one taunted by commandments to undertake deeds regularly seen as guided by the hand of Satan. Not wanting to be tempted by the fruits of atrocity or led by the foundation of evil, verbal messages persecuting residents' conscious would become a nightmare because those combating auditory transgressions routinely accept these words with no provenance as direction which must be adhered to.

Visual hallucinations—although much less common than their articulated counterpart—would need to be remedially pursued in a reality-based fashion as well, in order to assist the person whose senses are playing tricks on them. This lapse of reason where they genuinely see things that are not there can be very frightening for the resident because what is viewed can be an upsetting figment of their subconscious. Apparitions taking form by the mind's imagination, mental dissociation and a perceptual incoherence are but two of the evolutional elements contributing to this ocular disturbance. Like the fascinating "voices" being heard, attending to areas when nothing was there would be a favorite pastime denied as occurring by those observing illusionary phantoms.

An individual living with a schizophrenia disorder oftentimes has to overcome delusional thinking just so they would be able to function with some semblance of peace. Co-existing with these ordinarily outrageous false beliefs/fixed ideas inconsistent with logic generally preoccupies the one maddened by these fictitious perceptions mistakenly accepted as known fact. Steadfast beliefs formulated from thoughts with no origin or basis, the irresistible impulse to hold a non-compromising position would be manifested by the functional disintegration of one's ability to sift through and discard absurd ideas. The ruling passion to adopt a ludicrous proposal at the expense of a more reasonable one creates such an elevated infatuation that it practically borders complete mind-control. With this morbid drive to fixate on a preposterous sentiment being all-encompassing, the frenzy/furor generated from mythical presumptions could drive one berserk. And I wouldn't only be talking about the therapist who had to confront illogical conclusions about life in order to assist the person impaired by fantasy reasoning.

Inconsistent with ultimate truth, when a psychotic episode would occur, it would be essential to instruct the residents how to go about addressing this idiopathic development of their sickness upon its onset before it rendered some permanent, irreversible consequence. Healthy environmental techniques such as implementing functional/soothing dialogue one can say to themself to ease through one of these uninvited events when a person is no longer in total control of their senses would be a basic strategy which could prove beneficial, if adopted. Someone polluted by these irrational views of what is happening within their world may, for instance, whole- heartedly ascertain and conclude that three cloudy Tuesdays in a row would surely mean that the apocalypse cannot be far off. It would be imperative then to sensibly confront this ridiculous presumption, for fear that the one making the determination may act on this helpless/hopeless foregone conjecture.

Whereas the prescription of psychotropic medication by a psychiatrist is an absolute necessity for the treatment of those with a psychotic disturbance, it takes much more than a tonic of anti-hallucinogenic drugs to bandage the ills of those diagnosed with a personality disorder. Not to suggest that the symptoms of the two ailments could not overlap—because they frequently do—but the latter's developmental history influence requires much more than the administration of some pill regimen. With both genetics and environmental factors serving as ammunition, most often the residents with the personality disorder diagnosis would have their sense of practical orientation clouded by this nature/nurture dual compound.

Along with self-absorbed residents having narcissistic fragments dominating their character where, among other things, over-inflated opinions of themselves could make most anyone sick, and those with histrionic mannerisms characterized by hyped exaggeration/energy, this groundbreaking facility was traditionally overrun by natives possessing personality disorders with more severe, pathognomonical traits. It wouldn't be all that unusual to run into people who are egotistical or somewhat overactive, but when these two pronounced character non-conformities are so extreme they create significant turmoil in one's life, this is when it crosses from being an annoyance to a serious aspect of an illness. Exceeding troublesome, the treatment program had an abundance of residents possessing intrinsic personality disorders which were a core fiber of their everyday functioning.

Wound tight, for example, those with an obsessive-compulsive disorder would usually be disturbed quite significantly because many waking moments would be overtaken by the all-consuming nature of their illness. Obsessions are recurring thoughts or ideas which insistently intrude one's conscious. Compulsions are behaviors a person carries out because of an overwhelming, unwanted preoccupation/urge to perform various irrational rituals or acts. Concurrently drilled by these two forces, a person would be twisted by never-ending formations of what they are to do at any particular moment.

Ideas formed capriciously, because of their inability and/or reluctance to gear their focus on functional concepts, those stricken with the need to engage in impulsive behaviors such as checking, counting, cleaning, and hording are difficult to work with because they become extremely agitated/ dysfunctional, if they are guided away from acting upon their fleeting images of what's believed is their mind's instruction/directive. Conducting group where its fellow rationally-compromised members can feed into and heighten the confusion/anxiety of the one being sabotaged by OCD or any other kind of mental illness can, many times, confound the situation that much more. And, if there's one type of personality disorder which doesn't need anymore interference, it would be those pleasant individuals with a borderline diagnosis (301.83 DSM-III) who normally have a penchant of causing those whom they may be around to want to yank out their hair—one at a time.

Riding out the storm with a borderline, one would need Noah's Ark because the deluge of turbulence never seems to stop overflowing with these people. Just by what is said and the manner in which they go about delivering their scripted dialogue when interacting with someone, the person fortunate enough to be relating to the borderline could soon pick out this mentally ill population's deceptive motives, as their means of misleading through manipulation are very transparent. Learning not to be surprised what their mind comes up with next, these disoriented people are always seeming to be digging into their bag of tricks for something to make life difficult. Misery enjoys company.

Feeling as if they're justified, rarely—if ever—accepting responsibility for occurrences which they would be directly accountable, those with this type of discontented disorder would alter reality, so it appeared that they were endlessly victimized in a world designed to inflict hardship against these innocent souls. Utilizing the manipulative tactic of "shifting the blame"—where the gross negligence of others would be the reason why things weren't right—borderlines using this scheming mechanism could, therefore, attribute all problems to everyone but themself. Deflecting all liability and adopting a persona of innocence very possibly could occur with these conspiring people because a whopping 70% majority have been incestually abused and this acquired reflex of denying sponsorship serves as a means to avoid any further harm. Because it had proven to be an effective protection devise when they were molested as a child, refusing to accept fact or tampering with history seemed to be a favorite learned behavior many residents with a borderline personality disorder incorporated into their adult lives.

From the very beginning, a child rightfully accepts their parents as omnipotent because caregivers are equated with survival, being that the necessities of living are provided by these elder figures. Responsible for their maintenance, regardless of circumstance, a child will naturally view their guardian as ever-loving and perfect. Therefore, anything gravely cruel, heinous, and/or unthinkable inflicted upon the child by a parent will be received by the little one as something for which they are responsible because of the vision that they have of paternal and maternal symbols as being error-free. Firm beliefs having evolved into general acknowledged understanding, because caretakers are initially received as not capable of making mistakes, an innocent child will assume that if something "wrong" or "bad" happened to them, it must be their fault. Feeling as if they are inherently bad, these young victims will keep the sewage of being trespassed upon a secret.

In many cases, with the truth having been twisted by the attacker and sensing that this type of touching wasn't proper, little kids who have been sexually abused bottle a flurry of turbulent emotions inside, perceiving that what happened to them must be concealed. Torn between their inborn instincts of appropriateness and what they have come to comprehend as a given about their parents' standards, these children who have been violated are swamped with agony. Fire raging within them having concluded that the parental monster rendering harm surely must be justified committing this crime, these children survivors of incest with a borderline personality disorder diagnosis will often create upheaval within their surroundings which closely corresponds with the turmoil and confusion that's stewing within their emotions concealing what happened to them as a youth. As is any youngster's due expecting protection, security, and respect, a child betrayed customarily carries self-defeating, internal baggage with them for a lifetime.

Even if a father was physically and/or emotionally abusive, it never ceases to amaze that so many females search for a significant other romantic partner and lay claim to one who can "act out" the past paternal dysfunction experienced during childhood. The selection of a love interest occurs mainly because this choice strikes some emotional chord for the one looking for a match. Simply, for some, short-lived bubble gum excitement may be sparked solely because a person could see themself as a member of a couple, instead of being alone. But for others who have an unfulfilled/unconscious need—like those who pick a shadowy mate who can "fill in" for an unhealthy image from their history—the attachment to a similar experience or relationship one has struggled through before is, too frequently, very appealing because the opportunity to rewrite an irreversible script had erroneously been seen as having miraculously presented itself. The temptation to latch onto this deceptive representation of what one desires could levy an overpowering stranglehold on someone whose vulnerability is of a degree where they could be exploited.

This "comfort of familiarity" principle can commonly occur with an individual having a borderline label as they, often enough, try to pair their seemingly ingrained mood with those fortunate people happening to be in their "firing line." Striving to create an environment with which they are accustomed, those mentally handicapped with a borderline classification would manufacture situations which cause distress for others because the dissension being produced corresponds with the ever-lasting misery they're used to which boils within them. Being in a calm environment is just too unnatural for a person categorized as having a borderline malfunction, so they will habitually do what they can to spice things up with a little bit of strife. Having no conscience and stunted morally, there's one personality disorder taking up residency at this facility that's even light years worse than your ordinarily difficult, everyday, household borderline.

Sprinkle a "tried and true" sociopath or two into the group treatment mix, as well as a few who could pass for having this Antisocial Personality Disorder (301.70 DSM-III), and the blessed therapist who had to counsel this lovely batch of unseldomly reasonless people could have their hands full. Just as prone to pat one on the back as stab it, those finding it difficult obeying societal rules/norms deliberately behave in a deviate fashion because of a demented rationale where it is believed that they're deservedly justified undertaking evil deeds.

These non-conforming members of society discovering it is impossible to adhere to accepted standards of conduct, experience a demeanor of no remorse and this seems to be evolved from their crazed deduction that they are "owed" a privilege by the populace. No regard for others' welfare or property, these delightful Homo sapiens will engage in aggressive and irritable actions to such an elevated degree that it usually is grounds for, and warrants, arrest. As well as working with those suffering from perceptual incapacities and conduct disorders, I had the quasi-hypocritical task of assisting those smothered by the "blues."

Despite feeling as if everything had "closed down" on me in the head injury and comprehensive rehabilitation job market front, I couldn't give the appearance that I was so close to unhappily "folding up the tent" on any of my long-term pursuits because those residents with a diagnosis of a depressive disorder filling group would need all the optimistic, positive role-modeling impressions they could witness. I think there was a reason I survived that accident, making the world class comeback that I did "against all odds," and I doubt it was to assure people with schizophrenia that the "voices" being heard weren't real.

Undisputed, I believe that I was given a shot at cheating death and breaking free from the internment of a brain injury, so that I could give a little something to those head injury survivors less fortunate than myself who could gain from what I may be able to offer. I realize that I don't have nine lives, but I wouldn't totally discard that so many invigorating things falling into place for me like they did during my recovery weren't somehow designed to happen in order to reap benefits for others as well.

Hopefully, it was more than coincidence that I reached the promised land of restoring quite a bit of my physical health back and all my mental health. It would have been incredible if my continuing rehab efforts following a time when my brain would have been condemned as a "blighted area" could provide legitimate hope to similarly traumatized patients who may surrender tomorrow's dreams as dark, and despondently accept the passageway towards promise as nothing more than a bleak proposition. However, with New Medico and seemingly every other rehabilitation outfit that cares for those with head injuries casting stones at me, I had to set my sights elsewhere and carry on the best I could with minimal demonstration that I was being eaten up internally, not being able to convince rehabilitation executives of my competencies.

Quite a few with a diagnosis of Major Depression, Recurrent (296.3x DSM-III) or on the despondent side of their manic-depressive/bipolar disorder (296.4x DSM-III), often believed that there was nothing worth living for and wouldn't care if they were "snuffed out" by morning or not. Therefore, it would be imperative staff "keep their chin up" as an example for those who had been thrown more than their fair share of curves in life. Any suicide gesture needing to be taken seriously, bogus attempts abounded, which usually meant a need for attention or was a cry for help with this predominantly sound cluster of mentally-challenged inhabitants.

The legitimacy of residents wanting to be "rubbed out" being in question, professionals working with those possessing Rapid Cycling Disorders (296.6x DSM-III), for instance, still had to be very sensitive to the signals given off by this disturbed population because a resident may go from being jovial to affective melancholia within a matter of minutes. This drastic intermixing of emotional tones could be particularly worrisome, if the resident had a past penchant of engaging in abusive behavior. And it wouldn't help matters much for those who had enough to contend with, if I exhibited my pain.

On the flip side of the mood disorder chain, if one had a continuous and abnormally elevated affect, it would be essential to bring these racing/flighty, helium-inflated/turbo-charged roadrunners back down to earth before anything toxic may happen to them being on "Cloud Nine" (irritability, distractibility, invincibility, grandiosity, decreased sleep, psychomotor agitation, etc.). However, there were more than a few who took a toxic course of action in a misguided attempt to make their disease more tolerable and flee from this pathological nightmare.

Realizing that a chemical composition dysfunction within their neurological system would never permit them to experience life free from the bondage of haunting symptoms—only confounding matters—too frequently those with an undeserving mental distortion would resort to toxicity in the form of drugs and alcohol, as a means to escape an existence void of serenity/ fraught with self-deceptive illusions. This dual diagnosis of one of the mental illnesses and substance ab/use would be particularly harmful because the use of narcotics or any kind of liquor could limit prescribed medications' prophylactic effectiveness to the extent that an individual with mental illness who had been drinking or getting high could get "sick."

Although the residents could understand the counter-productive, long-term consequences of ingesting ill-advised chemicals into their bodies, the immediate relief from the pain of having a mental deficiency would often be just too tempting. Knowing what this "D and A" group facilitator wanted to see and hear, halos floating about their heads, these slick dual-diagnosed group sweethearts with the lofty recidivism rates would often just behave as long as they had to before disappearing into the land of "Wild Turkey" and grain alcohol.

Unless firmly entrenched in denial, the majority of the population with mental illness knew that they had significant problems and areas needing lifetime, individualized treatment. Those caught within this wrath of mental paralysis, require distinguished professional care in order to become disentangled from this psychotic web and I was grateful to have some seasoned pros to facilitate my understanding of this population.

Symbolic of society's general approach of trying to keep those with any kind of perceptual deficiency at a safe distance, tucked away about a hundred yards or so off this back country road was the treatment facility, housing these residents having the mental disorder. Far enough from any sparse traffic (the mainstream) where they could not bother or pose any threat to those living an ordinary existence—separating the special needs tenants from the outside world—two tree lines surrounded our program and the structure where the troubled youths resided. The woods confining these two specialty care outfits into their own little universe and their isolated placement closely parallel the "out of sight, out of mind" attitude citizens too often possess towards those who require some degree of designated therapy.

With the MH/MR payroll budget not anywhere close to being as abundant as the amount of duties required at this rural community living/therapy center, the limited number of staff working at this rustic locale usually had to wear at least two hats at any given time and always had to hustle, just to stay afloat. For instance, until some additional bachelor's-educated resident specialist staffers got hired, I'd have to drive a van of potentially white blood cell-impaired program dwellers to Mount Lebanon, so they could have their corpuscles checked to see if the sometimes miracle psychotrop, Clozaril, was eating up these infection-fighting/injury-healing leukocytes.

Thank God we have a program supervising manager who could serve as a nurse backup, because if our regular nurse would happen to miss a staffing day when meds would need ordered—not possessing the necessary medical qualifications—I wouldn't be allowed to make a call to a pharmacist, arranging for a stock of prescribed drugs to be delivered. Versatility being a prerequisite of the few staff occupying professional stations at this treatment boondock and the psychiatrist's medical demands a priority, this restriction would not work in my favor.

Nice meeting you too. My first day at this refuge for those bereft of reason was Monday, 6/22/92. By the afternoon—a whole three hours on the job—my character and competency were assassinated in front of about seven professional staff members by the Chief Psychiatrist, "Dr. Peon." Seeing facial hair stand on end and those whiskers of that paramount crew cut ruffling about—not exactly giving a good first impression to my fellow agency employees whom I hadn't been formally introduced to—those faculty attending this initial staffing of mine could have very easily thought I somehow burned down this conversion education establishment on my inaugural day, rather than not having a chance to review a forthcoming admission's medical chart thoroughly because I was yet to be situated and still being oriented to the various center's procedures. Hopefully, I had a bull's eye planted on my forehead because of my "rookie" status and not because this extremely observant physician accurately perceived that abnormal forward stroll of mine as one with neurologically-impaired origins.

Unpredictably volatile, these Russian Roulette conferences at this sanctuary seemed to be a source of power entertainment for this female most times fashionably clad in blue jeans, a nifty sweat shirt, and stained sneakers. Right from the "get-go"—not exempt being the new kid on the block—I had immediately been frost-bitten by the antagonistic climate of these discussions which, for the most part, would have a different adversary chosen each time. Not conducting formal therapy, I had been mistaken thinking I'd receive a little break from those who were apparently at war with images from their past.

With the welcome mat being pulled out from under this hemi-paralytic worker before I could even say "Hello," I figured this message was one with the intent of letting me know who would be running the ship at this place and, possibly, that the captain wasn't real pleased a male incorrectly perceived as being in regular need of sick bay had been selected to come on board. Once wearing a patch on me eye, a leg so close to being a wooden one, and a hook for a right arm, the die had been cast and the role of Pirate on this treatment vessel seemed to be mine. "Shimmer me timbers, looks like there be rough waters ahead," so I need to show I could weather the storm.

The types of group services offered at anytime were tailored for the specific needs/concerns of the particular attending members. Discharge rates varying, revisions of the treatment schedule would be made according to what areas needed focused upon. Over the course of a week's time, within a community congregation, a resident could expect to address a variety of issues ranging from medical, psychological, residential, and physical.

Along with the partial staff office, one spacious bedroom which was to be divided, a small sleeping quarter, and a dinky laundry room, the group treatment/partial hospitalization component of this two-story building's layout was located in a large downstairs area. Upstairs, were the residents' rooms, community space (kitchen, dining room, TV room), conference room, front desk, and the Unit Director's office. With the exception of Mondays and Thursdays when part-time therapist/agency "mind reading guru" and psychiatric staffing stenographer—Terry Whalen, M.A.—would provide her multitude of outstanding skills for a half-of-a-day on those she was assigned to come in, there were only myself and a Psych Nurse—Sue Besselman, R.N.—working 7.5 hours each day in the partial program, five days a week during the daylight shift.

Not much room for error or time to breathe, the administrative/residential/clerical daytime element of this multi-purpose operation was also lacking in needed bodies. At ground level, seated at the entrance of the top floor to this haven for individuals perceptually-challenged, Phyllis Matthews undertook her administrative assistant duties and a host of other tasks with E.M.T. (Emergency Medical Technician) precision. Last, but by no means least, was my incredible boss who not only got fascinating results, but did it with an incomparable human touch.

The essence of style—Janice Poole, R.N.—was a Unit Director whose goal-oriented approach reaped some tremendous rewards for this new facility because of her remarkable ability of getting things done with an altruistic flavor. Studying for her M.B.A.—overqualified for this agency—I think part of the reason this most compassionate health care provider took this post was so she could add to her already impressive resume that she developed a program from the bottom up and formulated many of its methods of operation. Conducive to her genial demeanor, almost unheard of in an organization which deals with a population fighting frayed mental functioning, Janice was able to assemble a program-wide atmosphere of cheerful respect with her contagious friendly disposition and energetic personality. With the building blocks for a foundation having been set into place, the construction of a fine-tuned establishment could be initiated.

Primarily business-minded and conscious of the agency's limited resource base, so that an additional secretary needn't be hired to dig into the already scant funds in the operation's treasure chest, Janice taught partial program staff how to use "Word Perfect" on the computer, so neatly type-written progress notes could be developed on a printer she also instructed staff how to manage. With this "Jack of All Trades" cap that had to be worn by the self-sufficient employees here at this rural residential organization, am I ever glad my brain had healed enough by the time I had reached grad school that I could quickly work the typewriter keyboard again. Taking precisely detailed notes on the sequence of steps needed, along with Janice's other grateful understudies, I was tutored step-by-step how to go about using this computer function.

For a few weeks at the beginning, before being shown how to use this "Word Perfect" operation on the computer, I had to write my various documentation on the residents with a pen. Still getting words down with my non-dominant left hand after ten years because this was the only way my brain felt comfortable gripping a writing utensil, I really struggled to localize words between the tiny margins of those pink, medical record progress notes. Legibility impossible and speed out of the question, the unthinkable proposition of controlling my left hand in order to produce daily and efficient records was a blessing in disguise, for I would stick a pen in my once-ruling right hand one day and just "go at it."

Fortunate the admissions hadn't started to pour in yet, I had enough time to torture myself and practice scribbling notes on the few people on my caseload until I trained my right hand how to write again. My right hand's surprising responsiveness to my brain's command to jot down letters would not be the only physical function that I was ecstatic to see return.

A "blip" on the radar screen, in the middle of the hinterlands, this facility had an abundance of acreage surrounding it. Unlike the concrete jungle of Monroeville, there was plenty of pasture to "let loose" and take advantage of the playground nature offered those in this corner of the universe. When I first began working here, I could only perceive this medical/ therapeutic treatment program as one being situated in a desolate "no man's land," without realizing the key to an amazing amount of my physical restoration had presented itself. In no time, I took a situation which was only seen as regression initially and made it work for me, turning it into an opportunity to heal.

If permitted, a good many of the residents would just as soon sit around, looking at each other, and have their muscles atrophy. On Thursdays for ninety minutes and Fridays for forty-five, I led an "Outdoor Activity" group which this therapist gladly took the role of an active participant because I viewed this as an opening to enrich my own physical capabilities. Not exactly having been made available to me this past decade since I had so much of my physical health taken from me, seizing the occasion to work on my motor-skill deficits would reap significant long-term profits for me.

Since my head injury, I had reluctantly—and as it would turn out, prematurely—accepted that participating in athletics in any way was something that I just couldn't do any longer because of the biting pain which shot down my right arm when I threw. During those years when I had been studying to get my college degrees and then working my previous jobs, I didn't have much of a chance to practice sports of any kind. However, the excruciating emotional pain of not being able to perform like I wanted and the subsequent competition stagnation didn't stop my brain from mending.

Quicker than I could have ever imagined, in large part because the fiery sting which exploded down my throwing arm when I'd toss disappeared, I would be shocked to discover that I needn't forego my sports passion entirely and the utter enjoyment this provided me. Figuring that my "sports days" were over and that playing ball of any kind had permanently "bit the dust," I couldn't have been more overjoyed making a mistaken assumption.

There was this one resident with a troubling diagnosis who was a tremendous athlete. Earning a full, free ride, football scholarship out of high school to a major university as a defensive lineman—one of the first occupants of the residential/treatment service—this huge guy and myself would not only talk individually about various dilemmas which had developed in his life when outside, but also we'd simultaneously throw a pigskin on the grounds when we could. While discussing sensitive items where I'd gather a good bit of information, we'd engage in concurrent play, so that his attention could be diverted from the fact that we were going over things. Normally affable until those times would hit when this physically-imposing ballplayer would think about how his illness forced him to leave college, believing that this was the only way I could whip a ball, I threw left-handed initially to this one-time interior lineman.

Pass-catching on a daily basis during different breaks from group and those times when I'd hang around a little after work—like the reincarnation of my writing right-handed once more—on those occasions which presented themselves, am I ever glad I decided to practice and bring to life again some of my right-handed throwing ability. This repetition designed in order to stop being a southpaw hurler, like the re-emergence of my ability to write with my dominant hand again, it was unbelievable how well my right arm responded pain-free to my attempts at reviving this extremity I had practically given up for dead.

Doing the rejuvenation rhumba, my ultimate happiness and self-esteem had grown by leaps and bounds. Ten years post, it felt positively awesome that my brain was still healing and responding to my demands of it to work for me after having done the "cerebellum shake." Possibly even in a sort of promotional type of capacity for this disability, I guess in a few respects, I could serve as a longitudinal case study of how an injured brain can respond to diligent effort over the course of time. Come to think of it, groundhogs are kind of on the cute side, anyway.

I'm not so sure this would be attributed as a positive trait of my character, but I wasn't thrilled I was employed again when I got this low-paying, MH/MR job. Providing reimbursement only pennies more than the Monroeville counseling position, I was actually a little disappointed I couldn't gear my focus on my autobiographical writing project, rendering it an unfinished product. While beginning my book, the hope that I could give a few head injury survivors a hand in their time of futility, served as the beacon to guide me through my hard times I experienced being unable to land a career position working with those at arms with the symptoms of a traumatized brain.

Sometimes it's funny how a seemingly decrepit situation actually can work in one's favor over time. If I hadn't gotten this particular countryside therapy post with its different cast of players and had remained in a suburban office building where this youthful employee's presence was symbolically flicked "the finger" by various senior therapists of the agency, the opportunity to relearn how to pen words right-handed again and develop some computer literacy abilities likely wouldn't have evolved. In paradise that I had recaptured and acquired these journalistic skills, I had the means to an end in order to produce an enhanced literary work.

I guess my brain is genetically wired in such a way that I'm to be right-handed because—even after a decade of doing so—I never developed into a skillful southpaw handwriter, as the final product took forever to complete and was very ugly. Attaining a therapy position in this farmland community therapeutic living arrangement enhanced my chances of finishing my book, for I no longer need to produce a rough draft with my non-dominant writing hand, like I had to starting the beginning of my self-disclosing project. Nor do I have to contend with the burdensome/time-consuming chore of messing with eraser paper when making one of my not-too-infrequent mistakes, or retype an entire section over again, because now I have many computer skills which can transfer over to a Word Processor. However, five months into my new job, the elation which I had experienced grasping functions again/learning new ones and developing an effective group counseling approach with those having a mental illness, would be replaced with rage.

Well, well, well. What do we have here? Stunned, the words spewing from the television set made my entire body numb. Emotionally anesthesized, my mind was barren and my heart became hollow when I watched the Cable News Network (CNN) newscast on November 12, 1992.

A sick chill shot down my spine when hearing the broadcast's highlight: "New Medico Industries, a brain injury treatment company in Massachusetts, is under federal investigation for fraud. They are charged with 'ambulance chasing,' and prolonging stays for additional revenue."

Heart pounding from what I just listened to and anxiously waiting for what facts would be reported next, I was beginning to get a little queasy and lightheaded. Gut growling and tossing around, I started getting pretty sick to my stomach by the time Anchor, Leon Harris, finished up his portion of this segment with, "Earlier this year, CNN's Special Assignment uncovered allegations that the industry has been riddled with fraud."

At this point, the T.V. camera showed Mark Feldstein, Special Assignment correspondent, when he said: "For the past two weeks, F.B.I. agents have been combing through documents seized during a raid at the headquarters of New Medico Associates, a nationwide chain of head injury treatment centers. Sources say federal authorities have issued at least twenty-three subpoenas and two search warrants in ten states, and may soon follow with criminal indictments. The grand jury probe is centered on allegations of fraud."

By the time this part of the federal investigation was announced, things started to sink in ever so slowly, as my shock and disbelief had systematically grown into anger. On the other side of the spectrum, I felt jubilant that these scandalous bastards got nailed because of how I was personally "done wrong" by the Corporation. But this self-oriented cheer quickly dissolved and the anger escalated into fury because of what would be divulged next.

Teeth clenched, I started seeing red when Feldstein revealed: "Earlier this year, CNN reported allegations that New Medico, which, last year, had some 400 million in revenue, mistreated its patients, holding them to collect private insurance or Medicaid, whether or not a patient's condition improved."

Wanting to tear the lungs out of those New Medico at Meadowlands administrative son of a bitches as it was, silhouette forming on the picture screen, when I saw the emotionally-drained face of that beaten woman whose trust had been violated by New Medico—hearing her talk of the extortion tactics this Corporation underhandedly used which added to and prolonged the suffering of her loved one—I boiled over because I know firsthand how much a patient is reliant upon their health care provider to operate within the bounds of regulated conduct. Weary from having her confidence diluted and destroyed fighting over this breach of faith, the man dear to this woman's heart then hit the high spots of the impossible discharge criteria he encountered as a New Medico patient before she summed up the situation that this criminal company was getting guaranteed money picking the pockets of taxpayers by holding patients for their hard-earned dollars.

Confirming this patient and family member's claim, the camera panned in on Feldstein again when he said: "In an internal memo obtained by CNN, New Medico employees were instructed to 'maximize client length of stay,' 'because length of stay directly affects facility and corporate revenues."

Leaning forward in the rocking chair and making a fist by now, eyes glued to the television screen, images of New Medico's Program Directors —Goyette and Micklow—reeked into my conscious as former congressional investigator, Marc Smolonsky, said that, basically, New Medico kept patients at their respective (not respectable) facilities as long as those dependent on the Corporation's care had the financial means to reimburse staff. Summarizing the unethical company's strategy with its inpatients, Smolonsky concluded: "Once their insurance runs out, they miraculously recover."

As I was cringing from the thought that Meadowlands' executives had the bravado and audacity to abuse fidelity right under a counseling intern's nose who was once a member of the very disability population they were cheating, Feldstein's image appeared on the air again as he disclosed: "Former employees say they were even told to scour the newspaper for accident victims, then pressure grieving families to sign up with New Medico."

Caught with their pants down, this news item made it known that Company officials naturally denied any wrongdoing and that a spokesman welcomes the federal probe, to show that the best care possible is being provided. "Well, uhhhhh. . . . ."

Not that two wrongs make a right, but the news program also made sure to highlight that: "Sources say the Justice Department is also investigating alleged fraud at other brain injury treatment centers. Officials predict more health care prosecutions once President-elect Clinton takes office." Absolutely delightful.

Once I flicked off the T.V., my mind immediately reflected on the peculiar aura of evasiveness which seemed to permeate Charles Goyette and Donna Micklow's New Medico Rehabilitation and Skilled Nursing Center at Meadowlands facility where I unfortunately served my academic field training. Not that I expected to get any kind of confirmation or admission, I decided to telephone my primary supervisor, Berkowitz, shortly after this New Medico expose aired in order to hear what he had to say and to get his "scoop" on things. Just to let him know that this former patient/trainee was aware of his felonious employer's alleged unethical maneuvers with patients suffering as I once did, I filled him in about what was excavated about the company which he collected quite a bit of pocket change abiding by New Medico's practices. Naturally unaware of any illegitimate tactics/ supposed abuses occurring within the saintly walls of Meadowlands Health Care Center, I wasn't the least bit surprised when this New Medico staffer claimed he missed that particular CNN segment on T.V. and had no idea what investigators could possibly find or what in the world they were talking about.

Infuriated, I regretted I hadn't learned about the suspicion which loomed over this unlawful Corporation's head at the start of the year when all this question about their sneaky procedures began. In time, I thought I'd take a deeper look at this company's supposed illegal misgivings and discovered that the following printed news report issues had an article about the undermining ways of New Medico: <u>Wall Street Journal</u> (Oct. 28, 1992), <u>The New York Times</u> (Oct. 28, 1992 Late Edition—Final), <u>The Boston Globe</u> (Oct. 30, 1992—City Edition), and <u>Modern Healthcare</u> (Nov. 2, 1992). No wonder my veteran New Medico primary supervisor told me to focus on strengthening my counseling abilities and not be concerned with patients' discharge criteria or insurance coverage. "Well, uhhhhh. . . . ."

With my primary objective being one where I'd want the best for patients and those who care about them—and that my loyalty would not be for the shareholders investing in Corporate stock—administration at the New Medico Rehabilitation and Skilled Nursing Center at Meadowlands had to have viewed the prospects of hiring me as an extremely risky proposition. Knowing how vital proper treatment is because of my own personal background with rehabilitation, the foremost concern of this once similarly devastated survivor would be focused on the care and well-being of those whose brain trauma yields little clemency.

Under normal circumstances, a job candidate possessing these altruistic/empathetic traits—such as myself—would more-than-likely be seen as desirable, but the villainous New Medico Corporation surely viewed me as a potential "whistle blower" of their wrongful operation. Mind floundering back to when I served my dreadful field training with New Medico at Meadowlands, like pieces fitting into a puzzle, the reason various events took place during my practicum/internship started making a whole lot of sense after learning of the company's corrupt dealings.

By the looks of things, it appeared my assessment that New Medico at Meadowlands never intended to give me legitimate consideration for a Family Counselor position was correct, but it looked like the reason for this lack of regard went a lot deeper than merely creating a job opportunity for a sorority girl. When bringing me on board to train, despite being the first student intern they ever had, Meadowlands' administration knew damn well that I was to experience the entire gamut of Family Counselor responsibilities. Making it difficult for me to understand why I was banned from attending Goyette's meetings He had with the Family Counselors, I can see now why I was being kept in the dark. Reading F.B.I. reports about the dastardly workings of New Medico, I could just imagine what took place in these concealed conferences now.

Responding to a Family Counselor's request that someone on their caseload be allowed to return home permanently for treatment, because this patient's despondence being away from loved ones had led to numerous setbacks, I could just hear Program Director Goyette barking, "Hell, are you crazy? We can soak another ten grand out of this gullible soul, if we keep him here another month!!"

This action would be consistent with a statement in the 10/30/92 issue of The Boston Globe which reported the House Committee of Government Operations' panel confirmed complaints filed by patients that some unscrupulous New Medico providers "deter patients against their will, provide unnecessary care and extend clients stays to generate revenue."

If the New Medico Rehabilitation and Skilled Nursing Center at Meadowlands had been firmly established in '82 when I was hurt, naturally, my parents would have elected to have me treated there because of the close proximity to home. If New Medico could have somehow convinced the government that my out-of-state academic home of Morgantown, W.Va. was also my permanent residence, and, of course, as long as my coverage would pay for my stay, I could have expected to be told by Meadowlands that I'd need continuing inpatient services indefinitely and to just forget about trying to attain my Bachelor's—let alone my Master's—anytime during the 80's, for I'd need New Medico therapy well into the new millennium. Before being discarded as exaggeration, this notion wouldn't be so far-fetched given what was being unmasked about the lovely Corporation. Feeling as if they could walk on water and were impervious to the sanctions of the law, New Medico would have essentially told me to forego my future in order to pad their pocketbooks.

In harmony with an edition of The New York Times two days earlier—10/28/92—where it was written that New Medico had been discharging patients "as soon as their insurance runs out" and The Boston Globe's report in the aforementioned 10/30/92 paper, stating that New Medico "dumped people still recovering back into the community when their insurance funds were exhausted"—being a fly on the wall during one of Goyette's sealed conferences—I could just imagine a dialogue based on the under-the-table facts currently being unearthed.

"That's too goddamned bad patient 'Joe Schmoe' won't get to experience significant progress with his paralysis, if he's not permitted to stay here a little longer," Goyette's hypothetical response would be to a brief moment of Family Counselor compassion where a patient's mental/physical health was actually being considered over dollars, "but we're not about to keep him because his coverage has expired. And Shirley's been eyeing up some diamond earrings, so I can't be strapped for cash!"

Also disclosing facilities in the New Medico firm "billed patients for therapies not provided," "misrepresented services available," and would "admit patients based on their insurance coverage, not their medical needs," The Boston Globe paper dated 10/30/92, gave an insider's view of the Corporation's discharge practices after determining the length of time reimbursement would be forthcoming. This unidentified New Medico employee, whose conscience must have been twisted, wrote: "We then figure out how long the money will last and immediately plan discharge based upon that. We rarely discharge before the benefits are exhausted and we absolutely discharge the minute funding goes sour."

Because of the compassionate staffs I've met "across the board" in my rehabilitation travels during school and my personal bout with disability, it was difficult to fathom professionals within this field mercilessly reeking mass havoc on defenseless folks enduring neurological malfunctions just for personal, monetary gain. During my own rehabilitation struggles, if I had been let go A.M.A. (against medical advice) or detained for anything other than what was in my best interests, the obstacles which I ultimately triumphed over would have surely conquered me, leaving me nothing but a fragment of a whole. Purposely keeping one from embarking on a path that could harvest enhanced restoration is sinister, but this appeared to be the backbone behind most everything New Medico did.

So that explains it. With families being such an integral part of a head injury survivor's recovery, I couldn't understand why this support wasn't encouraged and facilitated more by New Medico in the form of arranging demographic accommodations. Visiting hours would come and go when families could be with their inpatient loved ones at the New Medico center at Meadowfraud, but the place would look like a ghost town most often during these times because relatives lived so far away.

Unsettled being so removed—screams of isolation frequently scorching from their lips—many of those patients from South Carolina, New York, Kentucky, Ohio, and W.Va. I'd train with would be in the doldrums throughout their day and on the brink of giving up. This helpless/hopeless demeanor would occur not only because terrifying symptoms of a neurological impairment teased their every waking moment, but because those tangled within the mesh of a broken brain rarely got to see anyone close to them who could help ease them along in their horrific rehabilitation journey through the perils of a brain disorder. Concluding that the "Man of Honor" (Goyette) and "Florence Nightengale" (Micklow)—the two fiduciary ring leaders running the New Medico show at Meadowlands—were only being gracious and had a stellar restoration plan allowing long-distance patients to be rehabbed at their New Medico shrine, could not have been too much further from the truth.

Dedicating quite a few words to many of the Corporation's sleazy tactics, The Boston Globe's 10/30/92 copy also contained several paragraphs about the staggering mileage New Medico consumers regularly had to travel one-way just to get to the rehab destination where their loved one was being deposited. Not surprisingly, this ghastly inconvenience incurred upon survivors and their families was done in order to fatten New Medico wallets. Choking on my disdain, thoughts focused upon the New York resident I was assigned to work with at Meadowlands who tearfully begged daily to be transferred home to a New Medico facility in his backyard, the contempt within me overflowed because this New England gazette implied that the deplorable New Medico operation would keep these "Empire State" patients seeking treatment away from familiar territory—such as "Ben"—so that a substantial profit of over three times as much could be made. As an example, The Globe reported that New Medico would, "Manipulate the Medicaid system to place patients in out-of-state facilities, and thus gain higher reimbursement rates."

If my "home" rehab center had pulled such an awful stunt with me when I was suffering amidst my precipice, there would have been no way I could've survived. Chants of "executive privilege" falling on investigators' deaf ears, I could just picture Goyette and Micklow shitting themselves while the maneuvers of them and their employer were being inspected. Smelling a rat, detectives caught New Medico administrators in the center of a firestorm.

In addition, the 10/30/92 Boston paper divulged that this despicable Corporation would dispatch "ambulance chasers" to treatment sites where accident victims would be taken for care and how "New Medico marketers routinely made hospital rounds with physicians and had inappropriate access to medical and insurance records," making "recommendations to hospital staff that the patient be transferred to New Medico facilities." Personally understanding how treacherous a head injury disability experience can be, knowing that their company was inflicting massive suffering on those whose pain/torment could hardly be imagined and not doing "right" by survivors already suffocating with enough misery, it wouldn't be too hard to figure out the motives as to why staff members at New Medico's Meadowfraud Health Care Center approached me as they did.

From the onset, when Goyette didn't want to spare a moment of His time to interview this one-of-a-kind practicum intern, to my final day at Meadowlands when He let it be known that shaking my hand goodbye would be a chore, New

47TH STORY of Level 1 printed in FULL format.

WALL STREET JOURNAL

October 28, 1992, Wednesday

SECTION: Section A; Page 6, Column 1

LENGTH: 32 words

HEADLINE: HEAD-TRAUMA FIRM'S RECORDS SEIZED BY FEDERAL AGENTS IN FRAUD INQUIRY

BYLINE: BY RON SUSKIND

JOURNAL-CODE: WSJ

ABSTRACT:

FBI agents have seized documents of New Medico Associates Inc, a large head-trauma rehabilitation company that federal officials are investigating for health care fraud (M)

LANGUAGE: ENGLISH

Medico tried to tear down my walls. Naive, I just figured that Meadowlands going out of their way to be disrespectful and inhospitable was merely a reflection of their top henchman's "standoffish" personality. Believing it inconceivable that New Medico at Meadowlands' executive manpower's own agenda would interfere with my good Samaritan strivings to share with the head injury disability population the invaluable fraternal member's perspective I possess, I had no idea anything "fishy" was going on with this heavenly Corporation.

Using my professional standing and attainment of an advanced degree, I wanted to do what I could to disprove faulty stereotypes/preconceived notions which do too much damage to members of this population who have a reasonable prognosis. Belonging to the disability group that this Corporation claims to care for, New Medico turned their back on me and anyone who could have benefited from witnessing a real-life example of what quality head injury rehabilitation can achieve.

On a collision course with despondency, before the industry's crooked ways were uncovered, I assumed that Meadowlands' administration only wanted me to show my astounding recovery video to a select few and demanded that I be "gagged" from discussing my personal experience with trauma because these Corporate lieutenants didn't want to have to defend the hiring of a far less experienced applicant. It being far too easy to engage in nepotism, if the one being victimized not getting the work position has had a head injury, feminists would likely stand up and howl that "Woman Power" presided.

But this particular Meadowlands situation would not be a male vs. female one, rather, discrimination against a "disabled" person who had already proven his

45TH STORY of Level 1 printed in FULL format.

The New York Times

October 28, 1992, Wednesday, Late Edition - Final

SECTION: Section D; Page 3; Column 6; Financial Desk

LENGTH: 387 words

HEADLINE: COMPANY NEWS;
F.B.I. Seizes Records of New Medico

BYLINE: By PETER KERR

BODY:

Agents of the Federal Bureau of Investigation entered the corporate headquarters yesterday of New Medico Health Care Systems of Lynn, Mass., the operator of a national chain of brain-injury rehabilitation centers, and seized records.

The F.B.I. said the move was part of a national investigation of "alleged health care fraud."

New Medico, which until recently operated 42 rehabilitation and nursing home facilities in more than 15 states, has been accused by former patients, employees and Congressional investigators of promising near- impossible cures to emotionally devastated families, overcharging patients and discharging them as soon as their insurance ran out.

The company has denied such charges and says it provides the highest-quality care.

Federal Warrant Served

F.B.I. agents entered the company's headquarters at 7:30 A.M. yesterday, served a Federal warrant and asked to have access to company files, particularly those dealing with patient records, Jack Barrette, a New Medico spokesman, said. Mr. Barrette said he was unaware of the nature of the investigation.

"This process does not mean there are new allegations," Charles A. Stillman, a lawyer who represents New Medico, said. "This means they have decided to gather together documents. Our obligation is to be as cooperative as we can."

A spokesman for the F.B.I.'s Boston office said that he could disclose nothing more about the investigation of New Medico than to say it involved his agency, the Federal Department of Health and Human Services and criminal investigators of the Defense Department.

In Congressional testimony earlier this year about New Medico facilities, family members of former patients described rehabilitation programs that admitted and kept patients who could not benefit from treatment and that sometimes charged as much as $30,000 a month. A lawsuit by former employees in New York charges that the company systematically cheating Medicare and private insurance companies.

New Medico now operates 27 centers around the country, down from 42 a year ago, Mr. Barrett, the company's spokesman, said. Two of the centers are being shut down, he said, and others are being sold.

New Medico is a privately held company founded and operated by Charles Brennick, a longtime operator of nursing homes.

LANGUAGE: ENGLISH

LOAD-DATE: October 28, 1992

42ND STORY of Level 1 printed in FULL format.

The Boston Globe

October 30, 1992, Friday, City Edition

SECTION: ECONOMY; Pg. 67

LENGTH: 818 words

HEADLINE: House report finds head injury treatment rife with fraud, abuse; Mass.' New Medico is often cited

BYLINE: By John H. Kennedy, Globe Staff

BODY:

A congressional panel yesterday slammed Massachusetts-based New Medico and other head injury rehabilitation providers in a searing report on alleged fraud and abuse in the $ 10 billion industry.

The draft report said consumers and insurers are pouring millions of unnecessary dollars into head rehabilitation facilities that are inadequately monitored by state and federal government.

"The lack of regulations and cost controls in the head injury rehabilitation industry leaves the door open for some providers to take advantage of vulnerable patients with limited financial resources," said Rep. Donald Payne (D-N.J.), chairman of the Human Resources and Intergovernmental Relations subcommittee, which conducted hearings earlier this year on the industry.

"New Medico is an unfortunate example of what can happen when we trust an industry to monitor itself," he said in a statement.

A New Medico spokesperson said the company had not yet seen the report, but he defended the company's operations and criticized the committee's handling of the hearings on which part of the report was based.

The report by the House Committee on Government Operations was released the same week federal agents descended on New Medico's offices in Lynn and Goshen, N.Y., as part of a criminal probe of health care fraud allegations.

The panel said it confirmed complaints lodged by patients that some unscrupulous providers detain patients against their will, provide unnecessary care and extend client stays to generate revenues.

The report also claimed it confirmed complaints about facilities which billed patients for therapies not provided, misrepresented services available and dumped people still recovering back into the community when their insurance funds were exhausted.

"Unethical providers will continue to profit from the greatest hopes and fears of distraught families unless federal and state health officials and third-party payers examine alternatives to institutionalized care, and enforce greater accountability in the head injury rehabilitation industry," the report concluded.

Already, Rep. Ron Wyden (D-Ore.) has introduced legislation that would allow states to set standards and provide Medicaid reimbursement for home treatment of the head-injured. "We think that if you provide for home treatment you will give some of these persons higher quality treatment, and at a lower cost," said Steve Jenning, an aide to Wyden.

Insurers are taking notice, cutting down on the reimbursement level they pay to head injury rehabilition facilities, said one health specialist.

The Boston Globe, October 30, 1992

"Profits have been falling as a result of insurers shortening the lengths of treatment they will pay for," said John Reichard, editor of Health Business, a Washington-based magazine. "I think basically they concluded it wasn't medically justified to cover very long stays."

New Medico spokesman Jack Barrette said the company wasn't invited to subcommittee hearings chaired by the late Rep. Ted Weiss (D-N.Y.), nor were any of the patients who were satisfied with their treatment.

"But we know the vast majority of those people are satisfied with our company, our services and the way we do business," he said. "Those people have not testified to the subcommittee. The happy people have not been a part of that process. Therefore, people who were not satisfied are half the story."

While the report stopped short of directly accusing New Medico of fraud, it devoted vast portions of its 29-page report to the company and a handful of others.

Among the allegations were that some companies:

- Admit patients based on their insurance coverage, not on their medical needs. One unidentified New Medico employee wrote the panel about the company's exhaustive research of a client's insurance coverage.

"We then figure out how long the money will last and immediately plan discharge based upon that," wrote the unidentified employee. "We rarely discharge before the benefits are exhausted and we absolutely discharge the minute funding goes sour."

- Manipulate the Medicaid system to place patients in out-of-state facilities, and thus gain higher reimbursement rates.

Wisconsin paid a per-diem average of $ 73 for in-state services, but paid $ 550 per day to New Medico's facility in Slidell, La. New York state paid an averge $ 92 per diem for in-state, $ 300 for out-of-state treatment.

- Labeled recruiters for some facilities "ambulance chasers in the classic sense." New York officials found New Medico marketers routinely made hospital rounds with physicians and had inappropriate access to medical and insurance records and made "recommendations to hospital staff that the patient be transferred to New Medico facilities."

Some providers complained that because New Medico awarded a research grant to a hospital in Albany, N.Y., "the hospital showed preference in their referrals to New Medico."

LANGUAGE: ENGLISH

LOAD-DATE: October 31, 1992

40TH STORY of Level 1 printed in FULL format.

Modern Healthcare

November 2, 1992

SECTION: THE WEEK IN HEALTHCARE; Rehabilitation; Pg. 8

LENGTH: 254 words

HEADLINE: Feds seize New Medico records

BYLINE: Sandy Lutz

BODY:

Federal agents last week seized records from New Medico Associates, a Lynn, Mass.-based head injury rehabilitation company that has been the focus of congressional hearings on healthcare fraud.

''We're making it our job to cooperate fully with them,'' Jack Barrette, a spokesman for the privately held company, said about the search that began on Oct. 27.

He confirmed that the agents were from the FBI, HHS and the Defense Department.

Mr. Barrette said no charges or indictments had been filed against the company and that the federal agents were on an ''investigational action.''

FBI officials were quoted in published reports as saying the document seizure was part of a national investigation of healthcare fraud. The Defense Department was participating because some of the allegations involved treatment of military beneficiaries, one report said.

Allegations of fraudulent billing practices and substandard care at New Medico have been investigated by a congressional committee, the New York State Department of Health and a U.S. attorney's office (April 13, p. 29).

The company, which has about $ 200 million in annual revenues, has 27 facilities in 13 states. Only two of those facilities are hospitals, however. The remainder are long-term-care and transitional facilities.

New Medico has treated more than 15,000 patients, Mr. Barrette said. ''The vast majority of those people are very satisfied with the treatment they received,'' he added. "We will do anything to fix any errors we find.''

LANGUAGE: ENGLISH

proficiency despite numerous obstacles being laid before me by this seedy Corporation to minimize my effectiveness. This prejudicial course of action being a "no-no," I originally thought that maybe this might simply be a case of the "haves" prevailing over the "have not wannabes," once again. However, with the way this Corporation's unethical treatment of its patients had been unfolding, I could see how me and New Medico would have been a combustible pairing.

Like dropping an atomic bomb on a M.A.S.H. unit, corporations such as New Medico are primarily designed to maximize investor value, not necessarily what's in the best interests of its patients. Having worked and labored in the social services field which usually doesn't monetarily reward its workers all that tremendously, being underpaid for years, the New Medico skilled laborer work force likely thought it was their right to make a little money. And by the way things materialized, the squalid administrations at New Medico surely must have reasoned that if this cash collection came at the expense of "head injured cripples" who don't know what to make of things anyhow, so be it.

For the many mid-level New Medico counseling craftspeople aware of the Corporation's sordid executive tactics who tried to come across as this former patient's friend/advocate, their conscience must have abandoned them. To knowingly abide by evil Corporate procedures and not report it is not only shameful, but an accessory to the crime. The money must have been just too good, for cheating people needing the utmost in care and prolonging many patients agony was seen as a small price to pay for a bulging billfold.

Sacrificing survivors' already alarming condition for dollars, those New Medico staff members who recognized/implemented this firm's shenanigans and basked in the profits, need to do some serious soul-searching. Apparently viewing it as justification given their compromised salary over the years, it appeared as if more than a few New Medico rehabilitation authorities would forget about their obligations to stricken patients and discard what was proper, so they could "cash in" on "head injured invalids'" anguish. It's admirable when caregivers will go to great lengths to assure that their offsprings' lives are filled with happiness, but when some New Medico parents go as far as to violate the trust and care of head injury survivors in order to have the needed income to afford the latest line of expensive Hasbro toys, this would be taking things way too far.

Because I have had an injury which scares rehabilitation employers away, it was absolutely imperative that I get the good career reference I earned from New Medico in order to have a fighting chance to "get ahead" in this brain trauma disability field. Gored by the need to sustain their cover-up, this recommendation would never be forthcoming, all but killing my pursuit to start a mutually prosperous rehabilitation career where my role-modeling example could have been put to good use. Dishing out master lip service, self-proclaimed rehab "experts" will tell those having sustained a handicap to "turn that frown upside down" because those having a disability have as good a shot at landing that reputable rehabilitation job opening as someone who hadn't been hurt—but these well-wishers could not have been any more wrong.

In addition to the academic degrees I earned, thinking that my strength and fighting spirit would be advantageous in my pursuits to get a professional rehab job, I couldn't have been more mistaken. My one-time traumatized history was seen as a permanent hindrance, as my grit and determination have been discounted by stereotypical fear. Taking the traditional route of career attainment where one acquires an advanced degree and serves a productive apprenticeship, it's absolutely impossible to get a profitable position in head injury rehabilitation, if the job applicant was once in need of this treatment service at one time. Hoping that an employer of a top-notch rehabilitation program could set aside their personal biases and accept how valuable/unique a qualified former patient would be counseling this population, sadly turned out to be a fairy tale.

My one-time affliction has been an insurmountable barrier, putting me into a "funk" which prevents me from attaining a position where I could put my full-worth into play. The defeating attitudes which exist about people with head injury disabilities couldn't have been reflected any more perfectly than during my scholastic training.

Sandwiched in-between my icy New Medico arrival and the not-so-promising exit, were a number of disgraceful events which delivered a message not to expect any sort of a cheerful reception marking my placement at Meadowlands. With all the heinous tactics New Medico "pulled" with those dependent on them for honest care and to discourage me from trying to land a Family Counseling position here, no wonder staff had a "Well, uhhhhh..," say nothing, politician's dialogue when speaking.

For instance, always ready with some comeback, my primary supervisor would rarely give me a straight answer to any managerial inquiries or observations I'd make which weren't obvious. Either implying I'd need to prove my inferences or else would just reflect on what I had asked and chuckle as if to make it look like my deduction was ridiculous, when I'd say something to the effect that I didn't think I was being treated with the respect I certainly felt I deserved by administration, I could expect to hear parts of my statement repeated before being told—in essence—that this executive branch had a multitude of responsibilities which need prioritized over my sensitivity. I wouldn't be surprised to hear that, basically, I'd have to accept that I'm simply not the center of the brain trauma universe like Harmarville and grad school must have brainwashed me into believing.

Embarrassed to think my achievements after my head injury were somehow noteworthy and unique, feeling as if I had ungraciously pried in some way, I would think twice before pressing the matter anymore. Unfortunately for me, apparently as planned, this manipulation device worked to a tee, for I would be ashamed to think of—let alone mention—such a proposition again.

The lack of regard and disrespect which followed me around most every administrative corner at Meadowlands was much more than Goyette's style, but a means of survival that He saw as needing to be employed, so that the sneaky New Medico moneymaking machine could keep running. Serving as an advocate promoting that proper care for the head injury population be provided—viewing me as some kind of squealer—Goyette could have had nightmares of this spotless intern being interviewed by some Independent Counsel or an Attorney General, as I unknowingly would cry shame upon the Corporation's operation at Meadowlands.

Not having a clue as to what this would mean in relation to the overall scope of an investigation, I realized after having learned of the mischievous ways of the Corporation that I would not have made Goyette's day had I unwittingly told a federal agent how New Medico at Meadowlands: alleviated the essential Family Room to make it another patient quarters for someone not needing rehabilitation services who lived several hundred miles away, seemed to hold a few patients who had stagnated against their will, appeared to have overly-embellished the quality of some programs for staff would just seem to watch patients breathe, collected a good bit of money renting out lodging rooms to out-of-state families who needed accommodations for the night, often appeared to cause radical stress dysfunction for patients who were unable to get home, etc.

Now that the underground maneuvers of New Medico are getting dug up, it would be safe to assume being locked out of those reviews the Meadowlands' Program Director had with the Family Counselors was done in order to keep me from understanding illegal Corporate workings. With the objective being to deter me from pursuing full-time employment with New Medico—where I would be a righteous migraine—with this game plan becoming all too clear, I can see why Meadowlands stooped to such dark, subterranean levels to throw cold water on my vocational aspirations to join their staff and serve as a proponent for the head injury disability population, championing their constitutional rights. To put a damper on my longing for gainful employment here, with the Corporation's nauseous deeds unveiled, I can understand the motives behind the childish tricks which occurred at New Medico's Meadowlands brokerage.

Only working there several weeks in a practicum schooling capacity, I definitely would be hurt, but not completely undone when Meadowlands didn't hire me after having had an opening for a Family Counselor position develop during my internship when the center's operation increased to four teams. Knowing that they got a capable worker (Patton) and figuring I would be next in line for a psychological counseling job because of my previous Meadowlands' orientation/what I perceived as a potentially invaluable personal background with rehabilitation, I proceeded in a hopeful fashion. Despite never hearing so much as a peep that administration ever seriously considered one day employing me as a permanent, full-time counselor, I never surrendered my pursuit because I had trouble imagining that Meadowlands Health Care Center could find anyone more qualified than myself. If the walls of the New Medico at Meadowlands' administrative office could only talk, given the developments as they occurred, these partitions would no doubt tell me that my vocational perseverance had been cussed and sworn at by the directors.

Looking back on it, I wouldn't think it would be unreasonable to ascertain that when this law-abiding student intern didn't give any indication that he was about to give up on his desire to snare an employment position with Meadowlands—even after being overlooked for a Family Counselor vacancy during his internship—a sort of "Plan B" was devised by New Medico. Inevitably sending me back to the hospital, finangling methods to dissuade me from trying to attain the job I had deserved with New Medico at Meadowlands ambushed me from almost every professional corner. Those New Medico staff members who claimed to advocate for the brain trauma disability population—but carried out the Corporation's executive way of doing business—would have surely turned things around, accusing this trainee of suffering from existing trauma-induced paranoia believing that New Medico was the least bit dishonest. With illegitimacy being discovered as the fundamental supporting structure of this fraudulent-riddled rehabilitation treatment industry, schemes such as the ones employed at Meadowlands surely were a basis of the Corporation's operation.

Knowing that this survivor's primary motivations would be for the care of its patients and the likelihood of their getting "busted" drastically minimized having a spoiled osteopath's kid digging into their overflowing private-for-profit payroll budget, upon reflection, New Medico at Meadowlands crime moguls went about their deception with an all-too-transparent design. Aware of how extremely proud I was having a video documenting my startling recovery and realizing that it would take much more than being looked over for a Meadowlands' counseling employment slot to stop my assault on equal opportunity with them, Goyette made sure to drop another discouragement bombshell on me by demanding that I only share my rehabilitation videotaped drama with a limited few, who already knew about my experience with disability. Harboring gut-wrenching disappointment and resentment that I couldn't give my gift of experience after having almost taken a ride on a hearse with a brain contusion, preventing me from expounding on my one-in-a-trillion comeback, Goyette's plot to dissuade me from attaining staff membership would only be warming up.

Pertaining to the disturbing lunch break circumstance where this Program Director couldn't wait a minute or two until I got into the staffing office ready to present my video, if one would have asked Goyette how He could justify hiring a "cliff notes" student over someone whose amazing, related experience with head injury was captured on tape, all this chaste exec needed to say to cover His bases would be that He never saw this depiction of my recovery. Surely claiming that word of mouth was all He had to go by, Goyette thought He knew what steps needed taken to capsize a potential government informant's quest to sail on His New Medico merchant marine. Not one to give up easily, my not seeing these stunts for what they really were upon their detonation, it looked like more than opinion that infantile pranks were actually discharged to torpedo this aspiring Corporation employee off his navigational course towards a career in rehabilitation with Meadowlands. Because I would be more than capable of "snitching" on New Medico's blackmarket dealings upon learning of their unlawful strategies, other staffing options would need to be pursued.

To make it look like I was some sort of "head injured degenerate" who shouldn't have ever rightfully expected to be a paid staff member at Meadowlands and to "water down" this aspiration, Goyette's tricks occurred here at a breakneck pace. Not too hard to imagine with New Medico's mistreatment of its patients as I once appeared being hung out to dry, devastating another person with a history of brain injury would be no big deal because it had become "old hat." The wounds from my student history with the Corporation likely will always tear at me from time to time, however, the cuts dug that much deeper and the pain hurt that much more upon understanding the baby shit antics such as the ones Goyette pulled with me—largely engineered to disinterest me from working at Meadowlands—were only part of an organization-wide ploy to keep out those apt to report the operation's wrongful conduct.

Not wanting to believe a head injury health care establishment would further scar someone who symbolized much of what they supposedly stood for, from the moment I heard Goyette had become histrionically pissed that this inconsiderate subordinate had thought of doing something so sacrilegious as to present Him with an internship requests paper that wasn't typed, to the time this "pee-on" collegian signed off progress notes for His review as if I were established in the field of rehab, I still foolishly continued to have faith in the system.

Whole-heartedly surmising that New Medico's strivings were predominantly geared for the welfare of those reliant on their service provision, from that afternoon "The Boss" refused to pay this discourteous apprentice even minimum wage for my Meadowlands' counseling work which had the makings of being significant had the Corporation not been so concerned with hiding their true intentions from me, to the day this "head injured subservient" disgusted Goyette by balking at His request to pour lemonade and pass out name tags at the Meadowlands' summer picnic, I nonetheless remained hopeful things might still somehow work out for me.

Possibly always having a body in mind to fill any Family Counselor spot which may one day present itself, from the beginning when it appeared I would be hailed for my impeccable credentials after sustaining trauma, to when the unthinkable occurred and Goyette didn't even want to afford me with the respect of a farewell handshake, this rude ingrate was naive concluding that a rehabilitation industry wouldn't get the "willies" entertaining the idea of employing a survivor.

Fearing that I'd be a "whistle blower" on the New Medico Corporation—unless He initially saw my recovery experience as a means to somehow profit investors or to advertise His particular center—I had trouble figuring out why Goyette allowed me to serve my field practice at His facility in the first place. Upon review of this staffing situation where I would be dealt a destructive blow below the belt, given the sadistic way the New Medico Corporation was found to be run, it would be more than remotely possible that after Goyette saw my character during my training as one where I'd be focused on patient care—and that this attention would prevail over keeping quiet about the Corporation's workings—the Corporate administrator got scared and thought better of it to bring me on board as a full-time Family Counselor employee where I'd need to understand all aspects of a patient's program. Needing to keep the true intent of the operation "under wraps," New Medico saw it necessary to steal my dream of working professionally in rehabilitation.

New Medico ultimately exposed as a system of centers which were grossly insensitive to many of their patients' needs, some Corporate feathers surely ruffled when a head injury survivor—already familiar with some of the Corporation's protocol—wanted to serve in an advocacy role for their traumatized population. Prior to the firm's pretentious maneuvers being brought to the forefront, regardless of the accomplishments I had made afterwards, I mistakenly assumed that New Medico had victimized my future because of my past history where I was once in critical condition—and not for dollars. Blaming anything one doesn't understand or can't accept on a victim's head injury, I just figured New Medico held the generally accepted belief that all "brain injured" patients just aren't cognitively "with it" and that this Corporation's stereotypical presumptions about this patient population controlled their actions with regards to how this applicant/survivor was perceived.

I initially concluded that my head injury might not have killed me, but that it did claim any rehabilitation job pursuits as a casualty, and this was why I wouldn't be held in the high favor by New Medico that I thought would be a given and believed I had earned. Dependent on employers for further progress after my head injury, I would universally be flicked "the finger," putting a damper on my pursuits to make any more gains. Testosterone doing way too much hiring in this rehab field, trying to attain a professional Rehabilitation Counseling therapy employment position in the customary fashion of looking in the classifieds, applying, and interviewing, I could expect to find out that some female sporting a pair of size "D" cups was found to have more knowledge about the head injury disability population than this survivor. Not completely ruling out that my once mentally-disheveled condition didn't influence Meadowlands' execs, knowing that a multitude of other survivors had also been lynched of their rightful expectation of fair treatment by the Corporation, only fueled the flames of my spite.

Goyette's actions not being enough to send a message that I wasn't welcomed at Meadowlands—because I wanted to believe that any employment determination or judgment would be based on merit—other unsavory means needed manufactured to halt my attempts to catch a ride with the New Medico capital-mobile. With administration surely viewing someone on the level as a threat to hijack the price-gouging New Medico operation, every alternative would need exploited to divert my attention away from the syndicate.

Whether she was coached on what to say or else was simply a matter of a New Medico therapist wanting to brag a little and/or "rub it in" to someone not receiving as much as a dime of monetary pay for their efforts, I couldn't understand how a rehabilitation professional could so drastically contradict themself. I wasn't sure what to make of things when the female therapist I'd speak to at Meadowlands on occasion told me one thing during the early stage of my practicum training—that the New Medico cesspool really paid its employees well—and then later on, during the final leg of my internship practice when it was well-known that I wanted to be a permanent Family Counselor staff member, collecting a little slice of this reimbursement pie, claimed that they don't reward it workers. Implying that I should look elsewhere for employment, I got real suspicious.

Likely chalking this fleeting idea of mine up to paranoia manifested by my head injury, if I'd have suggested to the mid-level personnel I was exposed to during my field study that Meadowlands administration seemed to be approaching this TBI survivor as if I were some kind of paranormal phenomenon, I could expect to be told not to be ridiculous. With the distasteful practices so inherent of the New

Medico "out for a buck" organization getting the spotlight, if this former patient *had* been treated fairly by the Corporation, now *that* would have been unbelievable.

Her mocking snicker and sardonic grin having been forged into my memory, finding my struggles humorous beyond belief, the Program Director's lovely spouse/Meadowlands' Head Case Manager—Shirley Goyette—had a great time demonstrating the regard which existed at Meadowlands for me. Focusing my mind's eye and retracing my steps to the day when my balance deficiency/ unstable gait wouldn't permit me to steady a cup of coffee as I limped along out of the break room to an awaiting family, the head executive's wife's lack of compassion and disrespect would be a tell-tale sign not to expect any appreciation for my many potentially incomparable abilities with the head injury disability population I could empathize with all too well. Getting the "heebie-jeebies" knowing that if I were employed at Meadowlands, administrative manpower of this northern Washington County facility realized I could really mess up New Medico's unprincipled standard operating procedure with my conscientious striving to assist patients I could closely relate to. Therefore, given how the Corporation's true fabric wasn't found as one woven by the fundamental constructs of the law—to preserve the morally-offensive New Medico operation—it would be essential that this model survivor be "wronged," so as to force me to set my job attainment sights elsewhere.

Not realizing at the time that this message was related to my legitimate expectation to one day gain professional employment with New Medico—sneer barely visible—the Program Director's wife told me one afternoon "out of the blue" and not related to anything in particular that the word, "assume," is spelled, make an "ass out of you and me." Given this English lesson before it became general knowledge that many of the New Medico administrative procedures were in defiance of the law, the gleam defecating from The Boss' wife's eyes no doubt was an expectorant knowing what was in store for me. For her to "assume" that once my field training ended, she'd never have to worry about me reporting on her hubby's practices and other New Medico execs like Him who destroyed peoples' lives for riches, I guess I might just get the last laugh!!!!! "Ha, Ha, Ha, Ha, Ha, Ha, Ha, Ha, Ha, Ha, Ha, Ha, Ha, Ha, Ha, Ha, Ha, Ha, Ha, Ha, Ha, Ha, Ha, Ha, Ha, Ha, Ha, Ha, Ha, Ha, Ha, Ha, Ha, Ha, Ha, Ha, Ha, Ha, Ha, Ha, Ha, Ha, Ha, Ha, Ha, Ha, Ha, Ha, Ha, Ha, Ha, Ha, Ha, Ha, Ha, Ha, Ha, Ha, Ha, Ha, Ha, Ha, Ha, Ha, Ha, Ha, Ha, Ha."

Supposedly having a huge heart, looking at how the Corporation for which she collected substantial paychecks had been "pulling the rug out from under" so many patients as I once appeared for monetary enhancement, the compassionate female Family Counselor who didn't serve in a supervisory capacity with me (Thelma) likely balked because directly interacting with this former patient could have taunted her conscience—and not necessarily because she was intimidated by this intern's knowledge of head injury. Possibly aware of the Rich girl's imminent hiring and having inside knowledge that the reason I had to be approached with disrespect was so that the maintenance of this outlaw Corporation could continue, this W.V.U. Rehab Counseling graduate would likely rather not have to look me in the eye, if she could help it.

One noon lunch break in the psych doctor's office where the counselors and myself would gather to eat our mid-day feast and review patient care, the well-paid New Medico staff decided to have a snapshot taken in order to pay homage to this survivor's advancement up the ranks from comatose patient to verging professional. Sitting left to right, preparing to hear some accounts of how I had gone full circle from an unconscious Ranchos #1 patient to an aspiring professional primed and ready to work with the head injury population, my New Medico primary supervisor (Berkowitz), the new Family Counselor (Patton), the Neuropsychologist, yours truly, and the female Family Counselor (Thelma) were all decked out in our professional combat gear. Insisting that his masculine social worker's image adorn the pic as well, these Corporation counseling staffers wanted Butch to join in, but he adamantly refused; choosing instead to stay behind the camera, having fun with his photography hobby. Or, so he said.

Not about to take a backseat to anyone, given his extensive experience "caring" for those with head injuries—with all eyes focused on me while I was talking and accentuating a point with my left hand—I wouldn't be so sure that my being the central figure of this pic was necessarily why Butch didn't want to be included in this frozen portrayal of time, or if there wasn't a darker/more insidious reason. Could it have been he surmised that the rehab operation for which he harvested his bountiful fruit may very well be caught "red-handed" one day in patients' insurance cookie jar—profiting from their suffering—and this connoisseur of the New Medico firm's workings didn't want his face associated with a criminal organization, if he could help it?

Moonlighting as a National Head Injury Foundation group "leader" and wanting to pursue a long career counseling the head injury population, Butch surely wouldn't want his picture taken with several of his cohorts who attended Goyette's barred conferences every week, documenting a tangible record that he was a major player in a larcenous company. Fighting mad and wanting to reciprocate the respect I received from New Medico, this survivor would have other ideas, however.

A close environmental parallel, reflecting my heightened attitude counseling those with a variety of mental illnesses at this therapy/domiciliary body, the lot void of any commercial purpose next to this program would be cleared out to make way for a southern entrance to an attractive residential/recreational development. In the middle of nowhere when I began working at this establishment, the area slowly evolved into one sprawling with exciting activity and growth. Symbolic of my progress as a group counselor, the run-down farmhouse in the adjacent property was torn down in order to construct an entranceway for this costly suburban neighborhood of six-figure homes.

All pretty good signs that I had gotten the "hang" of things around this MH/MR place and that a sort of professional comfort level had started to settle in with me,

I would be asked to give an agency in-service on R.E.T. because my use of this contemporary/cognitive-behavioral psychotherapy method had worked pretty well for a good many residents, referred to as "The Master" by my "super" supervisor because of my apparent affinity for conducting productive counseling interventions with those struggling to grasp fact from fiction, complimented for my ability to create goal-oriented therapeutic movement by the seasoned agency mind-reading guru as she talked of how I could make the residents "jump off a bridge" if I wanted on more than one staffing, and having a few of the cognitive therapy approaches I'd traditionally use in group adopted by the skilled psych nurse in her own interactions with some of the residents. These professionals facilitating my performance/understanding and not routinely disparaging me, had led to my rapid development of an effective approach counseling those compromised by a mental disturbance.

Armed with a new confidence and reinforced by a refreshing structure of understanding, aided by several hours of group counseling therapy each day, these practice and support ingredients led to my instigating intervention methods which would reap quite a few benefits for those making fantasy interpretations of their world. Not going unnoticed by the administrative body of this provincial MH/MR organization—unlike the family counseling agency where this "crippled" employee's penchant for goal-directed therapy and ability to serve as a quality helper seemed largely overshadowed by the existing physical symptoms of this therapist's head injury—my professional skills were recognized/not constrained, as I was to share my ever-increasing counseling knowledge and train a graduate student how to productively go about helping those with perceptual/organizational debilities attain some semblance of operative functioning.

Having taken the Strong-Campbell Interest Inventory a couple of years ago, gauging both strengths and individual interests, the results of this personality background questionnaire indicated I would likely excel in a teaching capacity. Although guiding residents to discover what can be done to enhance the quality of their lives and counseling those experiencing other situational difficulties definitely takes on this desired instructional aspect of my makeup, supervising a Master's student from Duquesne University in Pittsburgh directly penetrated the core of my captivation and was an absolutely tremendous experience which provided me with an abundance of professional satisfaction and growth. Making the training that much more rewarding, Mrs. Joan Kaylar was an eager and receptive "Practicum" trainee, willing to learn and incorporate various dynamics of the group therapy approach.

Possessing a natural disposition where a good connection with those seeking her talents could be made, this aspiring master's-educated professional quickly learned to pick up both verbal and body signals in her initial growth as a group leader. Gaining increased cognizance what the signs given off mean in the general scope of things, as they relate to a resident's particular dilemma, Joan's ability to stay focused on the central meaning of issues and avoid being side-tracked by irrelevant/superfluous facts helped her begin to develop the ability to gather significant information and process how this fits into the overall picture of a situation.

Discerning nonsense from useful revelation, equating how disclosure molds into the general framework of a problem, Joan would be able to implement the various steps needed to carry out a resident's treatment plan by the time this introductory Practicum training ended and her "Internship" got under way.

Fortunate to have in my counseling armory both group therapy artillery developed by an accredited grad school program and the opportunity to practice using this weaponry several hours each day, I would be able to quickly consolidate these two elements into an approach seen as so effective that I was to train a student. Enhancing my own skills as a therapist effectively providing treatment services for a drove of perceptually-compromised residents having a variety of troubles, Joan's input forced me to examine my delivery and make revisions to better serve this population. Discovering that there's a fine line between making a sound judgment and "reading too much into things," while in the process of identifying factors which may contribute to a troubling circumstance, it would be essential to keep in the back of one's mind that being overly-analytical can stagnate the therapy process almost as much as not delving deep enough.

Either just being superficial or a ramification of their illness coming forth, it would be important to recognize when residents would have a legitimate concern and when they were merely seeking attention. While trying to clear up some of the pathological/situational confusion these disrupted program dwellers may be encountering, it would be beneficial to remember that service consumers *really want* assistance finding answers to their particular problem, or they likely wouldn't sit through a counseling session exhibiting a variety of self-disclosing behaviors. Tired of keeping skeletons in their closet secret—more times than not—underneath the overt demonstrations of resistance, those receiving treatment usually want the therapist to keep digging and "picking" their mind, so a resolution to their dysfunction may be found.

Needing some sort of reassurance that things will be alright despite the unpleasant circumstances of their history which can't be changed, the person seized by emotion would engage in certain actions, so a fairly accurate interpretation of their problematic situation could be made. Wanting encouragement, the resident would often seek reinforcement in the form of being told that it was quite natural to own the feelings they possess and that it *was* within their control to better their predicament, if they work hard towards a restoration goal.

No doubt, the traditional MH/MR approach with those irreversibly perceptually lacking had aided in the improvement of lives for more than a few residents; but for those who had felt that they had fallen into a sort of "rut" with the system and "between the cracks," it looked as if the addition of someone with a family therapy orientation might have energized a few who, otherwise, may not have been as receptive to treatment. Not to suggest that there aren't more than a few whose limitations are permanent—like people who have sustained serious brain contusions—stereotypical acceptance of what is and isn't possible with this perceptually-deprived group could definitely stunt the progress of those who have shown flashes that achievement would be within their reach.

Generally responded to favorably, using individual therapy utilized in the family counseling setting and applying quite a bit of the philosophy in a group treatment modality with residents having a mental illness worked well because they seemed to appreciate being approached as an individual whose specialized needs could be dealt with by a professional also accustomed to working with clients on "everyday problems." Especially for residents who had been in the system for years, it looked like a few could prosper working with a therapist operating from a different therapy orientation who utilized methods customarily implemented with the "adjustment disorder" population.

Either finding out through the treatment process or reading it in the overnight logbook that a resident was experiencing a certain difficulty, unless the issue was extremely sensitive/personal where the person needed to be taken aside and focused upon one-on-one, addressing troublesome developments in group using a methodology where a good bit of the attention was geared towards the individual needing the majority of immediate help seemed to be the philosophical plan of action which reaped the most benefit. However, because of their own limitations, soliciting assistance/support from the group assembly was something which needed to be done carefully—if at all—because this could often backfire. With this population's proclivities not exactly predictable, every now and then, a contentious environment would evolve because a resident would purposely avoid facing that which directly needed to be addressed.

Although it would often be advantageous to make a resident feel comfortable by utilizing less-evasive interventions initially, being a short-term treatment facility where resident stay would be limited to a few months, in order to set the brief treatment strategy wheels into motion and get to the "meat of a problem" quickly, there was only a restricted amount of time to supply optimal therapy. In order to provide maximum benefit in this time-constrained setting, the therapist would not only have to be sensitive to what was being said, but also needed to be attuned to what wasn't being conceded and observant of postures/non-verbal cues. Usually not pleasant, confrontation would often be necessary, if an unyielding resident would refuse to surrender their denial or intentionally skirt employing actions which very well could prove prosperous. Because of the emotional hardship involved admitting that the onset of a strange experience had derived from their perceptual malfunction, preserving their contradiction of the truth, residents would disaffirm any notion that was pathological in nature.

Like those who have sustained traumatic brain injuries, it's so easy to underestimate the abilities of people diagnosed with a mental illness, for most of these individuals that I conducted group with could conceptualize abstract principles and undertake complex behaviors. Important a therapist be aware of the motivations behind the manipulations, a resident being "investigated" might spew out aggressive dialogue or toxically juggle reality, so the detective/therapist "backs off." Done before the psychological inspector "gets too close" to discovering something a resident wants to remain hidden, those treatment carnivores accepted as universally challenged would twist the facts as a smoke screen.

On a few occasions in group, if a resident would see a cohort in a position where the one being inquisitioned felt inclined to reveal an aspect of their ailment they weren't 100% comfortable talking about—jumping to their defense—the therapist could find themself conversing with a pair of objecting resident buddies, instead of the one under the microscope. Weighing the urgency of the situation with the extent rapport/respect could be threatened, a judgment call had to be made where either deflection of outside interference had to occur in the pursuit of time-limited goal attainment, or else an olive branch had to be waved while in retreat.

Having troubles accepting or acknowledging symptoms of their illness because they didn't want to recognize the existence of a particular affliction, in order to back up the claim that a resident did indeed possess the certain malady they have been diagnosed with, characteristic behaviors or sequelae of their illness that they've exhibited in the past would need presented. So a point could be established and the issue at hand could be addressed, in more than a few instances, standing toe-to-toe with a resident and confronting their denial by getting their "goat" had to occur in order to "plow ahead" in the journey known as progress. Depending on their personality, those abreast to what was going on around them would either get histrionically agitated as a defense mechanism or make a concession, allowing for the possibility that maybe there might be something wrong beyond their complete control.

Viewed as some sort of confession by those needing to maintain their disallowance, discussing the delusion or hallucination clenching their conscious would be prohibitive because detailing what they were going through would be an admission that a mentally distorted view of the environment actually does exist. With the therapist not usually a beneficiary of a verbal confirmation, professionals of this nature have to "be on the lookout" and keep their eyes/ears open to what's really going on beneath the outward demonstrations. To get to the core of what's really being said, it would be mandatory that the therapist try to tune in on the same frequency as a "gun-shy" resident and search their therapeutic ammunition depot for the best counseling method to help the one incarcerated with fear and resistance divulge circumstances which would be "eating at them."

Body language frequently being the only means in which to begin making a conclusion in the neighborhood of what may be taking place with these people, assembling an accurate interpretation of an observation would need to occur. Often sending a deafening message almost as loud as any denial being screamed—with the "actions speak louder than words" premise boiling on the back burner of a therapist's intervention arsenal—sometimes what a resident *did not* divulge would be a crystal clear indicator, signaling whether or not they were enduring a psychotic episode or feeling uneasy.

For roughly half of the group, discussing matters associated with their particular difficulties would be seen as an unpleasant full-contact sport which needed to be avoided at all costs because reviewing issues just as soon forgotten would adversely affect how residents saw themselves at the moment. With long-term self-esteem directly corresponding with this self- perception—to those not "facing up" to the fact certain dysfunctions did exist—it would be vital to stress that maintaining their transparent facade of having natural experiences and disclaiming psychotic ones prevented progress from occurring. Not allowing for valuable insight, the stress created from withholding what was being encountered usually could not be hidden so easily.

More than likely a pronounced signal that topics being reviewed had substantial meaning to a group member or they were spinning in the funnel of a mind void of reason, it wouldn't be too hard to figure out someone was being bothered emotionally either by a subject being examined or a psychotic disturbance. When a resident would squirm in their seat, bounce their leg(s), rock back and forth, avoid eye contact by looking down or away, grind their teeth, cross their arms defiantly, or carry on a verbal dialogue with themselves, it would be a pretty safe bet that something was going on. Along with a hygienically-challenged appearance or heightened expression, twitching facial muscles and rapid eye movements would also be sure signs that something would be "hitting home" with those bothered by their stream of consciousness.

Whether it was helping residents to "talk through" their mind-altered state or knowing when to get tough, through demonstration and discussion, therapeutic nurturing and contesting chimerical pretenses were investigation methods the practicum student/trainee learned to fuse in her own approach. Unprofessional turbulence around this bomb shelter basically restricted to the majority of Monday/ Thursday "fire and brimstone" staffing days, developing techniques so effective I'd eventually be supervising a grad student really wouldn't be enough to provide me with any long-term sense of security. But my assignment to train this intern restored much of the confidence/thunder taken from me having the Monroeville agency welcome-wagon's bridle unhitched when I saddled up to join them and being flicked "the finger" by more than a few members of this organization's reception committee. Grasping a semblance of acceptance and some degree of comfort would be short-lived, however, for the progressive adoption of my new role would be substituted with upheaval.

What the hell's this? My mail has been opened!!!

Perseverant as ever, despite my growing tolerance working at this bumpkin therapy program and what New Medico did to me, I never completely relinquished my hopes of attaining professional employment someday with a rehab center treating patients and families who have been subjected to the ill-effects of a brain trauma disability. At some business organizations—with the employee's consent—it would be standard practice to give an envelope a swipe with a letter opener to save workers a little time; but because of the potential sensitivity of rehabilitation mail I would elect to have delivered at this yokel outfit, I never agreed to this control. But this apparently didn't matter.

Beyond stapled agency memos, I rarely received any correspondence, so I barely had any exposure to in-house policy when it came to postaged letters. Not abiding by the prudent rule, "It's better to be safe than sorry," I hardly put a moment's worth of thought into it that there would be any risk involved sending a job-search resume to a sunny rehab destination with my current employer's address enclosed. Assuming there would be a stamped return address on the envelope of a response notification didn't really concern me because, if I would happen to be questioned by management about my plans, I could just claim that this treatment center was one which had always appealed to me prior to my acceptance of my current workplace and that they were too late getting in touch with me.

Anxiously waiting for some kind of reaction from this Florida rehabilitation facility, I was shocked and infuriated to find the envelope had been ripped open. Upon reading this letter—like every other single notice I received from rehabilitation treatment programs—I would discover that there wasn't an opening for which I would be qualified, but that I'd be contacted should a position one day develop and become available. Like quite a few other rehab centers who wrote to tell me that I don't possess the credentials to be able to work for them in a disability counselor capacity, as a sort of consolation prize, this southern institute of care congratulated me on a fabulous recovery from my head injury.

Seeing an envelope with personal contents addressed to me sliced open like it was, believing I had to keep my head trauma history concealed from staff and not knowing what personnel might have read this congratulatory message, I wanted an answer as to why my mail had been trespassed upon. Thinking that this either was a violation where chief administration managing and developing guidelines of operation needed confirmation as to what exactly had happened to me, or an accident which occurred during delivery, I would be told not to worry because an executive order had been implemented by these higher-ups that agency procedure would be one where all staff mail would get opened regardless of approval.

Claiming that the contents would not be read, I didn't know if this would be an organization-wide tactic or just the branch of the agency where I worked. Having no idea if other staff's mail had been looked at, or if I had been singled out, my envelopes always would be customarily opened on a daily basis. Regardless of performance and effectiveness displayed, I wouldn't know how comfortable administrative generals at the executive headquarters would feel if they "got wind" of a therapist they were employing once had their brain injured. In time, I'd find out sure enough.

For fear that this would cloud my capabilities and nothing I'd say after this disclosure would have been heard, like the family counseling job audition in downtown Pittsburgh, I believed that if I were to be hired for this therapy position, I had to keep quiet about my personal history with brain injury when I interviewed. If the upper-echelon executive branch of this backwoods frontier establishment had the same administrative opinion about those having once sustained head injuries as most other employers, I knew I wouldn't have a shot at gaining employment. Nervous that I couldn't conceal the origin of my limp and bad hand, I could only hope that I'd be judged by my counseling knowledge and presentation.

Figuring that my disability history secret was now literally "opened up" for inspection by anyone who had the motivation to find out about me, before any degrading fantasy symptoms of my head injury evolved and feeling as if I had to prove that there really wasn't anything to hide in the first place, I reluctantly told my supervisor about my brain injury despite not ever wanting to do so. Understanding Janice's character as one of incomparable compassion and objectivity, deep down inside, I believed I really didn't have anything to worry about because I had more than proven myself as a proficient/reliable professional to her. This lack of certainty of how I'd be perceived after "confessing" that I had suffered a head injury would be an unfounded doubt, for my mid-management supervisor who interviewed me for this job, appeared to be sort of awe-struck about my standing after having a critical head injury and that much more impressed with the therapy inventory I had in my warehouse.

Confirming my security, detailing several aspects of my one-time trauma, Janice voiced her admiration about all the unbelievable accomplishments I had made since being so severely brain damaged. Not alone in her assessment of my achievements after almost "keeling over," I told this Unit Director of the public relations' video Harmarville shot of me as a patient and we then discussed if this portrayal of me could somehow be a valuable tool, benefiting the current cluster of residents without compromising my stature as a well-thought-of group leader. In addition to her multitude of exceptional executive talents—Janice having practiced as a medical nurse—this connoisseur of optimal treatment had the necessary background and experience to know that this resident fraternity could profit substantially witnessing a documentary such as this one, provided the material corresponded with their needs. Before the group would assemble for a showing, Janice wanted to review the contents for appropriateness. So, along with Phyllis, these two ladies were about to see that they had been working with a miracle these past twelve months or so, and didn't realize it.

Because it came from someone experienced in the field of medicine and was a reflection of how I carry myself, Janice gave me the greatest compliment I could ask for when she told me that she could have never guessed I was hurt so badly because—unless one were very sensitive to the mannerisms of the neurologically-impaired population—your everyday person simply could not tell that anything the magnitude of sustaining a severe head injury occurred with me. Having boys only a little younger than myself, Phyl was speechless when the video ended, but the shake in her voice spoke volumes.

Using this therapist as a kind of role-model example, after Janice received my assurance that it would be okay showing the depiction of my sturdy comeback to a gathering of individuals attempting a recovery of their own, we went about looking at how viewing a video so unique could best provide gains for the residents. My mental meltdown in '82 likely worse than most anything these residents have experienced with their illness, my status as a productive professional they've come to respect as an illustration, my supervisor and I believed it would help those group members feeling "down and out" to see a familiar representation of how determination can take one a long way. Stressing the importance of making "the most" of what one has in order to enhance a situation, for those wallowing in despair, we thought a V.C.R. presentation highlighting various achievements made possible by medicine and therapy could revitalize a few and create a general atmosphere of optimism. To brighten their outlook, it would be important to punctuate that one *can* indeed benefit from intensive care after a major setback.

Not having any idea how critically disabled I once was because I had never told anyone, possibly, increased therapeutic work which needed to be undertaken for residents to improve would occur at least temporarily because of my revelation. Hypothesizing that residents' confidence in treatment services had the potential of escalating in the short-term, my boss and I concluded that this heightened attitude had the capacity of being productive for more than a few who could process and conceptualize what this experience meant in relation to their own struggles. This facility not designed to treat the significantly psychotic population, even those mildly-challenged perceptually could appreciate how my restoration drama corresponded with their own predicament, often accepted as a quagmire.

Bellyaching that doctors, nurses, medicines, inpatient therapy, and the MH/MR system overall were generally useless, mentally ill pessimist complainers would use this bleak prospect standing as an excuse not to try different treatments which could benefit them. Accustomed to inpatient institutionalization throughout their life, the majority of these residents training to be integrated into society wouldn't want to concede that they were frightened of this independence transition and would try to convince themselves that prosperity/progress were simply beyond their means.

Afraid that their mind haunting them would be an insurmountable obstacle, preventing them from breaking free from their tragedy, more than a fair share of this flock of individuals with an aberrant diagnosis would give up their freedom ship before it ever set sail. Claiming that they were to forever be held with a lack of regard and stigmatized because their perception of reality was at variance with salient truth, those sensibly not congruent with unvarnished acknowledgment would frequently voice a desire to surrender virtues. Not necessarily an authentic opinion of this survivor's sense of the world's posture, I showed the videotaped record of my restoration largely with the intent of planting some seed in residents' tangled recognition that a future need not be foregone because of society's crippling stance.

Definitely damaging me not only in my pursuits to attain job satisfaction, but my self-concept as a potentially valuable participant in the rehabilitation work force, I calculated that the bias of employers was just too much of a prejudicial force to contend with and that I just had to accept that any respect or dollars offered for my counseling services would be "hard to come by" because of my history having sustained a head injury. With the New Medico influence still burning,

I unfortunately adopted the perspective managements of rehab centers apparently have of me being a lame "cripple" who's got to be hard-up for any work he can get his hands on and should just be grateful being offered the opportunity to do something better than volunteer work.

Although the family therapy agency where I was employed previously had a double standard when it came to addressing matters with popular veteran employees, as opposed to "handicapped" young ones becoming oriented, they at least offered an annual pay increase of a couple of percentage points. Interviewing for this therapy position where my group work would be for those deprived of their rational judgment, I took it for granted that a few more dollars would be coming my way after twelve months, but I was mistaken. The two interviewers not bothering to inform me of the "no pay increase" policy at this penury, it didn't do a whole heckuva lot for my ego thinking that maybe one of the reasons the Human Resources Department found me especially appealing was because of my below-sea-level salary requirement. Upon finding out one somber afternoon that—with the exception of a conditional bonus—my wage at this MH/MR center would never grow even by the smallest of increments or even keep up with the rate of inflation, I decided it was time to look at some other options. With a fixed income, no wonder this center for the treatment of those with faulty mental images of "what's what" would be so obliging to offer me a little more cash than my previous employer. I guess that Porsche is just going to have to wait.

Researching the Post-Gazette Classifieds section for any promising openings, I landed an interview with a psychiatric hospital in Ohio. Torn between my dedication to residents and the student coming in for her internship, I determined that earning a living wage and getting a raise before the year 2035 would provide me with more sustained satisfaction than knowing I kept an obligation that I would hardly be monetarily reimbursed for.

Trying to keep my head above water with an income and salary increase proportionate to my abilities at this "Buckeye State" psych hospital for adolescents, I sensed that I had given the executive and therapist questioning me about my vocational history what they were looking for during my hastened job hunt endeavor when asked if I could start immediately. Knowing that I had been working up to that point, by "immediately," I presumed the members of this established therapy facility meant after I gave my current employer the complimentary two weeks' notice that I would be leaving. Urgent to fill the position as quickly as possible with a qualified counselor, this organization was looking for someone to be ready for duty the upcoming Monday—in a few days.

Balancing the financial benefits with the cost of packing up and becoming situated practically overnight in an out-of-state rural community without warning, because the advantages of making a few extra dollars didn't outweigh the minuses of starting over again and uprooting myself by all that much, I elected to remain at the other countryside facility where I was already becoming established some. Intending to make a little bit of headway, I thought I'd just try my best and hope things work out to my advantage at the South Fayette Township center where I had gained a little bit of prominence already. Professional etiquette dictated that I couldn't announce that I was moving on "out of the blue," leaving the program short a body and angry partial staff (wanting to cut my throat) "hanging," without an immediate replacement.

Besides, having fulfilled my non-profit commitment to grad school, I thought I had developed at least a little bit of leverage when it came to any future contracting with an employer, since I was already entrenched within an establishment on a permanent/full-time basis; developing my therapy occupation with hours of daily group practice. Possibly exhibiting a little over-confidence when I made the final determination on my job site selection, I didn't take into account that sustained distinction at my workplace was equally dependent on performance, as much as mood fluctuation of key staff directorial members and the direction this spirit pendulum would be swaying on the emotion spectrum at any given moment. Sometimes gay and other times not, the atmosphere of this place would rarely be consistent, predictable, or conforming.

If I'd have known the 11th hour would be fast approaching on the quality progression of this center and my time as its premiere full-time therapist, I might not have been so quick to dismiss the Buckeye opportunity. The real world ain't always fair.

People who come to know me first as a person, and then subsequently as a former brain traumatized patient, can't believe the recovery I have made in the face of disaster and have an easier time seeing the attributes of my character. Accepted as a young professional with his fair share of pluses and abilities, I wouldn't be seen as having a dark cloud hanging over me to those unaware of my TBI history. But once "word" got out of my conflicts with disability, the thunderheads would usually start rolling in. Fortunate to have an empathetic nurse as a supervisor who was keen to the injustices people with disabilities are up against—a real trail blazer—Janice would be a tough act to follow.

A few short weeks after telling the warmhearted Unit Director of my bout with head injury, a closer match to her own individual identity, Janice would be leaving us to join a dynamic international organization which this MH/MR outfit couldn't hold a candle next to. Trying to fill some impossible shoes, an agency puppet whose strings would be pretty much guided by the directorial crew, a veteran "crony" of the agency would be next in line in an attempt to serve as the program's manager. Ordinarily operating as if she barely had an entrepreneurial bone in her body, going strictly "by the book" when it came time to make any kind of judgment and seeing to it that any moderately important decision would pass through commanding headquarters first—inveterately behaving as if she came from a military background—this woman would be the officer I'd have to answer to "here on out" at this base. If I would have known this administrative "changing of the guard" was going to occur before the fact, prior to "blabbing away," I would have definitely put more thought into it opening my "trap" before spilling my guts about the chapter in my life where my brain had taken a leave of absence. Too late to be careful, with my history an open book and the flood gates having been opened that I committed a *crime* sustaining a severe brain injury, I assumed that I'd be treading on thin ice and "butting heads" shortly.

With one resident commenting that I was an "inspiration," the overall sentiment of the group members upon viewing my video appeared to be one of encouragement and fascination. Shocking every resident that someone in a position of relative authority was once divest of his practical experience of the world and a few amazed at what the mind can overcome, if presented with no other option than to fight, I knew it surely wouldn't take long for "word" of my one-time sensory impediments to advance behind enemy lines and disperse out to installations occupied by the personnel policy planners of this foundation caring for those in want of stability. Although capable of identifying some rewards for this pack of residents habitually failing to detect "what is" from "what isn't," not being the disability group that could benefit most from my staggering passage through the dark time zone of rehabilitation after a head injury, I admittedly felt an overpowering sense of underachievement. Showing my filmed restoration escapades to a population void of any true appreciation as to the struggles encountered when a mind is numb to the world around it because of injury, I got mad thinking about how New Medico cheated me and hurt others as I once hurt. Approximating my champion boss's exodus and the intern's arrival, architect of my underemployment, the Company responsible for the "crash and burn" of my rehabilitation career aspirations would be extinguished.

With all hell having broken loose at the Massachusetts Corporate headquarters and indictments looming on the horizon, dangling from the gallows and gasping for air, New Medico would be taking its last breath because of their operation condemned as one where the infliction of suffering on so many had become standard practice. May God have mercy on their souls.

On page 18 in the "Business" section of The Boston Globe's City Edition dated August 9, 1993, the bold print practically jumped off the paper. A blessing for any patient and/or their family considering this rehabilitation company as an option for treatment, with the print as black as the Corporation's administrative workings, these six words and one numeral briefly summarized how a fraudulent organization got "busted" for their repeated offenses. Marking the demise of a deceitful era and telling the story of a deceptive rehabilitation "care" system coming to a close, the caption, "New Medico sells its last 3 facilities," would indicate that the F.B.I. found this rehabilitation organization as one universally engaged in profound wrongful activity. For trauma victims seeking compassionate care, this system of rehabilitation centers closing its doors would be a godsend of potentially life-saving proportions and a bonanza for their insurance carriers' pocketbooks.

Sitting in a state of dejected bewilderment at my cubicle in the Meadowlands' program office when this conscientious student should have been allowed to attend Goyette's patient review conferences, this image of me formed in my mind when reading three paragraphs down where it stated, ". . . . New Medico has been shrinking under the glare of complaints and lawsuits over its practices and a federal investigation into allegations of fraud." May God be with you, Charlie Goyette and Donna Micklow.

Before reading the sentence which let it be known that the owner of New Medico had "declined requests for an interview," ghosts of my field training began taking refuge in my conscious where shifty Meadowlands' managerial staff would turn a deaf ear to patients' merciful pleas to be moved closer to home soil. Becoming clearer and clearer, dwindling from more than forty health care facilities nationwide to zero, the fog of stealth secrecy surrounding this Corporate rehab operation had risen because of what detectives uncovered probing New Medico's records.

Sounding just a "wee bit" like a contradiction, after Globe staff writer John H. Kennedy reported that New Medico had "transferred operating responsibilities for all its remaining health care facilities to other organizations," this journalist noted how the double-talking spokesman for the owner of this shyster conglomerate wittingly refuted himself disclosing, "While New Medico continues to exist as a corporation, it no longer owns facilities, provides management services or employs personnel."

Either this impostor organization claiming to promote quality rehab treatment *con*tinues to function, or it doesn't. "Well, uhhhhh. . . . ."

Absorbing how New Medico was "mothballed" of its personnel base, once employing 7,500 workers around the country only about twenty months ago to a handful of employees helping to take out the garbage at the Boston executive headquarters, my relief was premature. Joyfully taking in the information before me, seeing the hyphen after the letters "ac-" in the word "acquired" on page 18 and needing to search page 19 for the remainder of the article, those goose bumps were sure popping up once I eyed up the "New Medico sells off its last three facilities" headline, because I wanted to see who would be acquiring this delightful organization and what extent inspectors saw it necessary to continue their federal exploration of—and descent upon—this lovely brain trauma company.

Heart chugging away with excitement because of what this could mean in relation to my impossible dream of finally attaining a professional job within head injury rehabilitation, was I ever "overjoyed" to discover that the proprietors of the New Medico operation taking so much heat by the feds lately would keep things "all in the family" making sure to sell the company to the cousin of New Medico's previous owner. Although presumably intending to strictly operate business from the public sector instead of the private, like its impeached forefather, the rehabilitation systems taking over New Medico more than likely made use of a few Corporate practitioners who were aware of their previous employer's means of revenue collection. It would be wise to keep your eyes open for any former New Medico rehab administrators in a treatment facility near you, because they walk amongst us.

Not suggesting this to be some prophetic sign, however, it seemed fitting this representative of the disability population that New Medico devastated and heinously trampled on directly would cheerfully grab the spotlight for a few moments the very month New Medico at Meadowlands would be sold. In May 1992—about a week or two before it was announced on Wall Street that Health and Rehabilitation Properties Trust (HRPT) purchased Goyette's/ Micklow's New Medico Rehabilitation and Skilled Nursing Center at Meadowlands, as well as seven other Corporate shrines to be managed by the Greenery—a picture of me pickin' my Fender Stratocaster on a Washington Park picnic bench adorned the local, hometown, Observer-Reporter newspaper. With this transaction of Meadowlands' ownership occurring at a time which approximated its parent base of operation being discovered as one engaged in widespread fraud, it certainly would be reasonable to deduct that the Goyette/Micklow New Medico consortium where I served my student field training had undertaken their fair share of embezzlement and misappropriation of funds activities.

Fielding complaints about New Medico and other operators elsewhere around the country, the 8/9/93 *Globe* reported that two Congressional panels have been flooded with accusations by a slew of sources about the operation of these organizations. Neglecting to follow through with their assurances to families that various remedial therapies would be provided to their inpatient loved ones, the New Medico Corporation still saw to it that they received substantial monetary reimbursement for these unfulfilled treatments, as well as other phantom services. A routine complaint by so many who had filed against this bill-collecting syndicate, for example, this official "Bean Town" journal also put in black and white that a couple from the nearby Chicopee, Massachusetts community "alleged in a Suffolk Superior Court lawsuit that their daughter was neglected and mistreated" by New Medico. Courthouses in this "Bay State" county would not only be booming with activity from those claiming New Medico had been unscrupulous in their practices with patients, set against the backdrop of these treatment charges, businesses contracting with this gold-digging brain trauma company would have legitimate allegations as well. Where there's smoke, there's fire.

On 8/20/93, with half of a million bucks nothing to "sneeze at," Plaintiff Insta-Care Pharmacy Services Corporation brought an action against the endearing New Medico Corporation for breach of contract. In early 1988, a couple of months before I'd start my memorable field practice of a lifetime with New Medico, Insta-Care verbally contracted to provide pharmaceutical products to facilities of this charming rehab organization. Not getting the agreement in writing, this drug company lacked the foresight required dealing with these righteous fellows and made an absolutely horrendous mistake trusting this Corporate managerial gang to keep their word of honor. Figuring New Medico would ethically "hold up" their end of the bargain because this system of seductive rehab outfits gratefully accepted all pharmacological goods supplied without reservation, Insta-Care naturally assumed (there's that word again) it would be reimbursed thirty days after delivery of their goods and services, as the terms of the oral agreement stipulated. But this wouldn't be the type of "holdup" the wonderful human beings of the New Medico Corporation had on its mind.

Until these rehab thugs had a change of heart, New Medico initially made the payments as outlined in the verbal promise. However, falling behind in payments for services rendered, the darling New Medico Corporation owed the lucky medicine company fortunate to get their business in excess of a million dollars as of July 1992.

Never disputing this debt nor any other monies due Insta-Care under the worded "gentleman's" pact, New Medico would be gracious enough to pay off some of the funds owed until deciding to stop altogether in April '93. With Insta-Care's repeated demands being ignored that New Medico pay up the remaining $504,349.37—plus four months' interest—some private-for-profit heads were gonna roll.

Believing it had contracted with a business which operated in good faith, having no intention of paying the remainder of their bills to this medical service provider, Insta-Care would be taking the lovable New Medico prima donnas to the Suffolk County Supreme Court. Trying to talk themselves out of yet another "jam" that breaking the oath of proper business graces put them into and attempting to convince impartial factions that they were the ones who had been cruelly victimized and enduring tumultuous difficulties, the enchanting New Medico racketeers would find themselves answering before a Justice of the Peace.

With the sensual New Medico Corporation apparently only abiding to contracts which would ultimately benefit them, these honorable deal-makers just decided one spring day to cease compensating Insta-Care for past materials and services delivered, forcing this medical supply distributor into a game of judicial "wild goose-chase" in an attempt to get what was justly theirs. As a result of Defendant New Medico's unfair/deceptive practices, Insta-Care suffered substantial monetary loss because of the investment/rehab company's willful peculating violation. Insta-Care wanting rewarded for damages plus interest/costs/attorney's fees, three counts against New Medico would have to be decided by a Court of Law. Needing to answer for their many suspect actions incurred over time, New Medico would be no stranger to the litigation process.

Trying to weasel their way out of the commitment to Insta-Care pharmaceuticals, New Medico claimed that no agreement with this pharmacy branch ever existed despite products/operations being provided in trust by this medicine establishment to a number of Corporate facilities over a lengthy period. Claiming that the arrangements with separate entities/agreements of individual centers do not constitute the workings of the "mother" New Medico Corporation—grasping for straws once more—these moneymaking rehab sweethearts flailed, trying to convey the preposterous message that the operations of their affiliates were something which they weren't at all responsible. C'mon New Medico, wake up and smell the coffee.

Identifying the facilities in question as separate and distinct, assuming the "spin doctor" role that they've customarily had to play since the less-than-straightforward antics of the Corporation have been excavated, this lovely New Medico rehabilitation body tried to pull another "fast one" by insisting that there were no instances where Insta-Care sent invoices directly to and under the precise name, "New Medico Associates Inc." Stating that there was never a circumstance in which a transaction was made by the Association via check with their specific name on it as a payee, these New Medico puritans tried to say that they should not be treated as if the operating syndicate had some kind of procedural relationship with their particular independent agents. Yeah, right. And grass isn't green.

Until proven within the bounds of the law, common sense apparently cannot dictate that a "mother" corporation like New Medico shall be liable for the performance of their subsidiaries. Knowing that the rules of the justice game are set up in such a way that criminal allegations must be shown to be a given without so much as a shadow of a doubt, New Medico wasn't about to "hang it up"/"fold their cards" and would embark on a litigation battle of "tit-for-tat" with Insta-Care.

Petitioning to reconsider, dissolve, vanish, etc., every last trick in "the book" would be played by New Medico in a last ditch effort to avoid sinking in the very swamp of financial chaos they attempted to drown many of their business and patient associates in. Listed in docket SJ 93-446 in the Suffolk County Supreme Court, an assortment of motions and counter-motions were filed by New Medico to "save their skin," not to mention a half-million of their almighty, private-for-profit dollars it was becoming increasingly more apparent they managed to get their hands on by swindling those who trusted them. But these strategic tactics to dispose and alter the evidence would be for naught because the preponderance of manifestations were just too much for this fiscally corrupt/driven, dollar-addicted rehab racket to contend with.

Emergency Motion for Judgment on the Pleadings, Memorandum in Support of Defendant's Motion for Judgment on the Pleadings, Emergency Motion of the Defendant to Dissolve Attachments, Supplemental Memorandum in Support of Defendant's Motion to Dissolve Attachments, Defendant's Emergency Motion for Reconsideration, and an affidavit by New Medico's Internal Auditor were simply not enough maneuvers to sway the rationale of The Honor presiding over this Court. With the abundance of facts Insta-Care provided and self-serving assertions basically all New Medico had to offer, it was quite evident that the heavenly head trauma Corporation's formal/written application for various requests of the Court would come up lame and be denied. Wow, what a surprise!

Long-term utilization of Insta-Care's services, prior penalty assessed of roughly 500 grand having already been paid, and various letters between the two managerial parties showing that an agreement had been consumed/did indeed exist, were all pretty clear signs that New Medico was just trying to illegally break and back out of their obligation. With the basis behind the New Medico Corporation's weak defense being that the "mother" New Medico Association Inc. institution was independent of the working of its satellite operations, these rehab scoundrels wanted to give the impression that their facilities and the Corporation were two distinct entities which had to be dealt with individually. Talk about nonsense.

Over the course of the proceedings, however, it was discovered that canceled checks stamped by different wholly-owned New Medico rehab operations and the parent company were found to be drawn from the same Bank of Boston account, meaning the forswearing trauma system with its "exclusive" factions were indeed in cahoots with one another. Leading to the venerative New Medico Corporation's lightweight petition being refused, monies withdrawn from the exact same site would be the clincher in the final verdict levied against New Medico. Despite New Medico's immaterial pleas of semantics where they unsuccessfully tried to make a case out of the fact that the designated names on the checks were not identical, the finding was a strong one and likely would stick, even to these slimy dudes. Having other ideas, New Medico would protest, "Not so fast!" Now, who would have ever guessed that?

Withstanding the attempt that the court change/modify its judgment, with New Medico tears flowing at the sidebar, the ruling would be in favor of Insta-Care and against the saintly New Medico larcenists. Borrowing from the dialogue of the legendary Pittsburgh Steelers' Head Coach, Chuck Noll, with the court system seemingly favoring the "criminal element," New Medico would give it one last shot to "save face" and a hefty chunk of cash. Well, if that isn't a shocker.

Not yet done reaching up their sleeve for a life preserver and trying to be sly, in an attempt to make "wrong" look "right," these New Medico foxes filed a Motion to Dissolve Attachments by the Trustee Process. New Medico's shifty motives able to be seen with half-an-eye, however, the conclusion that previous judgments/decisions remain in place would not be hard to predict. Considering materials filed in opposition and support of the ruling application, as well as hearing debates on both sides of the issue, the presentation of Insta-Care's tangibles (letters/checks) backing their position and the absence of any substantive/concrete evidence supporting New Medico's mythical claim were primary precursors pointing the determination in favor of Insta-Care. Nice going, New Medico.

With ill-gotten Corporate manners being disinterred and New Medico's character of pulling off heists taking center stage, these "for profit" rehab mercenaries' battles would no longer be with insurance companies trying to convince them that "eye-blinking" therapy was of paramount importance in the patient/policy holders' restoration. Rather, these New Medico rehab pricks would be finding themselves fighting wars in courtrooms across the country.

With so much of our great nation's patriotic history having taken place in this "one-hundred percent" American state and blood of patriot soldiers having spilled on battlegrounds here in the clash for freedom, New Medico running its base of operation out of Massachusetts almost bordered being sacriligious. This system of trauma centers found to be more concerned with the value of stock than the care of those who required their rehabilitation/ medical sophistication, these Corporate investors would find themselves on battlefields in this territory as well. However, instead of Revolutionary War Minute Men fighting for independence from the mother country England, patients and business establishments alike would revolt against the "mother" New Medico Corporation. Scratching and clawing for what duly belonged to them, these "little guys" were tired of being pushed around and having much more than lunch money taken by these New Medico Corporate bullies.

In addition to the Insta-Care trial occurring in the Suffolk County Supreme Court and legal action proceedings in a host of appellate courts scattered about this star-spangled commonwealth, many town halls elsewhere in the Boston metropolitan area alone would be "booked up" with arraignment hearings involving New Medico as the defendant. Summoned to appear before benches in this New England capital, New Medico Associates Inc. would be preoccupied for years to come trying to explain themselves in countless inquiries. In time, the Suffolk County Civil Superior Court by itself would hear a whopping forty New Medico cases where this rehab treatment bunch was being sued by plaintiffs and the Middlesex Superior Court would try in the neighborhood of twenty cases over time. With the Framingham County Courthouse refusing to release information, about the only courthouse around this port city which didn't conduct a trial on New Medico was the Cambridge County Courthouse and that was only because they deal primarily with domestic disputes, not universal fraud where executioners hang corrupt corporations.

Quite a few degrees longitude and plenty of points latitude, miles from the New England perimeter where they set up their sweat shop, New Medico would be finding themselves in hot water from sea to shining sea, trying not to be submerged under a wave of allegations of criminal activity. Stretching from the Canadian border to the crashing waves of the Gulf Coast, and reeking from fisheries along the Atlantic shoreline to the San Andreas Fault, tribunals about this great land would be filled with New Medico administrative powers sweating blood. Cold-blooded souls fearing pronouncements of "guilt" and sentences as punishing as the pain their patients had to endure being kept for extended stays until their insurance money had mysteriously been sifted, the crooked New Medico Corporation made a lot of lawyers rich. New Medico apparently viewing head injury survivors as "2nd Class" citizens with too many screws loose to be worthy of any kind of respect, verdicts flying every which way would be forthcoming in favor of those having anything to do with this salty rehabilitation crew.

In the same 8/9/93 Boston Globe reporting New Medico had sold its last three facilities—so these Corporate thieves would not get in too big of a huff—this herald quoted a federal source saying, "neither the company nor any employee has been charged, but the probe is 'ongoing.'" But federal criminal investigators would soon get the indictment ball rolling.

A little over two months after this "innocent until proven guilty" proclamation, the Wall Street Journal reported that a former Massachusetts public office representative admitted being involved in New Medico's scam to "rip off" Medicare of roughly a quarter of a million dollars and was sentenced to twenty-nine months in prison. With the conniving ploys New Medico utilized to line their pockets full of cash which rightfully didn't belong to them slowly coming to light, this Suffolk County Superior Criminal Court case would be the beginning of the end for this cheating Corporate operation, as a domino effect of rulings not favoring New Medico would cast its glorious head. Come to think of it, turns out the Rich girl and New Medico were a good match, after all.

Rather than trying to understand my deep anger towards these New Medico thieves for taking advantage of head injury survivors whose suffering I know all too well and for robbing me of experiencing a fruitful internship by purposely restricting my caseload/responsibilities so Penelope could get hired over this survivor, instead, sweethearts like the great majority of rehabilitation managements I've come across would take the "easy way out" by blaming my head injury for going after these Corporate rehab giants. Immediately, any perception, emotion, or behavior of a survivor not understood completely would sadly be attributed to their brain injury without taking into account that a wholly rational reason may be behind things. Equally, if not more distressing, is the fact that groundless explanations are usually accepted automatically as plausible with the "neurologically impaired" population because of people's general need for quick answers/resolutions. Assuming every nuance of a head trauma victim's character can be found and deciphered within the pages of a DSM-III-R/Neuro 101 handbook, usually head injury disability rehab "experts" feel they need not have to bother looking at the deeper picture.

Eyeing me up as if I were a "brain injured freak," needing to find some pathological cause and effect rationale for example, overly-analytical rehab "experts" occupying personnel executive positions would no doubt come to the conclusion that I had to have sustained significant frontal lobe damage for going after these New Medico safecrackers, despite exhibited sequelae indicating injuries had occurred elsewhere. As an illustration, serving as a workable excuse not to give someone who's experienced trauma to this segment of their neurological system an opportunity for professional advancement, all an employment supervisor need say would be that an injury to this portion of the brain "often" results in survivors experiencing impulse control deficits and having "someone like that" interacting with those seeking our services just wouldn't be worth the risk. Unfortunately, with very little known about the complexities of the brain, "often" is invariably interpreted as "always." Take my word for it, I've lived it.

After the hideous way in which New Medico took the wind out of my career sails, slaughtering any hope I had of joining the professional ranks as a rehabilitation head injury disability counselor, I would just have to pick up the pieces and try to get on with my life the best I could. For the most part, considering how badly I was hurt, I've been able to carry on and brush myself off reasonably well in a number of areas not believed possible. But sometimes it does get tough to move along in a positive fashion because of the physical disabilities (limp and paralysis) I know I've got to co-exist with for the rest of my life and the prejudice/discrimination which definitely hides around every employment corner. Like water under the bridge, I could have put the New Medico experience behind me, if the ramifications weren't so drastically profound and longlasting in my pursuits to be a part of the rehabilitation professional work force. With their criminal actions front page news in many areas, my employment resume stating that I had trained with "New Medico" might serve me better, if I just not mention this.

With former Corporate accessories scattered about different rehab facilities prospering, despite their criminal New Medico employer having been dissolved because of insensitivity to so many people's welfare, "brain contused" patients seeking conscientious care wouldn't be out of the woods quite yet. Having calculated the benefits of alerting patients and families falling under the care of former

New Medico execs with the likelihood of being "black balled" by these managements and their cohort rehab buddies who would no doubt protect them, because the provision of quality treatment could be at stake for helpless patients who need to be surrounded by professionals empathetic to their restoration concerns and not how many dollars are at their disposal, I felt it would be necessary to give the one-time New Medico lads I know about some no-cost publicity these bandits would just as soon rather not have. It's a sad review about the state of affairs when a survivor—truly dedicated to the head injury disability population—cannot get a professional position within a rehabilitation center because so many employment vacancies are filled by former New Medico laborers who knew about their Corporation's dishonesty, but purposely did not bother to stop the harm to patients because the money was just too good.

In the Pittsburgh area alone, from the Greenery at Meadowlands to the Greater Pittsburgh Rehabilitation Hospital in Monroeville, former New Medico personnel who were aware of and participated in the Corporation's iron-clad offenses of atrocity were gainfully employed, continuing to practice their witchcraft with the head injury disability population. Not missing a beat, from Micklow's start-up head injury program near downtown Bridgeville and a hospital in Morgantown, W.Va. to the neuro rehab east of Monroeville treating those with TBI, enamoring New Medico pioneer luminaries were busy with their voodoo, casting their magic on the head injury disability group again. Not adhering to a treatment philosophy of "survival of the fittest," rather, "survival of the richest"—for the sake of those auspicious patients they would be dealing with—one could only hope these New Medico scavengers had learned their lesson and developed a new appreciation where honest care would be seen as priceless. If they hadn't, may they burn at the stake. "Double, double, toil and trouble, fire burn, and cauldron bubble."

At New Medico, when I was a student intern, an old trailer served as Meadowlands Health Care Center's program office. However, getting income from needy patients encased in misery that these Corporate vultures double-crossed for their insurance dollars and charging exuberant rates watching the heartbeat of newly-admitted comatose policy holders, the Meadowlands' pallbearers would have the income needed to afford the construction of a substantial addition to the facility for their therapists to work. Based on the Corporation's past fiscally-oriented maneuvers and this individual Meadowlands facility's demand for comfort, surely no hesitation occurred when this treatment center discharged existing patients who were no longer covered by their insurance and eagerly replaced with new depositors having fresh revenue. Since New Medico's grave stunts have gotten mass media coverage, knowing She would get an earful from a member of the disability group Her Corporation devastated for monetary gain, no wonder Micklow tries to duck out of sight like a scared rabbit anytime She sees me out at the mall. Burning from just the sight of that pale face of Micklow's, I could just hear Her or Goyette saying, "He just didn't work out," upon being inquired by a Meadowlands' patient or family member on Penelope's caseload as to why I wasn't employed with them, given that

I had personal experience with the disability the Corporation treated and had served my field practice there. Not occupying the counseling position I proved more than capable of handling, New Medico struck again, fostering the detrimental stereotypes which are so prevalent with the head injury disability population.

My goal for going after the cowardly New Medico Corporation wasn't to engage in some kind of "witch hunt," but rather, to let these bastards know that they messed with one too many survivors to walk away scot-free, laughing all the way to the bank. Getting the ink they genuinely deserve, for those New Medico at Meadowlands' execs who surely "assumed" that this true grit survivor would slip off into the night and never be heard from again, I just wanted to come back and say, "Hello."

Regarding the Meadowlands' rejection letter I received signed with my mall buddy's name indicating Penelope Rich was found to be more qualified than this survivor for the available head injury counseling position for which I had already been trained, the New Medico Corporation would surely claim that my dissecting this notice for meaning had no merit because this was more-or-less a stamped response used in most every generic case involving a denied employment opportunity. Not exactly your run-of-the-mill job applicant and given that I had already served an unpaid, seven-month field training with them—unselfish in every aspect of this magical apprenticeship—I think it'd be fair to assume that neglecting to develop a speedy, personalized notification informing me of my status—considering all the good that I had done during my student initiation—was a sad commentary as to the lack of professionalism at the New Medico at Meadowlands treasury. Knowing this survivor as an intern trainee, with New Medico's lack of regard towards those having sustained head trauma getting the spotlight, familiarity seems to have bred contempt. Mixing savagery and barbarity into their treatment approach with patients needing the utmost nurturing, a truce with New Medico's administrative powers wouldn't be foremost on my mind. What's this world coming to?

With the unthinkable harm New Medico did to so many tangling with the treachery of a head injury, it wouldn't be conceivable for me to "let bygones be bygones" or to tolerate the inhumane treatment towards the disability population I once was a fraternal member. Because so many of the services provided to my fellow traumatized brethren were anything but "first rate," I felt compelled to devote a few words to the heinous New Medico Corporation and speak for a few of the multitude of their patients who were mistreated, but don't have the capability to communicate their hatred for this criminal, rehab outfit. Borrowing from the dialogue of the Meadowlands' Program Director's wife, thinking that New Medico was providing top-notch services for patients to the best of their abilities, they did make an ass out of me.

With the intent of picking myself up and proceeding in a functional manner, sometimes a very difficult premise because of all I'd been through, it would be essential to formulate my thinking in such a way as to not let things get to me. Trying to cognitively master negative occurrences the best way possible, I would need to remember cognitions which worked best for me and those I'd need to set aside, if I were to successfully achieve goals and "go for the gusto" in my work efforts. Malignant pictures of the past forming in my mind about how stigma had interfered with my progress, I'd just have to focus on concepts which minimized this distress and form healthy passages, so my outlook may be enhanced. Utilizing an approach based on the principal that behaviors are an aftermath of one's perceptions may not always be full-proof, but in order to make the most of a difficult situation and search for productive resolutions to a dilemma, one would need to develop a train of thought where the impact of interference could be stabilized, if not withdrawn altogether.

When my conscious would revisit the junction of my life where declined opportunities were based on prejudice or the widely-accepted perspective that if something is too good to be true, then there must be a "catch"—instead of manufacturing further ordeals in my mind that I didn't need or deserve—the motivation developed to find ways to "plug in" favorable images of my history in place of those which would only "bring me down." In '82, when I was comatose, nobody would have wanted my future. With a couple of college degrees under my belt and some pretty satisfying experience, a few might not mind possessing a little of my potential now, however. If what was going through my mind at a particular moment of time wasn't working for me, I'd just try to review how going from one end of this spectrum to the other, took quite a bit of character.

In April 1982, a little over two months after my accident when my thinking began to clear, shown the picture of me comatose on those mattresses and told what I was like during this condition, I absolutely couldn't believe it. Years later, after the disbelief had faded and reality took hold, if I would get angry/feel sorry for myself because of my permanent physical afflictions or how I had been approached with undeserved caution since my neurological impairment, I'd just try to reflect on my gutsy recovery and that what has been accomplished in my rehabilitation far surpasses what disability "experts" claim possible. However, presuming that my restoration was just some fluke and that being physically "messed up" must mean I'm intellectually lacking as well, I wouldn't be given much credit for my achievements by employers who knew of my medical history.

Attributes such as being professionally employed as a therapist, giving motivational presentations, supervising a grad student, asked to give an in-service on the cognitive-behavioral R.E.T. approach to counseling, getting a 3.81 G.P.A. in grad school, and in the process of writing a book would generally be overlooked by rehab managements because of my one-time aphasic state being presumed as a lasting debilitating predicament which supposedly will forever limit me and restrict my productivity. Because of the rehabilitation employment world's hypocritical stance that past acceptance of what is understood about head injury shall deny and overrule any new supposition of what's possible, I went from being extremely proud of what I've attained after surviving a brain injury, to being scared to death that my *FORMER* condition would be discovered.

Fully appreciating the need for a Higher Power, the level-headed belief that mom and dad instilled in me was that God will provide Craig Meyers with the opportunity to heal and that The Father allows people to find the strength within themself to prosper in the challenges life presents us. Given a shot at "getting back on my feet"—after accepting that my life would never be the same and I was just lucky to be alive—I set about on a mission to operate with what I had, so progress could be achieved. Not wanting to live a life constantly asking myself, "What if" I had put more into my restoration effort or hadn't been hurt, I had to embrace the fact that it was a miracle that I could even advance at all after sustaining a TBI and needed to experience just how far my rehab work could take me. However, not able to do without an objective viewpoint from rehabilitation employers, this would be where my reclamation journey would hit a dead end.

While feeling blessed that the chance to make some productive gains lie before me, logic would dictate that God wouldn't likely appear from the clouds anytime soon and intervene completely to make things "all better." Operating under this observation, I figured the amount of work I put into my refinement effort was up to me and I knew I had some sweat in store for me in the long recovery road ahead. Presented with a lifelong goal of abolishing horrid stereotypes, I realized defeating this nemesis wouldn't be easy. With this acknowledged appreciation for what I must do to thrive to the fullest and understanding from where I had come, I'd hate to accrue the losses of bookies who may have bet against me.

Though one's focus can take a person a long way, understanding and support by others are ingredients needed for the rehabbing individual to take their achievements to the next level. With the gift of life God gave me the opportunity to grasp, I feel as if I should share a little of my capabilities with others, so that they may also harvest some rewards from my rejuvenation experience. Furious that I was left behind to rot by New Medico and most every other rehabilitation establishment where I applied for work after having worked so hard in my own rehab to capture a glimmer of my former self—not feeling that I should have to hide the opportunity for recovery God presented me just because of Human Resource Director's ignorance that a "head injured" survivor couldn't possibly be a quality clinician—I decided to draw my sword and embark on a counteroffensive.

After having established a foundation of respect and dignified presence, if the circumstance proved to be an appropriate one, I'd even go as far as to inform a practical stranger that I was once in a coma after having sustained brain damage, in order to do what I could to minimize unfair/toxic judgments which no doubt exist towards most members of this disability population. Not intending to sound deserving or better than anyone else who has suffered through head injury rehabilitation where there is little "down time" if one wants to improve, I admittedly have given it some thought that maybe so many things having turned out in my favor during my personal rehab comeback wasn't somehow designed to happen due to my ultimate striving to assist others in a similar death-defying quandary. Suggesting that every survivor who had sustained damage to their brain shall possess the same degree of competency or won't be emotionally/intellectually compromised whatsoever would be foolish, but stigma frequently seems to levy more damage on the "head injured" disability group than the bruise itself.

Receiving rejection notification after rejection notification after rejection notification from those head injury/comprehensive rehab facilities where I had sought professional employment, stating that someone who had gotten an "A+" on their college "Fundamentals of Brain Injury" writing paper had been found who possesses more potential working with the head injury population than this survivor, I got a wake-up call as to the dysfunctional prevailing attitude which lingers towards those with disabilities. Praising my background, experience, and recovery as very impressive/inspirational, I sensed these rehab employers nonetheless viewed giving this survivor an opportunity as "going out on a limb" and wouldn't even consider the potentially invaluable proposition of allowing me to demonstrate what I could do.

Acknowledging the viewpoint of those who may see the repeated coverage of New Medico similar to "beating a dead horse"—feeling as though I ought to dedicate some time and effort to this serenity-robbing Corporation who were directly responsible for my adopting the attitude that "I'd rather be lucky than good"—I tried to convert the spite of being told "No" over and over in my quest for equal opportunity employment within the field of rehabilitation, into something which could light a fire under me and serve as a spark. In the perfect world, it would seem I'd have been welcomed with open arms into the disability counseling field right out of graduate school, profiting emotionally and monetarily from my unique knowledge. Not working out the way I had hoped, with my training site being a morally-removed operation, I'd just have to lick my wounds and keep plugging away.

With prospective rehabilitation employers apparently sticking their tail between their legs once they found out I had sustained a head injury, rather than assuming a "Why even bother?" position in my rehabilitation employment pursuits or working myself up that these "open-minded" personnel managements must have thought that I got my degrees prior to being a "brain injured malcontent," I constructed the incentive to prove various rehabilitation human resource bodies wrong and decided to give it my best. Hoping things would work out, before the refused rehabilitation employment strivings forced me to completely surrender my ambition to do some good for those traumatized by a neurological impairment, I'd just try to convince myself that there must be some "Master Plan" out there for me somewhere floating around with the way so many pieces of my reparation puzzle have fallen into place for me.

Like my continual struggles in rehabilitation, I'd just have to form a script in my mind where I take things one step at a time and try to remember that the degree in which a person can adapt to whatever they're confronted with in their environment, largely determines one's overall outlook/demeanor. For this applicant trying to gain belated admission into the world of prosperity, it would be truly essential to "keep at it" and try to make my experience since I almost died into something useful. Not wanting that split second where I was rammed into a telephone pole to be the end of my life, feeling as though destiny presented me with the colors to paint a masterpiece of opportunity, I sensed a greater purpose to create some intrinsic structure of significance and meaning from that harrowing Valentine's night which changed me forever.

Defining "fate" as it applies to the motions of everyday life, or even if this force exists, obviously would not be something that I'd have the capability to answer. Nor could I possibly know if the surface of my potential will ever be scratched, given the hard-line stance of society that victims whose understanding once was amiss, shall forever be a casualty. Comprehending the complexities which form tomorrow not within the bounds of reality, in this lifetime there could be no possible way to ascertain how events "come to be" and develop as history.

Whether there's a reason for occurrences or simply the "luck of the draw," since surviving that accident and achieving the unexpected, I have sensed that I need to fulfill some higher function. Grateful that February weekend in 1982 just wasn't my time to exit this earth, not thinking as if it's "me against the world" with God as my ally, I feel honored that I might have been selected in some minute way to carry out what I believe could be my intended duty to emancipate a few survivors from ill-founded assertions like those possessed by New Medico.

If significant gains are going to be made during one's restoration, a fine line exists where goals must be within reach, yet require maximum effort and output to attain. When I was striving to be more than merely functional during my acute and post-acute rehabilitation, if I'd have listened to many of the "experts" who scoffed at my aspirations as not being realistic, I wouldn't have attained the accomplishments I had following my head injury. Having to do more than just sit on my "duff" and watch the grass grow to pass my time, I aimed high and "went for it." Needing more, attaining the status quo just didn't "make it" with me, so I was set to put forth a fight which corresponded with my high-reaching hopes for the future. "Slumming" not an option, I'd be reaching for the stars.

Being a big dreamer who has been repeatedly laughed at and approached with skepticism by disability professionals, I have had the heightened goals I've set for myself snickered at as not being possible by most rehab execs. Time and time again, I've proven these rehab personnel "virtuosos" wrong, and I just hope one of these days I get an occupational shot at proving these "supportive" people incorrect once more. If I'd have believed these rehab "authorities" who thought attaining even my Bachelor's degree was a ridiculous proposition, I would not be in my "enviable" position of being qualified for Master'slevel posts at their respective centers and having them castrate me of my career aspirations.

If a psychological counseling position within a quality rehabilitation treatment establishment would one day be available for me, that would be great. But if such an offer from a prime, rehab managerial team would never be forthcoming because of my medical history, all I can do is try to accept this dream as something which just wasn't meant to be. I've been through worse—that's for sure.

Being a teen who didn't think anything could happen to him, I found out how "vincible," invincible could be. Having experienced extensive loss at a pretty early age, I had an "awakening" as to what's important in life and sort of became numb to that which didn't seem significant to the overall picture.

Believing that my adolescent name was "No" and feeling as if I were under house arrest wasn't easy, but in the general scope of what's meaningful in life, I'd learn that these are much ado about nothing. Using a little baseball jargon, with my support system more than in place providing anything I needed, I had the means to start "swinging from the ankles" in my attempts to regain what I had lost. With this foundation of love and reinforcement a given, I just "went at it" in my therapies because I had the freedom to concentrate on the fundamentals of my restoration effort. Letting the chips fall as they may, I knew that my chances for a profitable return were within reach because I could bring into focus what I needed to do to get better.

Needing to "take the bull by the horns" and "face the music," I learned a lot about myself during my war with disability. Liking what I saw in the mirror for perhaps the first time in my young life, I discovered that my character was one of astonishing strength. If one is not presented with any other choice and backed into a corner, it's incredible how the mind finds a way to get by. Because I don't throw a javelin, my face might not ever adorn any box of "Wheaties," the breakfast of champions, but that's okay because I now can appreciate the core of who I really am as something that most any "cream of the crop" gold medal Olympian wouldn't mind having in their own heart.

Able to make the serotonin in my brain fire off, this helped me to get the job done in my battle to get back some of what I had feared may not be retrievable. If I hadn't busted my tail in the midst of my recuperation struggles, there would have been no telling to what extent permanent, debilitating conditions would have influenced my capacity for happiness.

Intending to take a shirt off a hanger, but not able to because I couldn't keep from reaching for pants. Or unable to fill out something as simple as a library card because I couldn't remember how to write the letters of my name, permanent perseveration was a profound fear, and this terror would be all the coaxing I needed in my attempt to climb out of the grave, symptoms of a damaged brain tried to bury me in. Unfortunately, positioned at the summit of this death pit upon my arrival from Hell would be the scourge of rehabilitation employers' prejudice.

Until the pestilence of discrimination could be bound in captivity, I would have the increasingly difficult task of trying to put my heart into working for those whose thinking was unsettled. And the residents of this MH/MR treatment program had penetrating problems as well.

Scheduled to work 8:30 A.M. to 4:30 P.M. everyday, Monday thru Friday, it was utterly demanded of me by my follow-up supervisor that I not be at the facility engaged in therapy-related tasks more than 37.5 hours per week, apparently because the agency's policy handbook mandated this to be the set time-limit. Not about to reimburse full-time employees over and beyond an average of 7.5 hours a day during the week, I'd just have to adjust my schedule, if my time doing job-related duties during any one workday exceeded this restriction by taking a little "comp" time later on during the pay period.

Working a little overtime was not an issue with me, but it certainly was for the substitute Unit Director, because any guidelines in the organization's procedural manual would need to be adhered to as if etched in stone. This regulated time limitation was not a big deal from my perspective, nor was the fact that staff rarely got even fifteen minutes for lunch on Monday/Thursday "fire and brimstone" staffing days a problem because I just saw it as part of the job. Oddly enough, this survivor would get "hell to pay" because I complied with the mandates the new "king of the hill" was so emotionally attached to.

Not infrequently, a resident would have issues at their home-based residence which could only be addressed directly interacting with the parties involved. Understandably, for those on my caseload living with parents or other relatives, family conferences would occasionally need to be set up in order to best rectify matters occurring at the homestead. Because most family members worked and couldn't be reached during the day, I would have to make accommodations accordingly, so that these meetings could be arranged.

One evening, I had a session with a particular resident and this person's loved ones that lasted until 6:00 P.M. because the family members were having some significant difficulties coping with the side-effects of their "child's" illness and in steep denial about its long-term presence. Held an hour-and-a-half past my normal quitting time, I received clearance from the Unit Commander to start my weekend furlough ninety minutes earlier than usual and leave at 3:00 P.M. on Friday, so I would not overshoot my weekly time ration.

Being one of the objects of a vile attack earlier that day in staffing because I committed the foulest of crimes not pronouncing the name of a psychotrop correctly, upon making a call to one of the functions we would deal with, I wouldn't be in the most festive mood when some woman answering the phone either had trouble understanding or hearing what I was saying. Up to my grinding jaw with ill-will thinking about how my replacement supervisor passively sat watching as my professionalism had been sieged by the conductor of these staffings in front of the intern, my tolerance for anything but a quick response had all but evaporated. Having been "ragged on" in the morning as if I were incompetent, I got impatient with this lady over the phone when our communication broke down. Yet to attain the seniority required to have a "bad hair day" at the job site, as horrendous as this bleak February workday would be having my character hammered, things would get even worse when I got home.

My brother got a pretty bulldog puppy with champion bloodlines two years ago that I'd baby-sit quite a bit and had grown really attached to while I was between jobs. Playfully wrestling with him and playing "Hide 'n Seek" with his toys, "Baker" really liked his Uncle Craig too. Wanting a dog since Fritz died in '90,

Baker was my buddy whom I'd spend a lot of time with during those times penning my book when I'd get "writer's block."

Not knowing this at the time, but the night before the "hell or high water" staffing, Baker turned on Ug, gnawing his hand and side for no apparent reason. Normally a docile breed of dog, my brother couldn't risk Baker chomping into anybody else unprovoked or going after his next door neighbor's little, three-year old boy, so my gorgeous canine playmate was put to sleep. Seeing the facility for which I toiled systematically deteriorate into a concentration camp these past six months and the philosophical building blocks for a productive work environment now defunct, Baker dying would be the straw which broke the camel's back.

Having to rush off to my group engagement this Friday morning, the taskmaster in charge overseeing that the employment troops stay in line told me that she would "NEED" to see me this day. When my C.O. heard that I had gotten a little frustrated with the secretary on the phone yesterday, she saved the best of my workweek for last. Being "called on the carpet," my supervisor told me we were to meet a half-hour before I was to leave for my much-needed extended weekend—2:30 P.M.—to discuss how to best apologize to the kindly person I had gotten a tad short with. Figuring this tactical unit woman-at-arms would want me to write, "I won't be a bad boy anymore" two hundred times on the chalkboard, I wouldn't exactly be breaking a sweat.

Still fuming over what happened during staffing the day before and saddened by the loss of a pet, I thought I had finally gotten a little break this week upon finding out the commanding authority I was to report to about getting testy over the phone had left the premises and wouldn't be around at 1430 hours, the time when we were to meet. Not knowing where she went, it wasn't until later that I learned this disciplinarian who was going to scold me went to St. Clair Hospital in Mount Lebanon, presumably to prepare for the arrival of an emergency admission coming into the facility. And it would be here that I discovered the true essence of why prophets came up with the motto, "Never volunteer."

When residents would be brought in exigently on short notice into this stalag, all hell would usually break loose at the program because medications needed ordered/stocked, medical records gathered, residential regimens in place, staff schedules developed/altered, and behavior modification approaches implemented at the drop of a hat. With barely a warning, there would be an abundance of tasks which had to be completed normally by as few as two extremely busy people in the upstairs residential component getting everything organized. A time of crisis getting these previously hospitalized people situated at the treatment program, standing idly by wouldn't be an option because I knew my employee friends could use a little assistance.

The clock's minute hand several minutes past my quitting time today of 3:00 P.M. this afternoon, standing by my desk with my hands in my pockets with nothing much to do while the two residential staffers on duty at the time were running around like a chicken with its head cut off, I felt guilty. Despite wanting to escape this jungle for the weekend before my supervisor returned and while I still had a little of my sanity left, I made the ghastly mistake of asking if I could help out by keeping the natives in tow or answering the phone. Graciously accepting my good-will offer, this would be the last nail pounded into my coffin.

By 3:30 P.M., things had started settling in to the point where it wasn't such a wild free-for-all and I felt comfortable beginning my two-day sabbatical since I stayed, offering my services beyond the call of duty. Lending a hand to the residential staff for a brief time, I thought I had done my good deed for the day. But at this slowly sinking refuge for those deficient of accurate impressions, every man's for himself now.

My weekend having officially started a half-hour ago, after Phyl thanked me for helping out, I bolted out the front door wanting to get home A.S.A.P. because I needed to leave this place behind for a few days and just recuperate after another grueling week I'd just as soon forget. Lo and behold, at the precise moment I tried to make my speedy exit, marching in cadence down the sidewalk towards the main entranceway I was zipping out of would be none other than the brigade leader of this bunker. Headed for my parked car as fast as my left side could take me and assuming that if I didn't make eye contact then I'd be invisible, I lost my "cool" hearing those words spew from that woman's mouth for the billionth time.

"Craig," the executive program general said in her commanding tone which made me want to throw up whenever I heard it, "I NEED to see you—now!"

Burnt out from having been stampeded on for what had routinely become each day of the week the past half-year and with so much coming down on me at one time, I had all I could take when I told this commandant director that there was a death I had to deal with and, besides, my regulated time for the day/week ended thirty minutes ago. Adrenaline revving up and agitation souring, I leaned a bit on the argumentative side when I told this martinet to differentiate between the words, "need" and "want." With a head or two already having been severed in the short time she had occupied the helm, this warden's reputation that "crossing" her likely would result in termination had more than been upheld. Being a fresh face in the organization and veteran agency cronies which this director was familiar on "call" to flood the program, I figured I'd be moments away from being afforded the opportunity to tackle my long-planned writing endeavor "head-on," doing what I could to make it reality.

Before saying I'd see her Monday, in a voice not void of resentment, I told this adorable exec that I was the one prepared to meet at the scheduled time and that it was her who didn't bother to show up or inform me that our bogus discussion had been canceled. With the accomplished Unit Director serving as my staunch advocate gone, if I'd have exhibited the same compassion towards residents that directorial staff now regularly displayed with this survivor, I wouldn't have lasted a day into the new administrative dictatorship at this therapy/community service station.

Not even afforded the respect to grieve a death in the family, I lost the motivation to "stick it out" any longer at this detention camp. Driving home down 79 South, I kept hearing "taps" play in my head.

After leading the fifteen-minute "Community Meeting" group first thing Monday morning where residents' daily agendas and various other general matters were looked into, I answered the ringing phone in the partial office and my supervisor *asked* if I could "please" come upstairs to her office. Not hearing her infamous four-letter word, "NEED," I figured I was in trouble. Ascending the dozen or so steps from the partial program to the director's administrative control station, I felt as if I were walking a gang plank, but I was surprisingly apathetic about what was to come. The center having eroded into a disorganized mess these past half-dozen months, I didn't feel at all secure or content working here any longer, as the anticipation for continued progress had gradually withered since the solstice. The program's ameliorative standing having wilted away a little over a handful of months ago, since the good old summer time declined into dog days, the functioning of this facility regressed from being proficient to a "joke operation" under the new regime.

Limping my way into the program executive's command post this Monday morning, this Unit Manager and the agency's Human Resource Director were waiting for me, so they could play a game of judge, jury, and executioner. Calculating that it would be only a matter of time before this day would come being "shown the door" and given the "heave-ho" with my new supervisor arriving with the knowledge of this therapist's having once been seriously "brain damaged," even after having proven my efficiency, I had been counting my days since my orientation commentary about the preponderant influence of the agency.

From helping quite a few residents "flush out" some of the counter-productive garbage they had clung onto since childhood to talking group members "out of" doing stupid things which could only have hurt them, I surprised even myself with how indifferent I had become being "axed" and having the many productive results of my efforts overlooked/disregarded. As was the case with my previous employer who "cut me loose," every one of my work evaluations were rated "good" to "exceptional," but once an agency personnel member who had prior knowledge of my "brain injured" history became my mid-management supervisor, I'd be disposed of within six months. With this oligarchical agency's treatment/residential program going to "pot" being run by a "procedural handbook or bust" chief, goodbye and good riddance.

It would figure that the reason I was "given the boot" would be a word associated with the military. Tired of fighting with managements intimidated that I had injured my brain, sick to my stomach seeing this place evolve into a "dump," I wouldn't contest my dismissal despite having a legitimate defense. Because my so-called infraction officially occurred on my weekend, outside of the time scheduled for work-related activities, I would not think administrative staff would have all that much jurisdiction over me. With some of the higher powers apparently abiding by a sort of socialist frame of reference, if my mail hadn't routinely been confiscated, my privacy about my head injury likely would have been maintained and I ultimately wouldn't be joining the ranks of the unemployed. Terminated because of "insubordination," my increasing dissatisfaction with the state of affairs around this administrative bedlam had literally grown to the point of no return.

Management manufacturing the claim that I was disobedient within the bounds of work, they cleverly devised grounds as to why they weren't going to provide me with unemployment compensation. Symbolic of the position's overall regression, not only wasn't the new Unit Director trained in the field of medicine, but didn't even have a clue how to operate a computer system. Seeing to it that this understanding was grasped, she and the Human Resource Director combed through my desk drawers after notifying me I had been released from my duties and stole the detailed notes I had written on how to run the "Word Perfect" and "Lotus" functions on the computer, as well as how to operate the printer.

Maybe this idea's absurd, but given the amateur character of this operation, it wouldn't have surprised me for a moment if management staff didn't offer me unemployment and took personal belongings because they believed it was their right to be vindictive/angry with me for "pulling the wool over their eyes" not telling them about my head injury when I interviewed. As rationale for taking my instructions specifying the particulars involved to operate various computer functions, the Human Resource czar said that because these procedural steps were written on paper provided by the agency, my work was their property.

Because I had "words" with the woman who constantly would remind me of the "chain of command" at the agency officially after my work hours for the week had ended, I guess I could have caused a "stink," but I just wanted to get the hell out of there as fast as I could before I saw it go completely to the dogs. Not able to bear seeing this one-time promising facility go to "wrack and ruin" any longer, trying to flick off the chip employers put on my shoulder showcasing their short-sighted ignorance about people with histories of a brain injury, I thought I'd resume my "mission in life" and focus on working on the writing project I believe God had assigned me. Attaining gainful employment working with the brain injury disability population not about to occur because of rehab employers' prejudice, it looked like the only way I'd be able to get my "message" out for people encountering the effects of head injury would be to write a book.

About three months or so after I took pen in hand and bought a Word Processor, upon reading the Pittsburgh Post Gazette Classifieds section one sunny day, I not only learned that the agency hadn't found anyone to fill the "no frills"/"no pay" therapy position in which I had once manned, but that my less-than-independent supervisor who took aim at my employment status got court-martialed. Despite kissing company ass on the administrative front line for years, I would be informed that the fill-in Unit Director had been under the gun herself from the time she "tossed me out" until finally getting her pink slip. The "big cheese" of this wayward outfit not anticipating her tenure to be so short-lived, after following someone who was the true definition of "leader," the upper brass realized that a change had to be made before the spoilage spread too much more.

Like quite a few other positions assigned duty at the residential program since the stand-in exec took over, not able to find a body outside existing staff gullible enough to join this back-pedaling agency, a long-time nurse of the organization qualified to order Peon's demand of prescription meds would assume the therapist station I once held. With the way my vocational pursuits have been crumbling around me, I thought I could be useful and do a little something to maybe reduce some of the morbid cycle of misunderstanding and unfair judgments levied against people with head injuries by allotting some time to work on a written project which could have the capacity to change a few minds about this disability group's potential capabilities.

Our family being one where personal issues are essentially kept within the family, I barely scratched the surface of this historical project before I began working in Bridgeville because the very beginning deals with some highly sensitive items that I debated in my mind for a long time whether or not to include. Chipping away at the tip of the iceberg, not getting as far along in the book as I would have liked, I decided censoring ingredients would compromise the purpose of this assignment of revelation/self-examination because my experience could have the potential of benefiting a number of people with disabilities, as well as possibly levying some kind of worthy impact on a few who don't.

With the capacity to productively influence the lives of individuals, I felt the potential of enhancing the outlook and understanding of others was just too important to keep quiet about. On a personal level, hiding my rehabilitation recovery which I should be extremely proud, will wear on me no longer.

Writing left-handed when I started the early chapters of this book also hindered the number of pages that I had completed. Having returned to my dominant right hand after ten years as a southpaw writer, the physical ability exists to get my ideas down in written form within a realistic amount of time. As incredibly difficult writing left-handed would be physically, the emotional suffering was ten-fold because every word I'd struggle to put on paper would literally be a not-so-subtle reminder just how far I had fallen due to that accident. Also, learning a few computer/Word Processor skills, I have the mechanical means as well to finish my autobiographical duty before the 22nd millennium.

Lucky to possess a foundation already entrenched and available to me, I would be very fortunate to have the background in place where I could take a self-proclaimed sabbatical of sorts from jobs which didn't offer much in the way of career implications, and focus on recording my experience which could be seen as valuable in the eyes of survivors/family members searching for something in which to grasp. With the home situation having presented itself like it had, accumulating monies I had earned through my two therapy jobs and not having to pay tuition for grad school, I had a mechanism where I could take some time off from working formally and sustain myself almost adequately until I got a manuscript worked out/organized. Fulfilling the government's time-requirement working in the nonprofit arena, I could commit myself to working on my book.

I can at least gain a little satisfaction knowing that if Penelope continued to work in private-for-profit sanctuaries like New Medico and didn't bother slaving the specified number of years within a non-profit organization, she'd at least have to pay back the money awarded her at school, if the W.V.U. Rehab Counseling program did its mandated monitoring of its graduates.

With New Medico all but killing any hopes that I had of joining the rehabilitation employment ranks assisting those living with the effects of a brain impairment, I thought I'd meticulously chronicle some of my experiences, so that interested readers may gain a little insight upon reflection. Attempting to get some sort of "statement" out which could enhance the outlook of survivors trying to snare some semblance of promise, I thought I'd go at this book project with everything I had and "all guns blazing." From a self-oriented perspective, after New Medico clawed me of my vocational pursuits, being sad for so many years hadn't gotten me too far and I needed some type of cathartic expression to clear my mind in an attempt to get on with my life again.

Not being an author, with this work my only planned writing escapade, I thought I'd take my time and "do it up" right. With my exploits with brain injury and the ensuing circumstances not exactly something which happens everyday with everyone, I thought maybe my travels through the unknown could spark some interest in the general population who may just be enticed to read a different kind of human interest story. Rushing things and not paying attention to detail would only set me up—and the head injury disability population as a whole—for a stereotypical label of being "incompetent." For example, if I would be so careless as to use a past participle when a gerund would be more appropriate, rehabilitation personnel managers who may get ahold of my book and give it a scan would no doubt howl, "See? With this 'head injured' dude, you wouldn't know what to expect!"

Harping about employers' methods of hiring and general practices, with rigid opinions set upon questionable affirmations, the opportunity to climb out of minor-league jobs into a major league career very possibly may never present itself. Often, there's an unwritten understanding that what takes place within an employer's confines remains confidential, even if a worker leaves under unfavorable conditions. However, because New Medico back-stabbed patients as I once was dependent on rehabilitation professionals for my long-term well-being, I wasn't about to let what I knew about Goyette's Meadowlands tributary get swept under the rug and forgotten about without receiving a little advertisement.

Able to empathize with their patients' suffering, I couldn't begin to fathom how a system of rehab facilities supposedly designed for optimal treatment of those with neurological impairments could impose on the expected care of this population by churning out so much counterfeit treatment provision. Not trying to imply that I would've lapsed into a coma again if I'd have been treated here, but I thank the Lord every night that New Medico wasn't set up for operation when I was hurt, or I might have elected to receive treatment at one of their depositories.

Odds being that New Medico would counter any assault on them with case scenarios of ill-informed patients pleased with the treatment they were provided by this bunch, however, it would probably be safe to assume the smiles on their "happy camper" survivors' faces would have turned into clenched teeth grimaces had they known treatment of equal quality could have been delivered at a fraction of the expense, closer to home. Victimizing those suffering beyond belief not enough to play on New Medico's conscience, the infliction of pain wouldn't stop with their patients.

For too many years, because I felt New Medico had literally burglarized me of my future, I have been in a rage. I took Rehab Counseling in the first place because I thought getting a Master's in this field would afford me the opportunity to utilize my invaluable experience with head injury as a role model for those who needed to witness a real-life example of how treatments and medical technology could help survivors live to the fullest. Accepted as intellectually compromised and emotionally stunted, unable to proceed in a healthy manner because of the question looming over me as to why a Corporation seeming perfectly suited for my abilities would pass me over, I've been furious because my miraculous recovery has actually prevented me from landing a rewarding professional position serving this population. Earning my advanced rehab degree from an accredited academic program in 1988, affecting my relationship with subsequent employers, I haven't earned a dime or been employed a day working with those having disabilities because every rehab employer that I've encountered seems to possess a twisted attitude of bigotry about what a person with a history of a neurological impairment is capable of achieving.

Because any excuse will be fabricated in order to keep individuals having once sustained head injures out of the public eye, I wouldn't be the least bit surprised if influential members of the rehabilitation professional job market would claim that this accurate depiction of them scared them that much further away from ever providing a survivor with authentic consideration. With the real reason being that I made it known that they incriminated themselves with their close-minded tactics, rehab centers' Human Resource Departments would no doubt testify that I would have been given the benefit of the doubt/embraced as a courageous young man, but that my relentless pursuit to report the truth of their misdeeds made them suspect of me. If I wouldn't be received as a risk upon an employment search, then it would be a pretty safe bet that away I'd go in the first wave of any "downsizing" maneuver by an employer.

Not seeing it as being victimized by the devices of underhanded violations, but as biting the hand that feeds, the blame would certainly be shifted onto this survivor for ruffling feathers/whining about how cruel the employment world is for those with disabilities—and away from employers' predetermined notions—as the reason why unbiased consideration for employment could not be possible.

Defending their fellow rehab colleagues stationed at facilities where I had previously applied, sure to be accused that my brain injury must have robbed me of foresight, prospective employers wouldn't think twice of dreaming up some authentic-sounding explanation as to why one-time vacant positions needing filled by qualified applicants would no longer be available to me.

I realize it is considered taboo when one criticizes a former supervisor, but given what the two New Medico at Meadowlands' Program Directors and other Corporate generals around the country did to so many survivors agonizing with a head injury during their time of need, I still felt obligated to do my part for those trauma victims I could relate all too easily with and do some free advertising by reporting the facts. Not intending to be a smear campaign against Goyette or Micklow designed to vilify, cashing in their "blood money" paychecks as their reward for following the corrupt New Medico Corporation's directives, these two Meadowlands' execs slandered themselves. Willfully electing to engage in criminal activity, knowing full-well that those who put their faith and lives in their cash-groveling hands were being hurt and exposed to prolonged suffering for their monetary enhancement, using and taking advantage of survivors for personal gain caused these New Medico angels of love to be the objects of defamation. I believe people such as war hero and Pittsburgh Steelers' 1,000-yard running back, Mr. Rocky Bleier, would be encouraged that I'm "Fighting Back."

By August 1995, although I had constructed a healthy bulk of my book, I still didn't necessarily feel as though I was at a point in this penned adventure where I couldn't just "pack it up" and turn around. Wanting to experience "closure" on more than a few occasions in the midst of writing horrific accounts of my experience, I felt I needed to keep plowing forward and finish what I had started. My work status contributing to feelings of inefficiency and inferiority, to pick my spirits up out of the pit I dug for myself, I tried to believe that things ultimately turning out favorably for me during my recovery was somehow supposed to point me in the direction of a written expose. Trying to adopt this "holy order" mentality would definitely help guide me through the doldrums and my use of this "power of positive thinking" principle did ease a good bit of the emptiness, feeling as if I didn't have an identity.

Although this was a period where I "found myself" and continued to develop my confidence, I didn't write much detail about my undergraduate days at W.V.U. because there was really nothing all that unique to cover, for I was just like most every other college student. But maybe I should have written a few more paragraphs recapping my academic experience because this review may have benefited me emotionally being that quite a few of those times were my very best. With so many of the good opinions about myself after I finished college based on my professional standing and unheard of advancement after a brain injury—possibly selfish and unrealistic—I still combed through classifieds wanting the best of both the writing and rehabilitation worlds.

With attitudes of the latter very much predetermined, feeling as though a eulogy had already been read from the onset of my rehab job-hunting pursuits, I knew where the majority of my efforts and strivings needed to be geared. When it comes to employment objectivity for those having a physical deficit, had I known rehab employers possess a, "Why chance it?" attitude, I would've written my book right out of grad school.

One Sunday during this month of August 1995, in the Pittsburgh Post Gazette Classifieds, I discovered that my "home" rehab center of Harmarville was looking for someone with their Master's in Rehabilitation Counseling who preferably had experience with head injury. Feeling as though I had caught a break at long last because I possess this degree and my extensive experience with this disability had occurred within this treatment venue, I applied and interviewed for this position, only to find out later that a female more qualified than this survivor had gotten the job. With the Corporation which owned my "home" rehab center having employed at least one Goyette, it looked like opportunities would be non-existent in the rehabilitation field for a survivor. So much for identifying well with Harmarville.

During one of the first psychiatric staffings that I attended in that Monroeville counseling agency where my entrance into the family therapy arena was welcomed by being flicked "the bird," not knowing if this was done in order to make me feel good or else to reinforce my position that I "belonged," the doctor said to me in front of my "tenured" colleagues that once I get a few gray hairs, I'd be better able to understand the pitfalls life can deliver. Irritated that I had been deemed as someone not having experienced many of the scars in life which promote growth, knowing that I had likely been through more ordeals than probably the entire staff of "experienced" social worker therapists gathered around that conference table combined and had endured enough misery for ten lives, it was extremely difficult for me realizing that I had to bite my tongue. Life goes on.

Moving right along with my true account detailing the many challenges I had been up against since my head injury, still floundering in my search for equal opportunity objectivity, I randomly sent my head injury employment package and a column which came out about my book project to a variety of rehab facilities in the Pittsburgh area. Unceasingly turning their backs on me, my attempts to be monetarily reimbursed for my vast knowledge and experience with disability as a paid staff employee would incessantly be rejected. However, I did receive a phone call from one employee comfortably prospering in a TBI treatment establishment greeted by the sunrise moments before Monroeville. Informing me that all paying positions working with the "neurologically-impaired" population were occupied, but that I'd be more than welcome to give a freebie talk to their patients/family members, I politely declined Butch's gracious offer, citing the travel distance involved. Round and round we go.

Likely holding the review of my manuscript aspiration which I wouldn't have sent had I known he worked at this center, Butch then asked me a few open-ended questions about my writing project which I politely answered in a generalized fashion because I obviously wouldn't want to show my hand to a one-time New Medico Corporate employee who loyally followed the Meadowlands administration's directives for so many years. It would be a pretty safe call that "Mr. New Medico" would be at least somewhat curious how many—if any—words would be devoted to his corrupt, former employer which did so much to aggravate the conditions of those seeking their "care." Across the board, from patients to business associates and employees to interns, New Medico's wonted practice of operating without standards subjected them to founded complaints in courtrooms years after this Corporate Federal Reserve locked up their cash registers. Live by the sword, die by the sword.

Filed March 19, 1998 in the Middlesex Superior Courthouse, lies yet another complaint against New Medico. Recorded under docket #98-1282, levied against the executor managing the estate of New Medico's former owner, the plaintiff files suit for breach of contract. Accustomed to assuming the "Defendant" role by now, New Medico had been charged with failing to adhere to a guaranteed, five-year, financial agreement that they had consummated with one of their workers who saw to it that the bank vault be filled with stockholder riches. Finalized on or about 1/10/92, the former employee asserted that New Medico illegally revoked the written declaration of payment that they had made with him.

The plaintiff alleges that he was not paid the salary stipulated in the contractual understanding for a period of approximately sixteen months (3/21/92-7/30/93). Also, according to this one-time Chief Financial Officer, New Medico reneged on their written promise that, should termination be forthcoming without just cause, severance pay would be awarded in full for five years and benefits would coincide with this monetary compensation. Having developed as a kind of Corporation trademark since their greed put them out of business, New Medico wouldn't "hold up" their end of the bargain once again; failing to reimburse their employee in full as outlined in the agreement.

In August 1993, approximating the time these New Medico cash cows sold off the last of its three coffers, this budget manager was handed an eviction notice of his own. Apparently, conditions which should have caused his severance/benefits clause to kick in—still at it—one New England day this Corporate clan just decided that they weren't about to bother abiding by the terms of their employment promise. So, New Medico shit was about to hit the judicial fan one more time.

Ultimately, in court proceedings prior to this complaint, the plaintiff obtained judgment against New Medico; meaning these lily-white Corporate schoolboys had to reimburse their former employee a six-figure dollar amount for severance pay and benefits despite his getting "walking papers." Due monies from the day the agreement was completed (1/10/92) until June 30, 1997, the plaintiff had coming the 150 plus grand the sparkling New Medico Corporation tried to pretend was theirs. Within twenty-four hours of the ruling (7/1/97) through February 28, 1998, New Medico would owe their released C.F.O. $152,630 itemized in the form of severance pay, unpaid insurances, and automobile allowance. Hence, claiming for damages of their own, New Medico would yell for an arbitrator. As the world turns.

Not knowing for certain if things happen for a reason or not, maybe the plan for me was to do something a little more global in scope for the disability population than to limit myself working in a dinky rehab center somewhere. Possibly the writing has always been on the wall and simply tells a tale that the employment world just isn't going to allow for any exceptions to what is generally understood. In my longing to get on some professional track, with New Medico leading the charge in the rehabilitation job front, it appears I just may have to adopt an attitude that because my comeback deviates so far from what is generally accomplished, having this survivor's capabilities "lumped with" other members of this disability group looks like a prejudice I sadly have got to learn to live with.

However, like in my personal rehabilitation efforts, I'm just going to have to try and make that serotonin in my brain shoot around a little bit, so that I can finish this passage into my inscrutable history. With the hope that a few lives can be touched, maybe writing a book is the only way I can do service for those with histories of a TBI, given employers' stance. Getting perturbed being approached as if I had some kind of epidemic, I thought I'd break out my "Papermate."

Never intending to hire me or give me a chance at life, I hope this book can give New Medico at least a little glimpse of how their actions can destroy the life of a survivor who depended on them for a little respect and assistance. Possibly, New Medico bombarding this TBI spokesman off his career course was somehow designed to happen in order to get me so agitated that I'd feel compelled to write a smidgen about them. Not being excessively vindictive in nature, if I feel a principle is worth defending or I've been personally "wronged," however, I do bite back. Maybe things were supposed to materialize like they did, for if I'd have been associated as a wage earner with a corrupt Corporation who got their cash depot from hurting others whom I was once identified with, that would have "dragged my name through the mud."

Apparently a "head injured go-getter" requires having friends in high places, if they are to get that promising rehab position—even if their contributions had the potential of harvesting incomparable consequences. Because of their training and elevated "understanding," one could think that rehabilitation employers would be most appreciative of one who has made so many astounding gains following the onset of a severe brain injury disability, but empathy/entrepreneurial insight would be polar opposite of what would be demonstrated by managements.

With this enhanced knowledge, unfounded generalizations would develop and these stereotypical presumptions fed into a lasting suspicion. My trauma history making me prone to prejudice and discrimination, I don't feel as if I'm entitled in any way of preferential treatment because of my injury, but I would like to have seen a little fair objectivity. Not about to let my experience fall by the wayside again, I need to do more than just hope my dream of enlightening and benefiting survivors comes into play. Rehab personnel managements not affording me the consideration I'd need to have my abilities "discovered," other means would need utilized. There are more ways than one to skin a cat.

Acceptance and appreciation. As far as the onset of a disability is concerned, a sense of acknowledgment must settle in once the shock, denial, and anger stages have run their course. After this recognition sets in the forefront of one's understanding, a multitude of pathways can become available to guide one through the sludge of debilities and to the discovery of new strengths. Accustomed to "normalcy," it's tough to adapt to restriction and concede "loss," but in order to excel to the fullest given the condition, one needs to make options in the environment work for them. Truth's cruelties having harvested a genuine ideology for me, the impact of a perilous journey often can leave its traveler with a hunger for character or starving to be weeped for.

Attempting to make use of compensatory strategies to function optimally around deficiencies, to opening up the mind so one can be thankful for the capabilities that are within reach, different modes of behavior and philosophical practices must be assimilated into a survivor's everyday approach, if they are to progress in a healthy fashion. Sometimes, all a person can hope for is to have the willpower to tolerate those tasks that they can no longer do and just be grateful to be alive. If assistance is needed to avoid being hammered by a predicament, then it would be advantageous to form some kind of alliance with a strong network of support to help one through any tough times which may lie ahead.

Wishing to make the most of their abilities, one must realize that conceding the existence of limitations does not mean the expiration of happiness will occur next in the progression and that the dawn of an everlasting doom shall follow as its perennial substitute. Rather, ways around restraints need to be incorporated until they become as instinctual as breathing. And a fresh vantage point in which to look at the world needs worked on, so the livelihood of an individual with a shortcoming may be enhanced. Sometimes left with few other alternatives, if this labor becomes part of one's regular regimen of interacting with their surroundings, the fruits can be most bountiful to the extent that interference develops as something which seems to be overcome automatically.

Needing to accept so much at a relatively young age hasn't been easy, but if all that happened to this survivor on the rehabilitation and prejudice fronts wouldn't "get to me" on occasion, I don't think I'd be human. Knowing deep down inside that my days of engaging in most extremely fine motor skills right-handed with any kind of speed or spontaneity will likely forever be lost, sometimes cuts into the core of my passions. But I just have to move past that and be prepared to search for resolutions to whatever hurdles I may encounter next. Traveling many miles on this minefield since my accident, to avoid detonation and dismembering their emotional stability, one needs to learn that they have to accept who they are before becoming involved in other arenas.

Pretty early on during my inpatient recovery at Harmarville, I would be paid an unexpected visit by a neighborhood friend who lives a few houses down from me in Washington. In the line of work selling equipment for people with disabilities, this father of two—whose repeated attempts to show he was on a par with me when it came to sports were not successful—had some business at my "home" rehab center at a time I was struggling in therapies to make sense of the world. Stopping by my room to see how I was doing after being in "critical" condition and to wish me well, my mind not exactly cognizant of the surroundings quite yet, to this day I still have a dim sense of the embarrassment I felt being seen in a compromised state by someone who once knew me as an athlete.

Even though I don't have too much of a "clue" as to what else was happening around me at that time during my rehab, I can still appreciate the discomfort I experienced being witnessed during a circumstance when I definitely viewed myself as "no good." However, "pulling for me" with all of his heart, instances such as this demonstrated consideration/concern would help me to develop a self-endorsing attitude which would benefit me throughout my days.

With this experience only being one of the first of many more, I learned that if a survivor is preoccupied with what others think, then a life of sparse accomplishment can be expected, for there won't be time for anything else. Not wanting to be a self-absorbed/overly conscientious "basket-case," one must become secure with areas in which they are no longer proficient and try to embrace them as new challenges which must be mastered. Not "owning up to" the confined boundaries a brain injury will present one with could be one of the worst side effects of this disorder, for denial only prolongs agony to a slow burn. Compensation is not the most pleasant thing in the world, but if a symptom can be nullified or rendered ineffectual, the consequences would be well worth the effort.

Along with maneuvers to "work around" actions which pose one with difficulty, keeping busy can ease some of the damaging effects an injury of this nature is known to levy on its survivors. From the emotional scars of being traumatized to having been shit on by rehab employers not sitting with me very well, getting kind of annoyed, I thought I'd just "go at it" and hope things fall into place because that's about all I can do. Trying to put a "positive spin" on a situation sometimes being about all that one can do, needing to take the "high road" and be indebted that the short time I had been "living on the edge" didn't cause me to perish, I would just have to feel much obliged that I'm around to complain about rehab employers' true opinions of those with disabilities.

Maybe offered a job, but not a respectable wage, I'd be sure employers would line up to hire me for that prominent counseling position with their organization after learning that I had sustained a severe brain injury. Not knowing anything about therapy or disability, I haven't earned a penny in the rehabilitation field after all these years have gone by. Like riding piggy-back on a scud missile, unless masochistic behavior befit me and I weren't opposed to inevitably being destroyed, I would need to find a way to escape the poisonous images where prejudice turned out to be the executioner of my opportunity. My search having led me to the vitalness of keeping occupied by engaging in invigorating activity and replenishing the channel of the mind with productive film strips, one fragment of my conscious would not be so easy to divert.

Being in a car accident didn't do much for the remission of dad's cancer. In the process of gathering background information for this book, when reviewing my late father's memoirs he wrote the night I was hurt and how he wanted to die if I didn't survive, the shame/depression I experienced was tremendous. Feeling a deep guilt and selfishness about the agony dad went through fearing his youngest wouldn't make it, if I "let my guard down," the blame can "get to me" pretty bad. The majority of the time, I can either keep myself concentrating on priorities or try to convince myself that dad wouldn't want me to assume any responsibility for his dying. But during those not-too-infrequent instances when I want my dad, and he isn't there, I almost believe I should punish myself in some way for being so insensitive to such a great man after all he sacrificed on my behalf to ensure that I had a solid upbringing.

Trying to rationalize the situation by telling myself that dad didn't do his body any good never going to see a doctor for his smoking habit of over four decades, this self-talk helps me to put things in better perspective, so I don't carry through with this psychoanalytic pain principle; but I can only wish now that dad would've caught me that first time I smoked marijuana and taught me a "lesson" I'd never forget. Possibly resulting in his being with us a little longer, the circumstance leading to my "awakening" later on would be infinitely more harmful.

Since I was a little boy, I had a 4 x 8 foot piece of plywood in our basement where me and Danny Hobbs would play "war" with my 1/72 scale model tanks. Finally outgrowing this, I thought it would be great to convert this display from a World War II battlefield into a landscape with a locomotive "choo-chooing" around, so I asked for a train set one Christmas.

Making a long story short, my dream of constructing a "cannon-ball express" layout didn't turn out to be the fantasy that I had hoped, for after I tore the wrapping paper off the big present with *my* new railroad cars and track in it, my hands wouldn't get to touch this gift again during the evolution of this railway system. Saying he'd *help* me put together *my* electric railroad set—instructed to sit back and "watch how it's done" because I'd mess everything up, otherwise—I proceeded to observe dad lay down all the tracks, make a wire fence out of my Lincoln logs that could conduct electricity, and construct a control board. Hardly thrilled with the way dad customarily went about "teaching" me craftwork, not wanting to grumble because this would surely "stir him up," I'd just keep my mouth closed.

Telling mom "the mediator" of dad's take-over, wanting to keep the peace she was accustomed compromising for, I would be told that all I could really do was appreciate the nice arrangement I'm going to have. Oftentimes not possessing the patience for trial and error learning or willing to devote the time required while a novice will make mistakes, I just had to swallow my frustration. Angered at the time, not knowing how "good" I had it then, today when I revisit those rare days when I somehow thought I had it "rough" growing up, I can get a discomforting sense of uneasiness. Almost feeling shameful that I experienced distress over something so minor, what I wouldn't give to see dad do things for me now.

Having trouble accepting the premise behind the old saying which goes, "You don't miss what you never had," however, I will defer to the idea, "You don't know what you got, 'til it's gone."

Directing attention elsewhere, it's only human nature not to pay any "mind" to things when they're proceeding favorably and working out because it's merely assumed that the "good times" will keep on rolling. When meaningful people or events are gone that were taken for granted, this loss can leave a big void and renders a wound which hurts deep. In relation to the "A bird in the hand is worth two in the bush" position, striving for great heights occasionally can result in people not taking credence for what they do have, but when these unattended valuables are no longer around, one sure does miss that which has disappeared.

Although still attempting to bring about significant productivity, since I almost made a quick exit from this earth, I have found that I will stop myself from trying to reach some sort of zenith and focus more on the qualities around me I once overlooked/didn't bother to estimate their value. Accepting my limitations and not ignoring the goodness which life can offer, I will appreciate worth much better and all that I've personally done to reach a level nobody would have believed I could attain. No longer mourning those aspirations that it was necessary bidding farewell to, my conciliation has grown to the extent that I no longer see my injury as a permanently catastrophic downfall, and can take reverence in all that I've achieved since my life had changed. Possibly difficult to fathom, I'm generally not downcast about any of the permanent afflictions that my condition has left me to live with because I have confirmed their existence and have made accommodations, so that their hindrance on my functioning would be minimal.

Capabilities forever hampered within a moment's passing leaves its victims bearing a castigating reminder of the tragic impact an instant of time can have, if care isn't taken. Traveling through this Hell and having prospered to some degree amidst these flames of cruelty, I would like to think that I have the key to the makings of something influential. Given the general attitude of some segments of society, I wouldn't know for sure, but I can only hope that I have some ammunition to leave some relevant mark on this planet.

Overlapping into one another, I hear a prime example of the acceptance/appreciation principle quite often coming from mom when she'll comment that it's tough seeing me limp *around,* but it sure beats the alternative not having me *around.* Foregoing a blueprint of tomorrow's dreams in exchange for one not yet diagrammed will have its challenges, but it need not be an unfulfilled conclusion.

Apologizing to those readers seeking a fabulous ending, my struggles with discrimination being a "knock down, drag out" conflict—not being Hollywood—I simply wasn't provided with a script by rehab administrations to transform these pages documenting the harsh reality of bias into some kind of fairy tale. Feeling daily gratitude for the restoration doors that I have eventually been able to kick in which theoretically should have been bolted shut a long time ago, I can only wish upon a star that my story isn't over yet.

Not to savor the glowing tenderness of life, shall mean closing one's eyes to that which must be grasped to sparkle, for cherished dreams of the next light's prosperity, may fail to glisten on the horizon.

Chapter 9

Reflections

A light finally appearing at the end of the tunnel, this last segment of the book will be one where I'll try to tie up some loose ends. Designed to "wrap things up," I'll attempt to fill in some blanks and make some sense out of ambiguous events in these final pages of my work. Over the years, in both formal and informal settings, I have been asked a multitude of questions by people curious about what someone with a history of severe brain trauma goes through, and I'll give it my best effort to answer the inquiries that I haven't already in this closing portion of my chronicle.

Generally, writing a record of events is a significant undertaking as it is, but reliving so many deplorable/nightmarish experiences again sometimes made cataloging occurrences very trying on my capacity to remain composed. Figuring the benefits which may be reaped would make any personal pain a small sacrifice, I forged ahead the best I could. Glad that documenting happenings surrounding my tragedy is nearing an end, am I ever ecstatic my parents instilled in me the principle that one never achieves anything, if they quit. Tipping my hat to these fabulous parental teachers—being there for me every step of the way during my uphill battle with a brain injury where I would ultimately kick in some doors and violate the laws of nature—I owe them everything because of the instruction they provided which allowed me to hit "pay dirt" during my rehabilitation efforts. Possessing my fair share of mettle, when it was time to bust some ass and douse flames in the showdown with my head injury, this ingrained message would be the spark which would guide me along during my head trauma rehabilitation where neurological uprisings are more the rule than the exception.

Pit against this treacherous head injury disability where the brain goes through a wholesale change and overall functioning will initially undergo a swift decline, over the course of time, I have learned that "the show must go on" and one just has to bear down/exhibit a little "cussedness," if they are to right any wrong. In order that certain important aspects may get a little additional emphasis and inconclusive points are not left "hanging," I'll try to expound and recapitulate on a few items I think it would be essential to cover.

It was one of the strangest feelings I've ever had in my life and one that I hadn't had since. At Allegheny General Hospital on 2/1/83—the evening before I was to have the titanium rod removed from my right femur—I was in the shower cleaning myself up for the morning operation when a powerful emotion overcame me. It hadn't yet been one year since I was a comatose patient here, but my sanguinary condition at the time blackened all recollection of ever being at this hospital. With visions collected over the passage of time twisting in a maelstrom of mistaken recognition, my memory of ever having been present at Allegheny General draws a complete blank. Unable to identify anything upon admission this second time around, I just assumed that any images of my previous virulent stay here when I was on the throes of death were forever gone because my mind simply had been pillaged of its ability to process.

Although my room as an orthopedic patient preparing to have my leg operation was on an entirely different floor than the ones where I was as a non-responsive patient, oddly, I had this overwhelming sense that I had been here before. My awareness having "went on the lam" at the time when my neurological mechanisms were a dilapidated jumble—being a rational sort of person—I'd just tell myself that I had this sensation of receiving treatment here in my past merely because I had been informed of my prior placement at this medical establishment, and not from some indoctrination of deja vu. But still, because it was such an unearthly aura, a little part of me wondered if a glimmer of understanding hadn't been illuminated from the dark cavern of my subconscious. My accident in 1991 would have a vaguely similar "flashback" quality, but was nowhere near as overpowering.

On the bottom of the food chain and little more than a piece of flesh when I was profoundly unconscious on those mattresses, those billions of brain cells and trillions of synapses so close to dissolution would leave an empty void in my register of retrievable experiences. Embroiled in a fight for survival amidst a suffocating vacuum, if my family and the professionals who worked with me hadn't told me where I'd been and what happened to me, I wouldn't have any idea how things had developed as they had. Because of the venomous interference with my capacity to "take in" my environment, what occurred during the duration when my comprehension of the world was nothing shall be forever lost in this lifetime for, regardless of circumstance, time moves on. And not having any concrete perceptions when my senses were so close to being laid to rest is probably for the better because of the agony which had overtaken me.

Although I am absolutely positive the majority of people who claim to have met up with an "out of body" experience following a near death crisis firmly believe that it had happened, I'm not so sure what to make of such alleged occurrences. Unlike someone who may have had coronary or pulmonary distress leading to their supposedly experiencing "the other side"—giving them the benefit of the doubt—possibly because it was my neurological functioning which controls perceptions that was damaged, this could be why I had no paranormal sensation of ever hovering about the scene of the accident and witnessing paramedics extract my unconscious body from that destroyed Volkswagen.

Indicating that I just better straighten up, although I didn't hear late AC/DC singer Bon Scott singing "Highway to Hell" when I was teetering between life and death, maybe I should be a little more concerned that nor do I ever remember passing by any angels playing harps during a post-mortality journey amongst the clouds. Looking down on the earth from the heavens above, if my time had indeed passed, words alone couldn't possibly express how overjoyed I am that an opportunity had presented itself to make something positive out of my catastrophe.

Punished for being human, that albatross rearing its ugly head when I was living on the edge permanently deleted so much of my past. A substance in the brain which interferes with long-term memory—portasol—must have been leaking within my cranium from all fronts. Where short-term memory is stored within the brain, my hippocampus having been all but totally "wiped out," I have absolutely no knowledge of ever being in a room full of mattresses burning from fever. My guardian angel working overtime, I may not carry a four-leaf clover around with me, but wearing a cross around my neck 24 hours a day since I was about thirteen-years old sure didn't hurt my chances of coming out on top of this disability which will leave a mind wavering from basic understanding and one wishing to be physically whole again. Painted into a corner and praying that things would somehow "pan out" in the long run, I had no idea that fighting the wind with my neurologically traumatized condition would just be the beginning of my battle.

Possessing a sort of "crown jewel" recovery and on the "cutting edge" of a rehabilitation comeback not making much of a difference, because of the unknown nature of a head injury and the effects it will levy on its victims, this disability is one which had delivered—and will deliver—a punishing caveat towards this survivor. Going against the grain of what's routinely accepted and adhered to, I have learned not to be surprised the extent with which certain segments of society will go to avoid associating with a victim who has personally experienced catastrophe. Igniting feelings of uneasiness, the very thought of being around someone who has tangled with trauma can often be enough to give a person the "willies." Although having my fair share of successes with the ladies interpersonally since almost walking "through the valley of the shadow of death," on the flip side, the hemi-paralytic way with which I move unfortunately is not something that the professional work force has shown it can overlook.

As it applies to me, T.B.I. not only stands for "traumatic brain injury," but how the rehabilitation field I've been trying to get my foot in the door over the past decade has been, "the biased industry." Not about to give me a chance, rehab employers apparently view my "surreal" recovery as "unbelievable," and will go to whatever lengths it takes to maintain a hurricane-force avoidance of this head injury survivor. Their antics of skullduggery serving as the manacles to keep me in the dark, if it is my destiny to go down with the ship that the jaundiced attitudes of rehab employers have torpedoed me with, I'm not about to go down quietly.

Being a "thorn in my side," unable to start a rewarding career in rehab because of the stigma owned by those managing facilities, I have become so aggravated that I thought I'd just expose a few of the slanted actions in which I've been targeted. Unable to topple the court of public opinion, it would be highly unlikely that any administrations would need to answer for their skeptical personnel practices because this could open a Pandora's Box.

Writing this book, I don't know if rehabilitation employers or influential personnel supervisors will "stand up and take notice," but I hope that these cartels will think twice before discriminating again. Vultures circling, employers across the board would claim that my having sustained a severe head injury wouldn't impact their determination about filling a vacancy for an available employment position, but you better believe it matters.

Making a world of difference, informed that an applicant or employee once was in such critical condition, this revelation will forever become annoyingly lodged in the back of a human resource director's mind. Not regarded as "special" with incredible potential, but as a "catastrophe" needing to be shuffled off, rehab executives have subjected me to a panorama of misery.

In an industry claiming to be "people-friendly" and oriented for those who need assistance, there's no room for "bird flicking" short-sightedness and segregation within the human services field. Held at bay, claims that I would be regarded as a pundit couldn't be any further from the truth because I have been approached with guile by various "compromised" human resource directorial bodies along virtually every job pursuit I've undertaken. Having been violently victimized creating an unobtrusive revulsion, making personnel department's "gorge rise," it's looking more and more like the employment rat race is impossible, if one has had a traumatic brain injury. I'm not a whiner, but my being subjected to so much prejudgment and indifference has led me to believe that it would be easier to get a rehabilitation job, if I had been found guilty of being a serial killer, than to be a survivor of a brain contusion.

Capable of walking in some patients' footsteps not making a damn bit of difference, I'm inclined to think that the employment world's general attitude/opinion about people with disabilities isn't intended to change, and my strivings to be some kind of "voice" for this population just wasn't meant to be. This misunderstood and shunned disability population having to make their own "breaks" because none will be given to them, I always thought that life rewards those who work hard—but because I've sustained a brain injury—I guess anyone who once suffered through this condition receives an asterisk alongside this claim. Personnel Department's inability to detach the medical history from this survivor's outward manner being my "monster" I have yet to slay, I've just about "had it" being let down by rehab employer prima donnas who must assume that there's "nothing to it" going from a comatose patient to attaining the prerequisites needed to acquire professional status.

Not wanting my rehabilitation folklore to be one where I was unable to fulfill my potential because of employer's bent narrow-mindedness and twisted pettiness, I've tried to develop a thick skin and proceed as favorably as can be expected. Allowing for a one-time "ditsy" patient to prove that they're capable of efficiently handling a professional job within the rehabilitation work force apparently not the most enticing of propositions, such an opportunity wouldn't be forthcoming possibly because those doing the hiring at various establishments would be afraid that this would somehow lessen the significance/standing of their own place in the vocational world. Mistakenly thinking that the sky was the limit after earning an advanced degree, I would soon be doing battle with the harsh reality of prejudice and discrimination. Since getting my Master's in Rehabilitation Counseling, all I've ever wanted to do was to help those who have sustained a neurological impairment, but I've only found myself "swimming upstream" not getting the New Medico reference I worked hard for and deserved.

Unable to "cool my heels" because of what the New Medico pickpocketers did to harmless patients and their loved ones without batting an eye, having no business getting their hands on members of the head injury disability population again, a rogues' gallery of New Medico accessories can customarily be found comfortably employed at practically any rehabilitation setting across this great land. Its occurrence so widespread, it no longer amazes me when rehabilitation corporations gravitate towards former New Medico personnel who were aware of—and participated in—their employer's scandalous misgivings.

As a form of cathartic expression, maybe God didn't want me to completely get over what New Medico did to fellow traumatized brethren and myself, so that I'd get so perturbed, I'd write an account of this warm and cuddly rehab corporation for the broader population one of these days. Used as an outlet to shine a light on this disgraceful rehab organization, I could not know if things falling so badly out of place for me like they have by not getting a fair shake was somehow designed to happen in order that I'd have added incentive to be some sort of equal opportunity "point man," but I'm going to try to do what I can to "hammer home the point" that judgments influenced by prepossessed ignorance does far too much damage.

Unable to master any kind of "thought-stopping" counseling technique because the sweeping abuse New Medico levied was so extensive, affronting so many who were reliant on them for dependability, it wouldn't be humanly possible for many associated with the New Medico bunch to "tone down" their anger. Showcasing a chic look, children of New Medico accessories could usually be found modeling the most expensive pair of Loafers on the market, no matter how much suffering Corporate patients had to endure, so their parents could afford these and other "creme de la creme" material items.

Those rehabilitation centers familiar with my exceptional attributes and credentials could have been a torchbearer of sorts—universally demonstrating for the human services market that it can be profitable and advantageous to employ a formerly traumatized individual for a post of responsibility—but they chose not to engage in this exhibition of trust. Leading the charge, because these facilities knew of my unique capabilities and background—but did nothing to help me secure a means to enhance my livelihood—they only added fuel to the fire which is stealth bigotry towards those with a history of brain trauma. With the pen being mightier than the sword, it could not be considered exonerating those miasmic employers who would just as soon deprive a former rehab patient of their right to life, liberty, and the pursuit of happiness than to display courtesy.

The "mortality of disability" not being a comfortable concept to acknowledge, something so trite as my ugly left-handed writing could have presumably been viewed as an unpleasant, tangible reminder to interviewers/ employers that ones's permanent placement on this earth isn't guaranteed. Insolent dispositions and questionable attitudes needing to be kept out of sight, correlating physical debilities with one's professional makeup appears to be a fundamental practice within the employment world which would need to be denied.

With employers' consciousness of my disability history/subsequent physical ailments making this goal increasingly more difficult, I didn't utilize the Americans with Disabilities Act or the National Relations Labor Board for a variety of reasons. My post-acute limitations being so minimal, I never used the A.D.A. because I wanted to show that a survivor of a severe head injury could proceed in a "normal" fashion without needing to make use of any kind of specialized treatment. Assuming the NRLB wouldn't be an outfit interested in my case, I figured I'd just have to swallow my pride and "stew" upon discovering some blue-eyed, blonde hair femme fatale—sporting a pair of bouncing size "D" cups—was found to be more qualified to work with the head injury disability population than this one-time patient. Not always taking into account the impact of society's attitudes when assuming this ill-fated role-model assignment, unable to "rise above" prejudice/ discrimination and my getting "the shaft" too many times to count, this self-imposed duty of not soliciting any type of assistance would too often backfire.

The assortment of marquee achievements I had made leading up to the attainment of my Master's not exactly doing anything to taint my confidence, I thought I could catch the world on fire by simply resting on the rehabilitation/ academic laurels that I had earned and not concern myself with issues which regularly forsake those who have a chapter in their life consisting of some pandemonium. Hardly working in my favor, not worrying about outside factors such as the generally adhered to attitude that anyone once "kooky" will forever be damned to be "off their rocker," considering services for those with disabilities would not occur. Cemented in a pantheon of excellent comebacks, I couldn't fathom being cheated out of life after struggling so desperately to establish a foundation for a future. Ignorance is bliss.

Influencing my decision not to try utilizing the A.D.A., I would be told by a faculty member of mine and Penelope's graduate program that using the Americans with Disabilities Act in a hearing with New Medico likely wouldn't benefit me, whatsoever. This direction no doubt having its merits, this persuadable student would subsequently figure that he was up "shit creek" without a paddle.

Knowing that this provision for individuals with handicaps has been abused in the past by those who knew how to "milk the system"—although legitimately being in a sort of grey area—I wouldn't want to take away services/monies out of the finite resource pool from those who would have a greater urgency for this backing. Possibly selfish and maybe even defeating the purpose of this ignored "legislation," I wanted to get away from viewing myself as a "handicapped" person needing any type of assistance because I was damned proud to have busted my tail in order to attain a completely independent stature. Either simply not thinking about it or feeling that my former jobs just weren't worth the headache, I wouldn't see how using this recourse could enhance my chances for prosperity. However, if I could only see what was "around the bend," I might have thought twice about disregarding this support.

Interviewing in downtown Pittsburgh for the therapy position at the family counseling agency, as an enticement to accept this job, I would be told that I'd be working out of an office building in the contemporary professional's paradise of Monroeville the vast majority of the time. Working in such an attractive environment being a symbolic victory for the head injury disability population as a whole, my celebration would be premature. Evidently, filling a vacancy at this location was originally the plan, until it had been discovered within the first month or so of my employment that there was something that "just wasn't right" with the newly-hired therapist in town.

Confirmed later on by my second supervisor that staff wasn't fooled by my avoidance of the topic and could tell that something pretty severe must have happened to my neurological system because of the less-than-nimble way that I move, it would be practically impossible to prove that the transfer determination where I was to be permanently stationed "on the other side of the tracks" in a red-light district of vice and graft was done because of an educated hunch that something "bone-chilling" had occurred with me. Unable to gather enough evidence that this tactic was undertaken so I would be forced to quit, if this campaign for me to work full-time in the "hood" was all set to begin and I'd relent accepting this suicide mission, I would undeniably be viewed as dishonorable and grounds for a hasty dismissal could therefore be set into place.

Not wanting to "check out" a few years shy of my thirtieth birthday making little difference, the administrative powers-to-be would therefore have sufficient ammunition to give this wobbling novice the "heave-ho." With the ink having already dried on my signed employment contract which stated that I was to accept any assignment given me, I would be at the mercy of management.

In the "olden" days, any school marm who got married was disgustfully looked down upon by her supervisors, and would soon find herself moved indefinitely to a tenderloin area of squalor with the hopes that she'd resign. Unfortunately, it appeared this same outdated scheme was being put into play with me once it had been determined that I was keeping a "sinister" secret about a profound disability experience. But I wasn't about to make things easy for my new employer by "bowing out" because I foolishly wanted to prove to myself that, despite some of the sequelae from my injuries being noticeable/detectable, my performance on the job would not be overshadowed by my physical abnormalities. Convincing myself that someone with a disability could be approached with favor and objectivity being of primary importance, these strivings would turn out to be nothing but fool's optimism.

Without understanding the practice and life experience I had to endure to attain a counseling position of this level, it looked like the tenured workers could only view me as a limping, former greenhouse laborer/recent college graduate who was replacing trained veteran therapists. Definitely an indication of how I was thought of from the onset—this subordinate being in the awkward position of having to do it myself—not one "tried and true" therapist who had been associated with the organization for a prolonged period of time even bothered to welcome me into the establishment or even introduced themselves to this "new employee." The operation adopting an "out" with the old and "in" with the new philosophy of personnel management not doing a whole lot for this reception committee's spirit, not unlike my "knock down"/"drag out" escapades with disability and rehabilitation, it appeared that I'd largely have to "tough it out" on my own. From having my hometown repeatedly referred to as "The Great Wasteland," to a seasoned therapist laughing at me in front of a room full of little school kids when a classmate made a derogatory comment upon noticing my glass-shredded right ear —having to keep quiet about my status as a sort of "power broker" in the field of rehabilitation—respect for this "lame" therapist wouldn't be easy to come by.

A single parent conceivably having a substantially more profound diagnosis than an "adjustment disorder" slipping through the intake screening process, coupled with the question about the origins of my physical "peculiarness," my term working in the suburbs of a metropolis would be relatively short-lived. Learning until it was too late that the person whom I would mistakenly resort to as a confidante after my Monroeville accident seemed to possess a few features similar to that of one with a borderline ailment, a new chapter of unforeseen growth and healing would subsequently be written. Virginia, it looks like the skepticism and mistrust which notoriously shadows survivors whose thinking once sputtered continues to be a widespread virus.

Following my time at the rural establishment where I had expanded my knowledge of such conditions, with the hopes that my personal and educational experiences could help guide others down a more favorable path, I decided the time had arrived where I was to gear my efforts towards documenting many factors leading up to my staggering recovery following a severe head injury. Symbolic of how far I had deviated from my previous habits and associations, Paul used to refer to me and Kevin as the "Odd Couple." My roommate and I once very much alike until I started playing with "tea," this period of regression when distance separated me from many of the fundamental practices I had always complied with is where the true account of the events leading to my crisis would really "pick up steam."

Based on the premise that if something *can* go wrong, it *will* go wrong, considering Murphy's Law could not occur because of my adolescent frame of reference. Lifelong prosperity assumed to be a rite of passage, I'll be paying for the rest of my adult life observing this teenaged logic, and subsequently getting involved with the "wrong crowd" for that brief period of time when I strayed from discretion. Believing invinscibility as an owed grant could not have been any more off-target, nor would the subsequent efforts to be some sort of conquering hero set to slay the dragon of social acceptance be a concept that could possibly be attained by means not consistent with ambitious strivings.

Not giving enough credence to past direction, I made a near fatal presumption correlating income with moral fiber. When some people have been drinking, they can get rather boisterous and start swinging from the chandelier, while others just kind of "clam up" and withdraw into their own private stupor. Paul's partying demeanor being one where he'd look even-keeled and act level-headed, it would be tough to gauge as to what effect—if any—a few drinks may have on him. Paul's everyday laid-back personality making it that much more difficult to get a true reading as to whether or not he'd been altered in any way, I surely thought he was okay to drive the night I crawled into the car with him after the party

Unable to retrieve but a few dim pictures of that fateful February '82 night, I can only venture to guess that Paul had to have portrayed an outward appearance where he at least looked like he was in control and could manage to operate a motor vehicle. Supporting my belief that I could trust Paul getting me home safely, aforementioned reasons such as his having worldly professional parents and assuming he wouldn't put a friend at risk, only strengthened my confidence that I had nothing to worry about.

Not witnessing firsthand the number of drinks he downed because I wasn't around him—realizing that the "dulling" effect of alcohol is different for different people—what I had seen of him in college, I knew Paul wasn't a "light-weight" and supposedly could handle himself well. Unfortunately, various vital senses needed to maneuver an automobile like judgment, reaction time, and vision not being of the tangible nature, deficiencies in these prerequisites necessary for efficient driving cannot be externally observed. Assumptions all that I can go by because I had forgotten most everything about that Valentines '82 night, and little has returned to fill this absence—but knowing how I'd respond in such a circumstance—Paul evidently wasn't slurring his speech or staggering when approaching his car, or I would have found another way home. More than likely, if Paul had shown any visible signs that he was intoxicated, Wayne wouldn't have gotten into the car with him, either.

Able to effectively conceal how "tanked up" he really was when we left, one could deduct that undertaking the motor skills and engaging in the concentration required when driving an automobile were just enough to push Paul over the edge and make him light-headed. Getting "buzzed" to such a degree while behind the wheel that his decision-making and physical coordination must have abandoned him at the time when they'd be needed most, would spell "disaster" for the one seated in the projectile passenger seat—me.

Not having such a history at the time, if Paul would have been one of those people with two or more DUI's who had poisoned their mind so badly with repeated alcohol use that they couldn't do something—for example—so simple as to avoid confusing potassium for sodium any longer, there would have been no way I would've gotten into a car with him.

There has to be a mutual respect and openness between parents and their kids. Without taking into account the individual characteristics of their offspring, if age alone is the overriding factor which a parent bases various determinations, some undesirable outgrowths could result. Needing to give parents some credit for knowing what's going on as well, it would be important that children not be "out of touch" with their parental pilots, for this communication circuit "shorting out" can do some irreparable harm. Disregarding a family member's notion that they may actually be aware of something can create unwanted turbulence. Unfortunately, it wasn't until too late that I truly came to appreciate just how much parents really could comprehend.

Seen as a "no-win" situation, I was infuriated by dad's demeanor and subsequent actions pertaining to my driving situation, so I retreated much of the time and began to limit the communication with my folks. Tail jammed firmly between my legs, without considering their point of view, I saw my parental guardians as the core to my singular lifestyle and unhappiness as an aspiring grown-up. Feeling misunderstood and as if I was not being heard, I silently withdrew and this communication lapse was why my parents didn't know where I was going the night I was hurt.

Vague in most everything I told them as a teen, this penchant to be tight-lipped could have been disastrous had I "given up the ghost" and the two people who cared about me most wouldn't have had any idea the details surrounding their youngest child's demise. However, me being on "death's front door" wouldn't have much of an impact on those socialite "friends" whom I was at the party with that fateful February night I was so close to meeting the "Great Gatekeeper in the Sky."

From Paul's blatant lie that the party was at a residence in Canonsburg whom he didn't know, to Sam's sudden onset of amnesia regarding the specifics of the night in question, the details needed to compensate me fairly for the pain and suffering I had to—and will need to—tolerate for the remainder of my days would not be forthcoming. Due to the conspiring union of secrecy, given the misery my mind and body went through because no supervised guidance had been present at the infamous party, I received practically nothing for the permanent physical afflictions and prejudice which I must always contend with.

Unable to file suit against the distributor of the beer because this would be hidden so well by those who were associated with the purchase, feeling as if I had fallen off the brim of victory and tangled within a web of defeat, I was denied a healthy chunk of money that could've been coming my way. Held responsible for getting in the car with Paul after the party, for all intents and purposes, the crafty representatives from various insurance companies knew how to make me out to be some sort of irresponsible degenerate and keep the ante from going up.

Destined to be scrap metal only hours after my ass would be the last one to ever be planted here, ultimately ending up in the passenger seat with a driver who was able to disguise how "lit" he really was supposedly being of my own free will and volition, this accountability would translate into forfeited reimbursement dollars. Knowing what suffering I have already been subjected to and the grief I will need to endure contending with the therapy labor force's warped inclinations/hesitant tendencies aimed at those who once rattled their neurological foundation, it almost sickens me when I hear that some distressed soul had received millions of dollars for sustaining a hangnail in some comparatively minor mishap.

The pubescent code of silence being a principle largely adhered to, a good number of adolescent readers in particular—and maybe even a few sticky adults—might say that a writer isn't to report on friends about their acts of folly. But it was many of these so-called "friends" who prolonged me and my family's anguish by refusing to come forth and volunteer information which would have eased our despair during the time when I was on "deathwatch."

A time of unbearable hardship, those who elected not to render any help to my family and me when they could have been of the greatest assistance, was nothing short of sadistic and cruel. When a teen comes forward with incriminating information, this is perceived as heresy by their fellow adolescents. Nobody connected with the legendary party having the courage to break this unwritten oath, my parents would not be afforded the facts needed to extinguish the fire of their ordeal. Possessing a "tough as nails" fortitude, forced into a corner where one has to prove what they're made of, the Meyers clan demonstrated that their true character and fiber was one of incredible depth.

When visiting hours would end while I was in Harmarville, my not even owning good physical or mental health any longer, I'd tell my parents to be extremely careful on the way back home to Washington because I loved them and that they were all that I had. Always coming through for me when it really counted, my parental heroes would do whatever it took to see that I got the essentials required to beat this horrifying head injury disability.

Through both my personal and professional travels, taking the good with the bad and the "ups" with the "downs," I have learned that you can't change history, but if one has more positive marks in their file of experiences than negative ones, they can feel lucky and have the resources to proceed in a favorable fashion. Acknowledging how some counter-productive situations cannot be forgotten—but enhanced maturation and ripening can occur because of being entangled in less-than-desirable conflicts—I can now understand that one often just needs to "bury the hatchet" or else expect to flounder in past scripts of spite which cannot be edited. If a truce cannot be agreed upon, anger and even hatred could simmer throughout a lifetime.

Trying to be an R.E.T. role model, one needs to remember that nobody is perfect, as enough mistakes are going to be made during one's upbringing. Not immune to error, because of the unenviable status of being flawless in their little ones' eyes, parents have to be in touch with how the verbal and non-verbal messages delivered will impact their kids. Important to be aware of how the stressors of everyday living can influence their guardian's way of packaging this instruction—despite a few long-lasting images of their parents not exactly being loving—kids will usually be able to discard dysfunctional messages and develop from their caregivers' productive words of wisdom, if consideration has been the consistent/routine method of going about teaching values. Establishing a framework of their child's place in the world, a parent's style of interacting with these impressionable little people goes a long way towards how offspring see themselves. Erroneously thinking that I didn't "measure up," a lifetime's worth of growth and development nearly had been irreversibly undone.

The comforts of a nice home provided for me without lifting a finger and dad insisting that I play while I'm a kid because I'd have plenty of time to work as an adult, taking life for granted and not fully appreciating the years of sweat required to attain such a level of well-being, I wouldn't see just how good I had it because my isolated presence was all-consuming. Easy to overlook positive attributes when circumstances aren't going as one would like, omissions can weigh heavy on one's mind. Not having the means to be involved magnified to such a degree that I had trouble recognizing the many items in my possession, with freedom mine to glisten off away at college, I foolishly thought I'd make up for lost time and get involved with those who would be a counterpart while I dabbled with life on the "wild side." A recipe which almost led to my complete undoing, I practically didn't even make it into my 20's.

Hoping to project an accurate portrayal and authentic representation, I tried to make use of a few "quasi-witty" segments when depicting my first semester in college because the psychological preparation for my freshman year was one big joke. I thought conveying an impression with my interpretation of comical overtones—before turning lurid—was the best way to conjure an image of how my principles "slid by the wayside" because of marijuana, and subsequently found myself trapped "down in the dumps" like I had never been before. Having no productive payback whatsoever, use of the drug increasingly taking control over me, I quickly found myself "in over my head" and floundering in the pits before I knew what had hit me. Insidiously, like a riverboat gambler who thrives on the "kill" of hitting the jackpot, my values had been dispensed, with the hopes of reaching an illusionary apex.

Trying to "go with the flow" by way of enlisting with a "dead end" crew who liked getting "juiced" and dabbling with gunja, the means undertaken to grasp peer recognition would turn out to be a destructable one. Resulting in the death of a friend and me needing to expend a mammoth effort just to get back some of what I had lost, admission into a drug culture leads oneself to pay an enormous price for something which has absolutely no bountiful return. Impoverished of life experience, perceiving my surrounding adolescent environment as a condescending downward spiral would not be harmless, for not feeling worth my salt would make "escape" an inviting refuge. Manufacturing a more desolate circumstance, I would subsequently "imbrue my hands in blood" upon my riveting journey trying to overcome what a wound to my brain had done to me.

The discovery of my inner strength and identification of who I really am as a person truly came out after I was hurt, when my back was up against the wall and

I had to reach deep within myself to mitigate the symptoms of a disability where its survivors need to take their rehabilitation to a higher octave. Needing to assume a stalwart attitude in the face of this personal catastrophe, I knew that if I wanted the attainment of some semblance of normalcy to be more than a pipe dream, I had to tap into all the emotional firepower as I could in order to "bounce back" and battle this debilitating foe to the fullest. Realizing that it takes more than merely just having the will to fight or refusing to be denied, I don't know exactly why I was able to make the most of my comeback, but I'm not complaining.

Sending shock waves of dedication throughout my system, this brain injury at one time leaving my thinking "a quart low" and my physical presence thoroughly "dinged up," I knew it was "crunch time" if I was to make some sort of fabled recovery. Not willing to accept a stature where I would be permanently "out of whack," being tied down and feeling sorry for myself wasn't about to happen, so it was essential that I attack the effects of this head injury disability head-on and with everything I had.

Not about to turn "batty" if I could do something about it, before the time arrived where it was "lights out" and I was to dance with death, I had to address the onslaught of debilitating conditions with a mentality that I'm going to beat this thing and get on with my life. Understanding that a good many of my restoration efforts would be of the "trial and error" variety, I knew that I'd just have to "dig in" the best I could until I found something that worked, hoping different functions would eventually come around. Adopting a sort of "little engine that could" mentality during the early stages of my injury, kept me from being blinded of hope and having my spirit fizzle of all its virtue.

Acquainted all too well with the true essence of the saying, "Brothers will be brothers," I could never imagine that living with a heckler/bully could prove to be so salutary. Toughening me up, my brother, Ug, helped me immeasurably with my recovery. Being "picked at" constantly by an older male sibling would help me to assemble a tough outer shell which allowed me to develop a resiliency which aided me later in life with the many difficult situations I had to face in my struggles with disability. Had I been exposed to an environment throughout my upbringing which flattered me with tenderness, it's unlikely I would have been able to deflect troublesome circumstances as readily as I had after my injury, or generate the strong backbone necessary for achievements to occur in rehab.

"Lucky" enough getting the chance to participate in sports with a brother eight and one-half years my senior who took tremendous joy out of repeatedly rubbing it in how badly I'd be dominated, learning how to handle being psychologically bruised in such a fashion as a taunted youngster, actually would assist me with the turmoil I'd experience as an injured 18-year old needing all the deposited ammunition I could get my hands on. Having the "fortune" of being beat up by this fraternal rival, I'd have a lot of practice finding out how to deal with uncomfortable dilemmas, such as how to tackle the therapies needed to overcome a severe head injury disability.

Hearing continuous "trash talk" and feeling knuckles after they had found their way to my arm, I learned to proceed in a fashion where I could try to thrive to the best of my abilities with the least amount of discomfort as possible. Aspects of my history with my brother definitely having turned out to be quite advantageous, developing these traits of viscidity amidst my childhood practice would no doubt help me to prevail in my attempts to overcome the many symptoms that my head injury "tormented" me with.

Taught the lesson of acceptance and having the importance of viewing situations from a variety of angles role modeled for me, my parents way of addressing my displeasure being continually insulted would be to stress that if people don't like someone, they just don't bother pestering them. If getting "ragged" on" is a sign that one is thought highly of, Scott sure must like me. Thank you.

Like a shifty scatback in football who cuts and weaves in an attempt to break loose in the "clear"—with rehab employers' resistant consideration and forbidden acts of omission being my defensive front I've been unable to get around—I thought I'd just take a few twisting steps backwards and note in book form some of the improbable accomplishments which are part of my past, before time runs out and I haven't yet run all the plays from my playbook. In order to snatch victory from the jaws of managerial bias, like a bruising fullback, my attempts to "barrel over" and force myself into the rehabilitation work force utilizing the advanced academic standing most any healthy person can use to get a career position wouldn't be successful because of the fixed employer notion that those once disturbed of their capacities, shall be indelibly assigned as "unsound" propositions.

Viewed as going out on a limb, rehab execs everywhere would just as soon not "risk" giving someone a chance who doesn't meet the standard criteria of regular/routine. Employers being my "snake in the grass," I have been unable to make my reclamation experience following a severe head injury any kind of a "rags to riches" tale because managements have deemed my trauma history as leaving me unqualified to work in the fields of rehabilitation or therapy.

Trying to break down some walls, having been provided with the rare opportunity to attain some noteworthy resumption milestones and subsequently afforded the occasion to be a "voice" for the disability population following a critical injury, I have absolutely no right to think that I could quit and give up on this extensive writing endeavor anytime soon. Not about to "pack it up" or do a "rag-tag" job on this "magnum opus" of mine, I wouldn't necessarily want to suggest that God supplied me with the fabric to weave a design intending to expose some questionable human services providers, but that writing a book of this nature to serve a larger population with disabilities and their loved ones *WAS* in the back of HIS mind.

Not able to imagine He would want me to keep quiet about my revival because this autobiographical record could realistically serve as a tribute to the advances made in medicine and rehabilitation technologies over the years, I wouldn't think God presented me with a shot to make something out of myself after being so dangerously close to dying, just so I would have to keep my unthinkable recovery a big secret. Far from being a legend in my own mind, I just think that there may be a greater plan out there for me somewhere. Hope springs eternal.

Originally being a journalism major in college, I've more or less always wanted to make some sort of statement with the written word. Having worked a little more than the mandated number of years stipulated in my Rehabilitation Counseling grant—figuring it was just what the doctor ordered—I decided the time was ripe for me to get down to business and write a few words about my potentially inspiring rehabilitation recovery following a critical brain injury, before I headed off into the sunset. Prevailing attitudes towards those with disabilities being flagrantly guarded and infamously unwarranted, this far-reaching toxic stance would be a major player in my final determination to set aside individual ambitions and take the time to produce a work which could possibly revise the thinking of a few readers who might have previously been skeptical that any head injury survivor was intellectually capable of such a novel concept as writing a book about their experience. Enduring restless nights and frequently not coming up for air, I'd hope that taking on such a far-ranging project wouldn't necessarily mean that I'm eccentric, but I have gone "stir crazy" at times trying to organize the pieces to this literary storybook puzzle.

To avoid interfering with the flow of the story line as much as possible, while simultaneously providing real-life detail, consideration for the different names to be used depicting individuals would need to be undertaken. Whether real names, no names, or aliases, some thought had to be put into how exactly I was going to refer to various people in this profile of my trauma experience. On occasion, the assignment of what to call the figures related to traits consistent with that person's makeup, and others, the names employed were just picked at random.

For the sake of authenticity—primary people such as family, friends, professionals who worked with me, and select others—the utilization of actual names would obviously have to occur. To accurately record a particular circumstance, often, allocating a designation to someone wouldn't be absolutely essential; either because it wasn't a necessity towards getting the point across, or else the situation simply was not that significant. Whether it be in an adversarial or advocacy capacity, I'd frequently use a fake name if the character in question merely had some benign association with me. However, if offenses to the head injury population were massive and subject to public record, fictitious labels wouldn't be necessary. A few pseudonyms may have just been images which simply passed through my mind, while other pen names could have had a little more significance than something just popping into my head.

Sadly, because of the viewpoint so widely held by the rehab executive body that the entire brain injury population is one inefficient lot, it wouldn't be too far off-base if I would title this passage into the perils of my head injury disability, The Fantastic Comeback Nobody Knows About—and Never Will. An absolutely accurate depiction of my rehabilitation employment plight, I've grown tired of being kicked when I'm down, and made up my mind to do what I could to "level the playing field" for those with impairments of varying degrees. Trying to co-exist with physically healthy players in the vocational arena where there's two different sets of rules for people once stricken with an enervating condition and those who have not, is not only unfair, but a stealth crime the majority of those with handicaps can only cry "foul" about.

Similar to the W.V.U. Rehab Counseling grad school student who had sustained the C.V.A. and got flustered when the videotape depicting my rehabilitation "high drama" had been shown to class, some people may incorrectly believe that I am trying to somehow capitalize on the suffering caused by my trauma because I'm writing about events affiliated with my injury. Those mistaken souls who possibly think that I am trying to get self-serving attention or unilaterally profit from my accident/injury, don't realize my pursuits to attain a highly altruistic human services career position through less conspicuous means have been sabotaged along virtually every job front. Not being a helpful role model for those who could prosper from my example, the never-ending work that I have expended in my rehabilitation and ensuing academic effort to attain a significant level of intellectual/psychological efficiency after a brain injury has not been the satisfying experience for me that it should be.

Rewarding people for their exertion and subsequent performance being one benchmark of achievement that I have not been able to capture, unfortunately, my inability to snare significance within the disability counseling arena could have detrimental repercussions for individuals who stand to benefit from my unique status as someone who could provide a valuable survivor's viewpoint. Not trying to outdo anyone with my intimate interpretation of the world, "empathy" alive and well, I am hoping that this written portrayal proves meaningful to a few.

In an ideally-constructed planet, one might think that I wouldn't have to take a break from work and carefully mark down events of a personal tragedy in order to prove that I'm not a "head injured incorrigible," but rampant prejudice and discrimination would make this striving impossible. Ideally.

Having successfully "picked myself up by the bootstraps" more times than I'd like to remember since my brain repelled off the walls of my skull, I am extremely proud of how I assumed the individual responsibility needed to withstand a disability which has no rules as to what can be affected. Unable to count how often I've felt like Jimmy Stewart's character, "George Bailey," in the movie "It's a Wonderful Life," sometimes I can amaze even myself thinking of how I went from being a person with a mind in hibernation and a state of flux, to one where prolific advances would abound from its one-time dormant shadow.

Allowing me to achieve so much in my ongoing recovery efforts, those big dreams I never let go of that so many rehab connoisseurs deemed laughable, are what kept me going and propelled me to inconceivable heights. Approached as if unrealistic and inferred by textbook professionals more than once after I'd been hurt that I live in a "fantasy world," I wouldn't have been able to accomplish all that I did, if I would have just conformed because those rehab "experts" thought I'd be unable to attain what I set my mind to grasp. Brain injury rehabilitation being a combat zone where the surviving patient either sinks or swims, perilously close to being forever physically and cognitively brittle, I have been fortified with a balanced self-assuredness because of what I had been able to master again in the face of this head injury disability which takes no prisoners.

A renewed outlook providing me with a fresh and effervescent approach to an assortment of matters—from the time when the incomplete structure of my teenaged brain wouldn't allow me to fully appreciate that "my body is my temple," to my mind having shut down from its power outage, to my "awakened unconscious," to being "railroaded" by the employment world afterwards—recounting my experience has been far from being all bad. Serving as the rocket fuel I'd need to "turn the page," my growing adult appreciations of other perspectives would be the medicine needed to soothe some wounds.

In addition to having to accept the various physical aftermaths of my injury and wide-ranging prejudicial outlooks, vocationally and interpersonally, this brain injury history of mine has "put me through the mill." But I've tried to endure the best way I possibly could by taking the stance that it's always darkest before the dawn.

For instance, instead of viewing the opportunity to develop a nice friendship with that W.V.U. goddess in my freshman English class as "irreversible loss," I've just got to appreciate all the interesting dating situations I would have missed out on had I somehow been able to "hook up" with this healthy diva for any length of time. Hardly appearing overly- thrilled the one occasion our paths did happen to eventually cross on campus about two years after we last talked—not sure if she had much recollection of who I was or if "word" had filtered back to her that two parties with whom she knew had been associated with a serious accident and she just didn't want to get involved in any way—I'd just have to take the attitude that I avoided a lot of potential hassle because acquaintanceships which begin at the age of eighteen usually don't amount to all that much over the long haul.

Known for leaving its survivors as "chancy" investments to establish a long-term relationship with, I wouldn't think it would be too far out of the question to suggest that the physical symptoms of my brain injury disability has contributed to my "bachelorhood" standing. Rather than seeing my "single" status as some kind of omission, I need to assume the position that it's better to have my freedom than to be burdened in a marriage where I would take "roving eyes" everywhere because my wife's emotional and/or physical appeal had fizzled over the years. Not overflowing with much excitement on weekends, given what happened to me that Valentines '82 night I went out in Washington, I'm not so sure I'd want to have it any other way. Unless. . . . .

My limp and paralysis understandably rendering me uninviting to enough females—wishing upon a "lucky star" that good things actually do come to those who wait—unless I'd want to be hypocritical, I couldn't look at these womens' perspectives as a flaw in their character because operating from this avoidance posture has been something with which I have been guilty. Not easy to find a lady who can overlook physical peculiarities and look beneath the surface—recognizing that a pretty girl would normally find it embarrassing being seen with a guy who draws attention to himself because of his bodily "imperfections"—I have learned to be content being "my own man" and not depending on another's approval to keep me afloat. The pursuits to meaningfully "connect" not my only yearning to "take on water," my striving to secure a little income while recovering from a T.B.I. would also sink.

Appeal rejected as well because I can only assume that I was seen as not being hurt bad enough, trying to look at the bright side of things once again, I suppose never receiving disability payments indicates precisely how far I had progressed and just how damned spectacular my prognosis is. Needing certification from a variety of treatment professionals, I presume I ought to have dropped to my knees in gratitude that I had been viewed by someone as not being "messed up" that critically to need this social security provision. "Thankful" not exactly being one of the words which comes to mind when expressing how I felt about this judgment, with at least one unidentified fortune teller seeing some promise in me, I guess I shouldn't have gotten too upset. One report on my improvement apparently glowing—such an uplifting assessment that it prevented me from collecting any funds while still in therapy and incapable of the "work hardening" qualities necessary when undertaking the tasks of a job—I wondered which professional was holding the smoking gun. When it rains, it pours.

Admittedly, when I began to commit putting on paper various circumstances surrounding my tragedy, it cut so deeply going through the process of mentally reviewing select scripts of years gone by, that repressed feelings surfaced and made me question whether proceeding to "dig up" buried pain would really be worth the heartache. Buoyancy prevailing, am I ever happy to have worked myself through this discomfort, because resolution in different instances had come to the front while examining prior strife and kinetically placing on record a host of turbulences I initially had some trouble reliving again. Surveying the situations from the vantage point of their ultimate truth, things wouldn't turn out all that ghastly in the long run, after all.

Considering what not only "could" have, but "should" have happened to me, I can't complain about the few physical limitations with which I'll always have to contend. A spastic dominant right hand, hemiparalytic walk, a minute trace of post-op double vision, and a slight ringing of the ears would likely be catastophic to most, but I have adapted to the best of my abilities because I had no other choice. Compromise and compensation my only recourse for my bodily shortcomings, trying to savor my predicament as promoting significant enrichment in quite a few areas and enhancing my emotional/psychological development, I feel blessed that my comprehension and rationalization capacities are fully intact after having sustained an injury to the neurological system where the processes controlling awareness/understanding too frequently go completely "kaput." With an abundance to be registered, avoiding the thought of consequences as completely "damaging," accentuating positives won't be difficult.

The physical aggravation doing everything "ass backwards" with my non-dominant hand for a decade would be merciless, but the emotional agitation struggling to manipulate the world for ten years entirely as a southpaw was a ruthless cruelty because of its being a never-ceasing reminder of how I'd been butchered of my good physical health. "Regard" not easy to come by when one is not physically fluent in their daily operation, making different entries of how I regained the ability to write and throw a football righthanded again when I worked at the "Green Acres" mental health facility, brought about feelings of incredible happiness. Although gripping a small baseball and consistently releasing these hardball throws when I want remains a postmorbid fine-motor skill still too difficult to master, my ability to get words down on paper again with my dominant hand and fire a pigskin are joyous reminders that my brain continues to "rewire" itself in an attempt to make up for those damaged parts of my neurological processes normally accustomed to undertaking these tasks. Achievements I was doubtful would ever be experienced again because of my assumption that the pronounced sluggishness and pain of my bad right side would never subside, "acceptance" having been reluctantly anchored, documenting the occurrence of these grandiose accomplishments was exceptionally fantastic because of their joyfully unexpected appearance after all these years.

Because of my infatuation with the instrument and music in general, when I cast my eyes back to when I picked up a guitar for the first time since I was hurt, I became a little "choked up" revisiting how I completely lost all my playing ability. About two-and-one-half years of diligent practice for nothing, not only was my paralytic right hand disobedient to my brain's command to "pick," but I couldn't recognize the fretboard anymore, strike individual single notes, or recall how any chords were fingered.

Turning back the hands of time to the desolate evening a really good rock 'n roll band jammed in the Harmarville cafeteria, I had trouble reliving the profound depression I felt seeing those musicians belt out a few riffs I once tackled. Paralytic arm decerebrately held at a 90` angle, the fingers of my right hand curled and stiff while seated in my wheelchair, I couldn't bring myself to describing any of the circumstances I vaguely remembered about this heartbreaking concert in the beginning of my writing endeavor because it would have hurt too bad.

Possibly an indicator as to where some of my priorities have been mistakenly placed, I didn't feel the least bit comfortable noting how I forgot everything about my six-string obsession until I came to grips with how I systematically equaled—and then surpassed—my pre-accident capabilities playing guitar. Retracing my steps to the juncture of my rehabilitation experience where unyielding perseverance allowed me to relearn the instrument—this rehab center show and the one therapeutic weekend I was home listening to my proficient playing on that 8-track serving as the catalysts—I am much more than pleased with how I overcame a variety of tormenting memory and motor skill obstacles in order to regain my musical ability.

Like my guitar playing preoccupation which one day I suppose could be an avocational aspiration, the counseling trade I've had a good bit of training and experience has also reaped more-than-a-few rewards. However, the occupational

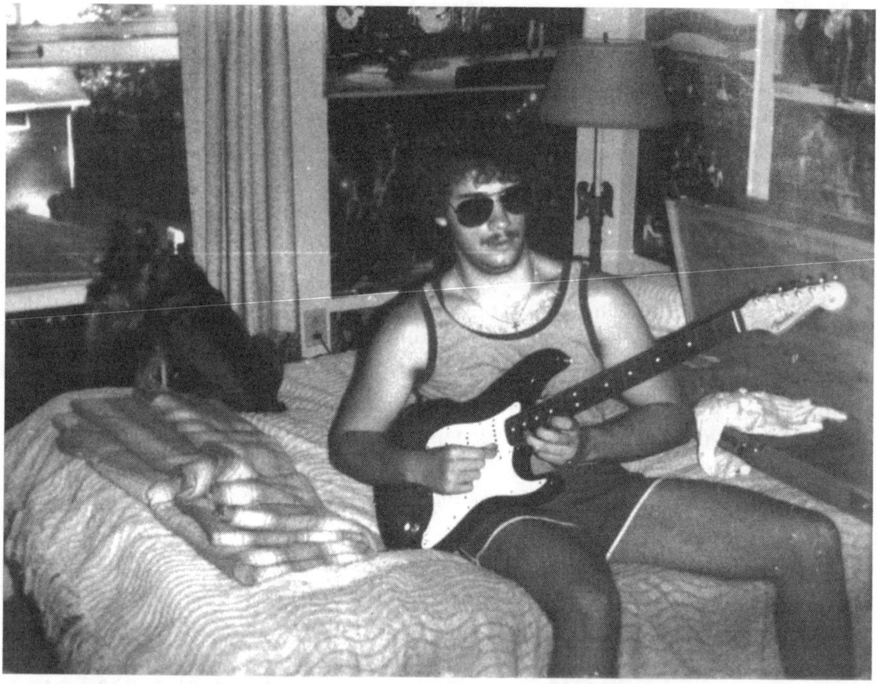

Back in the Saddle, with a little help from a thumb pick/flat pick compensatory invention, Craig's perseverance on his Fender Stratocaster has resulted in him currently playing better than before the accident.

plight of my post-traumatic condition hasn't emerged quite as successfully, pretty much because relentless dysfunctional attitudes have been a not-so-minor impediment I have yet to get the better of. Understanding and compassion not necessarily set to appear on the horizon, disability- conscious influences secretly lurking, I'll just have to try to take it upon my shoulders to recognize that the only opinion I can directly revise is my own. If past employer scrapes are any indication, I will need to extract a sizable portion of rational thinking in my reserve to combat the corporate world administrative ignorance which lies in waiting to pounce upon those with histories of handicaps.

Other than looking at my work history as one where I could have built a better foundation of consistency had so many of my supervisors not been fired, demoted, or—in the case of the New Medico hooligans—possibly arrested, I need to take solace in the fact that I have been afforded the opportunity to experience a broader array of therapy populations and corresponding treatment modalities because of these mid-managers' glaring inefficiencies. No matter how positive the "spin" used when trying to size up the uniform prejudice of the administrative labor network, I can't help but think that if an employer within the miscalculating rehabilitation profession advertised in the classifieds the need for someone—with my social security number and birthdate—who knew a little something about head injury therapy to fill a good-paying position, I still wouldn't get the job because my stock would take a not-so-subtle plunge once it was suspected or discovered that I had sustained this frightful condition at one time.

Given my past history, it looks like those presiding over rehab establishments have decided that hiring an applicant once critically injured is analogous to an epidemic needing immunization. Fortunately, I have some good friends and awesome family available to me should support be needed for most anything, such as trying to avoid being grappled by faulty preconceived inclinations which have absolutely no merit or basis with reality.

In addition to a few girlfriends over the years and some female acquaintances with whom I'd be able to talk to about things, neighborhood friends and a couple of former high school baseball teammates still around good ol' Washington have always been supportive of me since I was injured. Standing out, everybody could use a good friend like studly Kevin Brezinski to ride out some of the bumps of life with. Continuing throughout adulthood, childhood derelicts Frank McNamara and Craig Johnson have always more or less touched base to see that I'm still sucking wind. A day rarely passing that I wasn't involved in some sort of testosterone-induced athletic activity or war game endeavor with him during my developmental years—although no longer able to keep "tabs" because of more important commitments—I know Sgt. Dan Hobbs would always be in my corner of the bunker, heaving hand grenades at my foes, if he could. Like that which has been subjected to the magician's slight of hand, important not to dismiss uncertainties as "every rose having its thorn," events accepted as fact have been known to be nothing more than illusion.

So deeply focused on how I felt abandoned, being in harmony with the feelings of two buddies would not occur. Big and ugly enough to take care of themselves should I have happened to go "ballistic" on them, if they would have visited me during my therapeutic weekends home from Harmarville when I still was very much bewildered from a feral mind, good guys like Dave McClellan and Randy Boyer did not emotionally detach themselves from me once I got hurt, as I initially believed. Rather, their kind-hearted sensitivity to my perils would serve as the red flag which kept them away. Confusion and perhaps maybe even a little paranoia on my part having arisen—except for the proper cause—a gamut of reasons would cross my mind for their failure to come see me after I was almost put out of my misery and left for dead.

Not experientially developed enough to appreciate how my tragedy extended beyond a personal sphere, possibly because I was obviously aware of my generally cognizant state at the time as opposed to the hazard occupying the minds of my pals who are not fluent when it comes to understanding brain trauma, I couldn't figure out why these two slippery comrades didn't at least stop by and express their regard once I made it home after practically being killed. Unnecessarily taking it on the chin when I didn't need to—a phone call to these two compatriots demonstrating my coherence all that would have been required—my previous self-centered assumptions that their unfamiliarity with head injury conjured such harrowing images about my condition that they avoided me, would turn out to be foolish.

Almost embarrassed now when relaying how upset I felt when I'd see Dave cruising in his sports car around the neighborhood on my weekend breaks home from the rehab center when he didn't spend any time with me, or assuming Randall Vantine Boyer wasn't really all that "swift" when our valedictorian said that he'd come see me once he knew I was alright, my awareness having sprouted a little as time wore on has allowed me to grasp how difficult a circumstance paying a visit may actually have been for some. An individual's personality developed from the tokens of experience accumulated over the years, explaining how some could "stomach" seeing the damaged Craig Meyers while others could not, reactions could vary as much as the prints on one's fingertips.

Dave and Randy being absent during this time when my thinking capacities were thoroughly "out to lunch" wasn't because they feared for their safety, had other concerns/didn't want bothered, couldn't have cared less/weren't really that "tight" with me, or were in "cahoots" somehow with the characters connected with the party, as I had previously believed. Rather, it can be extremely trying seeing a friend forever disabled, especially when visions of them as healthy specimens seemingly enjoying the fruits of life are the preferred way one would like to remember a peer. Assumed to no longer even be sufficient with activities essential for daily living, acknowledging that someone who is liked will be permanently bound to restriction and omission does not come easy.

Confirmed some sixteen years after the accident when Dave joined me for a therapy lap around the neighborhood, he said that he *did* see me in '82 from a distance once, sporting this "wild look" in my eyes while seated in my wheelchair. Not being a scene he was sure he could bear, having fond memories of better days playing ball together at the Legion field behind his house, Dave told me that he was afraid he might have started to cry had he come up to talk with me and figured that "tearing up" wouldn't exactly make my day. Tomorrow not being guaranteed, knowing that one can be subjected to harm at a given moment not the most enticing proposition to consider, someone like Dave who tries to make good use of the pleasures life has to offer, would have particular difficulty coming face to face with unpleasant circumstances. Having had little exposure to me when I was physically whole, I was elated to discover that my post-traumatic condition wouldn't prevent me from being accepted by my fellow W.V.U. countrymen.

With the man, the legend, Mr. Kevin Brezinski always somehow managing to be a collateral fixture in my background at home and away at school, we were both able to thrive reasonably well in the interactive climate of college, after that shaky start. Developing a congenial core of Mountaineer companions whom I could count on for continued validation that I really did belong in a world overflowing with "normal" people, would be a personal milestone in my progression to maintain durable emotional health. "Let's go-oooo, Mountaineers!"

Particularly the two Daves (Stouffer and Schneeweis) and some of my other deranged roommates, I had formed a multitude of good friendships with residents at the Pierpont House apartment complex in Morgantown and established a solid nucleus of confidantes throughout my undergraduate days as a Psych major. With grad school a setting where I predominantly got down to the academic business at hand, W.V.U. would turn out to be a spectacular place, fostering intrinsic and interpersonal growth while on the mend from my injuries. Difficult to fathom just how important and valuable it was for me to generate affable relations in my restoration pursuits after being hurt so critically, the college triumphs I had attained "against all odds" would allow me to turn the corner and "set up shop" in society, for an unprecedented second crack at doing some good. Without a doubt, making quite a few quality friends to associate with during my scholastic rehabilitation effort was definitely a high mark helping me to get better. However, with the possible exception of the superb medical treatment and top-notch therapy instruction I received, the single most important factor assisting me with my recovery was the focused support I received at home.

Having a first-rate family that would be tough to beat, providing me with the wherewithal to intellectually and psychologically rebound so I could be myself again—always knowing impeccable support would be provided when needed—allowed me to have the security required to shift my rejuvenation efforts into high gear without interruption. Furnished with the necessary means to retrieve so much of what was in jeopardy of being completely obliterated, the peace of mind that I would never be left alone while confronting the symptoms of a head injury was priceless towards helping me get my feet back on the ground. Pulling together for the common cause of making sure any auxiliaries I might need would be provided, my sensational familial support system wouldn't refrain from seeing that I got everything necessary in order that I could recuperate from an injury which frequently leaves its prey forever mentally spellbound.

Afforded the opportunity to cultivate my strengths amidst a disability with which one's physical and cognitive capacities are usually set adrift, I would never have to worry about being a stranded castaway on some remote island, void of any reinforcements which could aid me in my attempts to reclaim my life. Seeing to it that I got whatever nourishment would be required to excel in my objective to regain some stature, my loving folks were keenly systematic when it came to supplying and soliciting care. Because of their lasting love and influence, to me, my parents will always be in a league by themselves.

Never leaving a stone unturned to assure that I received optimal care, mom and dad were a fantastic team. Making me their #1 priority after I was brutally wounded, my parents put aside their own life and any individual aspirations they had, so that I got whatever it took for me to recover to the fullest. Obsessed with the idea that I be functionally independent, their daily regimen revolved around my needs. In addition to both serving as guidance counselors, dad doing whatever manual labor was called for and mom's nose always seeming to be buried in paperwork of some sort, these two "battering rams" were going to make sure I could be as content and comfortable as possible. No way I could ever repay them or thank them enough with any kind of tribute, I want them to know that they're going to receive my love through all eternity.

Once in large-scale theatrical plays and other productions in school, my princess mom—who could pass as an identical twin of Queen Elizabeth of England—wouldn't have to act when demonstrating her love for her kids, because she would naturally treat her offspring like royalty. Never failing to be "there" for me and always making room in her heart for this undeserving soul no matter how stupid I might be, if the picture with mom sitting on those floor of mattresses next to me while I was comatose were placed in the dictionary alongside the words "understanding" and "nurturing," it would be tough to find a more symbolic or appropriate representation. Providing me with some immaculate company, a perennial "Mother of the Year" winner by my vote, anyone would be happy to have a mom as great as mine. "Forgiveness" a virtue with which she has unmistakably been blessed—not exactly thrilled reading just how far from a mama's boy I had actually become all these years—mom and I have needed to become especially close, so that the impact of losing dad may not be so intolerable.

Having paraded on the fault line far too long engrossed with his nicotine habit, witnessing the responsibility I assumed, mom would tell me that dad was lucky to have lived as long as he did because of the way he abused his body smoking cigarettes since he was fifteen. Hard-working, a strong man dedicated to doing what he thought was best with the resources available, and someone who could provide unparalleled comic relief are just a handful of the fatherly attributes which stand out in my memory about my buddy. Even years after passing away, provided a nice home environment in which to live and some monetary resources, dad's support is still quite evident. The spittin' image of actor Don Ameche, the quintessence of what made dad who he was, will forever have a bearing on me.

To this day, still hearing his words of encouragement/direction when taking on a seemingly impossible rehabilitation task and saying "Attaboy, buddy" upon showing improvement in some skill, dad's never-ending optimism continues to be a pre-eminent force coaching me along. Not wanting to imply that this reunion has to occur any time soon, with "people" time being a blink of an eye to God—if looked at from this vantage point—it won't be too long until my dad and I get together to have that non-alcoholic celebration, marking our being reunited.

The spirit of his backing very much alive and well, I hope this book can be received favorably, so that the stifling accuracy and magic underlying dad's ability to foresee tomorrow's affairs may continue. Wanting to make my pop proud, if this punctual account of events could gather a little solid exposure, my lengthy memoir could go a long way towards affirming dad's prophecy that, "God has some big plans for you, boy."

Suggesting my qualifications are not sufficient enough to work within the field of head injury disability, although I could do without the multitudes of rejection letters from rehab employers who can't wait to "shuffle me off" on my way fast enough, it's great to be back.